COMMUNICABLE MEDICAL DISEASES

A HOLISTIC AND SOCIAL MEDICINE PERSPECTIVE FOR HEALTHCARE PROVIDERS

R H van den Berg

BALBOA.
PRESS

A DIVISION OF HAY HOUSE

Cover art by BS [Bennie] Botha

Author Credits: Doctorate in Nursing and Masters in Higher Education

Balboa Press books may be ordered through booksellers or by contacting:

Balboa Press
A Division of Hay House
1663 Liberty Drive
Bloomington, IN 47403
www.balboapress.com
1 (877) 407-4847

ISBN: 978-1-4525-8772-1 (sc)
ISBN: 978-1-4525-8771-4 (e)

Library of Congress Control Number: 2013922150

Printed in the United States of America.

Balboa Press rev. date: 12/16/2014

CONTENTS

THEME III

THE HOST - THE ADVERSARY IN THE CONFLICT

DEFENDING THE BODY AGAINST THE PENETRATION OF PATHOGENS AND CARING FOR THE INDIVIDUAL AFTER INVASION HAD TAKEN PLACE

THEME IV

<u>VICTORY FOR THE PATHOGEN - THE HOST HAS LOST THE BATTLE</u>
THE CLINICAL MANIFESTATION OF COMMUNICABLE DISEASES AND THE SPECIFIC HEALTHCARE TO BE RENDERED

INTRODUCTION

As a health and medical phenomenon, communicable medical diseases/infections, just like all other medical conditions, have been known to humanity since the creation of man and the dawn of time. Although the first documentation of epidemics was only done at about 5000-4000 BC, several epidemics and/or pandemics occurred throughout the ages worldwide, often leading to the partial, sometimes the total erasure of populations. Regardless of the fact that communicable diseases have been declining as a cause of death in Europe and North America for nearly 150 years, communicable diseases are still the biggest killer in the developed, under-developed and developing world and are increasing at an alarming rate. Unknown and known communicable diseases continue to emerge or re-emerge due to drug resistant microbes, new patterns of travel and trade (especially food), new agricultural practices, altered sexual behaviour and overuse of antimicrobial drugs. Economic, social, and political changes have weakened healthcare systems while enhancing the effects of poverty and malnutrition. Thus, instead of claiming that communicable diseases are in irreversible decline, it has to be stated that every major change in society, population, use of land, climate, nutrition or migration is a public health event with its own pattern of diseases (especially communicable diseases). Although the impact of communicable diseases on the health of people has been reduced drastically over the past few decades (mainly because of the progress that has been made in the sciences of healthcare and environmental sciences), epidemics/pandemics can still occur on a large scale should the existing control regulations be relaxed. The resistance of certain pathogens against modern antimicrobial drugs heightens the possibility that communicable diseases can assume the magnitude of wide-spread epidemics and/or pandemics. Furthermore, modern means of transport today plays an important role in the spread of communicable diseases because communicable infections can now be spread within hours from one continent to another.

The prevention and control of communicable medical diseases is one of the eight basic components of a comprehensive healthcare service that needs to be delivered to the population in any country in the world by all the different healthcare systems that exist. Other services also to be implemented in the prevention and control of communicable medical diseases encompasses, among others

- the maintaining of a healthy environment by providing non-personal (environmental) healthcare services
- the provision of health information to individuals, families, groups and communities to take responsibility for their own health
- the upholding of all legislative measures supporting all preventive, promotive, curative and rehabilitative programmes and services
- the rendering of healthcare, at home or in hospital, to all healthy, ill, disabled and dying individuals within familial and community context

1

- the keeping of accurate statistical information regarding population demographical, mortality and morbidity statistics, and making it available to assist in the planning for the delivery of the correct and comprehensive healthcare services as well as the prevention and control of communicable diseases.

The prevention and control of communicable medical diseases, as a component of a comprehensive healthcare services delivery system, is focused on the total well-being of the individual, the family, and the community, and encompasses preventive, promotive, curative, and rehabilitative healthcare services delivery and healthcare rendering that is supported by legislation, as sporadic/endemic/epidemic/pandemic episodes of communicable infections must be prevented at all times. However, should a sporadic/endemic/epidemic/pandemic outbreak occurs, it has to be effectively controlled. Based on the principles of primary healthcare services delivery and healthcare rendering, the prevention and control of communicable diseases forms an integral part of the primary healthcare services delivery system.

In South Africa, according to the National Health Act, Act 61 of 2003, the rendering of healthcare relating to communicable diseases must be affordable and of the highest possible quality, and all services must be available and accessible to all individuals (whether healthy or sick or disabled or dying), their families and their communities within the population. All care rendering must also comply (as underwritten in this text) with the Constitution of the RSA, the Bill of Human Rights, the Patients' Rights Charter, and the Rights of Children, the Elderly, and the Disabled. Thus, in order to provide the expected and effective service delivery and healthcare rendering, it is imperative for all healthcare providers (professional, traditional and lay care) to be thoroughly conversant with communicable medical diseases as to protect and promote the health of all individuals, their families and their communities. Healthcare providers (professional, traditional and lay care) must also restore health by identifying all sick and suspect cases (individuals, or families, or communities); by applying control measures; by rendering compassionate, comprehensive, holistic and culturally congruent care to all hosts (individuals and/or families and/or communities whether healthy, or ill, or contact, or carrier) within familial and community context; by implementing the necessary legislative measures; and by giving health information to all individuals, families and communities as well as to all care-givers (professional, traditional, and lay care) about communicable diseases.

Based on the epidemiological fact that all communicable medical diseases are characterised by the existence of a dynamic and symbiotic relationship between three elements, namely, the human host, the environment and specific pathogenic microbes and that these three elements are inextricably interwoven in the causation, prevention and control of all communicable medical diseases, the point of departure of this book is based on Social Medicine and the Holism of human life and well-being. Because Social medicine describes all social, economic and other determines of health and disease, it is applicable to all healthcare practices to ensure a healthier society, and because the questions asked are bio-social in nature, the impact of all bio-physical, social, economic and other factors of importance on the health and disease patterns of individuals/families/communities must be determined when communicable medical diseases occur. The concept "Holism/Holistic/Holistically" is used because it refers to the wholeness of human life and well-being as it takes in account that all human beings live in relation to or having dialogues with himself/ herself, in relation to/with all other human beings, in relation to/with a Creator, and in relation to/with the universe and because it relates to the epistemological fact that the wholeness of human life and wellbeing are as such intertwined/interwoven with the environment and the infinite different systems which forms the environment. As the individual, the family and the community forms an integrated unit that can never be separated from one another and because the wholeness of the well-being of all individuals/families/communities and the environment is determined by the interplay and interdependence of all these infinite factors, the combined effect of all these factors that influence the state of health/well-being of all individuals/families/ communities and the environment they live in must be assessed and described when grounding the healthcare to be rendered at primary, secondary and tertiary level as to provide in the life needs of all healthcare users in familial and community context. This relational approach ensures that compassionate, **holistic and culturally congruent healthcare** is rendered to promote, to protect and to restore the wholeness of human life and well-being. The best practices for upholding the wholeness of human life and well-being, based on a combination of modern scientific diagnosis and monitoring techniques as well as healthcare practices practiced for millenniums, must thus be prescribed as to provide in the life needs of healthcare users within their familial and community context.

In the light of above, the specific educational exit level outcome of this book is as follows:

All professional and traditional healthcare providers/practitioners must render to all inhabitants (individuals/families/communities whether healthy or ill or contact or carrier), in a responsible and accountable manner, comprehensive (scientific fundamental and specific healthcare at primary, secondary, and tertiary level), holistic, compassionate, and culturally congruent healthcare that leads to self-caring and self-reliance within familial and community context, by

- ❏ having a full working knowledge of the symbiotic and dynamic interrelatedness and interdependence of the human host, pathogen (infectious agent) and the environment/milieus in the causation, control and prevention of communicable diseases
- ❏ preventing and controlling communicable diseases at primary, secondary and tertiary level by means of breaking the links between the symbiotic and dynamic interrelatedness and interdependence of the host, pathogen and the environment through compiling and implementing the necessary programmes
- ❏ understanding the defence mechanisms of the innate and adaptive physiological immunological systems of the body against the penetration of pathogens and the factors that improve or impair the immune system
- ❏ diagnosing communicable diseases and rendering healthcare which is compassionate, comprehensive, holistic and culturally congruent in nature and

that is based on a combination of traditional and scientific fundamental and specific healthcare interventions, to all persons suffering from a communicable disease within their familial and community context

❑ complying conscientiously with all standards and transmission-based precautions as well as with all legislative measures in the prevention and control of communicable diseases.

To achieve the specific educational exit level outcome, the book has been divided into four themes:

- In **Theme I** the point of departure, namely, **"The Epidemiological Triad of Communicable Diseases"** model is discussed. The symbiotic and dynamic interrelatedness of the human host system, the environment and the pathogenic microbe (infectious agent) in the causation, prevention and control of communicable diseases is depicted as well as a description given of all the characteristics/properties/attributes intrinsic to each element to be taken account of

- **Theme II focuses on breaking the links of interrelatedness between the human host system, the environment and the pathogenic agent to prevent and control communicable medical diseases.** A full description is given of the general principles underlying the prevention and control management of communicable diseases as prescribed in relevant legislation, programmes for the prevention of communicable diseases, and the control of communicable diseases as based on the Epidemiological process wherein the "Epidemiological Triad of Communicable Diseases" model is integrated

- **Theme III** focuses on **"the host as the adversary in the conflict"**. The discussion concern the body's defence mechanisms against the entry of pathogenic agents into the body and the reaction of the body to the pathogen after invasion of the body had occurred. The body is protected by the innate and adaptive immune systems consisting of the natural protective barriers based on anatomical, biochemical and mechanical factors, the inflammatory response and phagocytosis, and the antibody-mediated and cell-mediated physiological immunological responses. After gaining entry into the body, the local as well as the systemic inflammation reactions develop in the body which are manifested in a general clinical way. Vaccination programmes to prime the adaptive immune system as well as the comprehensive, compassionate, holistic and culturally congruent fundamental healthcare to be rendered in hospital or at home are also discussed

- In **Theme IV - "Victory for the pathogen - the host has lost the battle"** - the epidemiology, pathogenesis and clinical manifestations of selected communicable diseases are discussed as well as the specific healthcare (excluding pharmacological prescriptions) to be rendered and the specific preventive and control measures to be taken.

Please take note that this book is a complete re-writing of the original book "Oordraagbare Siektes - 'n Verpleegkundige Perspektief" published in 1989 with RH van den Berg and MJ Viljoen as editors

DESCRIPTION OF CONCEPTS RELATING TO COMMUNICABLE DISEASES

Address

An address refers to the physical residential address of a person, not a postal box address

Antibody (immunoglobulin)

Antibody or immunoglobulin is specialized soluble factor proteins that are mediated or synthesized by the B-lymphocytes of the human host. Antibody possesses the ability to recognize the antigen(s) of the infectious agent and then coats the infective pathogen with several adaptor antibody molecules to induce complement fixation and phagocytosis by the adapter antibody. Specific antibody (sub-classes) is mediated by the B-lymphocytes in reaction to the presence of the foreign protein of the infectious agent. Antibody, as such, circulates in the blood and help to destroy the specific infectious agent or inactivate it by

- complexing/bonding with the antigen whereby the resulting complex activates the first component of the complement C1 for neutralizing the toxic properties of the pathogen
- causing it to precipitate through lysis and opsonisation when antibody and complement act together whereby the rate of phagocytosis is thousand-fold enhances
- making it more vulnerable to phagocytosis
- causing the pathogen to agglutinate and to render the pathogen more susceptible to phagocytosis
- neutralizing toxic properties through blocking the microbial reactions of the toxin(s) on the body cells

Antigen

Antigens refer to the distinctive properties of the different groups of pathogens causing communicable diseases, namely, prions, viruses, bacteria, fungi, protozoa, helminths and arthropods. Each group of pathogens has distinctive properties such as structural and molecular make-up, biochemical and metabolic strategies, reproductive processes and living either intracellular or extracellular. These distinctive properties determine how the different infectious microbes interact with the human host and how the specific infectious pathogens cause disease/infection. After recognition by or priming of the specialized receptor sites for antigen(s) on antigen-dependant T-helper-cells, the B-lymphocytes are activated by the primed T-helper-cells to mediate/ synthesize antibody immunity with memory while simultaneously stimulating T-cells to differentiate and mediate T-cell-immunity with memory. Antigens not only select and clonally expand B-lymphocytes and T-lymphocytes bearing complementary receptors but also control the immune response of the adaptive immune system as the concentration of the antigen activates the immunity response and then switch off the response when the antigen is no longer present (when the antigen is eliminated by metabolic catabolism and clearance through the immune response, the stimulus to the immune system disappears). Pathogens evade/elude recognition by lymphocytes through concealment of antigens (remaining inside cells without their antigens being displayed on the cell surface) and antigenic variations (through mimicry, antigenic drift and antigenic shift)

Antiseptic preparations
Antiseptic preparations are chemical compounds that inhibit (retard) the growth of microbes without destroying/killing them

Arthropods
Arthropods are fleas, lice, bedbugs in any stage of development of the relevant species

Asepsis
Asepsis is the absence of living pathogenic agents and/or any infectious matter that cause an infectious condition

Bacteraemia
Bacteraemia refers to the condition occurring in the body when pathogenic microbes (excluded viruses) exist and multiply in the bloodstream

Barrier healthcare or barrier nursing care (Isolation/restriction)
Barrier healthcare or barrier nursing and medical care or isolation is the practice of seclusion of an infected person from other persons for the period of communicability (period the disease is transmissible). Barrier healthcare or barrier nursing and medical care or isolation measures refer to all those care measure put in place to prevent the spread of the causative microbe/pathogen to other human beings. Barrier healthcare/barrier nursing and medical measures/isolation measures can be classified as either routine barrier healthcare/barrier nursing and medical care/ isolation measures or high grade barrier healthcare/barrier nursing and medical care/ isolation measures

- In **routine barrier healthcare or routine barrier nursing and medical care or isolation** all Standard Precautionary Control Measures (including cough etiquette); transmission-based precautions; engineering control of ventilation; environmental hygiene; and waste control) are applicable and are put in place in general hospital units/wards to control the airborne transmission of infected droplets. For the control of gastro-intestinal communicable diseases enteric precautions and disinfecting of the environment must be instated
- **High-grade barrier healthcare or high-grade barrier nursing and medical care or high-grade isolation** is instituted for a specific group of communicable diseases that constitute a serious risk to all healthcare practitioners because they are transmitted via blood; fomites and airborne infected droplets (when seeding of the lungs had taken place and profuse growth of the pathogen in the lungs had occurred). High grade barrier/isolation care is **only** instituted in a specialized isolation unit for communicable diseases (**these measures can never be put in placed in general hospital wards/units**) and the care has

to be rendered by specialized trained healthcare personnel only. No visitors (family and friends) are allowed in this specialized isolation unit. All ccontacts (even entire communities) will be placed under quarantine. The service of the National Defense Force can be called in to enforce all quarantine measures

> **Note** Routine barrier healthcare or routine barrier nursing and medical care or routine barrier isolation as well as high-grade barrier healthcare/high-grade nursing and medical care/high-grade isolation can never be implemented when family members render care to the sick individual at home as the family members are not professionally educated to institute the above specialized isolation healthcare regimes

Carriage/carrier state
Donates a state of being a carrier of a particular communicable disease as identified by means of laboratory tests and/or other examinations

Carrier
A carrier is a person who does not show any clinical signs and symptoms of a specific communicable disease at a specific time although it has been proven by means of laboratory or other tests that the person is infected and therefore able to spread the disease. The carrier harbours the specific pathogen in his/her body, causing the person to become a source of infection. A person can become a carrier after having been ill and recovered (the pathogen is still harboured within his/her body) or the person may have become infected without ever having been ill at all (healthy carrier)

Case
A case is any person who actually suffers from the particular disease and has been diagnosed as such. The term does not refer to the infected person as such
- ❑ **Index case**
  An index case is the first person brought to the attention of the authorities as having contracted a communicable disease. It may not necessarily be the primary case
- ❑ **Primary case**
  The primary case is the first person who has been infected and thus spreads the communicable disease within the community
- ❑ **Secondary case**
  A secondary case is a person or persons in whom the disease develops after contact with a primary case
- ❑ **Suspected case**
  A suspected case is a person who has been exposed to other persons in whom the disease has already been clinically manifested. The person's medical history and symptoms indicate that he/she may have contracted the communicable disease

Chain of infection
The chain of infection is sequence of events or "links" underlying the development/ outbreak of all communicable diseases, namely, a specific infectious agent/pathogen

(mode of transmission; portals of entry and exits); a reservoir (the host [infected person or source of infectious agent]) and a new susceptible (uninfected) host

The route of transmission can be simple or complicated

- ❑ Heterogeneous chain of infection: Transmission occurring from a host of one species to a host of another species, for example, avian flu, measles in pigs (animals to human)
- ❑ Homogeneous chain of infection: Transmission occurring from a host to a host of the same species, namely, from human to human, for example, influenza (type B and C), pneumonic plague

Child

A child is any person under the age of 18 years (The Child Welfare Act, Act 38 of 2005)

Communicable diseases / communicable medical diseases / communicable infections

This group of medical diseases are caused by specific infectious agents that are transmitted horizontally (from one person to another person or from an animal to a person [directly] or indirectly by an intermediary such as either a vector or a vehicle) or vertically (from mother to child). A particular communicable disease is caused by a specific pathogenic agent and the signs and symptoms are characteristic of that particular disease. A person who has had contracted a particular disease is usually immune to that specific disease as the physiologic adaptive immune response (antibody-mediated and cell-mediated immunity with memory) had been elicited. Diseases transmitted from animals to humans as well as all sexual transmitted diseases are the exception to this rule as no immunity with memory is induced

Contact

A contact is a person who was exposed to the risk of infection as he/she has been in direct physical contact with a sick or infected person or animal, or has been directly or indirectly exposed to an infectious agent or a contaminated environment or fomites, and for these reasons the infectious agent could have gained entry into the body of the person. Depending on the mode of transmission of the infectious agent, specific persons will be considered to be contacts to that particular disease. Based on factors such as natural physiological resistance (innate and adaptive) as well as acquired physiologic immunity, the contact may or may not become ill. A contact that becomes ill is a source of infection

Contagiousness/Communicability/Transmissibility

Contagiousness/communicability/transmissibility refers to the ability of pathogenic microbes to retain their pathogenicity when transmitted from person to person or from an animal to a person thus causing the particular disease in a susceptible human host. A number of pathogenic microbes, however, lose this ability soon after the characteristic signs and symptoms of the particular disease have manifested. The disease can now no longer be transmitted by the sick person and susceptible hosts will now not contract the communicable disease

❑ **Period of contagiousness**
The period of contagiousness refers to the time period during which the pathogenic microbes retains their pathogenicity and are able to cause the particular disease in a person

Contamination

Contamination is the presence of an infectious agent on the body surface (skin) of a person (for example, on hands/fingers or under nails) or an animal, as well as on any inanimate substances/utility items such as clothing, bed linen, toys, medical equipment and supplies, and in other inanimate substances such as water, milk and food. The infectious agent is alive and able to gain entry in the human body and cause an infection

> **Note** Contamination differs from pollution as the latter refers to the presence of offensive, non-infectious substances in the environment. Contamination also differs from infection as the latter refers to the presence of the pathogen within the cells (intracellular or extracellular) of the human body where it multiplies/replicates, spreads from and is shed from

Degree of impairment/Gradient of severity/Degree of seriousness

The degree of impairment/severity/seriousness refers to the *severity* of the disease which may vary from sub-clinical to moderate to serious to fatal. It is also known as the spectrum of the disease

Disease

Disease refers to a pathological disorder or condition or infection of the structure of the human body, such as an organ or a system of the body, or to a pathological disorder or condition in the functioning of the normal body organs such as the syntheses of glucose in the body, that is caused by various causes such as pathogenic microbes, genetic factors etc. This disorder/condition/infection of the structure and/or function of the body produces signs and symptoms that affect the life/lives of the human individual or/and his/her family and its members or a community as a whole, especially when the disease is a communicable medical disease or infection. All known diseases as medical conditions are classified by the science of medicine in specific groups and then broken down into a list of diseases, for example, a group of medical diseases classified as communicable medical diseases or infections which is then broken down into a specific list of conditions listed according to the body organs affected/inflicted and/or according to the pathogenic microbe causing the particular disease

Disinfectants

Disinfectants are chemical agents which inhibit (retard) the growth of pathogenic organisms or destroy them

Disinfection

Disinfection is the process of eliminating pathogenic microbes by means of chemical or physical methods from the surface of the skin of the body (but does not penetrate the skin) or from utility items or from the physical surroundings

❑ **Concurrent disinfection**
Concurrent disinfection entails administering disinfection immediately or as soon as possible after a person has been in contact with secretions/

excretions of infectious material from the body of a person who suffers from a communicable disease, or the disinfection of contaminated articles which the sick person had any contact with

❑ **Terminal disinfection**
Terminal disinfection entails the cleansing of personal belongings, clothing and the immediate physical surroundings of a sick person who has recovered as the disease can no longer be transmitted

Disinfesting (de-lousing or de-flea-ing)

Disinfesting is the removal of lice or fleas from a person's or an animal's body

Educational institution

Educational institutions constitute all schools (pre-primary, primary, secondary – private and public [state-funded]), universities (academic and technological – private and public) and Colleges for Further Education and Training (FET) as well as hostels, homes or facilities maintained for the attendance, residence and care of the learners at an educational institution. Educational institutions also include any building or premises maintained or used for the attendance and care of more than six children of preschool age during any part of a day, or an entire day, on every day of the week or on certain days of the week only, and registered as an institution of care according to the Child Welfare Act, Act 38 of 2005. Playgroups and day care centres are also viewed as educational institutions

Endemic

Endemic refers to the phenomenon where there is a continuous presence of a communicable disease within a given geographic area

Endogenous infection

An endogenous infectious condition is caused by the normal flora (saprophytic microbes) living within or on the body of the human host

Epidemic

An epidemic refers to the phenomenon where a large number of persons contract a particular communicable disease within the same geographic area during the same period of time

Epidemiology

Epidemiology is the study of the nature and distribution of communicable medical diseases within the population. The study also includes all environmental conditions contributing to outbreaks of and contracting of communicable diseases; the lifestyles and health status of all human hosts as well as all other circumstances associated with the various states of health of the hosts, their families and their communities; and the characteristics of the different infectious agents, including the mutations of infectious agents. The principles of the epidemiological process are then applied in the control and prevention of communicable medical diseases

Erythema
Erythema is a diffuse or blotchy redness of the skin that becomes pale when pressure is applied. It is caused by congestion of the skin capillaries

Exogenous infection
An exogenous infectious condition is caused by the exposure to an external source of infectious agents such as pathogenic microbes (not by the natural flora living within or on the body of the individual)

Exposure
Exposure refers to the process by which an uninfected person is exposed to an infectious organism whereby the contraction of a communicable disease is promoted, for example, by being in direct contact with an infected or ill person, or by being directly or indirectly in contact with the pathogenic microbe

Fomites
Fomites are all infected discharges, excretions and secretions of an infected or a sick person, as well as all non-living intermediaries such as equipment, objects or/ and any matter contaminated by the ill/infected person as he/she was in contact with it. Fomites act as a vehicle because it provides a means to transmit the infectious agent from the reservoir to the host

Fumigation
Fumigation is the process by which poisonous gas are used to exterminate arthropods and rodents

Healthcare users/patients
Healthcare users or patients refer to all individuals, families, groups, and communities (whether healthy, ill, carrier or contact) who access the healthcare service delivery system, public or private, for any form of healthcare rendering by professional and/ or traditional healthcare practitioners

Healthcare providers
Healthcare providers refer to all <u>professional healthcare practitioners</u> registered with statuary councils or boards (for example, doctors, nurses, allied medical practitioners, environmental health officers, veterinarians, etc.); all <u>traditional healthcare providers</u> registered with a voluntary or statuary board or organization (for example, sangomas, herbalists, spiritual healers, traditional healers, traditional birth attendants etc.), and all <u>lay care givers</u> (for example, family members, voluntary care givers, care givers working for non-governmental organizations, etc)

Holism/Holistic/Holistically
The concept "Holism/Holistic/Holistically" refers to the wholeness of human life taking in account that all human beings live in relation to/having dialogues with himself/ herself, to/with all other human beings, to/with a Creator, and to/with the universe human beings live in. Hence, the individual, the family and the community forms an integrated unit that can never be separated from one another and the wholeness of human life is as such intertwined or interwoven with the environment and the infinite

11

different systems which form the environment or milieus. Therefore, the wholeness of the well-being of all individuals/families/communities and the environment is thus determined by the interplay and interdependence of all these infinite factors – the combined effect influencing the state of health of all individuals/families/communities and the environment they live in

Taking this relational approach of holism as point of departure, **holistic healthcare** (allopathic and traditional) promotes, protects and restores the wholeness of human life by taking in account all factors relating to the wholeness of and interdependence of these factors in the well-being of man. Therefore, holistic healthcare treats and care for the individual in totality within his/her family and community contexts by considering all aspects of the life and the needs of the individual or/and family or/and community through care rendering that provides in the **needs** (wellness, therapeutic, and/or high-risk) of all human beings (whether individuals, and/or families and/or communities). As such, holistic healthcare combines modern scientific diagnosis and monitoring techniques with healthcare practices practiced for millenniums to ensure the best practices for the upholding of the wholeness of human life and well-being and provision in the life needs of healthcare users within their familial and community context

Host
A host is any living person or warm-blooded animal required by microbes (saprophytic and pathogenic) to exist and to reproduce (multiply). As healthcare is the focus of all healthcare professions, the term "host" in this book, refers only to humankind/human beings as the client system that is affected by communicable diseases. Every human being is a potential host for any of the microbes that cause communicable diseases. Whether the person will become ill, depends on various factors such as a person's nutritional status, immune status and many more. As all human beings are members of a family and a community, the term "host" refers to the individual person, his/her family and the community they live in

Illness/being ill/being sick
Being ill/sick or illness refers to the subjective feelings/emotions and the coping mechanisms an individual or family experience or portray when the individual or family members become sick/ill from a specific medical condition/disease classified as communicable medical disease. The term "illness" is not seen as the same as "disease"

Immune status
Immune status refers to the level of physiologic resistance (innate and adaptive) the body of a person has against the pathogen/pathogenic microbe that causes a particular communicable disease. When a person's body has naturally mediated/ formed its own antibody-mediated and cell-mediated immunity with memory against the pathogen/pathogenic microbe that causes a particular communicable disease, the individual will usually have a high immunity status against the particular disease which will last as long as the person lives. When a person has been vaccinated, his/ her immune status may be high initially, but it diminishes with the passing of time (5 to 12 years) unless he/she receives booster dosages of the vaccine or is exposed to

the pathogen causing the disease or contracts the particular communicable disease. A high immune status can be maintained if the person receives booster dosages regularly, thus enhancing his/her adaptive immune system (antibody-mediated and cell-mediated immunity with memory)

> **Note** When mutation of a pathogen/pathogenic microbe takes place, the pathogen changes its genetic composition, resulting in a new strain (modified form) of the specific infectious pathogen. The host's body, however, has as yet not mediated any physiologic response [innate and adaptive]) against this mutant strain of the specific pathogen and therefore the person is susceptible to contract the mutant (new strain of) pathogen, thus becoming infected and sick. Only now can the individual's body forms/mediates the specific physiological immunological resistance against the new strain of the specific pathogen

When a person again becomes sick of a particular communicable disease he/she previously suffered from (sub-clinically or in a very light form) and there is no physical evidence that mutation of the pathogen had taken place, the individual's body has already mediated/formed a level of physiologic resistance (innate and adaptive) against the specific pathogen/pathogenic microbe during the first bout of the communicable disease but the level of resistance mediated is however not strong/high enough to combat the specific pathogen/pathogenic microbe at this stage in life when the individual is re-infected

> **Note** An individual's body very seldom mediate any level of physiologic resistance (innate and adaptive) against the specific pathogens/pathogenic microbes that are transmitted by animals to humans (zoonotic communicable medical diseases) as well as against the pathogens that cause sexually transmitted infections (STI's). Thus, individuals can be re-infected over and over time and again with either zoonotic communicable medical diseases or sexually transmitted infections or both and will become sick every time

Immunisation/Inoculation/Vaccination
Immunisation/vaccination is the procedure/process whereby a vaccine is administered to a person in order to stimulate the body to mediate (form/produce) its own physiologic resistance, namely, antibody-mediated and/or cell-mediated (sensitised T-lymphocytes) immunity with memory

Immunity and immune response
Immunity is the highly developed physiological resistance of the body against the influence and effects of any infectious agent (such as viruses, parasites, fungi, protozoa, bacteria and rickettsiae) after it had gained entry into the body. This highly developed physiologic resistance (immunological response) is the result of the innate (acute inflammatory response and phagocytosis) and adaptive (antibody-mediated and cell-mediated with memory) immunological reactions to the specific infectious agent that causes the particular communicable disease. The level of the physiologic resistance or immune status varies from one person to another

❑ **Natural/general/humoral/innate immunity** is the innate (born with) physiological resistance of the body consisting of external and internal defence mechanisms that do not require exposure to a specific pathogen for their development. The non-susceptibility of an individual to a particular communicable disease is mediated by the innate immune system

❑ **Acquired/adaptive immunity -** Acquired immunity, a homeostatic mechanism, is the physiologic resistance mediated by the adaptive immune system and is elicited by a specific antigen-antibody-response consisting of antibody-mediated and cell-mediated immune reactions with memory, both taking place simultaneously and complementing each other. Naturally acquired/adaptive immunity develops when a person has contracted the specific communicable disease (excluding the group of conditions where no immune response with memory is elicited) while artificially acquired immunity is elicited when the person has been successfully vaccinated against a particular communicable disease or when antibody are transferred from one individual to another individual. A particular communicable disease elicits its own specific adaptive immunological reaction

❖ The **antibody-mediated immunological (immune) reaction** is induced by the antigen-antibody-reaction whereby specific immunoglobulin is mediated by B-lymphocyte cells. The antibody (immunoglobulin) mediated against the specific infectious pathogen circulate in the blood plasma and lymph to protect the body against any further infection by that specific pathogen. The memory cells of the immunoglobulin **cross** (are transferred across) the placenta barrier, thus, providing passive naturally acquired immunity to the unborn foetus

❖ The **cell-mediated immunological (immune) reaction** is mediated when the production of specific sensitised T-lymphocytes with lymphoid characteristics are stimulated by a specific pathogen.

Note Some infectious agents do not stimulate an antibody-mediated immunological [immune] reaction that mediate immunoglobulin but only mediate specific sensitised T-lymphocytes with lymphoid characteristics. The specific infectious agent is destroyed or rejected when the T-lymphocytes make direct contact with the specific infectious agent (antigen) as the T-lymphocytes destroy the antigen's cell. The memory cells of the specific sensitised T-lymphocytes are continuously present in all of the body's cells where they monitor all cells for the specific infectious agents. The memory cells of the sensitised T-lymphocytes **do not** cross (are not transferred across) the placenta barrier

Incubation period

This is the time period (length of time) that elapses from been exposed to specific infectious agent and its gaining entry into the body until the appearance of the characteristic signs and symptoms of the particular communicable disease. This period may last from several hours to days. Every particular communicable disease has its own specific incubation period. During the incubation period the infected person is not ill/sick as such but possesses the ability to transmit the pathogen to other individuals

Infection

Infection follows/is caused by the invasion of cells and/or tissues of the body by living pathogens/pathogenic microbes such as bacteria, viruses, fungi, helminths (worms) and protozoa. The pathogen multiplies and produces effects that are injurious to the host

Infected person

An infected person is a person who harbours a specific infectious agent in his body and manifests the clinical or subclinical medical picture of the disease. An infected person transmits the infectious agent to other persons. Always keep in mind that an infected person can suffers from more than one communicable disease at the same time (simultaneously).

> **Note** As soon as a specific pathogen has gained entry into the body and has bonded with the tissue cells of the body, **the cells of the body become infected** (not contaminated) and the infected individual can now transmit the specific pathogen to other persons because the infected cells now shed the specific pathogen which then exits the body

Infection following gaining entry into the body

The process whereby an infectious agent penetrates into and attaches itself to body cells of a person or an animal is called "gaining entry into the body". To elicit the particular communicable disease, the pathogen must gain entry into the body through the right portal of entry. After gaining entry and binding with the body cells, the local and systemic inflammation reaction takes place in the body. As soon as the pathogen has overwhelmed the normal defence mechanisms of the body and begins to multiply/reproduce in the body, an infection had been induced

> **Note** The presence of pathogenic agents on the body surfaces [unbroken skin] and/or on articles and/or on inanimate surfaces does not denote an infection, but represents contamination of such areas and articles. As soon as pathogens gained entry into the body, the cells of the body become infected by pathogenic microbes [not contaminated], as the pathogens live in body cells only, multiply there, spread to other body cells and are shed from the body cells as to be transmitted to other uninfected hosts

Infectious agent/pathogenic microbe or micro-organism/pathogen/infective microbe

The infectious agent is the primary cause of a particular communicable disease. All pathogenic microbes (protozoa, rickettsiae, helminths, fungi, parasites, viruses, bacteria, and spirochetes) possess the ability to cause an infection in humans or animals

Infectivity

Infectivity is the ability of an infectious agent to invade the host's body and body systems and cause an infection. Infectivity is determined in part by the portal of entry and exit of the infectious agent and in part by the mode of transmission

Infested

Persons or animals are infested with arthropods when the arthropods are present on the surface of the person's/animal's body where they develop and reproduce. Infested articles (for example, clothing) or premises harbour arthropods or rodents

Inflammation

Inflammation is the complex reaction to injury or death of cells or tissues of the body. Inflammation is a non-specific internal defence mechanism initiated to control and/ or eliminate the offensive pathogen and to prepare a bodily environment conducive for healing and repair. The inflammatory process takes place in the healthy tissues adjacent to the injured or dead cells. Inflammation is always present with infection, but infection is not always present with inflammation (for example, myocardial infarction) as they are two separate processes

Insecticides

Insecticides refer to any chemical substance (powder, liquid, aerosol, or paint spray) which is used to eradicate arthropods

Intermediaries

An intermediary provides the means of transmitting the infectious agent from reservoir to host. Intermediaries are not infected with the specific pathogen nor suffer from the infection (does not possess the ability to propagate the infectious agent as this can only be done by the source of infection) but act as a go-between in facilitating the transmission of the specific pathogen. **Living intermediaries** are called **vectors,** for example, flies, fleas, mosquito's while **non-living intermediaries** are called **vehicles,** for example, water, milk, food, plasma, air, fomites, body fluids and secretions, clothing, toys, surfaces, toiletries, furniture etc.

International healthcare measures

International measures referred to in this book have only reference to situations where the World Health Organization **must be** informed by the National Department of Health of South Africa that an outbreak of a particular communicable disease(s) has/have occurred, and/or informing countries across the South-African national inland border that a particular communicable disease has broken out in South-Africa and may spread across the national border, and/or any information to be given to travellers to conform to the healthcare regulations of the country of entry

Learner/student

A learner/student is any person (immaterial of age) who attends or resides in an educational institution (pre-primary, primary, secondary and higher education) in order to receive some kind of education, counselling or training. (Children who attend play groups are also considered to be learners)

Legislative measures

Legislative measures are regulations which are contained in the National Health Act, Act 61 of 2003, describing measures to improve the health of the population of the RSA as well as to prevent the occurrence of outbreaks of epidemics. These measures are applicable to all persons and if it should prove necessary, a person can be taken to court for non-compliance. When necessarily (as soon as an epidemic or pandemic breaks out) these regulations/measures are given preference over the rights of an individual/group as imbedded in the Constitution of the RSA

Nosocomial infection
Nosocomial is an infection originating in or contracted in a healthcare establishment

Notification of cases
Notification of a case is a legislative measure whereby the health authorities is notified of an outbreak of a particular communicable disease in persons or animals and is done by means of an official report. According to law, it is the responsibility of all registered healthcare practitioners (professional and traditional) to report the legally notifiable diseases. Notification can be done by telephone or satellite phone (to be followed up in writing), by electronic mail/internet, fax or telegram

Pandemic
A pandemic is the phenomenon of an outbreak of a particular communicable disease world-wide over the same period of time, such as the Influenza-A pandemic of 1918, bird/avian flu in the early 21st century

Parasites
Parasites are microbes/animals/insects/arthropods/worms that live on or in the body of humans or animals and are dependent on the body tissues or blood of any human or animal for its continued existence. The parasite may be at any stage of development of that particular species

Parasitaemia
Parasitaemia refers to the condition of the presence of all types of worms developing, living and reproducing in the blood and/or body organs (most of the time in the intestinal tract) of humans and/or animals and are dependent on the body tissues and/or the blood of the host for their continued existence. Worms (or their eggs) living in the intestinal tract of the host are passed in faeces. The eggs of worms living in the bladder of the host are urinated. A biological vehicle (for example, a mosquito) transfers the eggs of worms living in the blood of the host to other hosts (human or animal)

Pathogenic microbe/pathogen/infectious agent/infective microbe
Pathogenic microbes/pathogens/infected microbes are infectious agents. A specific pathogenic microbe causes a particular communicable disease

Pathogenicity
Pathogenicity is the ability of an infectious agent to cause a disease in susceptible hosts. Pathogenicity is closely related to the attack rate which is the proportion of those hosts who eventually manifest the particular disease correlating to all hosts who were exposed to the infectious agent

Personal hygiene measures
These are the protective measures taken by an individual to promote his/her own health and to prevent the spread of communicable diseases which are mainly transmitted by being in direct contact with the infectious agent. These measures include

- keeping the body clean by thoroughly washing with soap and water on a daily basis
- washing of hands after using the toilet (urine and faeces)
- washing of hands after any physical activity inside or outside a home, hospital, work place, etc
- washing of hands after coming in contact with pets and garbage
- washing of hands after blowing the nose, coughing or sneezing
- washing of hands before preparing or eating food
- washing of the hands thoroughly after touching a healthcare user or his/her possessions or coming in contact with any discharge from any human or any animal
- washing of the hands before and after coming into contact with anybody who is sick or wounded
- keeping hands as well as contaminated articles and toilet articles away from the mouth, eyes, nose, ears and wounds
- avoiding the sharing of crockery, drinking utensils, towels, handkerchiefs, combs and brushes
- avoiding exposure to other persons who suffer from any infectious disease (speciality respiratory diseases) when coughing, sneezing, laughing, singing and talking
- using available material in public places to wash and clean hands or sanitize equipment before or after use
- covering of the nose and mouth when coughing or sneezing while disposing used tissues containing respiratory secretions in the nearest waste receptacle after use or incinerated it (if necessary) and washing hands after having contact with any respiratory secretions as well as any contaminated objects/ material

Portal of entry and exit

The portal of entry and exit denotes the point/site of entry and the point/site of exit through which the infectious agent causing the particular communicable disease, gains entry into the body and leaves/sheds from the body of the infected host. Portals of entry include the respiratory tract and system, the gastro-intestinal tract, the skin and mucous membranes. Infectious agents leave the infected host through/are shed from the body via the respiratory tract and body system in droplets, or through faeces passed from the gastro-intestinal tract. Blood and other body fluids such as semen, vaginal secretion, urine and saliva are also portals of exit for infectious agents. The skin acts as portal of entry as well as portal of exit for certain infectious agents. Portals of entry and exit are closely related to the modes of transmission of communicable diseases

Prevention

Prevention is the measures taken to prevent and control outbreaks of communicable diseases. The measures are aimed at the infectious agent, the source of infection and the environment. The necessary measures are instituted at all levels of prevention, namely,

- **Primary prevention (preventive and promotive)**
  These measures are taken to prevent an outbreak of a particular communicable disease by enhancing the health of all hosts (individuals, families and communities), maintaining a healthy environment and instating a comprehensive healthcare system that serves the population in totality

- **Secondary prevention (curative)**
  These measures are taken to control the spread of a particular communicable disease after an outbreak has occurred through early diagnosis and treatment. Also included are the interventions taken to care for the sick person/family/community. Other measures also included are those taken to remove/reduce any health hazards/risks in the environment as well as correcting any problematic factors in the healthcare system

- **Tertiary prevention (rehabilitative)**
  These measures are taken to assist those persons who have recovered from a communicable disease, as well as their family and community, to function as normally as possible. The measures are also intended to orientate communities regarding steps to be taken to prevent further outbreaks of communicable diseases. Other measures that are to be instated are to maintain a healthy environment and the strengthening of the healthcare system

Principal

A principal (Rector of tertiary educational institutions) is the person who is in charge of an educational institution, either permanently or temporarily, or, in his/her absence, his/her deputy

Prodromal period

The prodromal period is the time period between the appearance of the first non-specific/general signs and symptoms of a disease and the specific/typical/characteristic signs and symptoms of the particular communicable disease are manifested. During the prodromal period, the sick person can transmit the particular communicable disease to other persons. No specific medical diagnosis can be made during this period

Prodromal signs and symptoms

These are the first signs and symptoms of a disease of which a person complains or which are discernible before the typical signs and symptoms of the particular communicable disease manifest itself

Prophylaxis

Prophylaxis refers to the methods used to prevent the spread of a communicable disease. These measures are used by/on individuals and their families and/or on/by members in a community and/or on/by members of a part of a community. Chemoprophylaxis is the use of specific chemical-produced (pharmacological) drugs to prevent the onset of a particular communicable disease in exposed individuals. Vaccine-prophylaxis refers to the vaccination of all individuals (whether vaccinated previously or unvaccinated) with a specific vaccine after exposure has taken place and/or to prevent/control the spread of particular communicable disease. When individuals are prevented from developing the symptomatic disease, they are also prevented from spreading the disease to others

Public Health preventive measures
Public health preventive measures refer to those measures instated by different governmental bodies that deliver public services to combat communicable diseases in all populations. These measures include safe drinking water, a safe food chain, reliable sewage and garbage disposal, vector control, and vaccination

Pyaemia
Pyaemia is the condition that develops when the causative pathogen circulates in the blood of the infective person in small septic emboli

Quarantine
Quarantine is legislative measures that are taken to restrict the freedom of movement of individuals/families/communities or part of communities (whether healthy, carrier and contact) as well as of animals/birds/reptiles after they have been exposed to a particular communicable disease in order to prevent the spread of the particular disease

❑ **Period of quarantine**
This is the time period of restriction of movement of healthy people (animals included) as well as of contacts, and/or the exclusion of learners and/or educators who are contacts from educational institutions (schools [day care centres, preschools, primary and secondary schools], universities [academic and of technology] and colleges for further education and training). The quarantine period usually lasts as long as the longest day of the incubation period of the specific disease **plus two additional days**

Reservoir
A reservoir is the environment in which a pathogenic microbe exists and multiplies. A reservoir does not only transmit the infectious agent but is actually infected by the agent. Reservoirs can be human, animal or environmental. Human reservoirs are divided into two categories, namely, cases and carriers

Regulations regarding exclusion from schools and higher educational institutions
These regulations describe the listed groups of communicable medical diseases. When a learner/student and/or educator/lecturer and/or any other person employed by the institution of education as defined, contracts a listed communicable medical disease, he/she is not allowed to attend the educational institution for the full legally prescribed period. All susceptible contacts are also subjected to these regulations

Resistance of the body/innate immunity
Resistance/innate immunity of the body refers to the protection/defending of the body by the physiological immunological reactions of the innate and adaptive immune systems whereby the body is protected against pathogens from gaining entry into the body, or if invaded, prevented from being weakened by the pathogen self and/ or by its toxin(s). Resistance is grounded in the genetic make-up of a person, while

his/her level of resistance is enhanced or compromised by various factors, such as age, stress, the presence of other diseases, nutritional status, normal physiological functions and chemotherapeutic treatment (for example, antibiotics/anti-microbial drugs and/or other chemical drugs [such as immune-suppressive chemotherapy]); and/or natural substances (radiation)

Rodenticides
These are chemical substances used to exterminate rodents – mainly by ingestion of the substance

Skin lesions
Skin lesions are specific lesions that appear on/in the skin and are typical to the particular communicable disease. Skin lesions can be classified as primary and secondary lesions.
- ❑ Primary lesions are specific lesions that appear initially in the skin and are produced by the infectious agent or its toxin. Lesions may manifest as maculae, papules, vesicles, pustules, nodules or wheals.
- ❑ Secondary lesions are the result of changes which took place in the primary lesions and can manifest as squama (scales), scabs, crusts or scars

Sickness
Sickness refers to the phenomenon/state of being sick whereby an individual or family or community suffers from a specific medical condition/disease whether diagnosed by a medical practitioner or self or another person. In this book sickness refers to the state of being sick because of suffering from a particular communicable medical condition caused by a specific pathogenic microbe. The term "sickness" can be used synomous to "disease"

Social Medicine
Social medicine refers to the study of the social, economic and other determines of health and disease and its application to healthcare practices as to ensure a healthier society. The study of medicine in general, on the other hand, focuses mainly on diseases and the questions asked are mostly on a molecular level of the human body. The questions asked in Social Medicine is bio-social in nature as to determine the impact of all bio-physical, social, economic and other factors of importance on the health and disease patterns of individuals/families/communities

Source of infection
The source of infection can be any infected human, or any infected animal, or any spores formed in soil/dirt/excreta or any non-living material that is contaminated with the specific infectious agent, or any intermediary that provides a means of transmitting the infectious agent, or any environmental reservoir where infectious agents exist and multiply. Transmitting can occur by any mode of transmission

Sporadic
Sporadic refers to the phenomenon where a few or isolated cases of a communicable disease occur here and there

Sterilization

Sterilization is the process whereby all living microbes (saprophytic, pathogenic, and spores) are destroyed. Items to be used are now sterile

Transmission and Mode of transmission

Transmission is the transfer of the pathogen from one host to another (from an infected host to an uninfected host). Transmission occurs horizontally (from person to person or from animal/bird/reptile to humans or from reservoirs via intermediaries to humans) or vertically (from mother to child/foetus). The mode and form of transmission of a particular disease is the means/way by which an infectious pathogen that causes a particular disease is transferred from an infected person to an uninfected person. Communicable diseases are transmitted **horizontally** by several modes of transmission in different forms, namely, airborne (infected droplets); faecal-oral (infected faecal material); skin-to-skin contact (pus, crust, flakes, scabs); sexual contact (seminal fluid, vaginal secretions); inoculation (blood); animal or insect bite (saliva); as well as by any other means of being spread (for example, contact with spores present in soil or contact with inanimate objects). **Vertically** transmission occurs trans-placental when the pathogen is transferred via blood across the placental barrier to the unborn foetus

Toxaemia

Toxaemia occurs when the toxin (a by-product) released by the causative infectious agent is present in the blood.

Toxin

A toxin is a polypeptide (protein) or glycolipid released by an infectious pathogen to damage the body cells to such extent that it eventually leads to the death of the cell(s) of the body. Toxins are released with the aim to enter into certain body cells and kill off these cells, or to spread through the host's body killing off the body cells or to defend the bacteria against the host's defence mechanisms. Most of the bacterial toxins that are released act on body cells and body tissues but several bacteria release however toxins that affects the nerve impulses with a neurological impact such as Clostridium tetani toxin and Clostridium botulinum toxin. Toxins are classified as endotoxins, exotoxins and enterotoxins

❑ **Endotoxins**

Endotoxins are an integral part of the cell walls of the pathogen (especially gram-negative bacteria) and are only released when the host's reaction destroys the pathogen and the pathogen dies. Endotoxins consist mostly of glycolipids/lipopolysaccharides that are heat-resistant and insoluble. Endotoxins cause non-specific effects such as fever and inflammation but in large amounts they cause abnormal bleeding or clotting, hypotension and vascular collapse (septic shock/endotoxin shock because of the systemic spread of the pathogen). It is a weak antigen and elicits a poor immune response

❑ **Exotoxins**

Exotoxins consist mainly of protein and when actively released by the infectious pathogen, it is absorbed into the bloodstream of the host and then circulates to all the cells and organs of the body where they destroy the cells in the surrounding tissues. As exotoxins are powerful toxins, they elicit a good immune response which usually lasts life-long. An exotoxin can be detoxified or attenuated in formalin without changing the genetic structure of the antigen. Consequently, it is still able to stimulate antibody-mediated and cell-mediated immunological reactions with memory, whereby artificial actively acquired immunity is mediated. The attenuated exotoxin is unable to cause the disease or the symptoms of the disease

❑ **Enterotoxins**
Enterotoxins are released by pathogens in the digestive tract of the host where it causes local cell death. Should the enterotoxin succeed in penetrating into the small blood vessels around the digestive tract, it is absorbed in the blood circulation

Toxoid
Toxoid is a toxin-converted or toxin-inactivated product with antigen characteristics. The toxoid contains no toxicity since the toxin was detoxified by the addition of formalin. An immune response is mediated when administered to a person although booster dosages are necessary to maintain a high level of immunity

Vaccine (inoculant)
A vaccine is a suspension of a specific non-living (killed) or living attenuated pathogen (with reduced virulence) or the inactivated toxin (detoxified) of a specific infectious agent in a normal saline solution or glycerine. The vaccine contains some (or at least one) of the protective antigens of the pathogen. When the vaccine is injected into/ orally given to a person, the specific infectious agent is not virulent enough to cause the infection, but the attenuated/killed pathogen or toxoid or genetically engineered substance acts as immune response stimulant by inducing the body's physiological adaptive immunological response to mediate antibody- and/or T-cell immunity with memory

Vector (intermediary)
Vectors are living intermediaries that provide a means for transmitting infectious agents from reservoir to hosts. The means can be mechanical (a fly transmitting typhoid), or biological (a flea spreading plague or a mosquito transmitting malaria)

Viraemia
Viraemia is a condition where a specific virus circulates in the bloodstream

Virulence
Virulence refers to the specific pathogen's different genes and gene products involved at different stages in the process of pathogenesis. Virulence factors, for example, such as adhesion; penetration into cells; anti-phagocytic activity; production of toxins; and interaction with the immune system are coded by different genes and gene products of the pathogen. Some pathogens have a remarkable degree of antigenic variation whereby the pathogen can switch from one virulence gene to another to avoid detection. When a pathogen mutates (whether the result of an antigenic

drift or an antigenic shift), the virulence of the pathogen also changes (most of the time becoming more virulent) because the different genes and gene products have changed. The virulence of a pathogen is closely related to the severity/seriousness of the communicable disease and the case fatality (mortality) rate of the communicable disease. Infections caused by pathogens with very high virulence (extremely virulent infectious agent) results mostly in fatality (death) while pathogens with a low virulence cause a relatively minor illness

Note Do not confuse virulence with pathogenicity as the two terms refer to different characteristics of the infectious agent

THEME I

<u>THE ROLE PLAYERS</u>

The symbiotic and dynamic relationship between the host, the pathogen and the environment in the causation, spread and control of communicable diseases

Since time immemorial a symbiotic and dynamic relationship has existed between man and microbes. Within this relationship, the response of man (the human host) is grounded in the outcome of the complex interplay between man, the microbe (the specific pathogen) and the environment as most host-microbe-contacts do not result in disease, but when changes occur in either man or in the microbe or in the environment or in all three elements (man, microbe and environment), disease arises. Hence, communicable diseases/transmissible infections are thus a specific group of medical diseases/infections that are caused by specific pathogens/pathogenic microbes/specific infectious agents and the signs and symptoms (clinical picture/ clinical manifestation) the hosts (humans or animals) manifest, are characteristic of the particular communicable disease/transmissible infection. As communicable medical diseases/infections are transmitted horizontally (directly and indirectly) from one person to another (host-to-host) or from animals to humans or from environment to a person (host) and vertically from mother to child/trans-ovarially in certain animals, the host, the environment and the pathogen can never be regarded as single factors in the causation, spread and control of communicable diseases.

Based on the symbiotic and dynamic relationship that exists between man and microbe, the specific model that depicts the epidemiological triad/symbiosis of host-microbe-environment in communicable medical diseases is the **EPIDEMIOLOGICAL TRIAD OF COMMUNICABLE DISEASES Model** as it describe this specific host-parasite-environment-relationship or the specific interrelatedness of the human host, the infectious pathogen and the environment – each element characterise by specific intrinsic properties/attributes/characteristics. By using the "Epidemiological Triad of Communicable Diseases" model, all the multiple factors that contribute to the causation of communicable diseases can be identified and the "links of interrelatedness" can be severed as to prevent and control communicable diseases. The "Epidemiological Triad of Communicable Diseases" model is also directional in the healthcare rendering to all hosts (individuals, families and communities whether healthy, ill, contact, carrier) as well as in all healthcare interventions to maintain a healthy environment.

Chapter 1

"THE EPIDEMIOLOGICAL TRIAD OF COMMUNICABLE DISEASES MODEL" – AN EXPOSITION OF THE MODEL AS THE POINT OF DEPARTURE

As all living organisms use one another as habitat, all living organisms have formed symbiotic associations where one species lives in or on the body of another with no overtones of benefit or harm. Since time immemorial, humans and microbes co-existed in a specific symbiotic relationship with one another because man is also a living organism. Within this specific symbiotic relationship three broad categories of symbiosis can be distinguished, namely, commensalism, mutualism and parasitism.

Commensalism

In **commensalism** one species of organisms uses the body of a larger species as its physical environment and uses that environment to acquire nutrients needed for its own survival. As such, humans support an extensive commensally microbial flora on the skin, in the mouth and in the alimentary tract. This relationship of the microbes with humans is highly specialized, with the microbes having specific attachment mechanisms and precise environmental requirements. The commensally microbes benefit humans by preventing colonization of more pathogenic species or by producing metabolites that are used by humans, for example, the metabolites produced by enteric bacteria. Normally these microbes are harmless, but they become pathogenic when their environmental conditions are changed in some way.

Mutualism

In **mutualism** there exists a beneficial or mutual relationship in which reciprocal benefits are reaped by both man and microbe – for example, the health of humans and their resistance to colonization by pathogens depends on the integrity of the normal commensally enteric bacteria. The bacteria are highly specialized for life in the human intestine although no strict mutual dependence exist in this relationship.

Parasitism

In **parasitism**, the symbiotic relationship benefits only the pathogenic microbe as all pathogens are parasites. Parasitism is a one-sided relationship in which all the benefits go to the pathogen because man, the host, provides the parasites with their physical-chemical environment, their food, respiratory and other metabolic needs and even the signals that regulate their development. Most parasites/pathogens establish innocuous associations with their natural host (man or animal) and are not pathogenic under normal circumstances, for example, when the natural host is in good health. The state of *balanced pathogenicity* reflects the balance that exists between the competency of the physiological resistance of the host's systemic defences, (namely, the innate and adaptive immune systems and the intactness of the surfaces, skin, and mucosa of the host as to prevent infection because humans are host to normal commensally microbial flora as well as infectious pathogens) and the pathogenicity in the pathogen – the individual is in good health and the pathogen has establish an innocuous association with the host. In a state of *unbalanced pathogenicity,* __disease arises__ because the normal environmental conditions of the pathogen have changed in some way, and/or the pathogen has become established in an unnatural/ new host (for example, in man instead of an animal) resulting in disease, and/or the level of genetically determined resistance of the host has diminished or became compromised.

1.1   EXPOSITION OF "EPIDEMIOLOGICAL TRIAD OF COMMUNICABLE DISEASES" MODEL

Humans and microbes co-exist in a specific symbiotic relationship with one another because man is also a living organism. In a state of balanced pathogenicity man and pathogen live in an innocuous association with one another. When a state of unbalanced pathogenicity occurs, diseases arises that can lead to sporadic or endemic or epidemic or pandemic outbreaks of communicable medical diseases worldwide. Hence, the **Epidemiological Triad of Communicable Diseases model** depicts the dynamic and symbiotic relationship between the human host, the pathogen and the environment in the causation, prevention and control of communicable diseases. As such, the human host refers to the human client system (individual, or family, or community) affected by a particular communicable disease while the pathogen indicates the specific pathogen as the primary cause of the particular communicable disease. The environment includes all those factors in the physical, biological, social and all other environments/milieus that contribute to the causation, prevention and control of the particular communicable disease. Because the bio-complexity of this interrelationship of the three elements determines the outcome of the pathogenesis of the communicable medical disease, namely, a state of relative health or disease in man, and because each element in the relationship, man the host; the pathogen; and the environment possesses inherent or specific characteristics/properties/attributes that influence the health of all individuals, families, and communities as well as an individual's susceptibility to become ill and his/her response to the specific pathogen causing the particular communicable disease, data needs to be collected from all three elements in the model as to determine not only the bio-complexity of each specific element in the causation of communicable diseases, but also to plan the necessary measures to prevent and control the specific communicable disease. The dominant role that the environment (whether physical-biological, psychological, socio-cultural, political, religious, informational, economical, etc.) plays in the causation, prevention and control of the particular communicable disease(s) must never be under estimated.

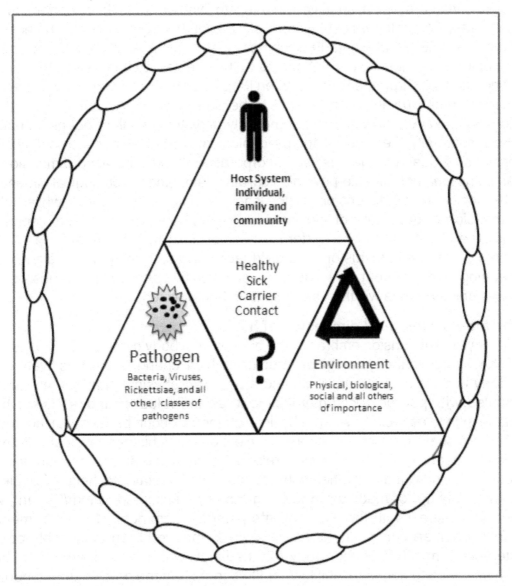

Figure 1.1 Depicting the interrelatedness of Man the human host, the Pathogen and the Environment man lives in through the schematic presentation of the "Epidemiological Triad of Communicable Diseases" model encircled by the Chain of Infection

The state of health of the individual/family/community is determined by the interplay of all the multiple factors of the different dimensions of health – the combined effect influencing the host's exposure, susceptibility and response to the infectious agent. To explain and describe the host-related attributes that determine the relative health status of a specific individual or family or community, the Dimensions of Health model is used. The Dimensions of Health model is grounded in the metaphysical point of departure that all persons are unique human beings and that as an unique individual, the baby's or toddler's or child's or adolescent's or adult's or elder's life dialogues/relations/possibilities/talents are unique to himself/herself and that the specific individual gives a specific meaning to his/her own life experiences and conduct himself/herself from out his/her Self/"I' in his/her life situations. In becoming the person an individual wants to become, must become and should become, all human beings live their life in relationship to themselves, to their fellow-humans, to the world and their Supreme Being, and on the strength of their choices they become the person/human being he/she wants to be and can be. As human beings, all individuals embrace a diversity and complexity of distinguishable (but not separate) dimensions, namely, the physical, the psychological, the social, and the spiritual. The Dimensions of Health Model, *per se*, incorporates all the embraced dimensions of human beings, namely, the bio-physiological dimension; the psychological dimension; and the socio-cultural dimension as the specific indicators of health whilst taking the dimension of behaviour of the individual/family/community; the environmental dimension and the healthcare system dimension also in consideration as further indicators of the health status of the individual/family/community. An explanation of the meaning of the different dimensions will be given first after which the host-related attributes of importance will then be described and/or listed.

1. **The bio-physiological dimension of health**
   The physical dimension embraces the bio-physical body of the person, consisting of the anatomical-physiological structure which changes progressively in an orderly and logical pattern. Because a person's physical changes are always coupled with psycho-social development, an individual changes his/her body image often, especially when physical changes occur because of ageing or through disease or disability. As a person experiences his/her physical self-image and the meaning of his/her body in relation to the world and fellow-humans, the body of the individual is his/her instrument (when, for example, he/she is walking, sitting, working) or mediator in fulfilling the roles allocated to him/her and with which to interact with the world or interpersonal communicator when meeting a fellow human being. In his/her relation to the world, an individual not only interacts from within his/her body (as mediator) with the concrete world, busy with its concrete goods to fulfil his/her life chores, but the person simultaneously constitutes his/her own psychological life world wherein he/she can actualize himself/herself as an independent identity (psychological self-image/the Self/the I).

   Health, disease, disability, death cannot be removed from the lives of individuals, families, and communities without robbing life of its meaning. Health, disease, disability, and death influence human beings in the totality of their personhood as these states change the essence of a person's being – his/her Self. To experience health problems, to be ill, to be disabled, or to die affects or disconnects a person's dialogues in his/her relation with himself, with his fellow-men and the community, with the world, and with his/her Creator. As the meaning of the Self/"I" of a healthy/ill/disabled/dying person is locked in the meaning of health and disease, health/disease/disability/death is conceptualized in different ways and different meanings are given to health/disease/disability/dying and death by individuals/families/ communities. As such, health and disease are dynamic conditions in the life span of every healthcare user - an individual is not statically healthy or statically ill but alternates between being healthy and being sick. Health is an instrument of self-actualization, enabling a person to be in dialogue with himself/herself, his/ her fellow-humans, his/her world, and his/her Supreme Being. Because disease, disability, or death endangers the existence of a person, and interrupts his/her life dialogues, a person has to change these dialogues, and reconstitute a new personal world leading to new relations with himself/herself, his/her fellow-men, his/her world, and his/her Creator. Because of these changed dialogues, the person's self-actualization may become retarded or may grow and mature through the meaning he/she has found in illness, disability, or death – the choice is made by the person himself/herself. And because no person is ever without a family, the healthy, ill, disabled, or dying person influences his/her family while his/her family influences the healthy, ill, disabled, or dying individual

2. **The psychological dimension of health**
   All human beings (infants, children and adolescents, adults, elderly) as individuals have a structured personality consisting of a unified systemic dimension (the bodily, psychological and spiritual systems) and a functional dimension (cognitive, will, and affective-emotional functions) that form a dynamic structural-functional multi-dimensional unity. In becoming themselves, all human beings live in relation to themselves, to other persons, to the world, and to a Supreme Being. On the strength of the choices they pursue, they become the person they want to become, and can become. From childhood to old age, all individuals conduct themselves from out of their Self or "I" as to become his/her own identity. The essence of every individual's being is constantly in a process of development because of the person's interaction with other humans and the world in which he/she lives. The Self or "I" is the driving force behind all the actions that the individual portrays while the individual's personality encompasses all the capacities, qualities, and possibilities of the individual as person.

   The personality of all human beings develops according to a specific pattern of unfolding; his/her inherent ability grows gradually and his acquired capacities are learned, undergoing changes throughout his/her lifetime. Within the unfolding of their lives, all persons go through different developmental phases that offer particular challenges and possibilities. All individuals are inseparably involved in their own development. They shape themselves because they themselves decide in what direction they want to unfold and how they will overcome their own limitations.

   All human beings live both in the physical world as well as in the socio-cultural world that is constituted by the members of the group they belong to. All individuals also live in the psychological world of their own making. This psychological world is the totality of the relationships the person enters in grounding his/her becoming or self-actualization through conquering the world with its horizons that ripple further and further outwards. And, because the psychological living world of all human beings is always multi-dimensional in nature, the individual experience his/her life in a historical way (past, present, future), in spatiality (boundaries and horizons), and in positive or negative ways while his/her living space is and remains secure, recognizable, and possessively meaningful to him/her. Because all human beings are body-psyche-spirit and, as such, possess a soul, all persons always live in relation to a Supreme Being. The individual thus makes choices according to his/her own values, norms, and conscience for which he/she takes responsibility.

The psyche of a person embraces his/her will, decision-making, actions, feeling/ emotions, aspirations, and intellect (thought, language, and learning ability). Although the intellect dictates how a person relates to other people in the world around him/her as well as to his Creator, the individual always participates through his/her feelings in any situation. As a person's emotions give meaning to his/her experiences, the individual's actions and aspirations are always influenced by his/ her emotions, thus contributing to the individual's mood, which is the foundation of his/her experiences. Therefore, the psycho-emotional health of an individual is a set of related phenomena describing the ways in which the individual copes with stress, adapts to personal and family losses, deals with problematic psychosocial-cultural situations or problematic bio-physical-chemical situations.

3 The socio-cultural dimension of health

In their origin as human beings, all persons are inseparably concerned with their fellow-humans, yearning for a community in which they find alliances, fellow sufferers, and fellow-companions to whom they are connected. Through and from his/her fellow human beings in the living world - the area where an individual's life drama takes place and his/her life is conducted - a person discovers himself/ herself and actualizes himself/herself as a human being. Thus, the self-esteem of an individual develops in his/her relation to others as he/she enacts the life roles allocated to him/her. All human beings are born into a family and a specific community. As a member of a family, all individuals live an intimate life with the other members of the family in the household circle, moulding one another's personalities. All individuals as a member of a family, a social group, and a community act according to the values and norms of the family, group, and community because, through the socialization process, the individual has internalized all the ideas (such as those concerning health, disease, disability, and death), norms and values, roles, attitudes, beliefs, habits and customs that are acceptable in his/her society. Throughout a person's life, a specific social status is imparted, based on a person's gender, age, household, and family status. While a person cannot change his/her specific social status much, he/she can bring about changes to his/her acquired statuses through his/her membership of voluntary groups. All persons explore the world according to the world-view of their specific social class while conducting their lives according to the standards and prescriptions of their respective families, groups, and communities.

By living a value-orientated life according to the ethos of their specific culture, all persons, their families and their communities are socio-cultural beings living in the socio-cultural world constituted by their family and community/society to which they belong, or the group to which the individual belongs. As such, the life of all persons is rooted in culture because culture encompasses both the material goods (money, equipment, art, clothing) and the non-material goods (values and norms, behaviour, laws, customs, practices, word-views, ideas, language and knowledge) that every individual has internalized as his/her own from childhood. Through socialization and education, cultural knowledge (the world-view that is held, the social values and norms that are shared, the categories within which reality is classified [including the meaning given to health and disease as well as to suffering, disability, and death]) is transferred from generation to generation, thus, ensuring the survival of the community. Although cultural diffusion does occur, and certain customs do change, certain behaviours (especially towards health, disease, disability, and dying, for example) remain traditional most of the time because cultural practices are habitual, and deep-rooted values and convictions change very slowly.

4 The behaviour dimension of health

Because the different dimensions obtain meaning only in conjunction with other dimensions and stand in a unity with each other, all human beings never act according to one dimension only (although an individual chooses a special dimension at a time). Therefore, all persons are always intentionally aimed, they are involved with something, focused on something as to answer to the appeal that life aims at them and therefore find the meaning of their actions outside themselves. Thus, all human beings do not exist for the sake of existing, but through their choices become what they can become, could become and should become because they live a norm controlled life. And because all humans are members of a specific group/community, all individuals direct their behaviour according to the rules (norms) that are laid down by the culture of the community they live in. As such, the normative component of culture embraces all norms, values and punitive measures, as well as the prescriptions of what type of social behaviour is acceptable and important, and how a person as a member of the community should behave. Furthermore, these norms can be sub-divided in formal norms and informal norms with the formal norms such as laws, written rules and regulations serving to maintain order within the society, while the informal norms such as social habits, national habits, traditions, morals, taboos, and etiquette of the culture set the unwritten conduct requirements for all group members. These informal norms are more permanent and change very seldom and any deviation from them is met with specific punitive measures by the community.

All individuals are socialized by internalizing the culturally-determined informal norms and values as their own, and although certain cultural customs do change, the behaviour of the members stay traditional because cultural practices are habitual and certain deep rooted values and convictions change very slowly (convictions are culturally based forming the basis of human thoughts and are reflected in human actions and behaviour). During the socialization process, all individuals learn the cultural view/orientation to health and disease as well as the role behaviour regarding being healthy/ill/disabled/dying. Because the meaning of health and disease is determined by culture, the health and illness behaviour individuals/families/communities display is also determined by their culture. As such, health behaviour reflects all those activities that healthy persons will participate in, with the exclusive purpose of prevention of disease or identifying disease during the a-symptomatic stage. Illness behaviour, on the other hand, reflects all those specific behaviour patterns that a person who feels ill will display to define the state of his/her health while looking for an effective treatment of the disease. Furthermore, the manner in which a person will seek help are also determined by a variety of factors such as the degree of seriousness of the symptoms, previous experience, motivation, knowledge as well as cultural values, accessibility and affordability of healthcare services delivery, and many other stumbling blocks - and the more the stumbling blocks, the greater the likelihood that the individual will ignore the symptoms.

5 The environmental dimension of health

The health of the individual host, his/her family and the community is influenced by not only individual behaviours but also by factors in the physical-biological, socio-cultural, psychological, economical and all other important environments/milieus wherein the hosts live. When the balance between host, pathogenic agent and environment is disturbed, it becomes a contributing factor in the causation of an outbreak and spread of communicable diseases. The environment consists of all factors in the physical and biological environment as well as in the psychological, economical, socio-cultural and other important milieus (for example, historical, political, religious, moral-ethical, judicial, working/occupational, etc.) that contributes to health-related conditions which increase or decrease the possibility for outbreaks and the spread of communicable diseases. When assessing the environmental and milieu conditions and their relationship "links" to the health of the host, the existence of all present environmental hazards/risks must be identified as well as the effect(s) these hazards/risks have on the health of the individual, his/her family and his/her community. The role being played by all environments/milieus must always never be under-estimated as the environment(s) plays a very important (sometimes the most important role) in the causation, spread and control of communicable diseases.

6 The healthcare system dimension of health

In reaction to illness, disability and death, all cultures/communities/populations develop structures and social actions to handle such phenomena. This led to the establishment of healthcare systems world-wide. A healthcare system is constituted of all resources (human and physical), all actors, namely, the healthcare users and the healthcare providers [professional, traditional and lay care givers]; all healthcare service delivery structures such as establishments/organizations/businesses/practices; all finances (private and public); and all management forms that culminate in the delivery of healthcare services to the population. There exist many different healthcare systems in the world and the different national healthcare systems vary in complexity, are not exactly the same and are constantly changing and being modified.

The dominant framework or "paradigm" of thinking regarding healthcare is based on two "models" – the biomedical model and the holistic model (psychosocial-environment model or traditional model). According to the bio-medical model, health is seen only in the biological context because the nature and causes of health and disease can directly be traced back to a specific aetiology (microbe, virus, etc) and treatment focuses only on the body of the patient (the patient's body is a machine and thus the patient is passive in his/her treatment). The nature of medical intervention is based on medical knowledge, technological engineering and chemical intervention because such treatment is sufficient to make the body of the patient better. Based on the above assumptions, a powerful image of the role of the allopathic medicine (professional medicine) in improving health had developed with emphasis on

- the treatment of organic diseases
- an orientation towards cure with chemical substances (based on the perception that disease is an autonomous and potentially manageable entity which threatens personal health in a temporary or episodic manner) because the specific individual is the site of the disease
- the belief that the medical environment (be it the hospital, consulting room) is the appropriate place of treatment because only professional healthcare practitioners can prescribe healthcare treatment.

The Holistic Health Model or Health Tradition Model puts health in a social context as it focuses on the promotion and maintaining of health through socio-environmental and behavioural changes. The point of departure of this model is that the life of human beings and their health status are determined by their behaviour, what work they do and how and where they live. Persons are seen not as passive victims of disease but as participators in their recovery from a disease and in the promotion of their own good health. Changes in society and environment contribute greatly to disease management as well as to the prevention of ill health and promotion of health. Underpinning the holistic model is the understanding that **culture defines the values, beliefs and meaning of health, disease, illness and sickness, as well as health behaviour, illness behaviour, sick role behaviour, and the established ways of maintaining health, preventing disease and treating the sick.**

The Health Traditions Model or Holistic Health Model aids in the understanding, assessment, and analysis of the beliefs and practices that an individual, a family, or a community follows to protect their physical, mental, and spiritual health, to maintain physical, mental, and spiritual health, and to restore their physical, mental, and spiritual health (see Table 1.1).

Table 1.1 THE INTEGRATED DIMENSIONS OF THE HEALTH TRADITIONS MODEL OR HOLISTIC HEALTH MODEL

Dimensions	Physical	Mental	Spiritual
Maintain health	Healthy diet Proper clothing Rest and sleep Personal hygiene Exercising	Social and family support systems Hobbies Occupation	Religious worshipping Prayer Meditation
Protect health	Special diets Symbolic clothing	Association with the right persons (avoidance of evil persons) Family and community activities	Religious customs Superstitions Wearing of amulets Talisman
Restore health	Homeopathic remedies Liniments Herbal teas Special foods Massage Acupuncture Other therapies	Relaxation Nerve teas and herbal remedies Traditional healers Dances	Religious rituals Special prayers Meditation Traditional healings Exorcism

Health maintenance refers to a person's or family's or community's beliefs regarding the daily or frequent activities that the individual, family, or community carries out to maintain health on an ongoing basis as well as the infinite number of substances or objects that may be used on a daily basis to maintain health, for example, diet, activities, rest, exercises, clothing, and much more.

Health protection refers to a person's or family's or community's beliefs regarding the use of specific strategies to protect the self from external harm as well as the infinite number of substances or objects that may be used on a daily basis to protect health, such as the wearing of objects of magical nature or hanging them in the home or erecting totem tokens in the community. Other forms of protective healthcare practices include the performing of certain rituals, prayers, diets (such as food taboos, for example), clothing for different seasons, exercises (such as hatha yoga and/or breathing), and meditation. The protection of health is grounded in the ability of individuals, families, and communities to understand the cause of a given disease or communicable infection and/or the set of signs and symptoms of the particular illness or communicable infection.

Health restoration refers to a person's or family's or community's beliefs regarding the use of specific practices to restore health as well as the infinite number of substance or objects that may be used to restore health. By adhering strictly to religious codes, morals, and practices, many persons believe that disease can be prevented and health restored. Religious healing and the use of traditional healers is another example of a very strong belief. The countless rituals guiding the dying process, including the Catholic ritual of "anointing the sick", are sacred practices involving the active participation of both the ill person and his/her family. The ritual washing of the deceased's body is a necessity for certain ethno-cultural groups. When disease is attributed to the forces of evil, various strategies for restoring health may be used, including the isolation of the ill individual, the chanting of special prayers for the ill person, the singing of incantations to cure the ill person, and/or the performing of sacrifices and dances in an effort to cure the disease or infection.

The provision of culturally congruent care mandates an awareness of, and sensitivity to, the socio-cultural background and health traditions of individuals, families, and communities (whether healthy, ill, contact, or carrier). To render culturally congruent healthcare to all individuals, families, and communities (whether healthy, ill, contact, or carrier), the healthcare brokering process must be used and adapted to assess effectively the health and disease beliefs, illness behaviours and practices of individuals, families, or communities (whether healthy, ill, contact, carrier), and to determine the impact of their cultural, ethnic, or religious values on the proposed scientific plan of care. Health beliefs and health practices must be recognized and respected, and, where possible, be integrated into the proposed healthcare interventions to be rendered.

In the light of the above, two definite and different healthcare sub-systems have developed regarding the diagnosing and treatment of disease, namely, the orthodox/ allopathic/professional/western healthcare sub-system and the folk/alternative/ complementary/traditional medicine sub-system. The allopathic healthcare sub-system is the sanctioned system in Republic of South Africa and it includes all professional practitioners, such as physicians, nurses, physiotherapists, and other practitioners. It is characterized by the application of scientific medical knowledge and technology to health and healing. Within this framework the sick person is removed from the family/community and placed in a healthcare setting (hospital). The practitioners of the allopathic healthcare sub-system are recognised and upheld by law. On the other hand, practitioners of traditional/complementary and alternative medicine or sub-system, approach the individual/family/community holistically, dealing with all aspects of the individual's/family's/community's life, including the persons' relationship with the supernatural forces and/or Creator, relationship with other persons, relationship with the natural world/environment as well as their relationship with themselves (any physical or emotional symptoms). The traditional (including alternative and complementary) practitioners provide culturally familiar ways of explaining the cause and timing of ill health and attempt to resolve them with culturally specific rituals or treatment.

Based on the two distinct paradigms of thinking, health and disease are differently constructed or defined by professional medicine and traditional medicine (including alternative and complementary medicine). The professional healthcare sub-system refers to disease as an objective condition in which the internal functioning of the body, as a biological organism, is impaired and can only be diagnosed by a licensed health professional. According to the traditional medical sub-system, illness refers to the meaning of the experience of the disease - thus relating to a way of being for the individual (meaning a subjective phenomenon in which the individual perceive himself as not feeling well). Sickness or disease, on the other hand, is defined as a social condition that applies to persons who are defined by others to be ill or diseased and thus lead to changed or altered behaviour. Health, as a socially constructed concept, is the result of the interaction between individuals and their social context. All communities integrate the concept of health into their total culture and what is experienced as health represents a complex, intimate and cultural understanding in a particular context – not a fixed set of physiological and biochemical facts.

Taking as point of departure the view point of Social Medicine whereby the Professional/Allopathic model, the Health Traditions Model/Holistic Health Model and other aspects/components/view points of importance are unified into an integrated wholeness and the discussion of the meaning of the different dimensions of health in the Dimensions of Health model, the following human host-related attributes of importance of the human host system, namely, the individual person, his/her family and the community he or she lives in will be described and/or listed. It must always be kept in mind that the individual, the family and the community forever forms an integrated unit and can never be separated from one another – when an individual contracts a particular communicable disease, both his/her family as well as the members of the community are at risk to become infected. Also, humans are multi-dimensional-unitary beings existing in dynamic relationships to the world, time and fellow beings and are as such living beings unlike any other living creatures.

1.1.1 ATTRIBUTES OF MAN THE HUMAN HOST

As all human hosts live a highly personalised life embracing opportunities and fulfilling the tasks that life presents while giving meaning the physical, the psychological, the social, and the spiritual dimensions of his or her being, the human host is far more than only his or her body. Although communicable diseases affect mostly the physical body and physical existence of the host, the living body of the host represents much more than anatomical structures, biophysical and biochemical processes and pathology. The physical body is unique as it is a subjective, experiencing, living entity which unconsciously contributes to the host's wholeness while maintaining the normal functioning of the organs and the biological processes through the meaningful, purposeful dialectic relationship with the environment.

1.1.1.1 Attributes of the individual as host

In elucidating the multi-dimensional existence of the individual host, attention will be given to the Biological-physiological dimension, the Psychological dimension, the Socio-cultural dimension and Behavioural dimension as the most important aspects to be clarified and incorporated into the individualized comprehensive healthcare interventions to be rendered.

- ✠ Biological-physiological dimension of the health of the individual
  The biological-physiological dimension of health refers to all the factors relating to human biology, such as age, genetics, and physiological functioning
  - genetic inheritance (race, gender, gene-pattern)
  - complex physiological functions (functioning of body organs and systems) such as
    - ➢ the person's basic state of physical health
    - ➢ the level of physiological maturity of the individual person's immunological system (premature and new borne infants have an immature immunological system [both the innate and adaptive immunological systems] while the immunological response of both the innate and adaptive immunological systems of elderly persons are impaired with age)
    - ➢ presence or absence of other disease states [for example, diabetes mellitus, HIV infection]
    - ➢ innate and acquired physiologic resistance (immunity) for example, natural immunity, acquired immunity, species immunity
    - ➢ the status of the immunological system – competent or compromised
  - physiological maturation and aging affect a person's risk of developing a particular communicable disease, for example, the young is more at risk for diseases such as measles, chicken pox, and whooping cough while sexually transmitted diseases are more prevalent among adolescents and adults.

- ✠ Psychological dimension of the health of the individual
  Good mental health (in its broadest biological, medical, educational and social aspects) is the ability of a person to live harmoniously with himself or herself, others, the environment and his/her Creator (Superior Being). When circumstances in these relationships changes in a way that it affects his/her life, the individual is still able to take appropriate steps to solve them. The following characteristics of good mental health are of importance
  - ❖ In relation to Self
    - knows and accepts him/herself as a human being, for example, own body shape, height, size, colour, etc.
    - loves himself/herself as a human being
    - possesses the necessary different coping skills
    - possesses the ability to adapt to change
    - knows own level of maturity
    - possesses self-esteem
    - knows own abilities and strengths
    - accomplished all developmental tasks (functional, interpersonal, psychosocial)
    - knows own levels of stress and anxiety

- has emotional support available (if lacking emotional support from family and friends the individual's mental/emotional health is at risk)
- has a specific attitude to life, health, disease, death and dying
- knows own cognitive and emotional status
- knows own emotional status (mood)
- knows own fears
❖ In relation to others (family and relatives, friends, groups and neighbours)
  - maintains lasting relationships
  - ends unhealthy relationships
  - trust others
  - likes to be trusted by others
  - accepts suggestions from others
  - voices concerns and opinions in a respectful way
  - accepts differences in opinions
  - respects other people
❖ In relation to the environment (whether physical, socio-cultural, economical, political, legal, historical etc.)
  - adjust to changing environment in a way that will suits him/her
  - is not afraid of the future and plans thoroughly for it
  - works hard to achieve his/her goals
  - Takes advantage of opportunities that comes his/her way.

✠ <u>Socio-cultural dimension of the health of the individual</u>
  - Desirable healthy behaviour to protect, to maintain and to restore health
  - Accepted modes of behaviour to protect, to maintain and to restore health
  - Adhering to social norms
  - Has social networks that can offer support
  - Has religious affiliation (including religious practices, religious health practices, religious beliefs re death and dying, and burial practices)
  - Prevailing social attitude re health and disease as well as to communicable diseases
  - Situational constraints in social milieu
  - Cultural aspects of health, for example, traditional health beliefs and practices to protect, to maintain and to restore health.

✠ <u>Behavioural dimension of the health or lifestyle factors of the individual</u>
  - Employment - some occupational groups, for example, healthcare practitioners or environmental health officers or waste disposal workers or police officers are more likely than others to develop particular communicable diseases, while sensitive occupations (for example, trash collecting/food industry/pest controlling) foster the spread of a particular communicable disease because of the contact that occur with fomites and intermediaries (vectors and vehicle); susceptible individuals; and environmental hazards/ risks due to the type of work that is performed. (The types of occupations considered sensitive for communicable diseases vary with the mode of transmission of the particular disease)

- The school situation has to be considered regarding the child (7-18 yrs); while for infants the day care facilities; and toddlers the pre-school facilities must be taken in consideration
- Consumption patterns – nutritional habits of the individual/family/community regarding the protection, the maintenance and the restoration of health that enhances or undermines the innate immunity of a person, while smoking, drinking and drug use predispose a person to several health problems, for example, influenza, HIV infection, tuberculosis
- Ability to perform activities of daily living
- Rest and exercise patterns to protect, maintain and restore health
- Language (mother tongue) in divulging information and comprehension of a situation
- Level of education and economic welfare of the individual
- Using/not using of drugs and injections during drug abuse (HIV infection can be transmitted in this way)
- Use of alcohol as it impairs the individual's immune system
- Leisure and other lifestyle factors such as
  - ➢ leisure activities (swimming or fishing in infected rivers can lead to bilharzias; farming with or keeping of parrots or doves can lead to the contracting of zoonotic diseases)
  - ➢ keeping of pets (dogs, cats, birds [whether domestic, wild, exotic] as zoonotic diseases can be contracted)
  - ➢ sexual behaviour of individuals (contracting sexually transmitted infections)
  - ➢ travelling and exploring (contracting of hemorrhagic fevers, for example, Ebola fever, Marburg fever)
  - ➢ friendships - visits received and visits made.

Based on the health status of the individual/family/community, the hosts system can be classified as healthy, ill, contact or carrier.

Healthy host

A healthy host is an individual/a family/a community who possesses a high level of innate physiological natural resistance (immunity). A very small possibility exists that such a person/family/community will contract the communicable disease at a specific time after having been exposed. A high physiological body resistance is the result of genetically-determined high immunity and/or vaccination and/or the fact that the person/members of the family/members of the community had contracted the particular communicable disease earlier in life and developed a resistance to it. The innate physiological resistance of a healthy host can however, diminishes with the passing of time, in which case the person/member of the family/member of the community becomes susceptible to any particular communicable disease.

Sick/ill host

The ill/sick host is an individual or a family or a community who has contracted the particular communicable disease and because they are infected, the disease is manifested, either clinically or sub-clinically. Attributes to be taken in consideration are

- ✪ the ability of the sick persons or the members of the family or the members of the community to transmit the disease to other non-infected hosts
- ✪ the incubation time frame, meaning the period during which the sick individuals/members of the family/members of the community are already infected, but the disease has not yet been clinically identified. During this period, however, ill persons/ill family members/ill community members possess the ability to transmit the specific pathogenic agent to other persons
- ✪ the clinical picture/clinical manifestation manifested by the ill persons/ members of the family/members of the community. As the clinical picture/ manifestation of a particular communicable disease is very specific, the particular communicable disease can be diagnosed based on the specific clinically identifiable signs and symptoms. When an infection is so mild that the signs and symptoms do not manifest clinically but can be identified by means of laboratory and other diagnostic tests, it is known as an infection of sub-clinical degree. A good example is the positive gamma-globulin test, indicating that a person has clinically contracted Rubella (German measles)
- ✪ the mode of transmission of the specific pathogen and its portal of entry and exit as it directs the isolation measures to implement and the specific healthcare interventions to render as well as all control and preventive measures to instate.

Contact host

Contacts are any individuals or families or communities who have been exposed to a specific pathogen as they had been in direct contact (that is, being physically present) with sick or infected persons/animals/reservoir(s) or indirectly been exposed to a contaminated environment or contaminated objects or intermediaries and thus now harbours the specific infectious pathogen in their bodies.

Contacts are classified as follows

- ❖ healthy contact – the healthy contact is an individual who has a high inborn physiological resistance and will not become ill, even though he/she has never been exposed to the specific pathogen before
- ❖ immune contact – the immune contact is an individual who will not become ill even after been exposed to the specific infectious agent, for one of the following reasons
  - the person has already contracted/had suffered from the particular disease earlier in life and an immune response was elicited; or

- the person has been successfully vaccinated against the disease and his/her immune status has not yet been diminished (that is, he or she still has a high immune status)
- ❖ susceptible contact - the susceptible contact is an individual who has a diminished physiological immunity status and, as such, possesses no physiological resistance at all against the particular disease and can therefore contract the disease. This diminished physiological resistance results from the fact that
  - the individual has never contracted the disease before
  - the individual's vaccination against the disease was not successful
  - the individual has been successful vaccinated but his/her immunity status has diminished with the passing of time
  - the individual's inborn physiological resistance had diminished for specific reason, for example, after a bout of flu
  - when taking immune-suppressing drugs, and/or
  - the individual's innate physiologic resistance is generally low.

  Note - All susceptible contacts are a source of infection.

Carrier host

A carrier is a child or adult or elderly (or an animal) harbouring a specific infectious agent in his/her body in the absence of any clinical manifestation of the disease, and is therefore able to spread the disease. A carrier harbours the specific pathogen in either the nose, or in the pharynx, or in the sinuses, or in the gall-bladder, or in the liver, or in the alimentary tract or in the urinal-genital tract. The specific pathogenic agent is found in the secretions and excretion of these body parts. Examples of diseases that are passed on by carriers are typhoid fever, amoebic dysentery, scarlet fever, poliomyelitis, diphtheria and meningococcal meningitis. The following attributes must be taken in account, namely,

- ❖ carrier state or carriage state - a carrier state develops after a person (child or adult or elderly individual) has recuperated from a communicable disease but still continue to harbours the pathogenic agent in his/her body. A carrier state, however, can also develop when a healthy person harbours the infectious agent in his/her body without ever fallen sick. A carrier is able to transmit the specific pathogen(s) which he or she harbours in his/her body (sometimes more than one specific pathogenic microbe can be harboured) to healthy or sick or susceptible persons or families or communities. The carrier himself/herself is immune to the disease. A carrier status is identified by means of laboratory tests and/or other examinations
- ❖ the classification of carriers, namely, healthy, convalescent, chronic, or transient
  - a healthy or symptom-free carrier is a person who has never suffered from the particular communicable disease. The person is immune to the disease, but as he/she harbours the pathogen in his/her body, the individual is able to transmit the pathogenic agent to other persons

- a carrier who had been sick (clinically or sub-clinically) and had recovered, but the person still harbours the specific infectious agent in his/her body. This type of carrier is subdivided into
  - ➤ a temporary or convalescent carrier who suffered from the disease but still excretes the specific pathogen for up to six (6) months after recovery
  - ➤ a permanent or chronic carrier who suffered from the disease but excretes the specific pathogen continuously for a period longer than six months after he/she had recovered
  - ➤ an intermittent or transient carrier who suffered from the disease but excretes the specific pathogen intermittently (from time to time) after recovery.

Note

Always keep in mind that certain communicable diseases do not elicit an immune response with memory despite the fact that the host has had or still suffers from the disease. Hence, all hosts are susceptible whenever they are exposed to these specific diseases

1.1.1.2   Attributes of the Family of the individual host

As the individual never stands alone, the family of the individual always forms part of the host system. A family (whether monogamous or polygamous) is formed by individuals or individual persons, namely, infants, children, adults, elderly - regardless whether the family is in nature a nuclear conjugal family; or an extended family; or a same-gender family; or a single-parent family; or a stepfamily; or a cohabiting family (living together); or tribal family (married according to traditional marriage laws); or a communal family (families living in communes); or an inter-racial family. Every family is a social system that has its own cultural values, specific functions and structure, and moves through recognizable developmental stages.

The following characteristics of the family are of importance
1.1.1.2.1   **Family composition and status** (unmarried, single, married {all forms recognized by law), divorced, traditional, same-sex)
1.1.1.2.2   **Type of family in view of support** (psychological, economic, social) that can be given when changes have to be made to lifestyle patterns and when care must be rendered; as well as the pattern of residence (who lives with whom)
1.1.1.2.3   **The family as a social system**
  - "open family with a open-hearted way of life" (without visible boundaries and minimal privacy with freedom of reporting on facts of life, tragedies and diseases) or a "closed family with a closed-hearted way of life" (physical and/or emotional boundaries and the maximum privacy between family members and reservation regarding facts of life, tragedies and diseases)
  - members of the family as a subsystem (existence of subgroups)
  - as part of the larger supra-system (community)

- communication patterns of the family, between family members and with the community
  - ➤ verbal and non-verbal communication
  - ➤ high or low contextual messages
  - ➤ contextual consideration
- roles, position and status of individual family members, namely, children, adolescents, adult, elderly
  - ➤ roles of family members and subgroups in the family
  - ➤ specific role expectations of family members
  - ➤ gender roles and gender inequities
  - ➤ role development of individual members
  - ➤ roles of family members in respect to health and disease and caring during sickness and health
  - ➤ extent to which and at what point in time the family will sanction the individual member to adopt the sick role
  - ➤ the effects of the acute sick role (member becomes sick and recovers fully with no changes in roles enactment) and the chronic sick role (individual becomes sick and does not recover fully resulting in the partial fulfilment of designated roles) on the role expectation and role enactment of the family as entity

1.1.1.2.4 The structure of the family (the organized pattern or hierarchy of members that determines how family members interact to form a family unit)
- the role of each family member and how the roles complement each other, conflict with one another and whether role overload occurs
- power hierarchy when decisions have to be taken

1.1.1.2.5 Family functions (activities a family performs to meet the needs of its members)
- tasks typically performed
- inter-changeability of tasks
- who assigns tasks
- gender specificity of tasks

1.1.1.2.6 Developmental stage of the family (newly-wed, child-bearing, empty nest, grandparents)

1.1.1.2.7 Extent of emotional support to family members, the emotional strengths and coping strategies of family

1.1.1.2.8 Family goals
- family goals for the family as system and different family members
- importance of individual versus the group goals of the family, for example, subordination of personal goals, independence and individuality to benefit the family's needs/interest/goals
- commitment to family goals and goals of ethnic grouping

1.1.1.2.9 Cultural values of family
- views and beliefs regarding health and disease (medical and folk sicknesses) and healthcare practices (professional and traditional)

- family's (as system) and individual members' attitude to body and physiological functions
- values and beliefs re
  - human nature
  - man-environment relationship (man's interaction with the physical environment)
  - time orientation (temporal focus of life, past, present and future, time scheduling [clock or sun])
  - spatial orientation (personal, interpersonal and social territorial use of space)
  - activity orientation (modality of human activities)
  - relational orientation (relation of human beings to each other, for example, between members of a family, individualistic or group-orientated, other persons than family)
  - material goals, success and competition

1.1.1.2.10 Religious and magic beliefs and practices

- experiential dimension of religion (emotional aspects)
- ritualistic dimension of religion (certain prescribed behaviour to be followed in sickness, dying and death, burial practices)
- ideological dimension of religion (spiritual beliefs re health, sickness, dying and death)
- consequential dimension of religion (standard of conduct expected during sickness, dying and death, funeral practices)
- religious practices and rituals
- influence of religious beliefs and magic practices on health and healthcare practices to protect, to maintain and to restore health

1.1.1.2.11 Lifestyle of the family

- consumption pattern and practices to protect, to maintain and to restore health
  - preference for specific foods
  - modes of food preparation
  - food consumption patterns (2 or 3 meals a day and times when food are served)
  - symbolism attached to food and meals
  - use of food items for prevention of disease and therapeutic purposes when sick
  - sharing of food
  - association of food with family sentiments [for example, during Christmas, Ramadan]
  - beliefs and practices regarding food preparation and serving when ill and during life events (death and dying and funerals)
- cultural and familial attitudes to and behaviours expected in relation to
  - health and disease
  - death and dying - for example, attitude to natural causes of death and death due to communicable diseases; place where

an ill family member must die (home or institution); rites that accompany dying and death; who has to take care of the body; funeral and burial practices; communication regarding death with regard to children and adolescents; grieving practices; elderly person(s) who should attend to dying person
> birth and parenting practices
- household and safety practices
- employment/school: nature and job-related factors – especially re sensitive occupations held by family members
- leisure activities

1.1.1.2.12 Social interactions of the family as system and the social interactions of individual members
- friends
- recreational activities
- art and cultural activities
- societies and voluntary work

1.1.1.2.13 Authority and decision-making in the family (linked closely to individual versus group orientation)
- authority vested in elders as the decision makers
- respect for authority – agreement and compliance may reflect respect for healthcare practitioner rather than genuine motivation toward healthy behaviour or it can detract efforts to enhance reliance on host's own abilities to resolve health problems
- decision-making process
  > authority figure(s) and equal inputs of members
  > primary decision-maker - for example, eldest male, mother of husband

1.1.1.2.14 The family's attitude to changes
- individual members' and family's attitudes to change
- individual members' and family's openness and resistance to change
- individual members' and family's attitude of resignation and acceptance

1.1.1.2.15 The family's relationship to larger society
- complementary – mutual supportive
- colonial – subservient or superior in attitudes and behaviour
- competitive – resistance to help one-another
- conflictive – do not comply with norms and values of society

1.1.1.2.16 Interpersonal relationships and behaviour
- rules governing interpersonal relationships between the individual members of the family and between the family and society
- social amenities to be followed before directing to area of concern or interest
- family believes and value on individual's behaviour (especially regarding to protect, to maintain and to restore health)

- appropriate demeanour of interpersonal relationships and behaviour (prescribe reticence, openness re personal matters, courtesy titles, epithets, gestures)
- accepted and unaccepted behaviour of family members
- relationships: family network; work colleagues/school friends and friendships

1.1.1.2.17 **Level of education/literacy** of members of the family in view of health information to be given as well as level of understanding of therapeutic and rehabilitative interventions

1.1.1.2.18 **External resources available to family**

1.1.1 2.19 **Economical welfare of family**

- economic status to larger society
- medical fund and income levels
- social security
- money available for transport to healthcare facility
- debtors (if relevant)

1.1.1.2.20 **The family and the healthcare system**

- health and sickness status as well as status of vaccination of everyone in the family household
- family's perception of health and disease as well as disease causation
- family's perception of "adherence to treatment programmes" as well as key factors in the ability/inability of family members to obtain, maintain and complete therapy
- family response to any disease (including communicable diseases) when
  - ➤ dealing with sickness/disease
  - ➤ dealing with communicable medical diseases
  - ➤ family's belief regarding whether a person is ill/sick enough to stay at home and to be cared for at home or whether a person is so ill that he/she must be admitted to a healthcare institution
  - ➤ family's belief who has to care for the ill person – a traditional or professional practitioner or both practitioners simultaneously
  - ➤ limiting factors in the social and economic environment beyond the control of the family, for example, poverty and/or economic inequity; racism; gender inequities; homelessness; overt political violence; civil disturbance; and war
- family's folk healthcare practices to protect, to maintain and to restore health
  - ➤ at primary level (practices to promote health and prevent disease:
    - ✓ utilization of preventative herbal medicine
    - ✓ knowledge of communicable diseases (causation, spread, treatment) and precautions to be taken to prevent communicable diseases

- ✓ magical rituals and other rituals such as meditation or massages to be practiced
- ✓ dietary practices regarding consumption or avoidance of specific foods during sickness
  - ➤ at secondary prevention (practices designed to diagnose and treat diseases)
    - ✓ diet (cold and hot foods)
    - ✓ herbs to be used as treatment
    - ✓ application of heat and cold treatments
    - ✓ exercise, rest
    - ✓ healing rituals such as singing
    - ✓ treatment modalities (cupping, punching, coining, steaming, acupuncture, touch, compresses)
- • beliefs regarding and attitude to the professional healthcare system
  - ➤ perception of care-givers and cooperation with care-givers
  - ➤ distrust of the professional healthcare system
  - ➤ under-utilization/over-utilization of the healthcare system
  - ➤ utilization of both traditional and professional healthcare system
  - ➤ utilization of healthcare services based on "who to consults, where to consults, when to consults"
  - ➤ the accessibility and availability as well as the economics of healthcare and barriers to obtain healthcare, for example, funds available, language barriers, distance to travel to a service delivery point, transportation available to travel to a service delivery point, etc.
- • point of departure regarding healthcare
  - ➤ the family's behaviour during sickness is influence by the differences in the point of departure between traditional and professional medicine - professional medicine emphasizes the worth of individual while traditional medicine emphasizes group goals, for example, if a philosophy prevails regarding the continued survival of the family, it takes precedence over the life and welfare of one family member
  - ➤ when poor - the high cost of medicine and care prevents the poor individual or family to seek help (help is only called in when complications have set in or the disease is in an advanced stage)
  - ➤ when wealthy, helped is sought during the early stages of disease and prevention of disease is emphasized.

1.1.1.3 Attributes of the Community wherein the host and his/her family live

A community is a system of formal and informal groups characterized by interdependence and whose function is to meet the collective needs of group members. As the individual host and his/her family are members of a specific community and because the possibility always exists that the community as an entire system or only specific members of the community can become ill, the community (as a system) also forms part of the host system.

The following characteristics of the specific community are of importance

1.1.1.3.1 The specific bio-physical attributes (demographical data) of community members

- maturation and aging - composition of the population (very young or very old)
- gender composition
- racial composition
- health problems (prevalent and incidence of chronic diseases)
- overall state of health of community (morbidity and mortality statistics)
- vaccination level(s) of community as a system and of individual members (herd immunity)

1.1.1.3.2 Environment – all factors (individually and in combination) in the physical, biological, psychological, socio-cultural and economic and other important environments of the community have to be taken in account as it influence the health of the individual, the family and the community. (Refer to section 1.3 for the discussion of the factors of importance in the environment - the third element of The Epidemiological Triad of Communicable Diseases Model)

1.1.1.3.3 Healthcare system - this refers to factors within the healthcare system that influence, either positively or negatively, the health of individuals, families and communities, such as the organization of the service delivery system, the availability, accessibility, appropriateness, adequacy and affordability of healthcare and the usage of the services by the healthcare user. For example, a factor such as no accessibility into the healthcare system, contribute to health problems which lead to the increased incidence of such problems

Factors of importance regarding the healthcare system are

- the availability, accessibility, acceptability, affordability and effectiveness of the healthcare service delivery system
- the type of services delivered and the adequacy of the healthcare services rendered
- the utilization of services by healthcare users (over-utilization or under-utilization of services)
- the level of education of the host (the individual, the family and the community) in view of health information to be given
- categories of healthcare providers (professional, traditional and lay care givers) and type of services to be delivered
- competency and attitude of healthcare providers in service rendering
- inappropriate actions of healthcare providers that foster communicable diseases, for example, inappropriate use of anti-microbial drugs (antibiotics) or vaccines that impair the immunity of the host

- economics of healthcare and funding of healthcare services and services delivery
- attitude of healthcare users to healthcare practitioners and healthcare services (professional and traditional)
- rates of occurrence - incidence and prevalence rate of specific health conditions; for example, tuberculosis, AIDS, chronic diseases
- the use of old trusted resources rather than "outsider" resources and services
- the internal healthcare system – local community healthcare service delivery systems and family-centred care service delivery systems as well as services delivered by non-governmental organizations
- traditional healthcare services to protect, to maintain and to restore health:
  - ➢ traditional healthcare practitioners - education of and services rendered
  - ➢ traditional health practices at primary, secondary, tertiary level
  - ➢ traditional treatment modalities
  - ➢ traditional health rituals
  - ➢ relationship of traditional healthcare models and professional healthcare models
- barriers to healthcare rendering, for example, language; distance to healthcare facility; availability of funds; transportation; and other deterrents to access service delivery
- accessibility and cost of transportation to healthcare facilities

1.1.1.3.4 **Resources** - Individuals, groups, and communities always strive to obtain, retain, and protect all resources which they value. A broad but finite set of resources are critical within a culture and more broadly within the society. Four categories of resources are identified, namely, objects (e.g. transportation, shelter, food, credible communication channels and sources); conditions (e.g. diseases, seniority, marriage, wellness); personal characteristics (e.g. personal competencies and skills of community members, self-esteem of community, developmental stage of community); and energies (e.g. money, credit, health insurance, healthcare system infrastructure for service delivery, healthcare informational programmes). Resources are of importance as objects can meet survival needs or if scarce have acquired value through demand, while conditions aid in the obtaining of other valued conditions or goals as it ensures stability. Personal characteristics of the community provide access to other valued states (e.g. safe and healthy environment, the ability to care for the sick, the frail and the young) while the energy resources are used to obtain objects (e.g. food), enhance conditions (e.g. wellness) and/or increase personal resources. As a specific relationship exists between individuals and all societal systems and between groups and organizations and larger social systems, a minimal level of a number of resources is necessary for psychological and physical well-being. Furthermore, resources as such plays a central role in a community as those community members who are empowered, do well because they have access to resources to control their lives and their environments are positively affected, while those community members who lack resources have limited access to opportunities to protect themselves or to gain access to the resources available to others in the community because these community members have more vulnerable resources. When resources are threatened with loss, or are lost, or no resources can be obtained following investment in other resources, acute stressful conditions result because these stressful conditions (e.g. an outbreak of communicable diseases) ebb away all resources, even chiselling away strong reservoirs of resources.

1.1.2 THE PROPERTIES OF THE PATHOGEN (INFECTIOUS AGENT/PATHOGENIC MICROBE)

A specific pathogen (infectious agent/pathogenic microbe) is the primary cause of a particular communicable disease. All pathogenic microbes, whether micro-parasites (bacteria, viruses, fungi, and protozoa), or macro-parasites (helminths and arthropods) possess the ability to cause an infection in humans or animals when the state of "balanced pathogenicity" is disturbed. A microbe possesses distinctive properties regarding its structural and molecular make-up, its biochemical and metabolic strategies and its reproductive processes that determine how the specific microbe interacts with man/animal and how it causes disease. The properties of the specific infectious/pathogenic microbe determine not only the nature and course of a particular communicable disease but also whether a given person/family/community will contract the disease. The properties of the pathogen also give direction to all interventions to be set for the comprehensive, holistic, compassionate and culturally congruent healthcare rendering to all hosts and for the prevention and control of communicable diseases in general.

To cause a disease, pathogenic microbes carry out the following obligatory steps when infecting a host (man or animal) (see table 1.2).

Table 1.2 THE OBLIGATORY STEPS PATHOGENIC MICROBES FOLLOW WHEN INFECTING, SPREADING AND BEING SHED FROM THE BODY OF THE HOST

Steps	Requirement	Phenomenon
1 Pathogen attaches itself to the body cells to gain entry into the body	Pathogen must enter through the correct portal while evading natural protective and cleansing mechanisms of the body and then attaches itself to cells	Entry of pathogen into the body of the host
2 Pathogen spreads locally or systemically in the body	Pathogen must evade the immediate local defences of the body	Spread of pathogen within the body of the host

3	Pathogen multiplies or replicates itself	Numbers of pathogen must increase as many die in the host or on route to new hosts	Multiplication of pathogen within the body of the host
4	Pathogen evades the immune and other defences of the host	Pathogen evades immune and other defences long enough for the full cycle of reproduction to be completed in the host	Microbial answer of pathogen to host defences
5	Pathogen is shed from body	Pathogen leaves body at a specific site (portal of exit) and on a scale that ensures the spread to new and fresh hosts	Transmission of pathogen to new hosts takes place
6	Pathogen causes damage in host	Not strictly necessary, but a certain amount of damage is essential for shedding	Pathology occurs as end result - disease pathogenesis occurs

Because man has developed highly efficient strategies for recognizing foreign pathogens as well as effective inflammatory and immune responses to restrain the growth and spread of the invading pathogens and to eliminate them from the body, the microbes have also rapidly evolved properties that enable them to overcome or bypass the host's defences and carry out the obligatory steps. Unfortunately, microbes evolve with extraordinary speed in comparison with their host, the human body.

Important properties of pathogenic microbes that affect the host are

1.1.2.1 **Replication within or on the host's body. All micro-pathogens replicate within the host** and therefore multiply to produce a very large number of progeny, thus causing an overwhelming infection. **Macro-parasites, even microscopic small, do not have the micro-pathogen's ability to replicate within the host**. After the macro-parasite(s) invades or gains entry into the body, the infectious stage matures into the reproducing stage, and the resulting progeny leave the host to continue the cycle outside the human body. The level of infection is therefore determined by the numbers of parasites that enter into or live on the body.

1.1.2.2 **The size of the pathogen or parasite.** Pathogens such as viruses and rickettsiae and chlamydia can only live inside the cells of the host (intracellular microbes) as they are small enough while the remaining groups of pathogens have adopted either the intracellular or the extracellular living habit (with the exception of a few who adopted both). Pathogens that live intracellular are protected from many of the host's defence mechanisms, especially the action of antibody mediators which poses problems for the host. Very different problems are posed by extracellular microbes because these extracellular pathogenic microbes can grow and reproduce freely and disseminate extensively within the tissues of the body and destroy body tissues.

1.1.2.3 **The outcome of the extent of exposure.** The extent of exposure to the specific disease-causing pathogen affects the outcome of the exposure, that is, whether the individual stays healthy or becomes ill. The outcome of the exposure is also influenced by factors such as whether the individual was exposed to few or many of the specific pathogenic agent, time period of exposure [exposed for a long period or short period], and whether entry into the host's body was gained through the correct portal of entry.

1.1.2.4 **Pathogenicity.** The pathogenicity of the infectious agent refers to the ability to cause the disease in susceptible hosts based on
- gaining entry into the host's body through the correct portal of entry;
- resisting the host's defence mechanisms, and
- causing an inflammatory/infectious reaction in the host.

1.1.2.5 **Virulence.** The virulence of the specific pathogen refers to the ability of the microbe to adapt to changes in the environment by controlling gene expression, thereby ensuring that proteins are only produced when and if they are required. The expression of many virulence determinants (virulence–associated genes) by bacterial pathogens is highly regulated as it is only activated by a cascade of activators when their particular property is needed. The virulence of a pathogen is determined by numerous factors such as adhesion, penetration into cells, anti-phagocytic activity, production of toxin and interaction with the immune system. Different genes and gene production are involved at different stages in the pathogenesis of the particular communicable infection. Because of gene mutations, changes in the virulence of the specific microbe occur constantly leading to either a heightened or a reduced pathogenicity. The higher the virulence of the pathogen, the more severe the infection becomes. The degree of severity of the disease now becomes of importance. An example of this kind of pathogenic agent is the influenza A-virus which can cause a more serious attack of influenza than the influenza C-virus

1.1.2.6 **Efficiency of infection** (infectivity) refers to the number of pathogens required to infect a fresh host. The efficiency of infection varies greatly between pathogens. High infectivity (small number of pathogens is required to cause infection) is not necessarily associated with the degree of severity of the disease. For example, the virus of Varicella (chickenpox) is considered extremely infectious, although the disease is self-limiting with few complications or none at all.

1.1.2.7 **Chemical composition and structure** of the specific pathogenic microbe determine the effects on the host, for example, the cell walls of bacteria are destroyed by certain anti-microbial drugs, while viruses have to attach themselves to specific protein structures in human cells when gaining entry.

1.1.2.8 **The reproductive cycle of the pathogen**. The **rate** at which the specific pathogenic microbe **reproduces itself**, influences the body's ability to kill off the invading pathogenic microbe before it overwhelms the body's defence mechanisms while the **reproductive cycle** of the specific pathogenic agent determine the incubation period of the disease. The reproductive cycle also affects the specific pathogenic agent's ability to cause the particular communicable disease as well as the natural history and course of the disease. The reproductive cycle also plays an importance role in the implementation of interventions to control communicable diseases.

1.1.2.9 **Portals of entry.** Infectious agents causing communicable diseases gain entry into the body through different portals, namely,

- the respiratory system – by inhalation of contaminated dust or infected sputum or saliva droplets. Entry into the body is gained through the mucous membranes of the Eustachian tube, the tonsils and/or the lungs
- the digestive tract – by swallowing pathogenic microbes, entry into the body is gained via the mucous membranes of the mouth, the tonsils and the stomach, small intestines and colon and then absorbed into the bloodstream
- the skin - via inoculation of the skin or via insect bites or stings or via open wounds or via the intact skin {rabies}
- the bloodstream - via wounds or via pricks with contaminated injection needles or via transfusion needles or via transfusions of contaminated blood or plasma
- the placenta - entry into the body of the foetus is gained via the placenta when the pathogens cross the placental barrier
- the urethra, vagina and rectum - via secretions of the genital-urinary tract and reproductive organs during sexual intercourse

Note Pathogens causing sexually transmitted infections (STI's) have adapted to also gain entry into the body via attachment to mucosal epithelial cells of the mouth and throat and via skin lesions

As pathogenic microbes cannot attach easily to the human skin because of the skin's natural physical, biologic and chemical protective barriers, infectious microbes mostly gain entry into the body via the respiratory, digestive and genital-urinary body systems. The mucosa of these body systems thus becomes the primary portal of entry where the pathogen attaches to and penetrates the epithelial cells. The portals of entry play a very important role in all care rendering interventions, all control interventions and all preventive strategies (also see table 1.3 for a detailed exposition of portals of entry and exit and related modes of transmission). To elicit a communicable disease, the pathogen must gain entry into the body through the correct portal of entry.

1.1.2.10 **Portals of exit.** Pathogenic microbes causing communicable diseases must be shed from the body through different portals of exit if they are to be transmitted to a fresh host, namely,

- the digestive tract - via faeces (the infected stools contaminate water and food with the infectious/pathogenic agent)
- the respiratory tract and mucous membrane of mouth and nose - via contaminated droplets of saliva and/or sputum and/or phlegm and/or mucous which are spread when sneezing/coughing/singing/talking

- the skin and skin lesions - via pus and secretions from skin lesions and wounds, as well as from pustule and crusts
- the urinary tract - via urine that is contaminated, for example, with bilharzia eggs or any other infectious/pathogenic microbes that causes cystitis or typhoid fever
- the genital tract - via the vagina or urethra, for example, HIV-virus in seminal fluid and vaginal secretions
- the circulatory system - via blood that leaves the body when sucked up by insects or by blood draining from wounds or secreted through the body's natural secretion organs (kidneys and bladder) or by blood being withdrawn mechanically from the circulatory system

The portals of exit play a very important role in all care rendering interventions, all control interventions and all preventive strategies (also see table 1.3 for a detailed exposition of portals of entry and exit and related modes of transmission).

1.1.2.11 **Transmission of the pathogen.** Transmission refers to the transfer of the pathogen from one host to another. For successful transmission, a **sufficient number** of pathogens must be shed, **the pathogens must be stable and able to survive in** environment and the **efficiency of infection** must be high. Pathogens are transmitted from human to humans (respiratory/salivary, faecal-oral, sexual) and from animals, namely, vector-borne reservoirs to humans (for example, biting arthropod [vector]; vertebrate reservoir [dogs, cats, primates, pigs]; and vector-vertebrate reservoir [rats and their fleas]). Transmission occurs either horizontally (direct or indirect) or/and vertically. Direct transmission horizontally takes place when direct contact occurs between an infected individual and a fresh uninfected individual. Indirect horizontally transmission takes place when intermediaries such as vehicles (hands, clothing, surfaces, air/dust, milk, water that is contaminated) or vectors (mosquitoes/arthropods) play a role. Vertically transmission occurs between parent[s] and offspring via sperm, ovum, placenta, breast milk, or blood. When vertically transmission in the animal species occurs, the infection(s) maintain themselves without spreading horizontally as long as the infection does not affects the viability of the host. In humans, on the other hand, vertically and horizontally transmission occurs simultaneously in sexually transmitted diseases/infections, namely, syphilis and AIDS. Transmission is furthermore also depended on three factors – the number of pathogens shed, the pathogen's stability in the environment and the number of pathogens required to infect fresh hosts.

The **modes and form** of transmission refers to the means by which the specific infectious/pathogenic agent is transferred from an infected person to an uninfected person. Communicable diseases are transmitted (spread/ transferred) by any of several modes of transmission

- airborne transmission from the respiratory and salivary tract via infected droplets – the specific pathogenic agent is shed when the infected individual coughs/sneezes/laughs/spits/talks/sings and because it is present in the air, it is inhaled by a susceptible host during respiration

- faecal-oral transmission from the gastro-intestinal tract via faeces – the specific pathogenic agent is present in the infected stool of humans/animals/birds.
- direct skin-to skin contact (for example, skin flakes that were shed) or direct contact with mucous membrane discharges (for example, saliva) between the infected person and another person (for example, when kissing)
- by insect or animal bites transmission -- when an infected/sick animal or insect bites a person(s) the specific pathogenic microbe is transmitted from the animal/arthropod source of infection
- sexually/venereal transmission – during coitus (oral or genital) transmission of sexually transmitted infections occur as the specific pathogenic agent is present in seminal fluid and vaginal secretions. Because during sexual activity all mucosal surfaces of the body can be involved, other body sites can also become infected if the antimicrobial defences are not intact. Other viral infections such as cytomegalovirus and hepatitis B-virus infections can also be spread in semen. When the mother is infected by her partner, vertically transmission of the infection (such as syphilis) to the offspring takes place when the pathogen crosses the placental barrier
- transmission by direct inoculation – direct inoculation occurs when a blood-borne pathogen (that is, the specific infectious/pathogenic agent is present in the blood) is introduced directly in the bloodstream of another person, for example, via transfusions with infected blood/blood product or through use of contaminated hypodermic needles or through a splash of contaminated body fluid on mucous membranes or non-intact skin. Inoculation can also occur between non-intact skin and wounds, crusts, and the exudate of wounds
- transmission by other means – some communicable diseases are transmitted through contact with spores (e.g. Tetanus spores) present in the soil or larvae/worms present in soil.

The modes of transmission play a very important role in all care rendering interventions, all control interventions and all preventive strategies (see table 1.3 for the detailed exposition of portals of entry and exit and related modes of transmission)

Table 1.3 TABULATION OF THE PORTALS OF ENTRY AND EXIT FOR THE SPECIFIC MODE OF TRANSMISSION

Mode of transmission	Portal of entry	Portal of exit
Airborne	Respiratory system	Respiratory system via droplets
Faecal-oral	Gastro-intestinal tract	Alimentary tract via faeces
Skin to skin contact	Skin, mucous membrane	Skin, mucous membrane
Sexual contact	Skin, mucosa, urethra, vagina, rectum,	Skin lesions, vaginal/seminal or urethral secretions
Blood (horizontally and vertically)	Across placenta barrier, bloodstream to other body sites	Blood, from infected body site
Animal or insect bite	Wound in skin	Blood, respiratory tract when lungs are seeded
Vertebrate-human transmission	Wound in skin, intact skin Gastro-intestinal tract when eating/drinking infected meat, milk	Animal faeces, eggs or infected faeces contaminating soil (spore forming), larvae in muscle
OTHER MEANS OF TRANSMISSION		
Breast milk	Gastro-intestinal tract	Faeces, blood
Urine	Mouth, respiratory system (Lassa fever) and skin (Bilharzia)	Urine (Although urine *per se* does not transmit pathogens, urine contaminate food, drink, water and living space)
Birth canal (peri-natal transmission)	During passage down the infected birth canal, pathogens are wiped onto the conjunctiva of the infant or are inhaled.	Eye, respiratory tract, cerebrospinal fluid, faeces
Bile	Gastro-intestinal tract	Bile in faeces

Inoculation	Blood via contaminated used needles and/or infusion of blood and blood product.	Blood

1.1.2.12 The ability of the pathogen to attaches itself to and penetrates into the cells of the body.

Pathogens have developed chemical or mechanical mechanisms to attach themselves to the surface of the respiratory, urinal-genital and alimentary tracts. In the skin the pathogens depend upon entry entry via small wounds or arthropod bites. At the site of entry, either on the body surface or in the tissues, specific molecules of the pathogen attach themselves to receptor molecules on the cells of the host. These receptor molecules have specific functions in the life of the cell and are critical determinants of the cell's susceptibility to becoming infected. When attachment of the pathogenic agent with the epithelial cells takes place, a specific superficial interaction occurs that is characteristic of the particular disease, namely,

- some pathogenic microbes only multiply on the surface of the epithelial cells without penetrating the cells lying deeper below the surface. The pathogenic microbes secrete an exotoxin which is absorbed by the mucosa, causing local as well as general tissue damage. *Corynebacterium diphtheriae, Bordetella pertussis* and *Vibrio cholerae* are examples of these pathogenic microbes
- some pathogenic microbes penetrate the epithelial cells where they multiply and destroy the epithelial cells. Some of these infectious/ pathogenic microbes also secrete an endotoxin which destroys the cells. The genus Shigella is an example of these pathogenic microbes
- some pathogenic microbes penetrate the epithelial cells and infect the deeper-lying sub-mucosa without destroying the epithelial cells. From the sub-mucosa the organism spreads via the bloodstream and lymph to other organs in the body. Viruses are example of these infectious/ pathogenic microbes.

1.1.2.13 The ability of the infectious pathogen to spread throughout the body.

Once the infectious/pathogenic microbe had gained entry into the body, it attaches itself to the epithelial cells and when it becomes clear that the innate defence mechanisms of the body cannot destroy the infectious agent, the pathogen spreads through the body as follows

- from cell-to-cell - this occurs in the skin or in subcutaneous tissue, or when spreading from the lungs to the pleura
- via the body tracts – when pathogens are shed into secretions and discharges, the infected discharges and secretions infect the mucosa/ epithelium/organs which they come in contact with. The spread of the infectious agent therefore take place from the kidneys to the ureters to

the bladder; and from the nose to the larynx; from the trachea to the lungs; and from the gall-bladder to the liver
- via the lymph nodes to the regional nodes and then to the blood
- via the bloodstream to all the organs of the body.

1.1.2.14 The ability of the pathogen to releases bacterial toxin. Toxins are secreted by bacteria to damage the cell leading eventually to the death of the cell. Toxins are mostly proteins (polypeptide) and are often not coded by the bacterial DNA but in plasmids or phages. Toxins form part of the pathogen's strategy for entry into the body cells, to spread through the body of the host, or to defend it against the host's defence mechanisms. Powerful toxins are generally secreted by extracellular microbes because intracellular pathogens that multiply within the cells of the host, cannot afford to cause serious damage at a too early stage. Such endotoxins tend to be less toxic in intracellular infections. Exotoxins cause, on the other hand, serious tissue damage, especially in bacterial infections. As such, endotoxins cause dysfunction in immune and phagocytic cells although they can kill host cells.

In general, the mode of action and consequences of toxins are as follow
- to promote their survival or spread, pathogens may release enzymes that break down the tissues or the intercellular substances of the host, thus allowing the infection to spread freely
- some toxins (haemolysins) damage or destroy cell membranes enzymatically through lecithinase or phospholipase or by insertion of pore-forming molecules that destroy the integrity of the cell, resulting in the death of the cell
- toxin molecules that are characterized by two subunits (the A-subunit being the active unit while the B-subunit being the binding component needed to interact with receptors on the cell membrane) enter the cells and actively alter some of the cell's metabolic machinery. When binding occurs, the A-subunit or the whole toxin-receptor complex is taken into the cell by endocytosis and activation of the A-subunit take place
- some toxin effectively blocks the protein synthesis of cells
- entero-toxins change the sodium/chloride flux across the intestinal epithelium cells, resulting in a massive outflow of water and electrolytes from intestinal epithelial cells to cause profuse diarrhoea
- the most potent toxins, such as the tetanus and botulinum toxins, affect the nerve impulses as it interferes with the synaptic transmission in inhibitory neurones by blocking neurotransmitter release in the central nervous system (spastic paralysis in the case of tetanus toxin) or affecting the peripheral nerve endings at the neuromuscular junction, blocking the presynaptic release of acetylcholine (flaccid paralysis in the case of botulinum toxin).

1.1.2.15 The specific antigen-antibody-response. The specific antigen-antibody-response that is mediated (takes place/is produced), is grounded in the ability of the pathogen to infect the host and the ability of the host's body to recognize the pathogen and defend itself against the specific pathogen. The body has both "innate" and "adaptive" immune defences in response to the infection. The innate defences that are already in place (a variety of biochemical and physical barriers, phagocytosis, the complementary system producing the inflammatory response) may well be sufficient to prevent replication and spread of the infectious agent, thus preventing the development of the disease. Should the innate immunity be insufficient to prevent the disease, the "adaptive" immune system comes into action (namely the cell-mediated and antibody-mediated reactions) to eliminate the infective pathogen, thus allowing recovery from the disease. A close synergy exists between the innate and adaptive immune responses with the adaptive mechanism greatly improving the efficiency of the innate response.

1.1.2.16 **The ability of the pathogen to mutate.** When a specific pathogenic microbe mutate, it changes its genetic composition, resulting in a new strain (modified form) of the specific infectious pathogen. The host is now susceptible to the mutant (new strain of) pathogen as the body has not yet formed a specific physiological immunological response to the new strain of the specific pathogen.

1.1.2.17 **Intermediaries.** Intermediaries play a very important role in the spread of a particular communicable disease. Intermediaries as such, are not infected with the specific pathogen nor suffer from the infection but acts as a "go-between" in facilitating the transmission of the specific pathogen. Intermediaries are classified as non–living or living intermediaries

- Non-living intermediaries or vehicles promotes the indirect transmission of the specific pathogen as the inanimate objects/things are contaminated (not infected) with the specific pathogen. The infected person contaminates the non-living vehicle(s) and when the uninfected host comes in contact with the contaminated vehicle(s), he or she is exposed to the specific pathogen and becomes infected. Non-living intermediaries or vehicles are
  - ➤ air and dust particles in the air and the air can carry infected droplets over long distances
  - ➤ clothing worn by infested persons containing eggs of mites
  - ➤ water, milk, food, serum and plasma
  - ➤ fomites
  - ➤ surfaces and inanimate objects
- <u>Living intermediaries or vectors</u> are invertebrates such as blood-sucking arthropods, for example, insects, ticks, fleas, and mites that have adapted to living or feeding on the human body. Arthropods cause disease directly by their feeding habits and indirectly by transmitting infections. Contact between man and arthropod can be temporary (as in the case of mosquitoes) or permanent (as in the case of lice) and

pathogens of all major microbial groups are transmitted. Transmission by living intermediaries occur as follows

➢ biological transmission by vectors such as fleas, lice, tsetse flies, ticks, and mosquitoes, which serve as a necessary host for the reproduction (multiplication) and development of the pathogen. The pathogen is reintroduced into the human host after a period of time when the next blood meal takes place. Transmission occurs via direct injection, usually in the vector's saliva or by contamination from faeces or regurgitated blood deposited at the time of feeding

➢ passive carriage by vectors such as insects, flies, cockroaches that carry pathogens passively on their mouth-parts, on their bodies, or within their intestines. Transfer onto food or onto hosts occurs directly as a result of feeding, regurgitating or defecating. Blood-sucking vectors have mouthparts adapted for penetrating the skin in order to reach blood vessels or to create small pools of blood. The ability to feed in this way provides access for pathogens to gain entry into the body via the skin or blood. The mouthparts act as a contaminated hypodermic needle carrying infection between persons

➢ many other invertebrates such as shellfish and slugs/snails used for food convey pathogens that have been accumulated in their bodies after taking them in from contaminated waste and transferring them passively. Many parasites such as worms must undergo part of their development in the invertebrate before being able to infect a human. Humans are infected when they eat the invertebrate host or come in contact with their cercaria.

1.1.2.18 **Mediums pathogens grow in or can be cultured in.** Pathogenic microbes grow the best in the blood and tissue cells of the body. Pathogenic microbes can also grow in

● discharges and excretion of the body such as pus and faeces (however, these excretions and discharges must be moist for such growth to take place)

● contaminated soil and street garbage

● water, milk, raw vegetables and fruit, raw meat, canned foods and previously prepared food left to stand.

1.1.3 THE CHARACTERISTICS OF THE ENVIRONMENT

The health of all individuals, families, and communities is influenced by all factors in the physical-biological, socio-cultural, psychological, economical, and all other important environments/milieus (for example, historical, political, religious, moral-ethical, judicial etc.) wherein the hosts live as they contribute to health-related conditions which increase or decrease the possibility for outbreaks and the spread of communicable diseases. When the balance between host, agent and environment is disturbed, it becomes a contributing factor in the causation of an outbreak and spread of communicable diseases. When assessing the environmental and milieu conditions and their relationship "links" to the health of the host system and the pathogenic microbe(s), the existence of all present environmental hazards/risks must be identified as well as the effect(s) these hazards/risks have on the health of the individual, his/her family and his/her community and their ability to propagate the growth or mutation of pathogenic microbes.

1.1.3.1 Characteristics of the Physical-biological environment

Hazards in the physical as well as the biological environment can lower the resistance of the body and making it thus easier for pathogenic agents to invade the body. As such, the risks/hazards in the physical and biological environment contribute to outbreaks of a variety of communicable diseases that affects a number of target organs and systems in the body such as the central nervous, respiratory, gastro-intestinal, genital-urinary and reproductive, reticule-endothelial, muscular-skeletal system as well as the eyes and skin.

- The **physical environment** consists of all factors that influence the health of the individual host, the family and the community such as
  - weather conditions and climate changes
  - meteorological conditions (day and night temperatures, periods of droughts, periods of raining or snowing, windy conditions)
  - humidity
  - seasonal conditions
  - terrain (e.g. the exploration of unknown terrain in equatorial forests)
  - buildings (e.g. air conditioning systems transporting airborne microbes, sick building syndrome)
  - density of living conditions and housing conditions (e.g. squatter camps, informal settlements, tent refugee camps)
  - soil composition (e.g. mineral deficits of zinc and selenium in soil may lead to a compromised immune system as the body is not supplied sufficiently through food consumption)
  - geographical topography (e.g. polluting of rivers, deforestation of especially the equatorial forests)
  - sensitive occupations as well as unsafe working conditions
  - natural disaster conditions (e.g. tsunami's; floods; droughts, landslides, earth quakes and earth tremors, volcanic eruptions)
  - agricultural, animal husbandry, and fishery practices for sustainable food supply.

Marked changes in the physical environment, such as a decrease or an increase in humidity and meteorological temperatures (very hot, very cold), affect the resistance of the mucous membranes in the respiratory tract - in much the same way the resistance of the mucous membranes in the respiratory system is lowered by smoke and air pollution. Certain diseases are seasonal, such as measles, chicken pox and poliomyelitis. Endemic diseases occur in specific geographic areas, for example, in the eastern geographical regions of South Africa malaria (Mpumalanga) and rabies (KwaZulu-Natal) are endemic communicable medical diseases. During the winter months large groups of persons congregate indoors, promoting the spread of communicable diseases, especially of the respiratory tract.

- The **biological environment** consists of all living organisms, other than humans, that influence the health of the individual host, the family, and the community. These living organisms as well as other aspects associated with, are, for example,
  - ➢ vegetation - plants and trees (forests)
  - ➢ animals and birds (wild, exotic and domestic) as well as insects
  - ➢ microbes (infectious and non-infectious), presence of reservoirs and intermediaries for infectious agents
  - ➢ vectors such as insects, birds, fleas, flies, mosquitoes, rodents and arthropods such as lice
  - ➢ water (including the contamination thereof and wastewater recycling, as well as the overuse of limited supplies)
  - ➢ food (all processes involved in the production, marketing, selling, storage, preparation and serving {food-handling practices} of all types of foods [for example, meat/poultry, fish and sea foods, oil, milk, fruit, vegetable, herb and spices] and in all forms [for example, fresh, frozen, liquid, canned, dry/powder])
  - ➢ systems for the disposal of
    - ▪ solid waste (sanitation, sewage disposal and treatment)
    - ▪ medical wastes
    - ▪ garbage
  - ➢ technology, for example, air-conditioning and heating systems.

Of concern are especially the biological hazards, such as infectious agents (bacteria, viruses, rickettsiae, etc), insects, animals and plants. Biological contamination of water and food sources with infectious agents (for example, bacteria, viruses), the use of reclaimed water, the lack of sanitation facilities, ineffective garbage removal systems as well as unhygienic habits and certain socio-cultural rituals (such as the disposal of bodies after death) of communities contributes to the rapid growth and spread of microbes. Diseases such as cholera, hepatitis and typhoid commonly occur in circumstances such as these. Many pathogenic agents are transmitted by water, for example, when contamination of drinking water occurs as a consequence of improper sewage treatment; or when solid waste is improperly disposed off; or when reclaimed water is used (waste water reclamation); or when medical waste is not properly disposed off.

Insects and animals serve as reservoirs and vectors for a variety of communicable diseases that affects human beings, for example, tetanus, rabies, bovine tuberculosis, ringworm, anthrax. As such, diseases spread by vectors require the geographical presence of the relevant vectors, which in turn depends on a favourable environment for reproduction. Insects such as flies, lice, mosquitoes, fleas, cockroaches serves as vectors while animals and rodents transmit various communicable diseases, for example, rodents such as rats transmit plague; exotic animals such as monkeys transmit hemorrhagic diseases; wild animals such as bats and meercats transmit rabies; unvaccinated domestic animals such as cats transmit toxoplasmosis; unvaccinated dogs transmit rabies; and unvaccinated poultry transmit avian influenza. Animal faeces provide breeding ground for flies and other insects that transmit communicable diseases. Solid waste not properly disposed off also provides a breeding ground for insect and animal vectors. Deforestation exposes mosquito-borne, tick-borne or rodent-carried communicable diseases. Monocultures of grain are mouse food, but if mouse eating predators are exterminated, the mouse (and rat) populations erupt with their own reservoirs of diseases.

Modern technology also contributes to the transmission of pathogenic agents through the air by means of improperly cleaned air conditioning units, heating systems, and closed hot water systems such as showers. Modern means of transportation, especially air traffic and super-fast train traffic, also promotes the spread of infectious agents from person to person and from one place/ country/continent to another place/country/continent when infected hosts and ill hosts and/or infected contacts in the incubation period, board these means of transportation. Giant hydro-electric projects and their accompanying canals spread snails that carry bilharzia and allow mosquitoes to breed. New environments such as the warm, chlorinated circulating water in hotels provide breeding grounds for certain bacteria (such as the pathogen causing Legionnaires disease) while the modern fine-spray showers provide bacteria with droplets that reach the furthest corners of the individual's lungs.

1.1.3.2 Characteristics of the socio-cultural milieu

The socio-cultural milieu (environment) consists of all the prescribed norms and values that guide and direct behaviour (including health behaviour), attitudes, beliefs, perceptions, demeanour and philosophical orientations. As such, the socio-cultural environment contributes to the development of health problems in many ways. Every culture has both direct and indirect influence/ affects on the health of individuals, families and communities. The direct affects stem from the specific culturally prescribed practices and behaviour related to health and disease, lifestyle, life-events and interpersonal relationships. For example, all cultures have prescribed practices that promote health, prevent illness and restore health when disease had occurred as well as dietary practices that contribute to the nutritional status and health status of their members. The indirect effects of culture result from cultural definitions of health and disease, disease causation, acceptability of healthcare programmes and compliance with health or disease treatment regimes.

For example, the cultural definition of health and disease determines the kind of health problems that is considered worthy of attention and the kind of conditions that are to be disregarded. Beliefs regarding the causation of diseases determine whether traditional healthcare providers must be consulted or whether both professional and traditional healthcare providers can be consulted. If recommendations of healthcare providers are too far removed from the normal cultural practices in a given situation, the host/ healthcare user is unlikely to comply with these recommendations.

The social milieu within a specific culture also influences health and health practices in many different ways. Culturally defined norms not only govern the behaviour of the members (including health and disease behaviour) but all the social interactions of its members as well, with rules that profoundly influence the health of the members of the cultural group. The place/class allocated to the family by the particular culture, the role the family has to play in respect to health and disease, and the extent to which the beliefs and values of the family influences the behaviour of the individual family member, are of cardinal importance. The role and status of individual family members have implications for healthcare, for example, what is the role status of children and the elderly? Who can make decisions regarding health and disease? Who has to render care to the sick? Health is also affected by religious beliefs and practices; beliefs and practices in magic as practiced by families and communities; fatalistic attitudes that prevail; practices that enhance or detract from health, and expectations regarding standards of conduct.

Characteristics of the socio-cultural milieu that are of importance are
- culturally determined behaviour and the meaning/purpose of such behaviour
- perception of health, disease and disease causation
  - differentiation between physical and mental diseases
  - perception of a diagnosis and treatment
  - folk illness/diseases and folk healthcare practitioners
  - folk designations of physical diseases
  - folk classification of and word usage for diseases, for example, high blood, bad blood, poison blood as well as their identification and treatment
  - traditional folk medicine for treatment of diseases
  - diseases caused by witchcraft and cured by magic
- value orientations
  - orientation regarding human beings
  - nature orientation (subject to or harmony with or mastery over)
  - time orientation
  - activity orientation
  - spatial orientation
- individual goals and norms versus group goals and norms
- authority and decision making (government, community and family)

- social environment
  - rules governing interpersonal relationships
  - accepted modes of behaviour
  - cultural affiliations
  - level of cultural acculturation
  - social structures and family structures
  - place of individuals in the family and the place of families within the culture
- role of the family regarding health and disease
  - language – verbal and non-verbal, contextual
  - beliefs and values
  - prevailing societal attitudes to health, disease and disability
  - media portrayals of healthy, altered and unhealthy behaviour
- religious affiliations – practices and rituals
- lifestyle factors
  - dietary and food practices and consumption patterns
  - rituals and taboos during pregnancy, birth and post-partum period
  - rituals and practices during early infancy
  - rituals and practices during death and dying and funeral rituals and practices
  - rituals and practices during illness and dietary patterns to be followed by the ill person
  - congregation of large groups of persons indoors during winter months enhances the spread of communicable diseases
- social phenomena, such as prostitution, promiscuity, drug abuse, alcoholism, also contribute to the spread of communicable diseases.

1.1.3.3 Characteristics of the Economic milieu

Economic influences not only effects the individual host's and his/her family's access to goods/resources and services that promote, maintain, and restore their health, but the economics of a community may limit its provision of services related to health, sanitation and protection.

Characteristics of the economic milieu that are of importance are
- the total amount of money available for healthcare services and the composition and distribution of services delivered
- rising cost of healthcare services delivery - the poorer the individual/ family is, the less money is available to spend on healthcare and a longer time elapses before healthcare is seek with the result that risk for complications increases exponently
- decreased access to healthcare services due to the rising cost and the reduced income experienced by segments of the population
- poverty often goes hand in hand with urbanization, resulting in poor housing, which in turn leads to overcrowding, unhygienic communal habits and poor environmental hygiene

- urbanisation leads to informal settlements with high density population which contribute to closer contact between persons, as well as between humans and animals (vectors). In this way, the spread of microbes are facilitated
- ratio of employment and level of income (high, low, average) in view of obtaining services and goods and spending patterns
- rising cost of food and availability of food.

1.1.3.4 Characteristics of the Psychological milieu

The psychological environment (internal and external) contributes to a variety of health problems.

- The factors internal to the individual host contribute to problems such as substance abuse, alcoholism, family violence, promiscuous sexual behaviour (mode of interpersonal interaction).
- Factors in the external psychological environment that affects the host, the family and the community include attitudes and beliefs, the importance of individual versus group gaols, modes of authority and decision making, attitude to change and the character of interpersonal relationships. Other aspects of importance are stressors (for example, crop failure triggered by weather conditions); lack of resources; poverty; prevailing economic climate; the prevailing feeling tone (apathy, anger, aggressiveness, violent, insecure, secure and safe); future prospects; the history and response to events; the relationships between subgroups (tension, distrust, and harmony); and the formal and informal communication systems (degree of trust).

1.1.3.5 Characteristics of other milieus of importance

Many other environments/milieus such as the legal, political, historical, religious, communicative, transportative, educational etc. exist but will not be discussed. Cognisance of these other environments must be taken as they do play a role (sometimes a very important role) in the causation, spread and control of communicable diseases.

1.2.   KEY NOTES

❑ Humans and microbes have co-existed since time immemorial in a symbiotic relationship with one another. All living organisms use one another as habitat and all living organisms have formed symbiotic associations where one species lives in or on the body of another with no overtones of benefit or harm. Three broad categories of symbiosis can be distinguished, namely, commensalism, mutualism and parasitism.

❑ The human host, the pathogen and the environment are interrelated with one another in the causation, spread and control of communicable diseases – as depicted in the model "the Epidemiological Triad of Communicable Diseases".

❑ Each element of the model "The Epidemiological Triangle of Communicable Diseases", namely, the hosts system, the pathogen and the environment consist of specific attributes/properties/characteristics that must always be taken in cognisance.

❑ The attributes/properties/characteristics of each element are directional in the setting of all interventions for the rendering of comprehensive, compassionate, holistic and culturally congruent healthcare to all hosts, the maintaining of a healthy environment and the prevention and control of all communicable diseases.

❑ When the balanced pathogenicity between host, pathogen and environment is disturbed, it becomes the most important contributing factor in the causation of outbreaks of communicable diseases.

❑ If the "links" of interrelatedness are not severed very quickly, sporadic outbreaks can quickly develop in epidemics and pandemics.

THEME II

BREAKING THE LINKS OF INTERRELATEDNESS

The general principles underlying the prevention and control of communicable diseases

The prevention and control of communicable diseases form an integral part of primary healthcare services delivery and all interventions to be taken must be at preventive, promotive, curative and rehabilitative levels of healthcare rendering. These measures are intended to prevent the outbreak of epidemics and should an outbreak occur the epidemic has to be controlled with the maximum efficiency. All interventions to be taken in the prevention and control of communicable diseases must take the hosts system, the environment (including the socio-cultural, economical and all other milieus of importance) of the community and the disease itself (that is the specific pathogenic agent) in consideration to prevent the spread of the particular disease. Furthermore, all interventions for the prevention, healthcare rendering and control of communicable diseases are supported by the necessary legislation that has to be enforced when necessary. Healthcare services for the prevention, care rendering and control of communicable diseases have to be available, affordable and accessible to all citizens of the RSA.

Chapter 2

LEGISLATIVE MEASURES

The National Department of Health is legally required to protect the health of the public of the RSA and the **protection of the health of the public takes precedence over the rights of the individual.** Health legislation furthermore empowers the authorities to detain ill healthcare users with communicable diseases "until the disease no longer poses a public health threat". Legislation *per se* is one of the eight basic components of a comprehensive health service delivery system as legislation supports the prevention and control of communicable diseases. The aim of such legislative measures is to prevent the outbreak of epidemics, and the instituting and enforcing of the necessary control measures to prevent the spread of the condition, should such an outbreak occurs. Legislative measures further help to prevent the introduction of communicable diseases into the country as well as its spread across the country's national and international borders (sea, air and land). Legislative measures have to be meticulously instituted and enacted. As certain communicable medical diseases are classified as notifiable, the incidence of communicable diseases, on the basis of the authorities being notified of these notifiable medical diseases, can be closely monitored.

Also bear in mind that legislative measures may be amended and that the onus is on all healthcare practitioners/providers to keep abreast of new/ amended legislative measures.

2.1   NATIONAL HEALTH ACT – ACT 61 OF 2003

The aim of the National Health Act is to provide qualitative and comprehensive healthcare (preventive, promotive, curative and rehabilitative) to all citizens of the RSA; to monitor the health of the citizens of the country and to render to all citizens a caring and effective healthcare service based on the primary healthcare approach. Furthermore, all healthcare interventions must comply and be in line with the Constitution of the RSA, the Bill of Human Rights and the Patients' Rights Charter as well as adhering to the caring ethos of healthcare rendering.

2.1.1   The functions of the National Department of Health, the Provincial Department of Health and the District Health Authorities

The functions of the various departments/authorities are, inter alia, as follow
◆ **The National Department of Health (NDoH) has the responsibility of**
   ✳ protecting, promoting, improving and maintaining the health of the population

* ✳ ensuring the provision of quality healthcare, on national, provincial and district levels
* ✳ funding healthcare services and procuring resources for healthcare services delivery
* ✳ establishing liaisons on international level and with the World Health Organization
* ✳ establishing national healthcare programmes at primary, secondary and tertiary level, such as for the prevention and control of communicable medical diseases, environmental (non-personal) health, epidemiological informational systems and laboratory services

◆ **The Provincial Department of Health (PDoH) is responsible for the**
* ▪ provision of regional and specialized hospital services
* ▪ establishing of specific provincial programmes under the auspices of a specific Directorate, such as the Directorate for Communicable Diseases that is responsible for all programmes regarding communicable diseases, for example, tuberculosis
* ▪ delivery of non-personal (environmental) healthcare services

◆ **The District Health Authorities (DHA) are responsible for the**
* o delivery of primary healthcare services[1] that include preventive and promotive, curative, and rehabilitative healthcare services as well as environmental healthcare services such as clean water, sanitation, housing, hygienic nutrition, vector control and garbage removal

[1]Primary healthcare services, *per se*, include the following services delivery
* ▪ health information
* ▪ nutrition and nutritional information
* ▪ vaccination
* ▪ the supply of essential drugs (medication)
* ▪ control and prevention of communicable medical diseases (including endemic diseases)
* ▪ water, sanitation and environmental hygiene
* ▪ epidemiological and health statistical services
* ▪ monitoring of the health status of the citizens of the RSA
* ▪ medical legislative services.

2.2 REGULATIONS REGARDING NOTIFIABLE MEDICAL CONDITIONS

The Minister of Health may promulgate regulations relating to the compilation of a list of notifiable medical conditions, including naming the persons responsible for notification, the circumstances under which and the manner in which the disease was contracted, the person or authority to whom notification has to be made, the written records of these notifications and the forwarding by District Health Authorities of such notifications to the Director-General of Health or the Minister of Health. The Minister also has the authority to enforce suitable treatment, when necessary.

2.2.1 Notification of medical conditions

The purpose of the notification of diseases is the prevention and control of communicable diseases. Several communicable medical diseases have been declared notifiable under the National Health Act, Act 61 of 2003. These diseases are to be notified at the office of the District Health Authority or any other relevant department of the District Health Authority involved, or the Provincial Department of Health concerned, or the Director-general of the National Department of Health. According to Regulation R703 of 30 July 1993, notification should be made by the medical practitioner or a healthcare practitioner who is registered with a healthcare statutory body as such, or any other person who is legally qualified to practice for gain and legally competent to diagnose and treat a person with regard to a notifiable medical condition. Where the notifiable condition is a communicable disease, notification has to be done verbally/orally without delay (in person or by telephone) and confirm within 24 hours in writing (fax, electronic mail or telegram). Other conditions have to be notified in writing within 7 days. According to policy and if necessary, the National Department of Health (NDoH) will notify the World Health Organization (WHO) that a particular communicable disease has broken out in the RSA. The WHO will help the NDoH to control the outbreak as well as to monitor the situation to prevent further outbreaks.

2.2.2 Information to be supplied with notification

Name, age, gender, identity number (when not available, then date of birth), physical address (not postal address), place of employment, proof of educational institution being attended by the person concerned, date of manifestation of the notifiable communicable medical condition and any other available information concerning the probable site and source of infection.

2.2.3 Notifiable medical diseases

The following medical diseases are notifiable by law
* Acute flaccid paralysis
* Acute rheumatic fever
* Cholera
* Congenital syphilis
* Food poisoning (outbreaks of more than four persons)
* Haemophilus influenza type B
* Haemorrhagic fevers of Africa (Congo fevers, Dengue fever, Ebola fever, Lassa fever, Marburg fever, Rift Valley fever)
* Influenza A-virus infections of avian and/or mammal origin in humans
* Lead poisoning
* Legionellosis
* Leprosy
* Malaria
* Measles
* Meningococcal infections

* Paratyphoid fever
* Plague
* Poisoning by agricultural or farm remedies registered according to the Fertilisers and Stock remedies Act
* Poliomyelitis
* Rabies (human case or human contact)
* Smallpox and similar small-pox-diseases, excluding chicken-pox
* Severe Acute Respiratory Disease (SARS)
* Tetanus
* Tetanus neonatorum
* Trachoma
* Tuberculosis (all forms as well as when any child younger as 5 years has a significant reaction following tuberculin testing)
* Typhoid fever
* Typhus fever (epidemic typhus fever transmitted by lice, endemic typhus fever transmitted by fleas)
* Virus hepatitis A, B, non-A, non-B and undifferentiated
* Whooping cough
* Yellow fever.

Note

Sexually transmitted infections (STI's, venereal diseases, STD's), namely, syphilis, gonorrhoea, soft chancre, venereal warts, venereal granuloma, herpes simplex II and AIDS/HIV+ are not notifiable. A person who has contracted a sexually transmitted infection(s) may not intentionally infect other persons or expose them to the specific sexually transmitted infection(s), and has to subject himself/herself to treatment until he/she can no longer transmit the infection(s). If the individual is treated by a private physician and does not report regularly for treatment, the private physician has to notify the District Health Authorities or the Provincial Department of Health who has to bring the requirements of the law to the attention of the person concerned. He/she is then ordered to report for treatment. If the person should withhold his/her cooperation, a warrant is issued by a magistrate on the recommendation of the medical health officer. This warrant compels the person to undergo treatment or to be isolated for treatment until he/she is no longer infectious. All court procedures regarding sexually transmitted infections are to be held *in camera*. The law also prohibits the publication of any advertisements regarding anything professing to cure sexually transmitted infections or anything else referring to the genital organs in the public media. Professional medical publications are exempted from this prohibition. The law also grants District Health Authorities the right to carry out mass examination of the inhabitants of an area in order to eliminate sexually transmitted infections (reduce the pool of infected individuals). Permission must be obtained beforehand from the Minister of Health

2.3 REGULATIONS REGARDING THE PREVENTION AND CONTROL OF COMMUNICABLE DISEASES

Should there be an outbreak of communicable diseases in a community; the Minister of Health has the authority to make special arrangements to prevent such diseases from spreading. The regulations set out under the National Health Act, Act 61 of 2003 and Regulation R703 of July 1993 will be discussed in this section.

2.3.1 General regulations regarding the prevention and control of communicable diseases

Under the National Health Act, Act 61 of 2003, the Minister of Health may issue regulations, inter alia, relating to

- ✠ anything which may or must be prescribed in terms of the Act
- ✠ communicable diseases
- ✠ notifiable medical conditions
- ✠ rehabilitation
- ✠ emergency medical services and emergency medical treatment, both within and outside of health establishments
- ✠ health nuisances and medical waste
- ✠ the import and export of pathogenic micro-organisms
- ✠ health laboratory services
- ✠ health technology
- ✠ publications re health research
- ✠ the national health information system
- ✠ when circumstances necessitate the immediate publication of a regulation, such regulation can be published in the *Gazette* without any consultation being contemplated (in normal circumstances a period of 3 months for consultation and commenting must lapsed before commencement takes place after publication in the *Gazette*).

To prevent and control outbreaks of endemic/epidemic/pandemic communicable diseases on an ongoing basis, many regulations are still in place that were decreed under The Health Act, Act 63 of 1977, as amended. Furthermore, the Health Act of 1977 had endorsed most regulations regarding communicable diseases decreed under the "Wet op Volksgezondheidt of 1918" – regulations that would likely not be repealed because of their applicability to situations of today, for example, sea and air port authorization called Pratique. According to these Acts and Regulations, the Minister of Health may issue regulations relating to

- the closing of any educational institution, whether public or private, for the purpose of preventing the spread of any communicable disease, and the regulation or restriction of the attendance by any person at any educational institution
- the duties of parents or guardians of learners who are suffering or have suffered from, or have been exposed to a particular communicable disease, and of persons in charge of educational institutions, in respect of such learners
- the imposition and enforcement of quarantine in respect of, or the subjection to medical surveillance, examination or surveillance of persons suffering or suspected to be suffering from any communicable disease, where such persons are not removed to a hospital or a place of isolation, the premises on which such person are accommodated, the persons in charge of or attending to such first-mentioned persons, and other persons living on or visiting such premises or who may otherwise have been exposed to infection with the relevant disease

- the conveyance by rail or public transport otherwise of any person suffering from a communicable disease or the bodies/mortal or bodily remains of persons who have died of specific communicable diseases
- the measures that shall be taken at inland borders, sea ports and air ports with a view to preventing the introduction of communicable disease into the RSA or the export from the RSA of any substance or thing likely to introduce any communicable diseases into any area outside the RSA
- the prevention of the transmission of any communicable disease from any vertebrate or invertebrate animal, animal carcass, animal product, animal parasite, plant or plant parasite to human beings. The prevention of the development of any communicable disease in any vertebrate or invertebrate animal, animal product, animal parasite, plant or plant parasite
- the prevention of the spread of and the eradication of malaria, the extermination of mosquitoes and the removal or remedying of conditions permitting or favouring the prevalence or increase of mosquitoes
- the prevention of the transmission of any communicable disease by flies or other insects, the extermination of flies or other insects and the removal or remedying of conditions permitting or favouring the prevalence or increase of flies or other insects
- the extermination of rodents and other vermin and the removal or remedying of conditions permitting or promoting the prevalence or increase thereof, and the disposal of the carcases of rodents and other animals suspected to have died of a communicable disease
- the clinical observation, examination and performance of an autopsy on any person when the origin of the communicable disease is either unknown or uncertain
- the compulsory vaccination of persons against communicable diseases and any matter incidental to such vaccination
- the prevention of the development and spread of any communicable disease as a result of the carrying on of any business, trade or occupation
- the prevention of the transmission of any communicable disease by persons who, although not suffering from such a disease, are carriers of and likely to cause the spread of infection of such a disease; keeping under medical surveillance and the restriction of movements of such persons
- the disposal of any refuse, waste matter or any other matter or thing which is in such a condition that it is likely to cause the development of a communicable disease
- the provision of equipment for disinfecting and the disinfesting of any premises or thing which is or is believed to be in such a condition that it will cause the development of a communicable disease and, where disinfecting or disinfesting of such a thing is impossible, the destruction thereof
- the inspection of premises or articles with a view to ascertaining the existence of or otherwise of unsanitary or other conditions likely to favour the spread, or impede the eradication of any communicable disease and, where such conditions exist, the remedying thereof

- the evacuation, closing down, alteration, demolition or destruction of any premises, the occupation or use of which is considered likely to promote the spread or impede the eradication of any communicable diseases; the circumstances in which compensation may be paid in respect of any premises so demolished or destroyed and the manner of determining such compensation
- the compulsory medical examination of persons suffering or believed to be suffering from any communicable diseases specified in such regulations and the compulsory hospitalisation and treatment of such persons
- the compulsory removal, cleansing and disinfesting of persons infested with fleas, lice or other similar external parasites
- the control, restriction or prohibition of the use of any premises for a funeral/ undertaker's business and the measures to be taken in carrying on such a business to prevent the spread of communicable diseases
- the control or closing down of any place used for public receptions, recreation or amusement and the regulation, restriction or prohibition of the holding of or attendance at any meeting, reception or other public gathering, with a view to preventing the spread of communicable diseases or controlling or restricting any communicable disease
- all measures to be taken (including methods and products which can be used) in order to prevent the incidence or the spread of communicable diseases or to control or limit such diseases
- all information which have to be given regarding communicable diseases as by notice in the Government Gazette, whether in news papers, over radio and television, notices to be distributed among the public and notices to put up in public or to be announced verbally
- the declaration of any region (according to international health measures) as being an epidemic or endemic area and implementing the necessary measures in order to control the condition
- the vaccination of all travellers entering or leaving the RSA if it should be deemed necessary
- the examination and treatment of all persons and/or goods coming into the RSA from a country where there is an incidence of communicable diseases
- the supply of the necessary medication, equipment or treatment of persons with a view to clearing up or curing the condition.

Note

1. All healthcare users must be treated with dignity and respect
2. All policies and programmes concerning communicable diseases have to be implemented and executed in accordance with international policies, norms and standards
3. All heath care practitioners/providers must strictly adhere to all legislative measures and follow all procedures to the letter
4. Managers of healthcare institutions (public and private) can be held responsible (under the National Health Act) when personnel becomes ill with a transmissible/communicable disease or nosocomial infection during employment

5. Health officers may enter any premises, excluding a private dwelling, at any reasonable time to inspect such premises to ensure compliance with the National Health Act, questions any person who may provide relevant information, ask for necessary documentation, and take samples of any substance that is relevant to the inspection. All situations that may constitute pollution detrimental to health or likely to cause a health nuisance, or constitute a health nuisance must be investigated. Health officers, accompanied by a police officer(s), may also enter any premises (including a private dwelling) with a court warrant, or without a court warrant when reasonable doubt exists that the delay in obtaining the warrant would defeat the object of the warrant, to inspect or/and seize, photograph, copy, test and examine any document, record, object, or material as well as examine any activity, operation or process carried out.

2.3.2 Specific measures in respect of the prevention and control of communicable diseases according to Regulation R703 of 30 July 1993

Regulation No R703 of 30 July 1993 was promulgated under The Health Act, Act 63 of 1977, as amended.

2.3.2.1 Prevention and restriction of communicable diseases

A District Health Authority, on having received notification that a communicable disease is present or has occurred in its District and if the authority is reasonably satisfied that the spread of such a disease constitutes or will constitute a real danger to health, may by written order and subject to conditions contained in such order

(a) close any premises, whether public or private, such as educational institutions, places of public entertainment, places used for public meetings, receptions, recreation, amusement, sport, or any part of such institution or place that is situated within its District, where the disease had occurred or where persons have been exposed or may been exposed to the disease

(b) regulate or restrict access to and/or attendance by any person at any such premises. If necessary, in order to prevent the spread of a communicable disease, be furnished on request, with the names and addresses of

* learners and educators at educational institutions by the principal
* persons presence at meetings, places of public amusement or public receptions, recreation or amusement by the person in control
* sick healthcare users, medical practitioners, nursing practitioners, employees and visitors at any hospital, nursing home, maternity home or similar institution by the manager
* employees on premises or residing on the premises, by the employer or person acting on his behalf

(c) regulate, restrict or prohibit the holding of or attendance at any meeting, reception or other public gathering within its District

(d) place under quarantine in order to prevent the spread of such disease or in order to control or restrict such disease

(i) any person or animal actually suffering or suspected to be suffering from such disease, in cases where such person or animal is not removed to a hospital or place of isolation

(ii) any person or animal that is in contact with or who has, within the period determined by a medical officer of health or a medical practitioner in the employment of the State, been in contact with any person or animal referred to in subparagraph (i), in cases where such person or animal is not removed to a hospital or place of isolation

(iii) any premises where any person or animal referred to in subparagraph (i) or (ii), as the case may be, live or stay, or

(iv) a specific area, as determined by a medical officer of health, where such disease occurs or has occurred

(v) any goods or articles that may have been in contact with the infective agent of a disease or may serve as a means of spreading the disease.

Specific procedures have to be followed by District Health Authorities regarding persons who die of or who have already died at the outbreak of a communicable disease.

(i) When it is suspected that a person died of a communicable disease or other medical condition, and more information or facts are needed regarding the disease or condition in order to determine the measures to be taken to prevent the particular disease from spreading, or the particular condition from reappearing, and it proves to be impossible to gather this information except by performing an autopsy on the body, the Director-General of Health or the magistrate of the district where the person has died, may instruct the performance of an autopsy by a medical practitioner. If the body has already been buried, the official may order an exhumation to be done. Such disinterment shall be carried out under the strict supervision of an environmental health officer and in accordance with the measures laid down

(ii) When a person dies of a communicable disease in a hospital or a place of isolation, the body may not be removed unless it is for the purpose of immediate burial or cremation. Any person, who removes the body for any other reason or without the necessary permission from an authorised official, is guilty of a felony.

2.3.2.2 Quarantine and isolation

(1) Any person who is placed under quarantine in terms of an order or who has been placed in isolation shall be obliged to satisfy the provisions of that order

(2) Any person who is present on premises or in an area placed under quarantine

- May not leave such premises or area before the expiry of the prescribed quarantine period without prior authorisation
- Shall subject himself/herself during such period to any medical observation, examination or supervision determined by an authorised medical practitioner
- Shall subject himself/herself to all regulations relating to quarantine and regarding restriction, regulating of and/or control of movement and stay
- May not remove or have removed any goods, articles or animal from the premises or the area

(3) No person shall enter any premises or area that is been placed under quarantine without the necessary authorization

(4) An officer may detain and isolate any person if he/she knows or suspects that this person has not complied with or neglected to satisfy the aforementioned provisions, or has left the premises or area without authorization. This person may then be handed over for medical observation, examination or supervision to a medical health officer.

Note

The compulsory/enforced isolation/detaining/quarantine of sufferers of any communicable disease(s), for example, extensively/extreme-drug resistant tuberculosis (XDR-TB) or completely-drug resistant-TB (CDR-TB)/totally-drug resistant-TB (TDR-TB), is justifiable because the protection of the health of the public takes precedence over the rights of the individual. Health legislation in the RSA empowers the authorities to detain sick healthcare users with diseases "until the disease no longer poses a public health threat" while the National Department of Health is legally required and responsible to protect the health of the public. As long periods of hospitalisation may be necessary to stabilise sick persons until they are not more infectious, all reasonable measures must be taken to provide the recommended healthcare and the sick person must adhere to it voluntary before any restriction will be instituted. When the sick person refuses treatment, justifiable isolation/detention becomes necessary until such time the patient is not infectious any more.

Enforced hospitalisation/quarantine of sick healthcare users suffering from XDR-TB and CDR-TB/ TDR-TB is therefore justified as the last resort after all voluntary measures to isolate the individuals have failed. Unfortunately, confinement can continue until death or, conceivably, indefinitely until the sick person has been cured/became not infectious any longer since at the present time XDR-TB or CDR-TB/TDR-TB remains incurable and untreatable.

The restriction must always take place
- with sufficient legal procedural safeguards in place
- within a framework of human rights (according to the Bill of Rights as enshrined in the Constitution)
- with the interest of a legitimate objective of general interest in mind
- based on scientific evidence
- with a view to limited duration
- be subjected to review.

2.3.2.3 The handling, conveyance and burial of the bodies/ bodily or mortal remains of persons that have died of communicable diseases

The bodily/mortal remains of any person who has died of anthrax, cholera, a haemorrhagic fever of Africa, rabies, meningococcal infection, plague, poliomyelitis, typhoid fever or Acquired Immune Deficiency Syndrome (AIDS) may not be transported/conveyed by train or on public transport or in any other way unless
- ✳ the bodily/mortal remains is sealed in an airtight container and placed in a non-transparent, sturdy, sealed coffin or sealed container
- ✳ the outer surface of the coffin or container is free from any liquid or any unhygienic matter originating from such body and any offensive odours are absent

✳ no bodily/mortal remains/bodies shall be imported to be buried in the RSA or exported to be buried outside the borders of the RSA without the body been embalmed, sealed in an airtight container and placed in a sturdy coffin before being conveyed.

2.3.2.4 Prevention of the transmission of a communicable disease to persons by animals, insects and parasites

In order to prevent the transmission or development of a communicable disease among persons, a medical health officer may order the owner or occupier of premises situated within the official's district to

- furnish the officer with all information relating to the occurrence, spread, extermination or decrease in numbers of any animal, animal carcass, animal product, animal parasite, arthropod, plant or plant material, plant parasite or microbe on such premises
- take measures to prevent the spread of or exterminate or reduce the above
- provide all reasonable assistance and cooperation to the authorities or private institutions with regard to preventing the spread or with regard to the extermination or reduction of such diseases
- remove or remedy conditions that permit or promote the occurrence or increase thereof
- grant an officer access to the premises and co-operate with an officer to undertake the monitoring of communicable disease in indicator animals
- remove the carcass of any animal (referred to in the notification) that has died on such premises.

2.3.2.5 Compulsory medical examination, hospitalisation and treatment of persons suffering from a communicable disease

Any person who, in the opinion of a medical health officer is or could be suffering from a communicable disease shall, when so instructed by the medical health officer

- subject himself at a time and place determined by the medical health officer to such medical examination and such treatment as prescribed by the person undertaking the examination
- report to or be removed to a hospital or other place of isolation as determined by the medical health officer in order to remain there under medical supervision and receive treatment
- subject himself to the medical treatment prescribed by the medical health officer or the person assigned by the medical health officer, until he is free of infection or may be discharged without in any way endangering public health
- A medical health officer may, when he is satisfied on medical scientific grounds that the danger exists that a sufferer of a communicable disease can transmit such a disease to other people, order in writing that such a sufferer
  - a) (i) may not prepare any food intended for other persons
    - (ii) may not handle any food or water intended for other persons

(iii) may not handle any container for such food or water
b) must comply with such other requirements as are deemed necessary by the medical health officer in order to safeguard public health
* A parent, guardian or person who has legal custody and control of a child who is a sufferer, shall render all reasonable assistance in the implementation of this regulation or of any order issued in terms thereof in respect of such a child.

2.3.2.6   Compulsory removal, cleansing and disinfesting of persons and animals infested with fleas, lice or similar parasites

A medical health officer who is aware of a person infested with fleas, lice or similar external parasites, may by written order direct that
(a) (i) the infested person cleanse or disinfest himself, or
    (ii) a person who has legal custody or control of the infested person must, under supervision of a health officer appointed by the medical health officer, cleanse or disinfest the infested person or have him cleansed or disinfested at a time and place as directed by the medical health officer
(b) any person directed by the designated health officer removes the infested person or animal to a place mentioned in the order so that he/she/animal may be cleansed or disinfested there by or under the supervision of a health officer.

2.3.2.7   Carriers of communicable diseases

(1) Any person suspected by a medical health officer on reasonable grounds to be a carrier of a communicable disease and who, as such, constitutes a public health hazard shall, when so instructed by the medical health officer, subject himself to a medical examination at a time and place determined by the medical health officer in order to establish whether such a person is in fact a carrier as is suspected
(2) Every carrier so instructed in writing by a medical health officer shall
* at all times comply with and carry out all reasonable and feasible instructions given to him by the medical health officer in respect of the disposal of his excrement, the cleansing of his body and of articles used by him, or other precautions to prevent the spread of an infection or to restrict it to a minimum
* inform such medical health officer of his intention to change his place of residence or place of employment and, after such a change, of his new place of residence or place of employment, and such medical health officer shall inform the provincial Head of the Department of Health of the region of the carrier's new address.
(3) A medical health officer may, when he is satisfied on medical scientific grounds that the danger exists that a carrier of a communicable disease can transmit such a disease to other people, order in writing that such a carrier
(a) report at or be removed to a hospital, or other place of isolation or area referred to in the order so as to remain there under medical supervision for a period determined in such an order
(b) report for medical examination and treatment at the times and places specified in the order

(c) (i) may not prepare any food intended for other persons
  (i) may not handle any food or water intended for other persons
  (ii) may not handle any container for such food or water
(d) comply with such other requirements as are deemed necessary by the medical health officer in order to safeguard public health.
(e) A parent, guardian or person who has legal custody and control of a child who is a carrier, shall render all reasonable assistance in the implementation of this regulation or of any order issued in terms thereof in respect of such a child

2.3.2.8 Compulsory immunization/vaccination

(1) If the Director-General of Health is satisfied that there is sufficient reason based on medical scientific grounds to suspect that the health of the population of the RSA or any part of the population may be affected by a medical condition against which humans can be vaccinated, he may, by means of notification in the Government Gazette
- demarcate an area referred to in the notice for compulsory vaccination of all inhabitants or of a specific group or category of inhabitants, as referred to in the notice, of such a demarcated area
- designate the government body, person or persons to carry out such vaccination, and determine the period during which the vaccination is to be done

(2) A governmental body or person referred to in sub-regulation (1)(b) may authorize any medical health officer or nurse as an vaccination officer under the control of a medical practitioner designated by such government body or person, to vaccinate persons in terms of this regulation
(3) The Director of Health in whose region an area (or areas) referred to in sub-regulation (1)(b) falls, shall coordinate all matters in regard to vaccinations carried out in terms of this regulation
(4) A governmental body or person referred to in sub-regulation (1)(b) shall determine in a manner deemed suitable, the place and times of compulsory vaccinations as well as the classification of persons for vaccination at classification points
(5) No person may disregard or fail to comply with an instruction from the governmental body or person or vaccination officer referred to in sub-regulation (2)
(6) Any person who, when instructed to do so, cannot or will not undergo vaccination for medical or any other reasons, may, by order of the Director-general/Minister concerned be placed and detained in a place of isolation for a reasonable period.

2.3.2.9 Specific measures relating to learners and educational institutions

(1) A principal/rector who is aware or has reason to suspect that a learner at the educational institution of which he/she is the principal, or a person who is employed at the institution or who happens to visit such an institution
 (i) suffers from a communicable disease as specified in the list of communicable medical diseases (see table 2.1)
 (ii) was in contact with any person suffering from such disease, or
 (iii) is infested with fleas, lice or similar external parasites

shall without delay inform the medical health officer or head of the District Health Authorities or the head of the Provincial Department of Health of a province, either by telephone, telegraph or telex of such a situation

(2) Except on the strength of a certificate of admission issued by the attending medical practitioner employed by the local board concerned or the District Health Authority, or a medical practitioner employed by the state, a principal may not allow a person whose condition was reported in terms of paragraph 1 to enter the educational institution in question, except according to the times and conditions contained in the list of diseases

(3) The parent or guardian of a child who attends an educational institution as a learner and in respect of whom (to the knowledge of the parent or guardian) a condition referred to in sub-regulation (a)(i), (ii) or (iii) applies, shall without delay inform the principal of the institution concerned of such a condition

(4) (a) Where, in the absence of an opinion given by a medical practitioner, a principal referred to in sub-regulation (1) is in doubt as to whether a learner or an employee or a visitor referred to in that sub-regulation is an immune contact or a susceptible contact in respect of a communicable disease referred to in the list of diseases, the principal has to act in accordance of the requirements of the listed diseases as if such learner, employee or visitor is a susceptible contact

(b) The provisions of paragraph (a) shall apply mutatis mutandis to a parent or guardian referred to in sub-regulation (2)

Table 2.1 LISTED COMMUNICABLE MEDICAL CONDITIONS AS PER REGULATION

Communicable disease	Infected person may return to educational institution	Contact may return to educational institution
Acute flaccid paralysis	On submission of a medical certificate	Immediately Susceptible contacts should be vaccinated against poliomyelitis immediately
Chicken-pox and Herpes Zoster	After the disappearance of the rash or on submission of a medical certificate	Immediately
Cholera	3-4 days after normal stools are passed	Immediately
Diphtheria	On submission of a medical certificate. A course of vaccination should have been started	Non-immune contacts: 8 days after removal of source of infection. A course of vaccination should have been started Immune contacts: Immediately
German measles (Rubella)	On submission of a medical certificate or four days after appearance of rash	Immediately
Haemophilus influenzae	On submission of a medical certificate, provided the necessary prophylactic medicine has been or is being taken	Immediately, provided the necessary prophylactic medicine has been or is being taken

Haemorrhagic fevers of Africa	On submission of a medical certificate or on recovery	Immediately, but must be kept under surveillance for 14 days
Haemorrhagic virus conjunctivitis	When conjunctivitis has cleared	Immediately
Hepatitis A	Seven days after appearance of jaundice or on submission of a medical certificate	Immediately
Leprosy	On submission of a medical certificate or after being on treatment for three days	Immediately
Lice infestation	After proper and complete cleansing and delousing, and the removal of nits from the head, body and clothes	Immediately, but must be kept under surveillance
Measles	On submission of a medical certificate or four days after appearance of rash	Immediately. Susceptible contacts should be vaccinated against measles immediately
Meningococcal infections	On submission of a medical certificate, provided the necessary prophylactic medicine has been or is being taken	Immediately, provided the required prophylactic medicines are taken
Mumps	Nine days after appearance of swelling	Immediately
Plague	On submission of a medical certificate	According to quarantine procedures
Poliomyelitis	On submission of a medical certificate or 14 days after beginning of the illness	Immediately. Susceptible contact should be vaccinated immediately
Scabies	After proper treatment	Immediately
Tuberculosis of the lungs	On submission of a medical certificate	Immediately
Typhoid fever	On submission of a medical certificate	Immediately
Typhus fever	On submission of a medical certificate	Immediately after delousing
Whooping cough (Pertussis)	21 days after the onset of paroxysms or on submission of a medical certificate	Immediately

2.3.2.10 Compulsory disinfesting and evacuating of premises

If a medical health officer is of the opinion that any premises or object is in such a condition that it as such can give rise to the development of a communicable disease, he may disinfest or have such premises or objects be disinfested after the owner or occupier has been given reasonable notice thereof

(1) If the Head of the Provincial Department of Health or the District Health Authority is convinced on medical scientific grounds that there is sufficient reason to suspect

that the occupation or use of a premises or any part thereof is likely to promote the spread of a communicable disease or impede the eradication thereof, he may, by written order, direct the evacuation of such premises

(2) No person other than a person authorised by the Head of the Provincial Department of Health, a medical practitioner in the employment of the state or an environmental health officer may enter the premises referred to in sub-regulation (1) during the period of validity of an evacuation order

(3) Authorized officers or persons may at any time enter any premises (except those occupied by the Department of Defence), to perform an inspection or to perform their duty as authorized. Anyone who refuses access to an authorized officer or obstruct the officer in his/her performance of duties or refuses to provide information or provides misleading information shall be guilty of an offence.

2.4 OTHER MEASURES RELATING TO COMMUNICABLE DISEASES

The following group of measures also pertain to the prevention and control of communicable diseases although promulgated under regulations or acts other than Regulation R703 of 30 July 1993.

2.4.1 Measures concerning harbours, airports and inland borders (regulation promulgated under the "Wet op Volksgezondheidt" of 1918)

It is the duty of the National Department of Health to apply health control at sea and air ports and at inland borders. The port health service is controlled by a medical practitioner. No ship or aeroplane may enter a port without the authorization of the port health officer. This authorization is known as Pratique. Any ship within the territorial waters of the RSA is considered to be premises and the captain as the head of the household. All legislation applicable ashore is therefore also applies to such a ship. The ship must be boarded and inspected by a port health officer who must authorize mooring. The port health officer may also examine any person aboard ship. The captain must report any sickness/disease and death on the ship to the port health officer. The ship must produce a certificate to prove that disinfesting of rodents has been carried out. A certificate is valid for six months. The above regulations also apply to the landing of aircrafts. Ships, aircrafts, cargo and/or passengers may be put under quarantine or refused entry. Passengers on ships or aircrafts, who do not meet the requirements of international health regulations for vaccination, must report to a magistrate, medical health officer or local health officer (if necessary).

2.4.2 Regulations relating to the prevention of Plague (regulation promulgated under the "Wet op Volksgezondheidt" of 1918)

- When it is suspected that a person has died of plague, the matter must immediately be reported to the District Health Authority who will immediately notify the National Department of Health
- Premises suspected of being infested by rodents such as rats may be ordered to be vacated, public gatherings may be prohibited and the movements of people may be restricted
- All suspected cases have to be kept under quarantine for seven days
- All premises (public and private) must be kept/made free from rats and mice. Openings must measure less than 10 mm
- Premises to be found to be in unhygienic conditions and therefore could contribute to the spread of plague, can be ordered to be cleaned/disinfected/disinfested
- A court order may be issued to demolish infested premises. When this happens, rodent disinfesting must be carried out 3 days before demolition starts
- All interspaces created between building must be made free of rodents
- All ships have to be free of rodents. Rats have to be periodically eradicated.

2.4.3 Measures to combating mosquitoes and the transmission of mosquito-borne diseases (regulation promulgated under "Wet op Volksgezondheidt" of 1918)

(1) An owner or occupier of land shall take all reasonable measures to treat any collection of water or any other habitat in which mosquitoes can breed or live in, in such a way that the breeding of mosquitoes is prevented or kept to a minimum

(2) An owner or occupier of land shall, if ordered to do so, in respect of any building or structure used by human beings
  - Spray such building or have it sprayed with insecticide as prescribed to him/her
  - Screen the outer doors, windows and other openings with gauze screens, containing no less than five openings per centimetre to the surface, and maintain the screens in good condition in order to prevent the entry of mosquitoes

(3) The owner or occupier of any building or structure that has been treated with a residual insecticide as referred to in sub-regulation (2), shall ensure that such insecticide is not plastered over, painted over, removed or rendered harmless during the period of effectiveness.

2.4.4 Regulations relating to vaccines, serum, cultures and rabies vaccine

Vaccines are provided free of charge by the National Department of Health to the public healthcare sector. The NDoH also provides the necessary health laboratory facilities regarding communicable diseases and vaccine testing. In the private healthcare sector, however, vaccines to be administered have to bought and the necessary fees paid for administering. If bought and brought to a public healthcare institution, no fees for administering need to be paid. Compulsory and/or voluntary vaccination for travellers according to the health regulations of the country of entry must be bought from and administered by a certified medical practitioner at a certified travel clinic.

2.4.5 Responsibilities as member of the South African Development Community (SADC) and signatory to the Protocol of Health

As a member of the South African Development Community (SADC), the Republic of South Africa underwrites the Protocol on Health whereby healthcare is promoted through close co-operation between the countries who signed the Protocol. The Protocol as such, deals with coordinated regional efforts in the prevention, control and eradication of communicable diseases as well as epidemic preparedness; the control of specific communicable diseases such as malaria and tuberculosis; and the sharing of resources to enhance the diagnosing and treatment of communicable diseases together with the notification of an outbreak of specific communicable diseases.

2.4.6 Signatory to the United Nations Convention of the Rights of the Child

South Africa as a signatory of the United Nations Convention of the Rights of the Child is obliged to comply with the following principles, namely, that the child has a right to
- life, survival and development
- equitable treatment and care
- participation in activities and decisions that affect him/her
- all actions should be based on the best interest of the child

Accordingly, the Children's Act, Act 38 of 2005, lowered the age of consent for treatment to 12 years of age and in cases where a child has sufficient maturity, the child below the age of 12 years may also give consent. The scope of who may provide consent has been widened grounded in the definition of caregiver and giving classes of persons certain legal rights, which include the right to consent to medical treatment. All healthcare practitioners are obliged to comply with the above.

Also note that, under the Children's Act, Act 38 of 2005, based on the "opt-out" decision (refusal of treatment) of single mothers/fathers, or parents (biological, foster or adopted), or guardians, medicines or vaccines may be administered to the infant/toddler/child/adolescent without the written or verbal consent of the single mother/father, or parents (biological, foster or adopted), or guardian if it is in the best interest of the child to receive the specific treatment (right of the child to has his/her health protected/maintained/restored). However, counselling of the single mother/father or parents (biological, foster or adopted), or guardian prior to instituting the Children's Act, Act 38 of 2005, must take place.

2.5   KEY NOTES

❑ The regulations decreed under the National Health Act have to be strictly adhered to at all times.
❑ When a person does not comply with these measures, he or she is guilty of an offence.
❑ Prevention and control of communicable diseases take place within the parameters set by the Constitution of the RSA, the Bill of Human Rights, and the National Health Act which describes the duties of persons suffering from communicable diseases and all healthcare personnel.
❑ Should an epidemic outbreak occur, control regulations relating to communicable diseases and public rights take precedence over any rights the individual have under the Constitution of the RSA.

Chapter 3

THE PREVENTION OF COMMUNICABLE DISEASES

In the course of the last two centuries, a demographic, health and epidemiological medical pattern transition has taken place. Not only are world populations getting older, but the improvement in economic patterns (though not in educational development) that has taken place, has led to communities adopting unhealthy lifestyles such as smoking, alcohol and drug use, and physical inactivity - culminating in high levels of obesity, hypertension, and diabetes mellitus - type 2. The epidemiological patterns of disease has changed from acute infectious diseases to chronic degenerative diseases, while the treatment shifted from cure to care – as a consequence, the mono-causative model of disease changed to a multi-factorial model in which comprehensive treatment must be rendered by a multi-professional team. At the same time, the provision of healthcare has developed into complicated bureaucratic structures with most of the healthcare professionals operating within these structures such as hospitals and clinics. Their activities are greatly influenced by overall governmental policies on healthcare and, in particular, the means of the government to finance it.

Because communicable diseases will never be fully erased from earth, it is imperative that communicable diseases should be prevented, as far as possible, at primary, secondary, and tertiary levels. The levels of prevention correspond with the stages of the natural course of communicable diseases (see figure 3.1). Since all hosts (healthy, ill, contact or carrier) are always a member of a family and belong to a community, the prevention and the controlling of communicable diseases are never directed solely at the individual. The family and the community must be involved in all preventive, promotive, curative, and rehabilitative interventions. At the same time, attention must be given to the environment (physical-biological, psychological, socio-cultural, economic, and all other environments of importance) as to maintain it as healthy as possible for human beings to live in.

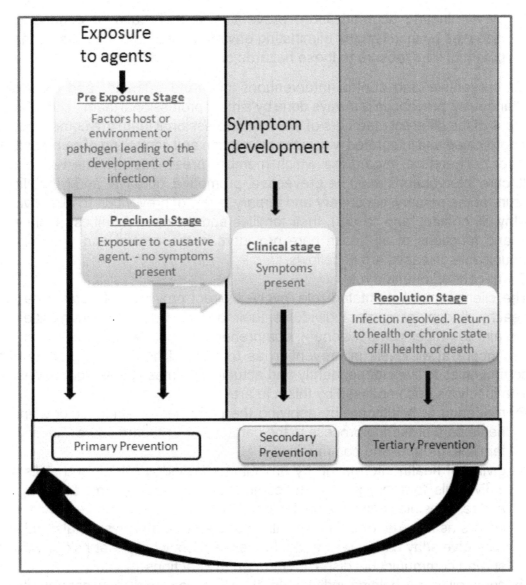

Figure 3.1   Schematic depiction of the levels of prevention corresponding with the different stages of the natural course of communicable diseases

The over-arching goal of all preventive healthcare interventions is to

➢ promote the wellbeing and protecting the health of individuals, their families, and their communities through ensuring safe conditions in which humans can live healthy

➢ prevent the consequences of preventable or treatable communicable diseases, that is, the prevention of complications through early diagnosis, treatment, and comprehensive, culturally congruent and holistic healthcare

➢ rehabilitate individuals (after recovery) to the highest level of functioning possible, and, at the same time help their families to cope with their disabilities (or their death, when individuals do not recover). Sometimes, it is necessary to rehabilitate communities also, for example, changing socio-cultural rituals and/ or health practices; or changing attitudes to sufferers of communicable diseases by eliminating stigmatization; preventing re-outbreaks of communicable diseases by modifying or eliminating environmental hazards/risks so that the potential for exposure to these hazards or risks is reduced.

As all preventive and control interventions go hand in hand, and take place simultaneously, prevention is always done by a multi-professional team. The roles and functions of the different members of the multi-professional team are complementary in a coordinated and integrated way in the prevention and controlling of communicable diseases. Therefore, regardless which member prescribes the interventions, all healthcare interventions must be preventive, promotive, curative, and rehabilitative in nature at the primary, secondary and tertiary levels of prevention to all individuals (healthy, ill, contact, and carrier), their families and their communities. Hence, the roles and functions of all health care providers in the control and prevention of communicable diseases are as follows

❑ Client-centred/oriented role

The client-centred/orientated role involves direct provision of healthcare to all healthy, ill, contact, carrier individuals, their families, and their communities with the aim to render compassionate, comprehensive, holistic, culturally congruent healthcare at all levels of prevention as to help all healthcare users/families/ communities to live independently and actualize themselves as human beings. The functions encompassed by this role are

◆ rendering of healthcare by applying the principles of epidemiology and the healthcare brokering process to the care of all healthcare users – individuals, families, groups, and communities

◆ giving of health information by providing knowledge (facts) and skills to all individuals, families, groups, and communities to make informed, appropriate, and responsible choices about their own health. The healthcare provider also serves as a guide for peers and all other healthcare professionals/traditional care givers/lay care givers and all other workers who are at risk or who can spread communicable diseases through their actions

◆ counselling by helping individuals, their families, and their communities to choose viable solutions to their health problems as to take responsibility for their own health and health behaviours, as well as for that of their families and their communities

◆ referral by directing healthcare users to the resources required to meet their specific needs. Referral also includes close cooperation between the multi-professional healthcare team members (professional, traditional and lay care givers), as well as cooperation with different departments of the governmental system, the private sector and non-governmental organizations (NGO's), to enhances health and well-being as well as preventing and controlling communicable diseases

◆ role-modelling whereby healthcare providers influence the health-related behaviour of individuals, their families, and their communities as well as all co-healthcare professionals, traditional healthcare practitioners and lay care-givers

❖ advocating by speaking on behalf of individuals, their families, and their communities to protect and enhance their well-being, for example, to advocate for the protection, maintaining and restoring of health and well-being at all levels of prevention, as well as lobbying for social, environmental, animal, educational, and labour legislation to prevent and control communicable diseases. Advocacy also includes the solving of problems that individuals, their families, and their communities may experience within the healthcare system

❖ rendering of primary healthcare by providing the essential healthcare that are based on practical, scientifically sound and socially acceptable methods and technology which is universally accessible to all individuals, their families, and their communities.

❑ Delivery-oriented role
The delivery-oriented role helps to enhance the functioning of the healthcare delivery system resulting in the rendering of quality care to individuals, their families, and their communities. The functions in this role category are

❖ coordinating and integrating the healthcare to be rendered as to best meet the needs of individuals, their families, and their communities because they receive services from a variety of sources and governmental departments or private sector or non-governmental organizations

❖ joint decision-making and collaboration between professionals (including traditional practitioners and lay care givers), individuals, families, and communities so as to resolve health problems by setting mutual goals and planning mutually acceptable action to achieve the set goals

❖ liaising between individuals, families, and communities by serving as initial point of contact between individuals, their families, their communities and healthcare agencies; by communicating, interpreting, and reinforcing healthcare provider recommendations; and to advocate, as needed, for individuals, families, and communities.

❑ Population-oriented role
Because the client-orientated and delivery-orientated roles relate mostly to specific individuals and families, the population-orientated role is primarily concerned with the wellbeing and health of the community and the population/inhabitants living in the community. The functions encompass the following

❖ case finding by identifying individual cases or occurrences of communicable diseases or other health-related conditions requiring healthcare services as healthcare professionals, traditional healthcare providers and lay care givers are skilled in detecting changes in the health status or the early signs of health problems and to carry out the necessarily follow-up

❖ identifying the needs of the community and coordinating actions to solve the health-related problems of the community

❖ acting as change agents by changing health behaviours of individuals, families, and communities, and by assisting populations to internalize the changes as well as to evaluate the effectiveness and quality of the healthcare rendered and services delivered

◈ initiating research on all negative factors in the physical-biological, psychological, socio-cultural and all other milieus of importance that threaten the welfare of individuals, families and communities as to contribute to the elimination/modification/diminishing of these factors in order to reduce the incidence of communicable diseases. The research must then be converted into health informational programmes and health promotive strategies related to the well-being of man, a healthy environment, and lifestyle modification behaviours that will promote the well-being of all individuals, families, and communities.

3.1 HEALTHCARE INTERVENTIONS AT THE PRIMARY LEVEL OF PREVENTION

The aim of primary prevention is the prevention of communicable diseases before the stage of pre-pathogenesis. Primary preventive interventions are aimed at the promotion of the health of and the specific protection against diseases in individuals, families, and communities; as well as the maintaining of a healthy environment (physical-biological {including the animal, reptile and bird kingdoms}, the psychological, socio-cultural, economical, and all other milieus of importance); and the establishing of a comprehensive healthcare system to deliver the necessary services.

3.1.1 Promoting the well-being of the host system

Health promotion and health protection focus on enhancing the level of wellbeing of individuals, families, and communities to protect, maintain, and restore health. As all individuals, families, and communities must accept responsibility for their own health, health promotion and health protection depend on behavioural changes in individuals, families, and communities. All promotional and protective health care interventions must be directed at achieving the following

- enhancing the biological-physiological health of individuals through personal hygiene, adequate nutrition, vaccination, and embracing a lifestyle that will not impair his/her health
- promoting the psychosocial health of individuals, families, and communities by enabling individuals and families to attain the necessary skills to optimize their mental and social health as well as cherishing the wellbeing of their family and community
- embracing a new approach to health and wellbeing by individuals, families, and communities whereby they take responsibility for their own wellbeing and the maintenance of optimal health. In so doing, individuals, families, and communities prevent diseases (physical, mental, and social) and when they should fall ill, accept help to adapt their lifestyle accordingly
- increasing the utilization, where necessary, of healthcare delivery services (the professional or/and the traditional or/and the lay care services). Individuals, families, and communities are to be informed about the signs, symptoms,

and treatment of communicable diseases as well as the prevention of certain diseases through vaccination and a healthy life-style.

The well-being of the host system (individuals, families, and communities) is promoted by means of health information, the aim of which is to enhance or alter the attitudes and behaviours of the individual, the family, and the community about health, thus encouraging a healthy life-style. Health protection is achieved by the vaccination of individuals as well as by the maintenance of a healthy physical-biological environment (for example, water safety, sewage and garbage disposal, building regulations, pest control, agricultural regulations and standards) and of all other milieus in which individuals, families, and communities live, together with the promotion and protection of the health of animals, reptiles and birds.

3.1.1.1 Promoting the well-being of the individual as human host

The healthcare interventions at the primary level of prevention pertain to the promotion and protecting of wellbeing of all individuals - infants, children and adolescents, adults (young and middle-aged), and elders. The persona of all humans embraces a diversity and complexity of distinguishable (but not separate) dimensions of being as an intricate unity exists between the physical, the psychological, the social, and the spiritual dimensions of being forming a unified being of mind-body-spirit. Although the wellbeing of the different dimensions is described separately, the unity of the dimensions must always be kept in mind because the health of one dimension has a profound effect on all the other dimensions of being, for example, when the dialogues of the individual with himself/herself, his/her fellow-men, his/her Creator, and his/her world are disrupted the unified well-being/health of the person is not protected and maintained.

➤ *Promoting and protecting the well-being of the bio-physical and the behaviour (lifestyle) dimensions of health*
The physical dimension of all human beings embraces the concrete and mortal body of his/her humaneness and personality and as such the person always experiences the corporeality of his/her own body. The mortal body of an individual is the anatomical-physiological structure which changes progressively in an orderly and logical pattern. The duration of an individual's life is divided into different stages, characterized by different physical changes which the person is not always aware of. The individual changes his/her body images often as physical changes are brought on by aging, disease, being disabled, or dying. Because a person's physical changes are always coupled with psycho-social development, an individual experiences his/her physical self image and the meaning of his/her body in relation to the world and his fellow-humans. In relation to the world, the individual experiences his/her body as an instrument or mediator (when walking, sitting, walking, etc.) and because of the body's perception value or greeting value, the person meets his fellow-humans as a person, and opens his/her human nature in a bodily manner.

To promote the health and wellness of his/her body (the bio-physical dimension of health), the individual must embrace a healthy lifestyle throughout the duration of his/her life. A healthy lifestyle is the key component of optimal wellness as it is essential for minimizing the incidence and severity of acute and chronic

97

illnesses (including communicable diseases). A healthy lifestyle is a way of living whereby a person engages in a specific pattern of positive activities on a daily basis. These activities act in a cumulative way to increase the individual's level of health and well-being. A healthy lifestyle is the result of all the thousands of choices an individual makes in the course of his/her life, and has its foundations within the family unit reflecting the family's unique cultural, ethnic, religious and socio-economic heritage and beliefs. Healthy lifestyle behaviours are powerfully reinforced each day as a child grows up and as an adult the individual practices them without supervision. The attitudes and interventions of healthcare providers influence healthy lifestyles by promoting routine health screening, prenatal and well child visits, and health information campaigns to make positive lifestyle choices. Episodic sickness contacts because of disease are important opportunities for providing health promotion information.

Although a healthy lifestyle includes a diverse range of topics, research suggests six personal behaviours that are associated with a healthy lifestyle, namely, (1) avoiding smoking, (2) limiting the use of alcohol, (3) engaging in regular exercise, (4) eating a nutritious diet, (5) maintaining a desirable body weight, and (6) getting 7 to 8 hours of restful sleep each night.

◈ Nutrition and diet to protect, to maintain and to restore health
  The relationship between nutrition, overall health, and the development of a wide variety of disease processes is well established. Good nutrition (in both macro- and micro-nutrients) enhances the general physiological resistance of a person. Sufficient Biotin (a B-group vitamin) and vitamin C decreases the body's susceptibility to infections. Sufficient Vitamin A prevents small epithelial lacerations while sufficient Zinc and Selenium strengthen the immunological responses of both the innate and the adaptive immune systems. Obesity, mal-nutrition, and underweight are major risk factors in disease causation and the diminishing of the body's defences against infection. Lastly, healthy eating is not just about disease-fighting nutrients – by sharing a meal with family and friends a bond is formed providing benefits far beyond those of the food on the fork.

◈ Sleep and rest to protect, to maintain and to restore health
  Getting enough sleep and rest also strengthens the immune system and the general wellbeing of the individual. Normal sleep cycles contain slow-wave, deep sleep, and REM (rapid eye movement) – sleep forms that are essential to health. The amount of sleep an individual requires varies significantly throughout the life cycle – infants and young children sleep more than older children, adolescents and adults while elders sleep less at night but nap more frequently during the day. Physical rest as such also plays an important role in health functioning as it restores adenosine triphosphate concentrations which is not actively stored by the body, and must be continuously produced.

◈ Exercise to protect, to maintain, and to restore health
  By doing regular exercise, the immune system and the general well-being of the individual are enhanced. Regular exercises enhances the physiological

health by improving blood circulation, increasing vascular fitness and stamina, maintaining or increasing strength and flexibility, maintaining bone mass, increasing glucose tolerance, increasing the proportion of high-density lipoproteins, and lengthens periods of deep sleep. Exercise plays an important role in weight control and in helping the elderly to sustain independence. Both aerobic and non-aerobic exercises are beneficial as it helps to prevent and manage a wide range of medical disorders. Of importance is that the individual does what he/she love, exercises whatever time-period works, and does not overdo exercising.

❖ Protecting health through vaccination
By vaccinating the individual, the immune system is primed with memory so that the first infection induces a rapid and effective secondary immune response

❖ Self-responsibility to protect, to maintain, and to restore health
A healthy lifestyle does not just happen - it must be enforced, consciously and unconsciously, through the choices made by the individual and his/her commitment to specific daily behaviour. The list of self-responsibility issues is endless, so most individuals make the easiest choices that are available to them. A pattern of health promotion and self-responsibility must be ingrained from early childhood so that the individual will adhere to a healthy lifestyle regimen.

➤ *Promoting and maintaining the well-being of the psycho-emotional dimension of health*
The psyche or psycho-emotional dimension of the persona of an individual embraces his/her will-power, decision-making and actions, feelings/emotions, aspirations and intellect (thoughts, language, and ability to learn). Not only dictates the individual's intellect how the person relates to other people in the world around him/her and to his/her Creator, but all individuals always participate through their feelings in any situation with their emotions giving meaning to their experiences, which in turn influence their actions and aspirations. Also, the feelings of a person contribute to his/her mood which is the foundation of the individual's experiences. All persons are constantly confronted with certain decisions and they must make choices according to their own values and norms, their conscience for which they must individually take responsibility. Because the persona is body-psyche-spirit, all persons exists in relation to their Supreme Being and have a conscience with a transcendental nature that enables the individual to behave in a responsible manner and living a responsible life in freedom and with responsibility.

Although the unity between the psycho-emotional dimension and the bio-physical dimension of being has for years being negated, today it is recognized that when an individual experiences any form of stress, his/her body reacts to it by initiating a chain of events to help the individual to either defend himself or to beat a hasty retreat. Because stresses cannot all together be dispelled from life, this "fight or flight" reaction is nature's way of challenging the body of a person to escape immediate danger. But, when chronic stress kicks in, the immune system of the individual is impaired, making him/her more susceptible to infectious/communicable diseases because fewer active CD8-and CD4-cells become available to help to destroy bacteria, viruses and cancerous cells. Anger and stress raises the blood pressure leading to heart-diseases; chronic skin diseases occur because of the release of corticotrophin-releasing-hormone; and wound healing is slowed down because of significantly lower levels of interleukin-1 and interleukin-8. Increased levels of glucocorticoids (the stress hormone) inhibits the functioning of neurons in the brain cortex and hippocampus resulting in slower thinking, trouble in handling of complex tasks, a racing mind or apathy, and memory failure.

To promote the psycho-emotional health of all human beings physically, a well balanced diet must be eaten as describe in *Promoting and protecting the well-being of the bio-physical and the behaviour (lifestyle) dimensions of health.* Other physical aspects of importance are exercising; avoidance of substance abuse (alcohol, illegal drugs, and addiction [especially prescribed and over-the-counter medication]); regular screening of own bio-physical health and vaccination against diseases; using family planning to prevent unwanted pregnancies or to do child spacing; avoiding unnecessary trauma by living a responsible life within a healthy physical environment and by taking responsibility for own sexual behaviour.

To further promote the psycho-emotional health of all human beings, the individual must be helped to develop and unfold his/her own Self in his/her own living world as to enrich his/her own personality through all the relationships he/she helps to shape. To enhance an individual's positive attitude to life, health and death, the individual must not only relate to his/her Creator but also to his fellow-men, lives and behaves in a responsible manner, learns the necessary role functions and acts accordingly, develops and implements life goals, becomes a productive citizen, maintains family relationships, and formulates a own philosophy of life. And because an individual never acts in one dimension only, all human beings never exist for the sake of existing, but live aspiring to a fulfilling life as their existence is the answer to their task of becoming whom they can become, should become, and must become because they lives a norm-controlled life.

To maintain the well-being of the psycho-emotional health of all human beings, the individual must be helped to feel good about himself/herself as the ability to love and be loved gives a person's life a sense of purpose and deep fulfillment. A person can bolster his/her own self-worth or self-esteem by keeping his/her body healthy to look great; by taking time out for himself/herself, by taking and maintaining control of his/her own life; by developing a life attitude of seeing molehills rather than mountains; by playing hide and seek through side stepping the things that cause stress and seeking activities, such as hobbies, to provide a refuge from stress. Gardening especially offers a connection with nature and focuses attention on other living things. Stresses of life can also be handled by guarding one's brain health and recharging one's memory; by managing one's moods; by keeping a journal; by getting a massage and learning to relax; by getting organized and de-cluttering one's world; and by laughing a little the feel-good brain chemicals, endorphins, are released. Leaning on other people for social support is sometimes necessary as family and friends (both human and furry) afford powerful protection against stressed-related diseases. There is also no shame in getting help from professional practitioners when experiencing more stress that one can handle – it shows strength of character when taking control of the situation by getting the help that is needed.

➤ *Promoting and maintaining the well-being of the socio-cultural-spiritual dimension of health*
All human beings live in a socio-cultural world, living a value orientated life according to the ethos of their specific culture. Because culture defines the specific word-view in which a person's way of life is rooted, a person's view of health/disease/disability/death and his/her role behaviour regarding being healthy/ill/disabled/dying, is prescribed by the cultural values and norms that are laid down by the culture of the community he/she lives in. Thus, every culture has both direct and indirect influence/affects on the health of individuals, families and communities. The direct affects stem from the specific culturally prescribed practices and behaviour related to health and disease, lifestyle, life-events and interpersonal relationships. Therefore, all positive prescribed practices that promote health, prevent disease, and restore health when disease or disability had occurred as well as dietary practices that contribute to a positive nutritional status and health status of all members, must be promoted. The indirect effects of culture result from cultural definitions of health and disease and disease causation, acceptability of healthcare programmes and compliance with health or disease regimes. Because the cultural definition of health and disease determines the kind of health problems that is considered worthy of attention and the kind of conditions that are to be disregarded, and because beliefs regarding the causation of diseases determine whether traditional healthcare providers must be consulted or whether both professional and traditional healthcare providers can be consulted, all negative views of health/disease/disability/dying as well as negative prescribed beliefs regarding health/disease/disability/dying need to be changed. Recommendations of healthcare providers must also not be too far removed from the normal cultural practices in a given situation as the host/ healthcare user will be unlikely to comply with these recommendations.

As the self-esteem of all persons develops in relation to other human beings, all human beings are in origin inseparably concerned with their fellow-men, yearning for a community in whom they find alliances, fellow sufferers and fellow-assistants, as no person stands alone in life. Social relationships with family and friends confirm human connectedness while promoting the well-being/health of all humans. By staying connected, persons who are socially connected, live longer and stay healthier than those who are socially and emotionally isolated. By making fellow-men a priority, an individual can maintain and strengthen established friendships and make new ones through initiating casual interactions; by reawakening dormant relationships; by not forgetting to write or phone or visit or use social internetting; through leaving home to venture into the unfamiliar by travelling, by joining different clubs, by taking different classes, by doing voluntary work or by attending religious services and by doing many more activities. Through engaging one's heart, mind and soul, a person can stay young at heart and say yes to life. By being actively involved in different culturally and educational activities that the community offers, a person becomes a lifelong learner while expanding his/her horizons. By embracing one's belief in a Supreme Being, an individual can deal better with life difficulties and enhances his/her health – bodily, emotionally, socially and spiritually - positively affecting the course of disease. And by caring for a furry or feathery friend, a person can have fun, feel adored and have someone to talk to – thereby staying in love with life. By finding satisfaction and pride in work-related accomplishments, a person's role in life and sense of Self are reinforced through the humans the individual meets and the work he/she does/had done.

3.1.1.2 Promoting and protecting the well-being of the family

The family is the oldest and the most enduring of all social institutions. Consequently, the individual is never a man or woman alone on an island because the individual's family always forms part of the host system. Therefore, the health of the family must be protected, maintained, and restored for the continual procreation and socialization of the next generation as well as for the continuation of all cultures of society. Regardless of the form and living arrangements of the family as a social system/ institution, every family has its own cultural values, specific functions, structure, and recognizable developmental stages – elements that have to be protected and nurtured as to protect and to maintain the health not only of the individual members of the family but also of the family as unit. Because the family as unit also serves the growth and health of the community and society, this mutual interdependence of individual, family, and community must be maintained and protected because what happens to an individual member affects the family as well as the community, and vice versa.

Seen in the light of the above, and because of the fact that families are an intergenerational social system with kin networks consisting of three to four generations, the health of all individual family members (infants, children, adolescents, adults [young and middle-aged], and the elderly) must be protected and maintained, as has already been described in Section 3.1.1.1. The family unit's different dimensions of health (biological, psychological, socio-cultural, and lifestyle) also need to be protected and maintained by helping families to take responsibility for their own health and well-being, and for the health and well-being of individual family members as well as for the health and well-being of their communities by living healthy lives.

Regarding the biological health of the family attention must be given to healthcare practices that protect, maintain, and restore the health of individual family members and the family as unit, such as housing; clothing; the provision of food; maintaining a healthy environment; and looking after the health of domestic, exotic, and farming animals, birds, or reptiles. The psychological health of the family can be maintained and restored through crisis interventions while simultaneously strengthening the family's existing healthy emotional strengths by reinforcing coping strategies; communication patterns; marital and family relationships and dynamics; and lifestyle regarding child-rearing practices and discipline. The socio-cultural health of the family must be promoted through the strengthening of the structures and functions of the family; the cultural and religious values and norms of the family; the affined and affiliated relationships of the family; the formal and informal role enactment within the family; and the family's interaction with the greater community.

3.1.1.3   Promoting the well-being of the community

As the individual host and his/her family are members of a particular community, and because the possibility always exists that the community as an entire system or specific members within that community can become ill, the wellbeing of the community (as a system) should also be promoted. Furthermore, the health of the individual, his/her family, and the community is influenced not only by the behaviours of individual members of the community but also by factors in the physical-biological, socio-cultural, psychological, economic, and other environments or milieus in which the community lives. It therefore becomes of the utmost importance that all negative and harmful factors in the community to be identified in order that they can be corrected because, when the balance between host, agent, and environment is disturbed, that imbalance becomes a contributing factor in the causation of outbreaks and spread of communicable diseases. In addition, healthcare providers must be well informed concerning communities' cultural customs regarding birth; becoming ill or disabled; dying/death; life-events; traditional healthcare practices and folk diseases; different lifestyles; dietary practices; beliefs, perceptions, behaviours and attitudes; and interpersonal relationships. Healthcare providers thus need to know and be alert to how these customs and practices can cause and/or promote and/or prevent the outbreak and spread of communicable diseases. Consequently, all healthcare practitioners have to alter the behaviour and attitudes of all communities regarding health (if these pose a threat) by means of health information.

At the primary level of prevention, interventions promoting the well-being of the community pertain to the following aspects of health
- enhancing the biophysical dimension of the health of individual community members to protect, to maintain, and restore health
- enhancing the psychological dimension of the health of individual community members and their families as well as the community's ability to function effectively and resolve identified health problems. Attention must also be given to strengthening the relationship between subgroups within the community as to create a psychological climate conducive to concerted community actions as well as to ensure the adequacy of the protective services provided by the law enforcement and emergency services to create feelings of personal safety and security
- enhancing the social dimension of health in the community by strengthening the commitment of government and other authorities as well as power

and authority structures in the community as to implement the necessary programmes designed not only to solve community health problems but also to maintain healthy lifestyles within socio-cultural, community, and familial contexts

- strengthening the arts and culture of the community as arts and culture form an integral part of the spiritual, material, intellectual, and emotional aspects of human society and are fundamental to all learning.

Based on the fact that the loss of resources leads to resource depletion which is always more powerful and more potent than the generation of resources and initial loss begets future loss, any situation that may lead to the possibility of loss, must be identified (before or as soon as it occurred) and the necessary measures be put in place as to protect and maintain the health of the community.

◈ Whenever new communities are established or existing communities are changed or relocated, healthcare providers must preserve and reinforce the value systems and cultural life-styles of the community as far as possible. Possible risks regarding all hosts (individuals, families, communities, whether healthy, ill, contact, or carrier) and the environment must be identified, and interventions planned accordingly

◈ Civil and guerrilla wars as well as natural disasters (for example, tsunamis, earthquakes, torrential rains leading to floods and mud slides) and cyclones/hurricanes/typhoons lead to the displacement of thousands of people from their natural homes and environment and their placement in refugee camps or shelters. Due to the stresses the displaced persons experience, their physiological resistance is not only impaired, but being crowded together in circumstances like poor environmental hygienic conditions, the rapid spread of communicable diseases is facilitated. A range of relief plans needs to be in place (for example, food, health, environment) and implemented over a long period of time on a very large scale to protect and maintain the health of these persons-in-need. Through cultural-based performing arts (dancing, singing, poetry, painting, cultural play by children, acting and performing of plays and operas, etc.), the psychological health of the stressed persons can be maintained

◈ Migration - an increase of migration (particularly of illegal migrants) can be a reason for the spread of communicable diseases (for example, tuberculosis) between regions. Poverty in a country also enhances illegal migration to more affluent countries, spreading communicable diseases across borders and regions. The necessary healthcare plans must be in place to prevent and control the spread of diseases as well as to treat sick illegal immigrants. Cross-border healthcare plans and co-operation between countries and regions must be promoted

◈ Poverty and unemployment may limit the ability of an individual to seek prompt medical care when disease occurs, resulting in more serious consequences of infection or disease. Families may not take their ill members for prompt medical care when necessary, or be ignorant of the advantages of vaccination for their children. Language barriers and lower educational levels under impoverished families and communities may prevent individuals, families, and communities not to use the healthcare services provided. Consequently, the general health of individuals, families, and communities is at risk, because they are impoverished. This makes such individuals, families, and communities more susceptible to communicable infections.

3.1.2 Promoting and maintaining a healthy environment

All healthcare providers must cooperate closely with team members and health authorities who are in control of the environmental health, as well as the other authorities - for example, agriculture, labour - that safeguard the health of individuals, families, and communities. The provision of a healthy physical and biological environment involves consideration of all the environmental factors and hazards that affect the health of humans. This is why attention must be given to factors such as housing, sanitation, garbage disposal, pest control, the consumption of safe water and food, the prevention of contamination and pollution of water and air. The beautification of the environment is of equal importance as it enhances the psychological health of man. Special attention must also be given to the ecology of the agricultural, animal husbandry and aquatic (fishery) food supplies as to ensure the sustainability of the global food supply chain because nutritional insults (malnutrition and hidden hunger [micro-nutrient deficiencies]) have a negative effect on all human beings, especially infants and children, with effects that can last through generations. Therefore, whenever the different environments pose any threat to the wellbeing of man, healthcare providers must bring it to the attention of the authorities.

Maintaining a healthy physical environment must also include all veterinary strategies to prevent zoonotic diseases by complying with the vaccination programmes for domestic and farming animals, including both small and large wild game. Healthcare providers must encourage individuals, families, and communities to protect their domestic animals; and should also ensure that all legislative requirements are met regarding animals, birds, reptiles as well as all animal, avian, and reptilian products (import, export, product manufacture, storage, and sales). Healthcare providers must also give health information to individuals, families, and communities about zoonotic diseases, its signs and symptoms, the identification of sick animals, and the immediate treatment of affected animals, birds, or reptiles and how to care for sick animals. Information should also be provided about the climatic and seasonal factors that are likely to bring humans into contact with sick animals. When keeping exotic animals or farming with small or big wild game, animal lovers must inform the healthcare providers about these practices as the diseases of these animals are not well known, and these animals may be the source of infection for zoonotic diseases.

Individuals, families, and communities also need to live in healthy socio-cultural and all other milieus or environments like the psychological, economical, legislative, religious, political, educational, labour, and recreational environments. These must also be promoted and maintained. Each of these different milieus has its own specific dimensions of importance that need to be promoted and maintained so as to prevent any negative impediment to the health of individuals, families and communities. Communities must also be empowered to gain resources or to prevent their loss or/ and to invest in other resources through mobilizing the available resources or add resources from outside the system as to create a balance in resources in order to offset loss and insure gain.

3.1.3 Establishing a comprehensive healthcare system for service delivery

The health of individuals, families, and communities is influenced by the way in which healthcare services are organized, and by their accessibility, affordability, appropriateness, adequacy, availability, and usage. Consequently, healthcare systems vary widely in performance and differ equally widely in their ability to attain key health goals. To promote the well-being of individuals, families, and communities, all health care systems must consist of the following major components

1. The production of human and physical resources for services delivery
2. The creation of programmes using these resources to deliver healthcare at primary, secondary, and tertiary level according to eight different programmes that include, among others, the following
   ✠ maintaining a healthy environment that includes, inter alia, agricultural, animal husbandry and aquatic practices for food production, safe water provision, safe waste and sanitation practices
   ✠ prevention and control of communicable diseases (including vaccination)
   ✠ health information to promote, to maintain, and to restore health
   ✠ community-orientated healthcare providers (professional and traditional). The healthcare manpower (healthcare practitioners like physicians and nurses, as well as traditional practitioners like sangomas, traditional birth attendants, and herbalists and lay care givers) must be competent to provide the necessary healthcare
   ✠ statistical information - health statistics such as mortality rates, morbidity rates, and fertility rates, together with population statistics such as gender, educational, income, and age distributions, etc.
   ✠ legislation to support the above – health, social welfare, labour, environmental, agricultural and animal health, economic, etc. Since legislation for social welfare and health well-being are of utmost importance in the prevention of communicable diseases, healthcare providers must not only be well-informed about existing legislation, but must also draw the attention of legislators to those deficiencies in the existing legislation that are threatening the welfare of individuals, families, and communities
3. Economic support to finance the procurement of healthcare resources and the provision of services by both the free market healthcare services as well as by the public healthcare services (national, regional, and district health departments).
4. Management methods to achieve the best services in the different organized programmes, for example, government agencies such as the National

Department of Health or the Provincial Departments of Health, non-governmental organizations (NGOs), and the private healthcare sector. Other governmental agencies also carry certain health responsibilities, such as social security programmes vested in the Ministry of Social Welfare, occupational health and safety programs vested in the Ministry of Labour, health informational programmes vested in the Ministry of Health, the education of healthcare practitioners vested in the Ministry of Education, food production programmes in the Ministry of Agriculture, and so forth. Of smaller proportions are the healthcare activities of non-governmental bodies, such as business enterprises that operate healthcare programmes for their employees. Religious bodies, social organisations, and philanthropic foundations may also run healthcare activities or support healthcare programmes. Service delivery must be integrated so that healthcare users can be referred to or transferred between different service points, depending on the type of service delivery needed to render holistic, comprehensive, and culturally-congruent health care to healthcare users and their family

5. The delivery of diverse services such as hospitals, clinics, private practices, and long-term care units to healthy and unwell individuals by both the public and the private sector.

Both the Allopathic medical sub-system as well as the Traditional healthcare sub-system must protect the physical, mental and spiritual health, maintain the physical, mental and spiritual health and restore the physical, mental and spiritual health of individuals, families and communities as to prevent and control outbreaks of communicable diseases. Furthermore, by providing comprehensive, holistic and culturally congruent healthcare an awareness of and sensitivity to individuals or/and families or/and communities (whether healthy, ill, contact, carrier) socio-cultural background and health traditions are mandated. Also, when rendering culturally congruent heath care to all individuals or/and families or/and communities (whether healthy, ill, contact, carrier) the healthcare brokering process must be adapted to effectively assess an individual's or/and family's or/and community's (whether healthy, ill, contact, carrier) health and sickness beliefs and practices and to determine the impact of their cultural, ethnic, or religious values on the scientific proposed plan of care. Health beliefs and health practices must be recognized and respected and where possible be integrated into the proposed health care interventions to be rendered.

3.2   HEALTHCARE INTERVENTIONS AT THE SECONDARY LEVEL OF PREVENTION

Interventions at the secondary level of prevention (during the stage of pathogenesis) are directed at

❑ the early detection of communicable diseases/infections as well as the diagnosing and treatment of the ill individual

❑ interrupting the transmission of infection from source to susceptible host (breaking the chain of infection); and

❏ eliminating and correcting the negative factors in the physical-biological environment and socio-cultural milieu so as to prevent the spread of communicable diseases
❏ instituting the necessary legislative regulations and enforcing it when necessarily.
In order to detect and diagnose communicable diseases and to do the necessary case finding, healthcare providers (professional practitioners and traditional providers) must have the appropriate knowledge of communicable diseases. Healthcare practitioners must also be able to implement the epidemiological process in order to break the links of interrelatedness in the epidemiological host-pathogen-environment triad, and the healthcare therapy (as grounded in the healthcare brokering process) has to be carried out in such a way that the physiological resistance of the body of ill and contact persons is enhanced. The necessary legislative regulations must also be put in place and enforced when necessarily.

According to the Epidemiological Triad of Communicable Diseases model, all health care interventions at the secondary level of prevention pertain to
✠ the healthcare rendering to all hosts (ill individuals, contacts, carriers and potential hosts) within their familial and community context
✠ the control and prevention of the spread of the specific pathogen (infectious agent) by interrupting the transmission of infection from source to susceptible host
✠ the elimination or rectifying of risks or hazards in the environment (physical-biological, psychological, socio-cultural and other milieus of importance)
✠ instituting all necessary legislative measures.
The roles of the different health care team members are complementary to one another in healthcare rendering to ill hosts (including the healthy, contact, carrier hosts) and their families; in the reconstruction and the maintaining of a healthy environment, and in the prevention of the spread of the particular communicable disease.

3.2.1 Caring for the ill, carrier and contact hosts within familial and community context

To be unhealthy, or to be ill, or to be disabled, or to be dying constitutes a life crisis – the not-healthy, ill/sick, disabled, dying individual is an individual-in-crisis (whether infant, child, adolescent, adult or elder) confronted with a crisis situation compelling him/her to change his/her relationships and dialogues. Thus, the healthcare user enters the healthcare situation as a human being and as a person-in-crisis - not as a health problem, or a disease/infection, or a disability, or a deceased body, but as a human being whose personhood or Self/"I" has been changed by health problems, or disease, or disability, or dying and who is reaching out to the healthcare provider for help. Therefore, the healthcare user and his/her family do not meet the healthcare provider(s) as physical bodies, but as healthy, ill, disabled, or dying human beings who must give meaning to health, disease, disability, or death from within the boundaries of their own possibilities in answering the choice of self-actualization by living meaningful lives or by capitulating to life.

Although the medical sciences have advanced through the years, infectious/ communicable diseases still continue to emerge or re-emerge, and, as such, remains the top killer, causing the greatest number of deaths in the world – in developed, developing, and under-developed countries. To suffer from a communicable disease or to become a contact or to be a carrier constitutes a life crisis for the individual (regardless of whether he/she is an ill, disabled, or dying infant, child, adolescent, adult, or elder) through which he/she has to confront his/her own mortality. As the meaning of the "Self" of a person is integrated with the meaning of health and disease (including disability and death), all individuals, families, and communities conceptualize health and disease in different ways, giving meaning to health, disease, disability, and death in their own unique ways. As unique human beings, all healthy, ill, disabled, or dying persons and their families give a uniquely specific meaning to all their life experiences, and constitute their own world in order to create their own safe place in which to live a meaningful life. Hence, their need is to be understood and cared for according to the unique dialogues and uniquely constituted world of the healthy, ill, disabled, or dying individual and his/her family.

3.2.1.1 Healthcare rendering to the ill individual at home or in hospital

The aim of healthcare rendering to all ill individuals (infants, toddlers, children, adolescents, adults, and elders) suffering from communicable diseases is to enhance the defense mechanisms of the body of the ill individual, prevent complications, and rehabilitate the convalescent individual or if the ill person dies, help the bereaved family to adjust to individual, family, and community life. All ill individuals must be cared for as a member of a family and a community, whether he/she is cared for at home or in hospital. All healthcare rendering interventions must be compassionate, comprehensive (promotive, preventive, curative, rehabilitative), holistic (need-orientated within family and community context), and culturally congruent in nature to maintain, protect, and restore health. (A full description of the fundamental and specific healthcare interventions to be rendered to the ill individual within his/her familial and community context is given in chapter 8 and Theme IV).

3.2.1.2 Tracing of contacts and placing them under quarantine

As soon as a particular communicable disease has been diagnosed, the contacts of the ill person must be traced and informed that they have been exposed to the particular communicable disease (infectious agent), that they must undergo certain test(s), and if necessary, submit to the appropriate treatment. Depending on the health status of the contacts (healthy, immune, or susceptible contacts), they will be
- kept under observation or
- kept under observation and receive prophylactic medication or
- kept under observation and be placed under quarantine.

Healthcare providers must instruct all contacts (even healthy ones) to report for treatment as soon as they begin to feel ill. Providers must also ensure that the required diagnostic tests are carried out, for instance, obtaining sputum specimens for testing for tuberculosis. When individuals, families, and communities or a part of a community need to be placed under quarantine, for example, when an outbreak of Plague occurs, it is up to all healthcare practitioners and traditional healthcare providers to prevent chaos by explaining to those involved, the reasons for the quarantine measures put in place, the specific healthcare measures required to treat the particular disease and the legislative measures applicable to prevent the disease from spreading. This strategy must also be followed when families or communities who are regarded as contacts, are immediately put on a prophylactic treatment programme.

Whenever contacts are subjected to a prophylactic treatment programme such as re-vaccination or the administration of medication/chemotherapy (anti-microbial or anti-viral drugs), healthcare practitioners have to ensure that all contacts receive the prescribed treatment. Healthcare practitioners must conduct the necessary observations and interpretations of all vaccination programmes, for example, the administering of polio vaccine, and provide support to the individual and his/her family and, where necessary, to the community. In tracing and treating contacts, healthcare practitioners must cooperate with employers by informing them about the particular communicable disease and encouraging them to retain the individual in his/her post. Employers must be encouraged to be actively involved in the prophylactic and therapeutic treatment programmes of their employees. The same strategy is also applicable to school children. Parents (biological or foster), legal guardians, and single mothers/fathers must also be encouraged to be actively involved in the prophylactic and therapeutic treatment programmes for their pre-school and school-going children.

Regarding healthcare providers and supportive workers as contacts, the following are applicable, namely,
- ◈ when healthcare providers and supportive workers become contacts themselves, the above applies to them also
- ◈ healthcare providers and support workers should undergo regular health checks, and know their post-vaccination status when employment vaccination(s) is/are offered before carrying out exposure-prone procedures
- ◈ all healthcare establishments must have policies in place for blood-borne viruses and other microbes in the management of healthcare employees (line-, support-, and staff functionaries) and other individuals when they become contacts.

3.2.1.3 Tracing of and commencement of treatment for carriers

Communicable infections can be introduced into families and communities by healthy carriers as well as by a convalescent, chronic, or transient carrier. Despite the fact that carriers are compelled legally to undergo treatment, to comply with hygienic measures, and to report to local/district healthcare authorities, these regulations are often ignored. For this reason, while implementing the epidemiological process, healthcare practitioners must visit all identified carriers and investigate possible carriers by having tests done on all who have been sick and have recovered but may still shed the specific pathogen. When a carrier is the source of the infection, the practitioner must point out the legal requirements to the individual and, when necessary, refer him/her for further treatment. He/she must also be instructed about his/her contribution to the prevention of the particular communicable disease, for instance, with regard to personal hygiene and/or a change of occupation. Parents are responsible to abide by these regulations when their children are carriers. Healthcare providers themselves must be tested on a yearly basis to detect whether they are healthy carriers and whether they have spread communicable diseases to their families and their communities.

3.2.1.4   Introduction of prophylactic measures

To prevent communicable disease from spreading, it is sometimes necessary to introduce prophylactic treatment, such as the administering of antimicrobial treatment, to all healthy and ill persons (including contacts and carriers), to ill healthcare users and healthcare employees (line-, support-, and staff functionaries) in hospitals, to members of families, and to the members of communities. Further, healthcare providers must always bear in mind that

- ✠ whenever mutation of the pathogen takes place, the body is no longer able to recognise the new strain of the specific pathogen and activation of the memory cells can no longer take place. Consequently, the healthy person becomes ill
- ✠ whenever the antigenic virulence of the specific pathogen changes, the human body is not always able to withstand the infection, despite the physiological resistance that has been built up. The person thus becomes ill
- ✠ drug-resistance (mono-drug-resistance, multi-drug-resistance, extreme drug-resistance [XDR], or completely/totally drug-resistance [CDR/TDR]) shown by many pathogens to chemotherapeutic interventions resulted in a situation where communicable diseases are not always treated successfully or cannot be treated at all (completely/totally drug-resistance). The abuse and over-use of vaccination and antimicrobial drug interventions also lead to the mutation of infective microbes and the development of new strains of a specific pathogen (most of the time, these are more virulent)
- ✠ certain pathogens elicit no immune response with memory at all, and the person becomes ill with every exposure.

3.2.2   Interrupting the transmission of infection from source to susceptible hosts

To break the chain of infection, the specific infectious pathogen must be eliminated through antimicrobial drug therapy. Thus, healthcare practitioners must have a thorough knowledge of the specific causative infectious agents with reference to

- the properties of micro- and macro-microbes
- modes of transmission of different pathogens
- portals of entry and exit, and spread within the body
- intermediaries - vectors and vehicles
- reservoirs and sources of infectious pathogens
- clinical manifestations of the different communicable diseases
- diagnostic tests and investigations to be done

- different methods to eliminate infectious agents (drug therapy, sterilization, and disinfection).

To confirm the diagnosis of a particular communicable disease, the necessary specimens have to be collected for laboratory investigation. Of utmost importance is the safe-keeping of the specimens and the protection of all healthcare providers and laboratory staff against the infection. Meaningful interpretation of laboratory reports has to be made in order to accordingly adapt the fundamental healthcare and specific healthcare that need to be rendered to the ill person, to his/her family, and to the community.

Attention must also be given to the structural and human elements in the chain of infection. Regarding the human element, all factors that promote or inhibit the spread of the infectious agent (such as crowding of potential hosts) must be identified. For example, if the mode of transmission is airborne via infected droplets, the crowding of potential hosts must be prevented. Therefore, it is recommended to insist on the closing of schools and the prohibition of certain recreational activities and meetings. In hospitals, the care behaviour (preventing and controlling the spread of the particular communicable disease) of healthcare providers must be facilitated through strict compliance with/adherence to all Standard/Universal precautions, bacteriological effective hand-washing and precautionary isolation measures. Healthcare providers must also take the necessary precautions to prevent themselves from becoming a source infection, for example, providers must enhance their own wellbeing, prevent themselves from getting infected and becoming ill or becoming a healthy carrier, or becoming a vehicle in the spread of the particular communicable disease. Careful attention must be given to hand hygiene, both before and after contact with the ill person, by using gloves, gown, mask, face shield, plastic apron, and eye protection within one metre of the ill person. Airborne precautions must be adhered to by placing the ill person in an airborne isolated room, ensuring the ill person wears a particulate mask when transported or moved, and adhering stringently to respiratory hygiene and cough etiquette. In laboratories, virus-isolation studies and biological-isolation studies for blood-borne and airborne pathogens in respiratory specimens must be conducted under the most stringent protection. **Strict adherence to Standard Precautions (including cough etiquette) by all healthcare providers is a must.** As such, Standard Precautions apply to blood, all body fluids, secretions and excretions (regardless of whether or not they contain blood), non-intact skin, and mucous membranes. Although Standard Precautions are appropriate to be used with all ill healthcare users, regardless of their diagnosis, as to protect both healthcare providers and ill healthcare users by reducing the risk of transmission of communicable diseases (diagnosed and non-diagnosed), Standard Precautions are effective only if implemented and used regularly. When the ill person is cared for at home, healthcare practitioners must give information to the caregiver about adhering to hand-washing protocols, food hygiene and general hygienic measures.

Other aspects under the human element of the chain of infection include that healthcare practitioners must ensure that all ill individuals (including contacts and carriers) take the prescribed antimicrobial or antiviral drugs. Practitioners must thus be knowledgeable about the therapeutic action of chemotherapeutic drugs in order to observe their effectiveness, and to identify allergic and/or toxic signs and symptoms. Practitioners must also understand how chemotherapeutic drugs modify the signs and symptoms and the natural course of the disease. The task of delousing of individuals and the extermination of vectors such as mosquitoes, flies, and rodents are not the healthcare providers' responsibility but the responsibility of environmental health officers. Nevertheless, healthcare providers, however, must provide guidance in this respect. The cyclic recurrence of certain diseases must also be borne in mind in order to locate the reservoirs/sources of infection as soon as possible and to keep high-risk population groups under observation. All healthcare practitioners and lay care healthcare workers as well as all administrative staff in healthcare institutions must undergo in-service education regarding the transmission, prevention and control of communicable diseases as well as the importance of strict adherence to policies and control measures.

Regarding the structural element in the chain of infection, attention must be given to the structure of the healthcare establishment where ill individuals are cared for and the equipment used as these play a role in the spread of communicable diseases. The airborne dissemination of pathogens occurs via the ventilation systems and air flow in healthcare institutions as well as by the carrying of microbes on/in the body of the staff (for example, on hands, in noses, on rings and other jewellery) and their clothing into the rooms of ill healthcare users suffering from non-communicable diseases must be prevented. Consequently, ventilation systems in healthcare institutions must be properly installed and maintained to prevent the ingress of contaminated air and to minimize air currents carrying microbes to other ill healthcare users. The effective isolation of ill healthcare users (both protective isolation and source isolation) not only reduces the airborne transmission of microbes via other routes by limiting access to the infectious patient. By facilitating aseptic practices and adhering strictly to Standard Precautions by healthcare practitioners and other healthcare providers as well as reminding staff of the importance of minimised contact in the spread of infection (by wearing the necessary protective clothing and masks), further reduction of transmission can be accomplished. All structural interventions must be backed-up by administrative controls in the form of the necessary policies, infection control plans, protocols and committees, and occupational health monitoring plans.

Housekeeping and sanitation practices must be strictly observed to reduce environmental reservoirs of pathogens, especially in high-risk areas in hospitals like nurseries, intensive care units, and operating rooms. Linen should be handled properly and waste should be disposed off according to law. However, the architectural design of taps, soap dispensers, and other washing facilities can influence human behaviour only to a limited degree. Education and regular reinforcement of the appropriate behaviour by healthcare practitioners and other providers is therefore essential. The exclusion of inanimate sources of infection can also be achieved by the provision of sterile instruments, sterile medicaments, clean linen, and uncontaminated food. However, it is more difficult to exclude inanimate objects contaminated by humans. Nonetheless, all precautionary measures must be in place, and adhered to, by practitioners and lay persons.

3.2.3 Modifying/reducing of risk factors in the environment

Healthcare practitioners and all other providers have to maintain the physical-biological, socio-cultural, economic, and other important environments when promoting the health/wellbeing of the individual, the family, and the community. The physical-biological environment is maintained in collaboration with environmental health officers and officers of other Departments by attending to factors such as housing, ecological disturbances (contamination of water, air, and food), water, milk and food hygiene, sanitation, garbage disposal, and pest control, for example. All healthcare interventions must modify or eliminate environmental hazards and risks as to reduce the potential of impairment of health and the exposure to infectious agents. Existing health problems (such as communicable diseases) caused by environmental conditions have to be resolved. Environmental conditions that also need attention, for example, are

- tourism and modern transport systems that can spread diseases easily and quickly from one continent to another or from one region to another or from one person to another person or group of persons. An example of this phenomenon is an outbreak of pneumonic plague in Asia that is carried to Africa by persons who were exposed and then travel by air
- importation of goods between countries can cause vectors to be spread from one region to another; for instance, the import of retreaded tyres to South Africa brought the mosquito, the vector for yellow fever, into the country
- droughts followed by high rainfall in areas where malaria has a high incidence, cause a proliferation of all mosquito populations (including the vector for malaria). The normal preventive and control measures may become insufficient with the result that the incidence rate of malaria increases drastically
- the exploration of unknown/uninhabitable regions and tourism to these areas such as the tropical forests of Africa and South America, exposes people to unknown pathogenic microbes, for example, the Ebola virus (a virus of unknown origin). When infected persons from these areas come into contact with other humans, epidemics develop rapidly.

Because of the fact that all risk factors in the social and other environments wherein individuals, families, and communities live, are of such magnitude and are so multi-faceted, it will not be fully describe. Of importance however is that attention must be given to all risk factors in the different environments where healthy, ill, disabled, or dying individuals, their families, and their communities live, and to reduce or modify them when they negatively impede on the health of individuals, families, and communities. Furthermore, when planning and implementing these interventions, attention must be given to any resistance shown by individuals, families, and communities to the modification or rectification of environmental conditions.

In addition to these interventions, attention must also be given to the care environment in which the ill person and his/her family and community are placed. The care environment encompasses all age groups, and includes healthcare interventions for the prevention of communicable diseases in the home and in the clinic environment;

disease management in the home or in the hospital environment; rehabilitation of the convalescent individual and his/her re-integration into the home and community environment; and adjustment to life by individuals, families, and communities after the ill individual has died of the particular communicable disease he/she was suffering from. The interventions applicable to the prevention of communicable diseases in individuals, families, and communities have been fully described in section 3.1.1 as well as the measures to be taken to maintain a healthy environment. As the services delivered in primary healthcare clinics also includes the care rendering for minor medical conditions, healthcare practitioners must always be mindful that many individuals and families when becoming ill, seek help at the primary healthcare clinic - the first point of entry into the allopathic or professional healthcare system. As these individuals are already ill (see chapter 7 about the stages of pathogenesis – pre-clinical or prodromal or clinical), these ill individuals become or are already the source of infection in the chain of infection in the clinic environment. Therefore

♦ all healthcare practitioners and all workers in the clinic must strictly adhere to all Standard Precautionary Measures as well as to all measures pertaining to a healthy medical institutional environment, especially regarding the handling of general and medical waste, abiding to housekeeping rules and practices, and the handling and washing of clinic laundry

♦ as the airborne transmission of pathogens to both healthy and ill healthcare users attending the clinic, as well as to practitioners/workers working in the clinic, poses a huge problem in clinics, the following must be implemented as a component of Standard Precautions

  ✠ placing posters in appropriate languages (including sign language) instructing individuals and accompanying friends and family members to inform healthcare personnel of any symptoms of respiratory infection and fever with/without a rash when booking in as to prevent the initiation or expansion of an epidemic or outbreak in primary healthcare settings that can have far reaching public health consequences

  ✠ posting visual alerts in appropriate languages (including sign language), instructing individuals who present with flu-like symptoms to cover their nose and mouth when coughing or sneezing; to use tissues to contain respiratory secretions and dispose it in the nearest waste receptacle after use; and to wash their hands after having contact with respiratory secretions and contaminated objects/material

  ✠ handing disposable masks to persons who are coughing while waiting

  ✠ ensuring that, when space and chair availability permit it, all coughing persons sit at least one (1) metre away from other persons in common waiting areas

  ✠ providing tissues and no-touch receptacles for used tissue disposal while all used tissues must be incinerated

  ✠ providing conveniently located dispensers of alcohol-based hand rub/ antimicrobial soap and water/antiseptic hand wash and ensure that supplies for hand washing and disposable towels are consistently available in all primary health care clinics

  ✠ ensuring that gloves and masks are worn by all health care professionals/ workers during all healthcare user-contact

✠ ensuring that a complete and thorough history is taken to rule out any possibility of communicable diseases

✠ doing a thorough investigation on all ill healthcare users returning with respiratory complaints or fever with/without a rash within 10 days after the previous appointment and on all staff becoming ill within 10 days of attending to ill healthcare users with respiratory complaints or fever with/without a rash for the possibility of exposure to a communicable disease(s).

The same measures must be instituted in all emergency care units, in all private practices run by both professional and traditional healthcare practitioners as well as in all out-patient departments such as lung clinics and paediatric clinics.

Regarding the management of the particular communicable disease, the ill person can be cared for at home or in hospital, based on the criteria where the ill person must be cared for (see section 8.1.2.1). When the ill person is cared for at home, the physical and emotional home environment becomes important as the caring is done by the family themselves. When the ill person has been admitted to a hospital, the physical, psychological, and socio-cultural hospital environment plays an important part in the caring and recovery or dying processes of the ill individual within his/her familial context. All healthcare renderings in the hospital must not only include the healthcare interventions to care for the individual and his/her family comprehensively, compassionately, holistically, and in a culturally-congruent manner, but also include all measures to create a therapeutic environment in which to render care to the ill person as well as to prevent and control the spread of the particular communicable disease (see sections 8.1.2.2, 8.1.2.3 and 8.1.2.4). When complications set in and the ill person is disabled or is chronically ill for the rest of his/her life, interventions at the tertiary level of prevention must be implemented as described in section 3.3.3. When the ill person dies because of the pathogenesis of the communicable disease suffered from, the family has to be supported to adjust to individual, family, and community life without the deceased family member.

As many medical establishments (hospitals) are low resource facilities (not build to prevent communicable infections transmitted by airborne infected droplets), the following control measures need to be implemented as Standard Precautionary Control Measures as to prevent other hospitalized ill healthcare users and healthcare practitioners as well as other hospital employees contract any communicable disease transmitted by infected droplets

✠ the placement of ill healthcare users must be planned within a nursing unit, with all ill healthcare users suffering from respiratory infections grouped together as far as possible. When the infected person is cared for in a room with other ill healthcare users suffering from any other medical condition, the infected individual must be cared for behind curtains

✠ medical practitioners in both the private and the public sectors must divulge the necessary information about the healthcare user's condition or suspected condition so that the necessary isolation/barrier healthcare arrangements can be made

✠ wearing of particulate masks (N95) by all attending staff and other ill healthcare users. Staff must also wear medical gloves, paper caps (to cover hair) and plastic aprons when working directly with the patient behind curtains. The protective clothing must be discarded prior to leaving the curtained area - the mask, gloves, cap and apron to be discarded in the medical waste container after which the hands have to be washed. When a plastic apron is used, it must be wiped down with a chlorine-based disinfectant solution and hung up

✠ engineering control must be attained and maintained through improved ventilation management. When a separate air conditioner is used for the room, it must be switched on and set to allow fresh air in from outside where possible. When an air conditioner is not available, the windows must be left opened to allow air flow through the room. The infected individual(s) must be nursed next to the window(s) or closest to the air conditioner. The curtains around the infected person's bed must remain drawn to minimise the spread of any infected droplets throughout the room

✠ superior cleaning of the room must be maintained as a mandatory measure

✠ on admission, screening of all ill healthcare users must be done. Lung x-rays must be done and an extensive cough assessment history and a health assessment history must be taken as to identify suspected or confirmed infection with *M. tuberculosis humanis*. A history of haemoptysis, lung x-rays suggestive of pulmonary Tuberculosis (TB) and a history of signs and symptoms suggestive of extra-pulmonary TB must be treated with caution. The ill healthcare user must be physically isolated until an alternative diagnosis has been made or diagnostic tests results indicate that the individual is not infected with TB

✠ health information must be given to all ill healthcare users regarding cough etiquette and sneezing hygiene to prevent the spread of infected droplets by using paper tissues only once when coughing; to safely dispose of all used tissues by putting it in a plastic bag destined for incineration; by not putting used tissues or handkerchiefs back into a pocket or a handbag; to safely dispose of sputum by spitting in sputum containers and to report any bloody sputum; by not coughing and spitting in public places and to wash/disinfect hands after coughing

✠ medical waste must be correctly disposed off

✠ used linen must be bagged in a colour laundry bag and the staff must be informed not to shake or mishandle the bedding as to dislodge any dried sputum flakes and infectious pathogens into the environment

✠ hand disinfected gel must be available at the patient's bedside

✠ mobile infected healthcare users must be informed to use the bathroom facilities after the other non-infected healthcare users have already used it. The bathroom and toilet windows must be left open to ensure adequate airflow and any bodily spills have to be reported to the staff as to immediately clear it away.

3.2.4   Reforming or correcting factors in the health care system

As health care systems do contribute to health problems, a structural analysis of the healthcare sub-systems and healthcare services delivery must be done to scrutinize for factors enhancing the incidence and spread of communicable diseases. The following factors need attention and must be reformed or corrected where necessary.

Analysis of the allopathic healthcare sub-system

❖ The economics of healthcare delivery – if the cost of healthcare services is too high, the ability of many persons to take advantage of the service offered is limited. This results in persons becoming ill without going for treatment whereby the spread of communicable diseases are enhanced

❖ Availability and accessibility of services delivered – if the number and the correct type of services are not enough and users cannot make use of the services, the incidences of communicable diseases can increase. Tuberculosis is a good example

❖ Service appropriateness – if the service does not provide the appropriate service to cater for the needs of the healthcare user, the user will not use the services delivered

❖ Acceptability of services delivered – if a level of congruence does not exist between services provided and the expectations, values, and beliefs of the target population, users will not make use of the services

❖ Adequacy of services provided – if the quality and range of services do not provide for the needs of the user, the service will not be used by the user

❖ Control of service delivery programmes - when an outbreak of a communicable disease occurs for which a vaccination programme exists, healthcare practitioners must examine the relevant vaccination procedure (storage, transport, reconstitution, and administering), the vaccine itself, and the diagnostic tests/investigations to determine whether persons have been adequately vaccinated. It often happens that a vaccination procedure is carried out incorrectly, that the vaccine is not up to standard, and that diagnostic tests or investigations are interpreted incorrectly. These factors contribute to a very low physiological immunological resistance in the individual or a weak (or absent) immune response being elicited after vaccination. These factors must be corrected and re-vaccination of all population groups at risk or of the entire community must be carried out.

Analysis of the practice of professional health care practitioners

❖ The level and appropriateness of the education of practitioners – when healthcare practitioners are not educated appropriately, they will be unable to detect and diagnose communicable diseases and do the necessary case finding. Healthcare practitioners must be able to implement the epidemiological process in order to break the links of interrelatedness in the Epidemiological Host-Pathogen-Environment Triad, and the healthcare therapy (healthcare brokering process) has to be carried out in such a way that the physiological resistance of the ill person is enhanced

❖ Actions taken by healthcare practitioners – when the actions taken by practitioners are inappropriate, they can actually contribute to the incidence of communicable diseases, for example, the over-usage of anti-microbial drugs contributes to antibiotic-resistant strains of gonorrhea and syphilis

❖ Adherence to all legislative requirements - healthcare practitioners must never lose sight of the legislative aspect of the care programme(s). When notification is required, practitioners must ensure that it is done. Practitioners must also ensure that the school exclusion regulations, as well as any other measures implemented by a District Health Authority or the National/Provincial Department of Health are carried out meticulously. While complying with these legislative requirements, practitioners must provide emotional support to the ill person, his/her family and, if necessary, to the community as a whole.

Analysis of the traditional healthcare sub-system

◈ The concept of health and disease/sickness, and theories of disease causation as well as the "explanatory model" that defines the nature of health, disease, disability, and death; the treatment of disease or disability; and the type of relationships that should be build between the healthcare user and healthcare provider

◈ The categories of traditional practitioners and the health–related services provided

◈ The education, skills, and competencies of traditional healthcare providers

◈ The methods employed by traditional healthcare providers to diagnose diseases (including communicable diseases or infections); the different diagnostic techniques used; and the treatment regimes prescribed for different diseases (including communicable diseases or infections) such as dietary allowances or restrictions and special foods/drinks; herbal and medicinal medicines and preparations to be taken; prayer, and magical interventions to be followed; and other treatments or alternative or complementary modalities to be administered like acupuncture, acupressure, poultices, cupping, and reflexology

◈ The specific ways in which healthcare users make use of traditional healthcare services, for example, whether only traditional healthcare services are rendered by family members, friends or traditional healthcare providers; whether the traditional healthcare provider/folk healthcare practitioner is consulted first before the allopathic/professional healthcare practitioner; or whether the allopathic/ professional healthcare practitioner is consulted first, followed by the traditional healthcare provider/folk healthcare provider

◈ The practices employed by the traditional providers in health and disease or disability at primary, secondary, and tertiary levels of prevention in meeting the specific needs of the healthcare users and the meaning and importance attached by the users to these culturally prescribed health practices. Regarding primary preventive practices (health-promoting and disease-preventing practices), the following are of importance: diet; herbal and other medicinal preparations; the wearing of religious or magical amulets/charms; cleansing or detoxification practices employed; and measures to prevent the transmission of communicable diseases, such as inoculation, isolation, burning of fomites, or washing of contaminated articles and waste disposal methods; as well as the manipulation of the environment to control and prevent the spread of communicable diseases. Curative measures of importance are diet prescriptions, herbal and other treatment prescriptions (including different orientations to medication use), and religious/ magical rituals to be adopted. The role of the extended family members, friends and community organizations in the care rendering process to the disabled person as well as the manipulating of the environment must be explored during the rehabilitation phase

◈ The mixing of traditional healthcare practices and allopathic healthcare practices in the promotion of health and the prevention of disease, the treatment of disease and the rehabilitation or cure of the disabled individual

◈ The potential for adverse interactions between therapies, especially herbal medicine and chemotherapeutic drugs (counteracting one another or potentiating one another, for example, both the herbal and chemotherapeutic drug has antihypertensive effects resulting in severe hypotension), and unhealthful treatment or harmful therapies (the over-use of antibiotics leading to drug resistance)

◈ The existence of a referral system or system of cooperation between traditional healthcare providers and professional healthcare practitioners

◈ The prevailing attitude of the community members and professional healthcare providers towards traditional medicine and traditional healthcare providers

◈ The expectations involved in the healthcare user-professional healthcare provider relationship, the healthcare user-traditional healthcare provider relationship, and the healthcare user-professional healthcare provider-traditional healthcare provider relationship

◈ The degree of individual and group participation in traditional healthcare practices

◈ The degree of acculturation of the individual and the group to the dominant healthcare system, and the degree of familiarity with the language and terminology used by the allopathic healthcare providers.

3.3 HEALTHCARE INTERVENTIONS AT THE TERTIARY LEVEL OF PREVENTION

Healthcare interventions at the tertiary level of prevention (during the resolution stage) are directed at the rehabilitation of the convalescent or recovered individual, and at the prevention of a future outbreak of the same communicable disease. The rehabilitation of the disabled convalescent or recovered individual includes

❑ social security
❑ vocational training or schooling of the disabled person
❑ functioning of the family as a unit
❑ independent functioning of the chronically ill or disabled individual and his/her family in all spheres of life
❑ reconstruction of the home milieu and the community.

Health care interventions at the tertiary level pertain to the rehabilitation of the chronically ill or disabled individual, the maintenance of a healthy environment and the strengthening of the healthcare system for service delivery.

3.3.1 Rehabilitation of the disabled or carrier individual within familial and community contexts

Because the western culture tends to be cure-orientated, healthcare for acute conditions is often valued more than the healthcare for the chronically ill or disabled individual. As not all communicable infections always have a positive outcome, the prevention and control of chronic medical conditions and disability as outcomes of a particular communicable disease constitute a major challenge to all healthcare providers. The basis for the prevention of complications and rehabilitation during the recovery phase of the disease is situated in the comprehensive therapeutic care of the ill individual during the acute phase of the disease. Healthcare providers must thus commence all rehabilitative actions as soon as the disease has been diagnosed. When complications have affected the individual's abilities (whether infant, toddler, child, adolescent, adult, or elder), the provider must support him/her to regain his/her physical, emotional, and social independence and provide support in the process of social integration. By developing the individual's remaining abilities to their highest level, the individual is enabled to live his/her life to the full to an advanced age, and to make the greatest possible contribution to his/her own welfare and social security.

When the ill or contact individual has been removed from his/her family because of the particular communicable disease, the re-integration of the convalescent individual into the family must take place as soon as possible during the recovery period. As the disabled or chronically ill person and his/her family have to deal with great personal and emotional losses, the practitioner must prepare and support the family to receive back the disabled or chronically ill family member. The practitioner must also contribute towards the reconstruction of the family routine, relationships, roles, and ego-boundaries to the extent that all individual members will be able to function at an optimal level and so prevent the dysfunction of the family as a unit. Family members must also be informed about the chronically sick role the disabled family member will fulfil and the adaptations that family members have to make. Of cardinal importance is the introduction of health practices, behaviours and routines that are congruent with the context of the disabled individual's and his/her family's cultural values, beliefs and symbolic meanings.

To help the disabled/chronically ill individual and his/her family to deal with their losses such as self-esteem, loss of status within the family and in the community, loss of independence, feeling of rejection and isolation, feelings of helplessness and the devastating effect of economic deprivation, the participation by the disabled/chronic ill individual and his/her family in community life is essential to their self-actualization. Therefore, the healthcare provider must, when necessary and in collaboration with other healthcare providers, motivate the employer to retain the disabled individual in his/her employment and to utilize him/her in an appropriate job situation where he/she will be able to use his/her remaining skills. Should the disabled or chronically ill person be unable to return to his/her previous occupation, he/she must be assisted in entering either the sheltered or open employment market by undergoing vocational training. The parents of a disabled or chronically ill child must be encouraged to allow him/her to continue his/her education in order to prepare him/her for employment when he/she leaves school. Social isolation of the family and of the disabled person must be prevented. A support network system composed of persons external to the family must be established so as to help the disabled or chronically ill individual and his/her family to carry out their tasks, to give emotional support and to help them to re-integrate into community life.

The purpose of rehabilitation is to develop self-care abilities and skills as to maintain the current condition and preventing further disability while improving of the condition of the disabled person for employment/re-employment or schooling. Since one healthcare provider cannot possibly manage all these rehabilitative tasks on his/her own, the provider has to refer the convalescent or disabled individual and his/her family to the relevant community resources or to a member of the healthcare team who will best be able to assist them. The specific healthcare provider remains responsible, however, for the coordination of the rehabilitative actions, as well as for the motivation and support of the disabled individual and his/her family.

A carriage state is a complication of certain communicable diseases whereby the individual may become a permanent or intermittent carrier. In such cases as this, the healthcare practitioner must assist the individual and his/her family to come to terms with this situation. All adult carriers as well as the parents of child-carriers must be informed about the procedures to be followed to prevent the carrier from spreading the disease. They should also be informed of the legal obligations with which they have to comply in this regard. When the carrier has to change his/her occupation, the practitioner must support him/her and his/her family until they have overcome the crisis and the individual has settled into a new occupation. Regarding the child-carrier, educators must be informed of the carriage state of the child as the school principal must prevent an outbreak of the particular communicable disease in the school.

An important aspect of the rehabilitation process is the reconstruction of the home and community milieus. Reconstruction services are directed at the improvement of the circumstances in the home and community milieus in order to provide a better opportunity for adjustment and recovery rather than having a restraining influence on the disabled person, his/her family, and the community. Reconstruction services are rendered by the healthcare team and are commenced as soon as the disease has been diagnosed. The role of healthcare providers in the reconstruction services comprises the following

- <u>supporting the family of the disabled or chronically ill individual</u>
  Because disease disrupts family life, healthcare providers must assist the members of the family of the disabled or chronically ill person to come to terms with the reality of their situation and/or the disease. The provider must also assist the family in coming to terms with their feelings of guilt, anxiety, hostility, and/or lack of involvement to enable them to accept the situation as well as the disabled or chronically ill family member. Services providing both social and material aid must be utilized
- <u>motivating the family to become actively involved in the process of support</u>
  As recovery remains a possibility, healthcare providers must motivate the family to cooperate and remain actively involved in the treatment of the disabled person. By giving information and clearing up uncertainties, providers help the family to demonstrate understanding and tolerance towards the disabled or chronically ill family member. Because the interest of his/her family is a strong motivational force, the importance of the family maintaining contact with the disabled or chronically ill family member must be strongly emphasized. Healthcare providers must also help the family to establish contact with other groups or families in similar circumstance is so that they realize that their situation and problems are not unique

- <u>re-instating the disabled or chronically ill individual and his/her family in the community</u>
  Because of the particular disease, the disabled or chronically ill individual's relationships and responsibilities in the community had to be temporarily suspended. Healthcare providers must support him/her and his/her family in their attempts to strengthen their social ties and to fulfill their social obligations
- <u>rendering after-care to the disabled or chronically ill individual within familial context</u>
  The services to the family cannot continue indefinitely nor be discontinued abruptly upon completion of the reconstruction services. The support of healthcare providers has to be continued but should be replaced gradually by after-care. Hence, it is the task of the provider to motivate the disabled or chronically ill person or the parents of the disabled or chronically ill child, to take his/her medication and to keep his/her follow-up appointments. The provider must also observe the disabled or chronically ill individual for signs and symptoms that may indicate deterioration of his/her condition so that the necessary interventions can be instituted timely. Because after-care can also not be continued indefinitely, therefore, the disabled or chronically ill person and his/her family must be prepared for its termination while healthcare providers must gradually withdraw their support
- <u>giving health information to the community regarding disability</u>
  It is of the utmost importance that all healthcare providers should disseminate information to the community regarding disability or chronic diseases and the positive contribution that disabled persons can make to the community.

3.3.2 Maintaining healthy environments in the community

Interventions at the tertiary level of prevention regarding the environment pertain to the promotion of a healthy biological and physical environment as already described under section 3.1.2 and the surveillance of the environment after it has been rectified as described under section 3.2.3. Attention must also continuously be given to all other environments in which individuals, families, and communities live as to prevent risks or hazards develop that may lead to conditions that influence their health negatively. Prompt interventions must be taken to correct these conditions before individuals, families, and communities become susceptible to communicable diseases attributable to environmental factors. Vulnerable community members must also be helped to gain the necessary resources they lack as to improve their well-being and health as well as their ability to face everyday challenges.

3.3.3 Strengthening of the healthcare system for service delivery

Both the allopathic and the traditional healthcare sub-systems must attain the key health goals that have been set. To promote the well-being of individuals, families, and communities, all components of both healthcare sub-systems must be strengthened. Among others the following components must receive attention

1. Enough human and physical resources must be available in both the professional and the traditional healthcare sub-systems. The production and procurement of general and medical stock and equipment must benefit both the allopathic and the traditional healthcare sub-systems while the medical stock must include a constellation of physical, natural, herbal and chemical commodities as professional required for treatment

2. Programmes must be organized in such a way that the delivery of healthcare at primary, secondary, and tertiary levels is of the highest quality

   ✠ a healthy environment must be maintained to prevent the environment becoming the source of infection or promote the outbreak of communicable diseases. Attention must especially be given to the physical-biological environment and the socio-cultural milieu to prevent and control communicable diseases

   ✠ service delivery programmes (including vaccination) focusing on the prevention and control of communicable diseases must be expanded and strengthened. Research regarding communicable diseases must be encouraged, especially on the negative factors in the physical, psychological, economical, socio-cultural and all other milieus that threaten the welfare of individuals, their families, and communities. In conjunction with other team members of the healthcare team and healthcare establishments, healthcare providers must contribute to the elimination, modification, or diminution of these factors in order to reduce the incidence of communicable diseases

   ✠ all mother and child care programmes must emphasize the benefits of vaccination in the protection of health as well as beneficial health practices to maintain health through a healthy life-style

   ✠ health information to be given to promote, maintain, and restore health is of cardinal importance. Healthcare providers must commence health information as soon as the diagnosis of a particular communicable disease has been made. The objective is to enable individuals, families, and communities to maintain and protect their health by making appropriate health-related decisions regarding personal health behaviours; the use of available healthcare resources; and social health issues of importance. To maintain optimal health, health information has to promote human biology; environmental health (physical-biological, psychological, social-cultural and all milieus of importance); a healthy lifestyle; and the proper use of the healthcare systems (allopathic and/or traditional). Of cardinal importance is the adaptation of healthcare informational programmes for individuals, families, and communities with low literacy skills, and/or who are low proficient in the English language, and/or who are illiterate

   ✠ facilities such as hospitals; general ambulatory care units; health care centres; special categorical clinics; long-term care facilities; environmental health protection facilities; and other specialized health units (blood banks, laboratories) in which personnel provide their services through structures outside the healthcare user's home must be available

   ✠ both professional and traditional healthcare providers must be community-orientated and culture-care competent. All healthcare providers must be able to render the necessary preventive, promotive, curative, and rehabilitative healthcare as well as maintain, protect, and restore the health of individuals, families, and communities. Multi-professional cooperation and referral between professional and traditional providers must become common practice in the prevention and control of communicable diseases

✠ accurate statistical information must be kept and be available as to assist in the planning for the delivery of the correct and adequate healthcare services

✠ the necessary legislation (health, social welfare, environmental, agricultural and animal health, economical, educational, etc) must be in place to support all healthcare interventions at primary, secondary and tertiary levels to maintain, protect, and restore health. All healthcare practitioners (professional and traditional) must not only be well-informed about existing legislation, but should also draw the attention of legislators to deficiencies in the existing legislation that are threatening the welfare of individuals, families, and communities

3. The necessary finances must be available for the procurement of health resources and the provision of services

4. The healthcare sub-systems, both allopathic and traditional, must be well organized and well managed as to render holistically, comprehensive, empathically and culturally congruent healthcare to all individual healthcare users, families, and communities

5. Diverse services must be delivered to both healthy and unwell persons - institutional, community-centred and home-based. All services to be delivered must be available, accessible, acceptable, affordable, and effective to all healthcare users (whether healthy, ill, contact, or carrier), their families, and their communities within their cultural context.

All health care interventions at the tertiary level of prevention are directly linked to those on the primary level. This cyclic phenomenon occurs because the skills taught to the individual, his/her family and the community by healthcare providers during the rehabilitation phase will contribute to the maintenance of their well-being, thus rendering them less susceptible to communicable diseases. Where the milieu has been reconstructed, the provider must assist the individual, his/her family, and the community to sustain the milieu in order to eliminate, modify, or diminish any harmful, negative, or hazardous risk factors.

3.4   KEY NOTES

❑ The responsibilities of all healthcare providers regarding the prevention of communicable diseases at the primary, secondary, and tertiary levels are comprehensive.

❑ Professional and traditional healthcare practitioners fulfill client-centered, delivery-orientated, and population-orientated roles in the prevention of communicable diseases.

❑ Although healthcare providers share many of their responsibilities with other team members, they remain primarily responsible, nevertheless, for the development of a particular attitude to health in individuals, their families and the community which will contribute, in turn, to their acceptance of their responsibility for their own health.

❑ Healthcare interventions at the primary, secondary and tertiary levels of prevention must be comprehensive, holistic, empathically and culturally congruent in nature, encompassing the host-system (individual, family and community - whether healthy, ill, carrier, contact); the environment (physical-biological and all other milieus or environments in which individuals, families, and communities live); and the healthcare system (including both the allopathic and the traditional sub-systems).

❑ There exists a relation between the interventions at the primary, secondary and tertiary levels of prevention and the different stages in the natural course of a communicable disease (see Table 3.2).

Table 3.2 THE CORRELATION BETWEEN THE DIFFERENT STAGES IN THE NATURAL COURSE OF ANY COMMUNICABLE DISEASE AND THE INTERVENTIONS AT PRIMARY, SECONDARY AND TERTIARY LEVELS OF PREVENTION

Stage of infection in the natural course of the disease process	Pathogenesis of the course of the disease process	Level of prevention	Specific interventions
PRE-PATHOGENESIS (PRE-PATHOLOGICAL STAGE)			
	• Interaction between host, infectious agent and environmental factors bring host and infectious agent together • Disease causative infectious agent gains entry into the host – depending on several physiological factors, the individual will become ill or stay healthy	Primary prevention	✓ Promotion of the biophysical, emotional and socio-cultural well-being of individuals, families and communities, for example, hygiene, healthy lifestyles, adequate nutrition, adequate rest and exercise, coping skills, vaccination ✓ Complying with legislative measures ✓ Promotion of environmental and animal health ✓ Promotion of the health of all milieus in which individuals, families and communities live in ✓ Creating a comprehensive healthcare system for service delivery
PATHOGENESIS			
Incubation period (pre-clinical stage)	• Local and systemic inflammation reactions takes place	Secondary prevention	✓ Awareness that the infected individual can already transmit the disease

	• The course of the pathogenesis of the disease commences • Non-specific signs of the disease have not yet appeared – the person seems to be healthy		✓ No specific interventions can be planned if no knowledge exists of the specific disease that had been contracted
Prodromal stage (pre-clinical stage) (non-specific signs and symptoms can be observed)	• Pathogen has invaded the body of the host and multiplies • Pathogenic process are taking place in body cells, tissues and organs due to physiological interaction between the immune system of the host and the pathogen	Secondary prevention	✓ When non-specific signs and symptoms of communicable diseases are diagnosed, the individual should be placed under quarantine until such time that tests yields specific results ✓ Non-specific medical treatment and fundamental healthcare should commence
Characteristic clinical picture (clinical stage) specific signs and symptoms can be observed	• The disease can be diagnosed based on the clinical manifestations • Laboratory and/or other tests confirm diagnosis • Ill individuals may show signs and symptoms of complications	Secondary prevention	✓ Modifying risks/ hazards in environment/milieu ✓ Treatment commences to prevent causative pathogen to spread to susceptible hosts (eliminate pathogen) ✓ Fundamental and specific healthcare rendering to the ill individual at home or in hospital within familial and community context ✓ Tracing of contacts and placing them under quarantine together with treating them prophylactic ✓ Tracing and treating of carriers

			✓ Implementation of prophylactic measures to prevent healthy individuals becoming ill ✓ Implementation of all measures (barrier healthcare and legislative measures) to control the spread of the particular communicable disease ✓ Rectifying/correcting factors in the healthcare system that promote outbreaks of communicable diseases
CONVALESCENT STAGE (RESOLUTION STAGE)			
	• Resolution of disease take place - acute signs and symptoms disappear and the process of recovery or convalescence starts • Disability or chronic illness or carrier state is either of a temporary or a permanent nature	Tertiary prevention	✓ Rehabilitation and retraining of disabled or chronic ill or carrier individuals for maximum use of physical and psychosocial abilities ✓ Reconstruction of home and/or community milieus to re-integrate disabled or chronic ill or carrier individual into family and community life ✓ Management of carriers to live a self-actualized life ✓ Strengthening of the healthcare system for service delivery ✓ Health information to be given and research to be done as to prevent further outbreaks of the specific communicable disease/infection

Chapter 4

THE CONTROL OF COMMUNICABLE DISEASES

Faced with one of the main contributors to death and disability, healthcare providers must prevent, identify and control communicable diseases. Communicable infections as such can be controlled by drugs, vaccination and a healthy environment. In general, chemotherapy controls infections in individuals whereas vaccination and environmental improvement control communicable diseases in populations/communities. The role and responsibilities of healthcare providers in efforts to control communicable diseases fall generally in the categories of case finding, referral, treatment and supportive healthcare as well as contact notification, chemoprophylaxis, health information, vaccination, complying with legislation and/or advocating for mandatory legislation and ensuring access to healthcare. To provide an accurate basis for the assessment of all risks and for planning the necessary interventions, detailed epidemiological studies must be done to determine the links between the host system, the pathogen and the environment in the causation, spread and control of communicable diseases.

4.1 USING THE SCIENTIFIC EPIDEMIOLOGICAL PROCESS IN THE CONTROL OF COMMUNICABLE MEDICAL DISEASES

Epidemiology is the scientific study of the occurrence, spread and control of medical diseases. Epidemiologic data is use to record the diseases (including communicable medical diseases) affecting a population, and when communicable diseases occur, to identify their causes and modes of transmission. The more complete the data, the more fruitful the analysis is likely to be. Accordingly, it is necessary to record not only data relating to the communicable infection itself, but also demographic, geographic, climatic, socio-cultural and socio-economic, behavioral and personal data, and all other data deemed important.

Understanding the epidemiology of a communicable infection helps to define the correct strategies for control at the population, the familial and the individual level. The understanding of and decisions about control measures depend heavily upon the ability to recognize outbreaks of communicable medical diseases, to follow their progress and to identify the causative pathogens concerned. Detection and diagnosis are therefore key activities in the control of communicable medical diseases as they are for the treatment of infection at the level of the individual.

All intervention strategies pertaining to the control of communicable medical disease are determined by the nature of the disease. All programmes designed in the control of communicable medical diseases are based on the epidemiological process as it is a systematic way to

- identify the strategic points of control
- design the necessary intervention strategies to minimize the effect of the disease on the health of the population
- implement the designated programme of control
- evaluate the results of the control strategies to prevent the re-occurrence of the disease
- promote research regarding the control and prevention of the specific disease and communicable diseases in general.

Note

All interventions planned must not only include the individual person, but also his/her family and the community wherein they live (as described in chapter 1) as well as the following epidemiological perspectives - the different dimensions of health (physical-biological, psychological, socio-cultural, behavioral), the environment (physical, biological, socio-cultural {including the healthcare system}, economical, educational and all other milieus of importance as described in chapter 1) and the specific causative pathogen concerned (as described in chapter 1)

The epidemiological process *per se* involves the following series of steps to be executed

❑ **Step 1 - Detecting and reporting a case or outbreak by defining the condition/ disease**

The particular communicable disease, for which control interventions are required, must be professionally defined based on the diagnostic tests that had been done and/or clinical picture manifested. The case definition (professional) must include the signs and symptoms of the disease as well as the individuals involved (contact patterns or mixing matrixes) and the timing of the event. All healthcare providers (professional and paramedical, traditional and lay care) must be able to detect and report a suspected case suffering from any communicable disease.

The lay definition of the particular communicable disease must be readily recognized at the community level and the signs and symptoms must be simple and clear and understood (where necessary, translated into the local language spoken) by the community. Community health workers, traditional birth attendants (TBA's), traditional healers, traditional and religious leaders, teachers, police officers, and other persons who are respected in the communities, who serve and who knows the families and their children intimately, must be informed to identify the ill individual and to inform the nearest healthcare facility immediately.

☐ **Step 2 - <u>Determining the natural history of the particular communicable disease by investigating the index case or outbreak</u>**

This comprises the identification of all factors (host-related, pathogen-related and environmental-related) that contribute to

- the development of the particular communicable disease
- the signs and symptoms (pre-exposure stage, pre-clinical stage, clinical stage and resolution stage) of the particular communicable disease
- the effects of the particular communicable disease on the human body
- the typical outcome of the particular communicable disease and the factors that may affect those outcomes.

The Epidemiological Triad of Communicable Disease model serves as bases for this information (See table 4.1 and chapter 1)

Table 4.1 DATA TO BE ACQUIRED PERTAINING TO THE HOST, PATHOGEN AND ENVIRONMENT

☐ **Human hosts (patient–related factors) Individual persons, family members, community members whether healthy or ill or carriers or contacts as well as the family and the community as an unit/group**
- The following dimensions of the health of the individual must be taken in account
  - ➢ the bio-physical dimension of health
  - ➢ the psycho-emotional dimension of health
  - ➢ the socio-cultural dimension of health
  - ➢ the behaviour (lifestyle) dimension of health
- Attributes of the family as a unit/group to be taken in account
- Attributes of the community as a unit/group to be taken in account

☐ **Pathogen (infectious agent)**
- All properties described in chapter 1 including the classification of the specific pathogenic microbe, the specific antimicrobial/antiviral treatment and/or immunotherapeutic products and other healthcare interventions applicable and the availability of vaccines
- Of utmost importance is the understanding of the biology of the infectious agent – micro-parasites and macro-parasites
  - ➢ Micro-parasites (viruses, bacteria, fungi, and protozoa) reproduce within the host and are typically transient. Recovery from infection usually elicits immunity against re-infection. In defining the epidemiology of these diseases it is useful to divide all hosts in classes of individuals
    - ✓ Susceptible
    - ✓ Infected but latent (i.e. non-infectious)
    - ✓ Infected and infectious
    - ✓ Recovered and immune

    The incubation period in terms of the latent period (time between infection and infectiousness) and the generation time (sum of the latent and infectious period) must also be taken in account

> Macro-parasites (helminths and arthropods) do not reproduce directly within the host, but produce transmission stages that pass to the exterior (environment) to complete their lifecycle. Macro-parasites are typically large and their generation times are often a significant fraction of the host's lifespan. Immunity tends to be of a relatively short duration once the parasites are removed, and hosts may be continually re-infected

> The spread of infection is related to the reproductive rate of the infectious agent (the biological success of the pathogen is measured in terms of transmission potential - for microbes it is the average number of secondary cases of infection produced by one primary case in a completely susceptible population, and for macro-parasites is the average number of female offspring produced throughout the lifetime of a mature female)

> The influence of behaviour on the spread of infection as the transmission of horizontally directly transmitted infections requires contact between already infective and susceptible persons. The degree of contact is determined by the density of susceptible persons in the community which exceed a critical value. Based on this value, the target vaccination cover for mass campaigns can thus be calculated with the aim to reduce the density of susceptible persons in the community. The behavioural factors are of particular importance in sexually transmitted infections since the rate at which individuals acquire different sexual partners varies (persons who have many sexual partners are more likely to acquire and transmit infection). As these individuals play a key role in the persistence of such infections in sexually active individuals in communities, they must be targeted for treatment and health information about safer sex practices

> Patterns of population mixing are of importance in designing policies and control measures. The intensity of transmission differs within different groupings (school children, sport fans, clubs for the aged, etc.) but still plays a key role in determining patterns of infection and disease. Patterns of mixing are also influenced by the timing of school terms and vacations (young children [3-5 years] and school-going children [5-15 years]) serve to seed infection via family contacts to younger and older persons). Targeting vaccination at young children before they enter school is an effective way of minimizing between-group transmission

> Many common horizontally directly transmitted viral and bacterial infections show regular peaks in incidence with the result the inter-epidemic period (the time period interval between major peaks in incidence) can be calculated. Regularity of peaks of incidence are a striking feature of many common directly transmitted diseases for example, seasonal (winter - common cold; spring - chicken pox and measles; spring - meningococcal meningitis) and longer term (poliomyelitis – 3-5 yrs and pertussis 3-4 yrs). These intervals are determined by interactions between the pathogen and its host. At the start of an epidemic cycle the pathogenic agent spread rapidly and as the susceptible persons become sick, the incidence starts to decline. This decline continuous until the pool of susceptible persons is replenished by new births, with the density of susceptible eventually rising to a level sufficient to trigger the next epidemic

> The transmission success of an infection vary between communities because of differences in demography (net birth rate); behaviour (patterns of mixing); and age distribution of the population. As such, vaccination alters not only the incidence of infection but also affects the age distribution of cases and the pattern of fluctuation, for example, measles is now becoming a disease of the adolescent and young adult age group, taking on epidemic proportions with a high ratio of complications leading to disabilities

❏ **Environment – physical-biological, psychological, socio-cultural and economic as well as all other systems/environments the community is composed of**

- All characteristics of/factors in the abovementioned environments/milieus as described in chapter 1 as well as
  - ➤ Physical-biological environment
    - ♦ location and topography (for example, rivers, woods)
    - ♦ type (rural, urban, suburban)
    - ♦ size and population density
    - ♦ climatic and seasonal conditions
    - ♦ soil conditions and food supplies
    - ♦ type and adequacy of housing
    - ♦ water, milk, meat and other food supplies
    - ♦ systems for sanitation and waste disposal
    - ♦ hazards and nuisance factors
      - ▪ physical – pollution and poisons, heavy metals
      - ▪ biological – insects, pollution of water and food sources
    - ♦ animals and birds (wild, exotic and domestic)
    - ♦ farming activities
    - ♦ unsafe working conditions and sensitive occupations
    - ♦ vegetation and vectors

  - ➤ Socio-cultural environment
    - ♦ demographic composition of population – adults, children, gender composition (male and female), and age distribution
    - ♦ community government and leadership, for example, authority structure, how decisions are made and who the decision makers are, who holds the purse strings
      - ▪ informal community leaders
      - ▪ business leaders
      - ▪ key informants in the community
    - ♦ language – formal and informal and whether it presents a barrier to health information and health service delivery
    - ♦ cultural affiliation of healthcare users – including cultural healthcare practices that enhance/impair health
    - ♦ religious affiliations, beliefs and practices that enhance or impair health of residents as well as the acceptability of healthcare services
    - ♦ marital and family composition (for example nuclear-, extended-, single parent, cohabiting-, step-, communal-, interracial-, same sex family)
    - ♦ transportation, for example, utilization of trains, taxi's, motors, bicycles, walking
    - ♦ type and adequacy of goods and services (for example, industries, services, facilities {such as recreation, shopping} and social programmes)
    - ♦ lifestyle patterns
    - ♦ consumption patterns:
      - ▪ general nutritional status
      - ▪ specific dietary pattern (for example, 2–3 meals a day)
      - ▪ symbolism and cultural aspects

- foods as medical therapy
- traditional foods
- use of harmful substances

    ↓ occupation – type and health hazards, sensitive occupations (poultry farmers, waste disposal workers, etc), unemployment

    ↓ leisure pursuits, for example, camping, outdoor activities

    ↓ other behaviours – promiscuous sexual activities, needle sharing (drug users)

    ↓ cultural beliefs and practices

   ➤ Psychological environment

    ↓ history of community in resolving health problems (tension and distrust between subgroups)

    ↓ relationships in community

    ↓ community prospects – growing (vibrancy) or declining (apathy) or economically depressed (apathy)

    ↓ community strengths and how the community deals with health problems

    ↓ communication networks (informal and formal)

    ↓ common sources of stress in the community

   ➤ Other systems/environments

    ↓ Political environment

    ↓ Historical environment

    ↓ Rural and urban environment

    ↓ Informational system (formal and informal; communication channels and sources)

    ↓ Trade and commerce system (including informal, small and big businesses)

    ↓ Seasonal and migratory patterns of employment and unemployment patterns

❑ **Contextual factors to be taken in account when doing an ecological analysis of the impact of potential risk factors in the prevention and control of communicable disease**

- Other healthcare user-related factors - the level of education and educational resources; purchasing power, preference for the private healthcare sector (private healthcare practitioners, traditional healers and private pharmacies) and out of pocket expenditure for health and disease

- Healthcare system factors - availability and adequacy of traditional and professional healthcare services; number of cases coming for treatment, functionality of the healthcare system (disability adjusted life expectancy–scale) and the responsiveness of the healthcare system relative to people's expectations and fairness, "hot spots" as indicated by treatment case ratio's, morbidity and mortality rates and patterns, extend of overused or underused of available services, and economics of healthcare

- Other factors - availability of resources, gross domestic product (GDP), health expenditure (expressed as percentage of GDP), human development index and the poverty index, resource-rich and resource-poor settings

❑ **Legislation – National and international measures to comply with and enforce (when necessary) to prevent the particular communicable disease from spreading across national and international borders**

The investigation into the natural history of the particular communicable disease, **MUST** provided answers to the following questions

> ➤ **When** did the outbreak occur?
> ➤ **Where** did the outbreak occur/
> ➤ **What** is the nature of the outbreak?
> ➤ **Who** is affected by the outbreak?
> ➤ **Why** did the outbreak occur?
> ➤ **How** can this outbreak be controlled/prevented from spreading/a single case be prevented becoming a cluster? **How** can an outbreak of the same disease in the future be prevented?

The answers to the above questions provide the basis for selection and planning of the appropriate response activities. It is crucially important to investigate an outbreak or index case as soon as possible to ensure a prompt outbreak response in order to reduce or prevent the occurrence of further cases. This is especially relevant for all highly contagious diseases because the rapid implementation of control strategies allows disease transmission to be interrupted. The investigation must include the examination of the identified index case (if possible) as well as interviews with close relatives and friends/co-workers/teachers/co-students or co-learners; an active search for additional cases (primary, secondary and suspected); and a visit to the site to identify all physical-biological and other factors contributing to/sustaining the outbreak. Also be included in the investigation are private healthcare practitioners such as doctors and physiotherapists; hospitals (investigation of admission diagnosis and other records to be done); and community sources/reporters such as pharmacists, private clinics, village leaders or anyone else likely to come in contact with such diseases.

❑ **Step 3 - Determine the extent of the disease through the analysis of diseases patterns and trends**

The extent of the disease is determined by means of obtaining the necessary morbidity and mortality data. Epidemiological and statistical data required are

- incidence rate – number of cases of infection at a given point in time or over a given period (endemic, sporadic, epidemic, pandemic)
- prevalence rate – the number of new cases arising in a population over a defined period of time (attack rate)
- age-specific/gender specific/ethnic specific/social group specific prevalence or incidence rate (infection within a particular age group[s], gender group [male or female], ethic group[s], social group[s])
- mortality rate (cause-specific death rate or case fatality rate)
- geographic distribution (urban, rural, highland, lowland, grassland) of the particular communicable disease
- time relationships (specific times of the year; particular seasons such as dry or wet seasons, summer (hot) or winter (cold) seasons, cyclic time periods over a time span), and

- trends and patterns (for example, increasing/upwards, declining/ downwards, periodic fluctuations over time, seasonal).

Note

A single as well as a cluster[s] of disease outbreak must be described in terms of person[s], place[s] and time[s]. The assumption that the reported cases constitute all the cases which are occurring must be avoided as underreporting does occur. The analysis of the disease pattern and trend of the particular communicable disease forms the basis for the control strategies to be planned as to prevent the situation getting out of control. Notification reports must therefore be promptly sent to the appropriate office/ authority for rapid action response

❑ **Step 4 - <u>Responding to a case or outbreak by planning strategies for the control of the disease</u>**

In designing programmes for the control of the spread of the particular disease, the strategic points of control must first be identified (such as water purification; sewage disposal; improved housing; improved nutrition; control of vectors, control of a reservoir of animals; chemotherapy and vaccines; changes in personal habits; screening of transfused blood and organs; and food hygiene). Healthcare programmes to minimize the effects of the communicable disease on the health of the population must then be designed, taking in account the following principles and aims

- all control programmes must have the following aims, namely,
  - ➢ to contain the disease in a timely and effective manner
  - ➢ to prevent the spread of the disease, and
  - ➢ to enhance the resistance of all hosts (individuals, families and communities whether healthy, ill, carrier, contact)
- all appropriate interventions to control the spread, must be aimed at the specific infectious agent (pathogenic microbe); as well as at the source of infection (both human hosts [individuals, families, communities who may be healthy, sick, contact, carrier] and animal hosts [warm-blooded {such as dogs, fleas} or cold-blooded {insects such as mosquitoes}]); the maintaining of a healthy environment; and the enforcement of the necessarily legislation. All appropriate responses should be
  - ➢ <u>rapid enough</u> to prevent or reduce the further spread of the particular disease or outbreak in the population
  - ➢ <u>extensive enough</u> to cover the entire geographical area at risk for disease spread or a re-occurrence of the disease
  - ➢ <u>complete enough</u> to protect the entire population-at-risk for the spread of the disease or the re-occurrence of the disease
- all persons who have been exposed to the communicable disease regardless of being healthy or sick, must be identified. They must be informed of being exposed, tested for the particular disease and then treated. Contact referral and contact follow-up must be carried out, where necessary

137

- chemo-prophylaxis must be given to prevent the onset of the disease in exposed individuals. When individuals are prevented from developing the symptomatic disease, they are not able to spread the disease to others
- all interventions planned must be based on the Epidemiological Triad of Communicable Diseases model (host, environment and pathogen) as well as the inclusion of the following epidemiologic perspectives, namely, the different dimensions of health (bio-physical, psychological, socio-cultural, behavioral), the environment (physical-biological, psychological, socio-cultural, economic and all others of importance) and the healthcare system (accessibility, affordability, appropriateness, adequacy, availability and usage). The strategies/responses/interventions set must
  - ➢ be in line of the objective[s] set for the control and prevention of a re-occurrence of the particular communicable disease
  - ➢ include all specific activities to be carried out to contain the outbreak
  - ➢ specify the geographical area where the activities must be carried out
  - ➢ specify the persons-at-risk (healthy, ill, contact and carrier) who are targeted for the outbreak response
  - ➢ specify the healthcare personnel and volunteers who are to be involved in the outbreak response and the training required by the healthcare personnel
  - ➢ specify the resources required, such as manpower, vehicles and fuel; vaccines and/or chemo-prophylactic medicine; funds; partner agencies
  - ➢ include the timetable of activities (starting and completing time)
  - ➢ include the criteria set for the evaluation of the outbreak activities and correctional activities to be implemented if the outbreak has not yet been fully contained
  - ➢ specify which other community institutions and organizations are to be involved in the outbreak response, such as National departments (Water Affairs, Agriculture, Environmental Affairs, Labour); the police and military services; educational institutions (including teachers and students/learners); non-governmental organizations (NGO's); local leaders; and many more
- the preventive measures to be taken to prevent a re-occurrence of the disease must also be put in place simultaneously. (Remember - The control of the spread of the disease and the prevention of the disease goes hand in hand, taking place at primary, secondary and tertiary levels simultaneously [see chapter 3]). The measures to be taken to prevent the spread of the disease, such as legislation, enhancement of the resistance of the human hosts and maintaining a healthy environment, encompass promotive, preventive, curative and rehabilitative healthcare interventions which promote the general

health of all persons, their families and their communities whilst preventing and rectifying all hazards/risks in the environment/milieus.

All control strategies to be designed, **must include the following**

❖ **Policy aspects regarding notification** - A national policy must be in place regarding the notification of an outbreak of a particular communicable disease. The procedure for notification must be standardized. The data required must be easy to obtain and must be taken down as accurately and completely as possible. Data has to be obtained from all relevant sources and be processed at a central office. This policy has to be carried out to the letter of the law by all members of the health team (including private healthcare practitioners and traditional providers). The necessary channels must be created in order to enable notification to reach the central office or authority within 24 hours or according to the set protocol. A sound reporting system is characterized by

➢ promptness – all benchmark cases must be reported within 24 hours of occurrence and investigated within 48 hours of being reported

➢ completeness of information needed – reports must include every aspect of information that is needed, or could be needed, and cover all cases seen

➢ accurate diagnosis – an accurate diagnosis must be made based on signs and symptoms characteristic of the particular disease, with or without bacteriological/virological and/or urine/stool/blood results

All healthcare practitioners and providers must thus be fully knowledgeable regarding the signs and symptoms of communicable diseases as described in the standard case definition (professional and lay) as well as being skilled in the diagnosing (detecting) of the particular communicable disease and the reporting of cases.

❖ **Execution of the necessary investigations and interventions**
Within 24 hours of notification of an outbreak, the necessary investigations have to be set in motion (clinical, epidemiological and virological/bacteriological). The purpose of these investigations is to

✓ identify sick persons whether individuals, or families, or communities as well as all contacts and carriers

✓ identify the specific infectious agent as to implement the necessary strategies of treatment and other interventions to be executed; and

✓ rectify/correct all adverse factors within the environment (physical, biological, socio-cultural and other milieus) that promote outbreaks of communicable diseases.

All healthcare practitioners must be able to collect and ship fecal, urine, blood and other virological/bacteriological specimens required from index, primary, secondary and suspected cases as well as vaccine and/or other specimens from a case of adverse events following vaccination/immunization.

❖ **Mopping up and reporting back** - When the outbreak has been brought under control, a mopping-up action (for example, by doing visits from house to house, from building to building, from street to street) has to be carried out in order to prevent any further outbreaks. The results of this operation must be communicated to all healthcare personnel to enable them to rectify those factors which caused the outbreak. Following this, a **surveillance programme** must be implemented to prevent a further outbreak of the particular disease.

❑ **Step 5 - Implementation and monitoring of the designed programme of control**

The overall responsibility for ensuring the quality of the control measures (case investigation and outbreak response), the preventive measures (prevention of a future outbreak and the enhancement of the resistance of all persons) as well as the measures for the surveillance of diseases in a specific Health District lies with the District Health Authority in cooperation with the Provincial and National Health Authorities. It is of utmost importance to check the performance of disease control activities at least every month (ideally weekly) against the set indicators. The six most useful indicators for disease surveillance and response information are

➢ timeliness and completeness of disease notifications (within 9 days after the reporting week [Sunday to Saturday])

➢ timeliness and completeness of the monthly immunization statistic form (within 10 days after the end of the reporting month)

➢ timeliness of case and outbreak reporting (according to protocol)

➢ percentage of reported cases and outbreaks investigated within a specified period (for example, 100% within 48 hours)

➢ percentage of reported cases and outbreaks with appropriate response (for example, 100% of all reported cases)

➢ percentage of suspected cases investigated with the necessary stool/urine/blood/other virological or bacteriological specimens (collected and shipped) and follow-up examinations performed (for example, 100%).

Should the outbreak of the particular communicable disease[s] is still not contained, re-evaluate steps 2, 3 and 4 and plan anew. Implement the new outbreak responses and re-evaluate the situation. Furthermore, feedback has to be given on a regular basis to all personnel/volunteers as well as institutions/organizations/services/departments and communities and groups involved. The feedback must always be clear, honest, informative and encouraging. Feedback can be given in several forms such as newsletters, newssheets and on-site visits. The role of the media and the internet must never be left out as they are effective tools to get public health messages to all persons.

❑ **Step 6 - <u>Disease surveillance (supervision of diseases for disease prevention and control)</u>**

The purpose of disease surveillance is to

* trace, as soon as possible, any change(s) in the natural course of diseases
* observe any change(s) in the host and in the environment which may promote an outbreak; and
* monitor the safety and effectiveness of the control and preventive measures implemented.

Disease surveillance is a public health management tool that provides a baseline for the assessment of all preventive and control measures. As a tool, disease surveillance helps to

➢ trace the natural history, clinical spectrum and epidemiology of a particular communicable disease
➢ identify individuals/families/communities-at-risk
➢ identify the geographical and seasonal occurrence of the disease
➢ identify the exposure and risk factors that are critical to its occurrence
➢ improve measures for disease control and prevention.

As disease surveillance encompasses the collection, collation, analysis and interpretation of information on <u>where</u>, <u>when</u> and <u>in whom</u> a particular communicable disease occurs, it is extremely important that all the necessary information must reach the authorities so that they can take the appropriate steps/actions as to prevent further outbreaks of the disease. Disease surveillance as such can either be passive or active. Passive surveillance refers to the process when ill persons present themselves to healthcare workers and the information is collected using routine reports. Because of under-reporting of disease, lack of representativeness of cases, lack of timeliness of reporting and lack of accuracy of the diagnosis, passive surveillance has many limitations and constrains as a useful tool. Active surveillance on the other hand, refers to the process where cases of diseases **are actively** looked for, case investigation are done regularly and regular analysis of disease patterns and trends are done on district, provincial and national level to monitor disease activity and detect any unsuspected changes in disease patterns and trends. In the light of these findings, future responses and control and/or preventive measures are planned and implemented.

The responsibilities for the different aspects of surveillance are assigned to the different levels of service delivery in the healthcare system. At the health facility level, records have to be kept and analyzed to detect patterns and trends as well as outbreaks; the necessary investigations must be conducted together with the necessary notification and reporting to the District Health Authorities. At the district level, the reports of the healthcare facilities must be analyzed to detect trends and/or outbreaks; further investigations must be conducted if necessarily; high risk areas or groups have to identified and the appropriate responses must be taken; feedback must be given to healthcare facility personnel; reporting must be done to the province within the set time limit; supervisory visits must be done and defaulters (healthcare facilities not reporting or responding) must be followed up and personnel must be trained. At provincial level, all cases must be followed up; districts-at-risk must be identified; supervisory visits must be done and defaulters (for example, silent districts) must be followed up; feedback has to be given to districts and reporting to national level must be done. At national level, all surveillance reports that were received must be analyzed to detect trends and patterns as well as possible outbreaks of disease[s] in the country; the appropriate actions in response to the reports must be taken (for example, amending or changing protocols/procedures/policies); feedback must be given to provinces; and reporting to the national management and international agencies such as the World Health Organization (WHO) and the United nations International Children's Educational Fund (UNICEF) must be done.

❑ **Step 7 - Promote research regarding the control and prevention of the particular disease and communicable diseases in general**
Research must be conducted into negative factors in all environments/milieus of importance that threaten the health of individuals, families, and communities as well as into all factors that enhance or diminish the health status of all individual hosts, their families and their communities. This research must be an ongoing process that should be carried out in co-operation with other healthcare practitioners and providers and institutions in order to eliminate certain factors as to lower the incidence of communicable diseases.

Note

The research findings must be converted into health informational programmes and health promotive strategies related to human biology, a healthy environment and lifestyle modification behaviours and the development of coping skills as to promote the well-being of all individuals, families, and communities. All health informational programmes and health promotive strategies must be culturally appropriate based on the group-specific values and behavioural patterns of social scripts (not a translation of health promotive strategies already in place for a different cultural group/community) as to make the interventions acceptable, relevant, effective, moral, familiar and credible. The availability and accessibility of healthcare services at all levels of prevention must also be instituted

4.2.   KEY NOTES

❑ Despite the use of vaccines and anti-microbial medications as well as improved sanitation measures, communicable diseases still continue to contribute to the morbidity and mortality experienced by human beings.

❑ The control of communicable diseases through specific control and surveillance programmes are of the utmost importance as communicable diseases will never be fully erased from earth.

❑ By using the Epidemiological Process integrated with the Epidemiological Triad of Communicable Diseases model, a systematic way is created to design, implement and evaluate designated programmes in order to prevent and control communicable diseases (where humanly possible).

❑ Chemotherapy, vaccination and environmental control measures all have their place in the control of infectious diseases. The appropriate interventions will depend on the relevant factors identified.

❑ Different epidemiological approaches are under taken when dealing with infections by micro-parasites or macro-parasites and in sexually transmitted infection

THEME III

<u>THE HOST - THE ADVERSARY IN THE CONFLICT</u>

Defending the body against the penetration of pathogens and caring for the individual after invasion had taken place

Humans live in an environment filled with pathogenic microbes. Subsequently, the human body is continuously exposed to a large variety of pathogenic agents and their toxin. The human body, however, is capable of protecting/defending itself against these pathogenic microbes in its environment. This protection of the body occurs in an innate immunological and in an adaptive immunological way. Without these defense mechanisms, the interactions of humans with pathogenic microbes would lead to lasting impairment of their health.

The body protects itself against all pathogenic microbes through the first-line and second line defenses of the innate immune system. The first-line defense consists of formidable anatomical, physical, biochemical and mechanical barriers that are genetically determined and are not depended on contact with a specific pathogenic agent. These natural defense barriers are already present at birth but are influenced by factors such as age, nutrition and hormones that enhance or diminish its level of physiological resistance. After a specific pathogenic agent has gained entry into the body by overpowering the body's natural defense barriers, the specific pathogen binds with the tissue cells of the host and starts multiplying. The innate immune system, the second-line defense mechanism consisting of phagocytes and circulating soluble factors, immediately kicks in and may be sufficient to prevent the replication and spread of the specific pathogen, thereby preventing disease/infection. Phagocytosis and activation of the complement system as well as other innate processes take place to kill off the specific pathogen. If the innate immune system is insufficient to parry the invasion by the specific infectious pathogen, the adaptive physiologic immunological response is activated to eliminate the infective pathogen, allowing recovery from the infection/disease to take place. The adaptive immunological response is the most highly developed physiological ability of the body to resist the influence and effects of the specific pathogen. The adaptive immunological response as such is only activated when the specific infectious pathogen bypasses and overwhelms the innate immune system and spreads through the body. The adaptive physiologic resistance (naturally acquired immunologic memory) protects the body against a subsequent infection of the same specific infectious agent as the body had developed an immunological antibody-mediated and cell-mediated resistance with memory to the specific pathogen.

Faced with the antimicrobial defenses of the host, microbes have evolved and developed a variety of properties that enable them to bypass or overcome these defenses. Because the host's defenses are not completely effective, pathogens do invade the body resulting in disease/infection. Whether an infection is a surface infection or systemic infection depends on a variety of factors. A surface infection is characterized by the multiplication of the infectious pathogen in the epithelial cells at the site of entry into the surface of the body but the pathogen fails to spread to deeper structures or through the body. A systemic infection, on the other hand, spreads systematically through the body via lymph and/or blood by a complex or stepwise invasion of various tissues before reaching the final side of replication and shedding to the exterior. The signs symptoms of infection/disease are produced either by the pathogen or by the host's immune responses.

Chapter 5

THE BATTLE

The body's innate and adaptive immunological responses to the invasion of pathogens

Because humans live in an environment filled with infectious agents, their bodies are perpetually exposed to a large variety of pathogenic microbes. Most pathogens establish a parasitic or innocuous association with their natural host (man or animal) and are not pathogenic under normal circumstances when the natural host is in good health. This state of "balanced pathogenicity" reflects the balanced level of genetically determined resistance in man and the pathogenicity in the pathogen. In a state of "unbalanced pathogenicity" disease arises as the normal environmental conditions of the pathogen have changed in some way and/or the pathogen became established in an unnatural/new host, for example, in man instead of animal, resulting in disease. The human body, however, possesses the ability to protect itself against infection/disease cause by pathogens in the environment by means of different defence mechanisms – innate and adaptive.

5.1 THE DEFENCE MECHANISMS OF THE BODY TO PREVENT "IMBALANCE PATHOGENICITY"

To prevent "imbalance pathogenicity", the body are defended by the innate immune system and the adaptive immune system - the integrated defence mechanisms of the body (see figure 5.1). The life-long resistance of the innate immune system is based on soluble factors and cells as no memory is imprinted during an infection. The humoral/natural immunity of the innate immune system is therefore non-specific and the resistance of the innate immune system does not improve with repeated contact with the same pathogen. The adaptive immune system, on the other hand, is lymphocyte-based and mediates antibody (soluble factors) and T-lymphocyte cells with memory. The immunity of the adaptive immune system is specific with memory to the specific antigen and resistance enhances with repeated contact. Both the innate and the adaptive immune systems are activated when primary contact with the antigen takes place. The innate and the adaptive immune systems always act in close synergy/integration with one another, with the adaptive immune system greatly enhancing the efficiency of the innate response, although it takes time for the adaptive immune system to reach its maximum efficiency. Both the innate and the adaptive immune systems are influenced by various factors leading to an enhanced (high) or a diminished (compromised) status of physiologic resistance of the body.

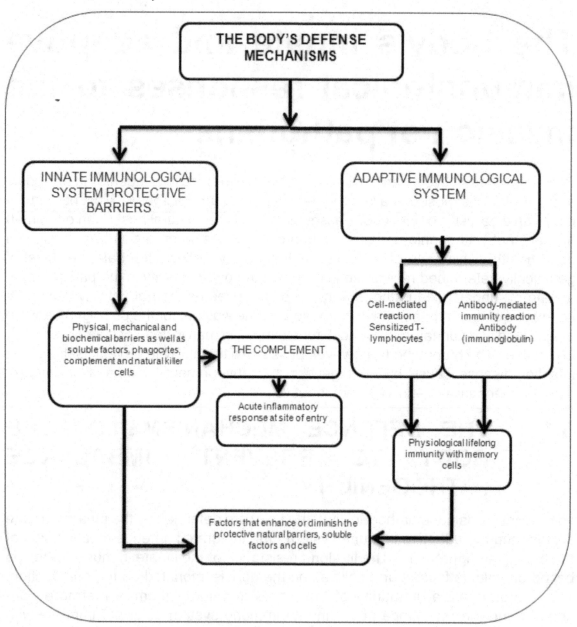

Figure 5.1   A schematic presentation of the body's defense mechanisms

5.1.1   The innate immunological system

The innate immune system consists of the natural protective barriers and the elements (soluble factors and cells) of the innate immunological defence response that is genetically determined and already in place before birth. When pathogens infect the body, the innate immune system already in place may be sufficient to prevent replication and spread of the pathogen, thereby preventing infection/ disease

5.1.1.1   The natural protective barriers of the body

The natural protective barriers of the body (all body surfaces) are essential to the survival of all human beings since they offer resistance against the gaining of entry into the body by pathogens which are always present in the environment, on the skin and in the respiratory and digestive tracts. The natural defence/protective barriers of the body consist of all the natural physical and mechanical barriers and biochemical substances in the skin, mucous membranes, respiratory and digestive tracts, urinary-genital tract and the eye. The protection of these defence barriers against pathogenic microbe is based on anatomical, biochemical and mechanical factors and is not dependent on contact with any specific infectious pathogen. These natural defence barriers are also **non-specific** since they are able to resist a wide spectrum of pathogenic microbes. Although not much attention is traditionally given to the natural defence barriers of the body, it is of utmost necessity that the health of these natural defence barriers is continuously enhanced so that their resistance can be upheld

Before an infectious agent can penetrate the body, it must overcome biochemical, chemical and physical barriers that operate at all body surfaces. One of the most important barriers is the skin which is impermeable to the majority of infectious pathogens. The membranes lining the inner surfaces of the body secrete mucus that acts as a protective barrier as it inhibits the adherence of microbes to the epithelial cells. The adhesive mucus traps microbial and other foreign particles that are then removed by mechanical means through ciliary action, coughing and sneezing. Another defence barrier is the phenomenon of microbial antagonism that is associated with the normal indigenous bacterial flora of the body. The commensally flora suppress the growth of many potentially pathogenic microbes and fungi at superficial sites by virtue of, firstly, their physical advantage of previous and active occupancy, and secondly, by competing for essential nutrients. Lastly, the commensally flora produces inhibitory substances such as acid and colicins - bactericides that kill off pathogens. Infants only acquire the normal indigenous bacterial flora of the body during and after birth as their body surfaces in uteri are bathed in sterile fluid. After the rupture of the membranes, the infant is exposed to large numbers of microbes and within hours the infant's body surfaces becomes colonized by organisms from his/her mother's vagina, skin, and respiratory tract. Any other persons involved in the care of the newborn infant also contribute to the infant's developing indigenous flora. The colon of the infant is usually colonised within 6-12 hours after birth (if breastfed with bifidobacteria, if bottle-fed with Enterobacteriaceae). Once the indigenous bacterial flora of the body has been established, it is more difficult for new species to become established – colonisation resistance. The normal indigenous bacterial flora of the body is, however, subject to change throughout life

❑ **Skin**

The skin is one of the most important natural defence barriers of the body as the intact skin effectively protects the body against invasion by pathogens because it is very difficult for any pathogenic microbe to penetrate the intact skin

The protection of the skin as defence barrier occurs as follows

❖ the skin has a horny layer (consisting mainly of keratin) which cannot be penetrated by the majority of pathogenic microbes. The living cells of the epidermis are thus protected by this horny layer against pathogenic microbes gaining entry into the body

❖ the skin is relatively dry and the proliferation of infectious microbes is inhibited by the high concentration of salt which is left when perspiration has evaporated

❖ the fatty secretions and perspiration contain germicidal and fungistatic fatty acids which protect the skin. This protection varies with age - for example, protection against ringworm (fungi) becomes more effective as a child grows older as older children secrete more fatty secretions than younger children

❖ the natural acidity of the skin also prevents the proliferation of microbes

❖ the skin also contains natural indigenous micro-flora which is non-pathogenic in nature that secretes a germicidal substance which destroys microbes.

❑ **Respiratory tract**

The protection offered by the mucous membranes to the structures of the respiratory tract is as follows

❖ **The nose**

• Cilia in the vestibule filter microbes inside the nose while the turbulence of the inhaled air causes the microbes to be trapped over the large surface of the nasal turbinates

• The trapped microbes are transported to the base of the tongue by the ciliary movements of the cilia of the epithelial cells, from where they are either swallowed or coughed up

• The nasal secretions also contain

➢ muco-polysaccharides which can inactivate some viruses

➢ specific phagocytic cells contains lysozyme, a mucolytic enzyme with germicidal properties that destroys some Gram-positive microbes

• The natural indigenous micro-flora in the nose also prevents infections

❖ **Smaller airways and alveoli**

• Microbes which have been inhaled and had landed on the walls of the smaller airways and alveoli, are phagocytosed by specialised cells, namely, the alveolar macrophages

• The mucous membranes of the respiratory tract secrete lysozyme, a bacteriolytic enzyme.

❑ **Digestive tract**

The gastro-entero (digestive) tract and the organs associated with ingestion (eating and drinking) and digestion (breaking down for absorption) of food such as the mouth, stomach and intestines, contribute in different ways to the protection of the body as follows

❖ The bacteriolytic enzyme, lysozyme, is secreted by the mucous membranes of the digestive tract

❖ The mouth contains large quantities of residual indigenous microbes which are continually decreased as they are swallowed with saliva

❖ Saliva also contains muco-polysaccharides that inactivate some viruses

❖ In the stomach, the stomach acid and pepsin destroys most of the pathogenic microbes

❖ In the intestine the normal indigenous bacterial flora destroy pathogenic microbes – in the small intestines the relatively high motility of the duodenum and jenenum keeps the number of microbes down while the slow-moving and relatively anaerobic conditions in the colon favour fermentation and anaerobic growth

❖ Enormous quantities of microbes are excreted daily in the faeces during the mechanical evacuation of the bowels. More or less 50-60% dry weight of faeces consists of bacteria and other microbes.

❑ **Urinary-genital tract**

The protection offered by the natural barriers of the urinary-genital tract is the following

❖ Urinary - Under normal circumstances the urinary tract contains very few microbes. This is ascribed to
  • the acidity of the urine which is bacteriostatic
  • the phagocytic cells in the mucous membrane of the bladder wall
  • IgA (an immunoglobulin) which is secreted in the urine, and
  • the continual mechanical voiding of the bladder

❖ Genital
  • The vagina
    The vagina has a unique defence mechanism - under hormonal influence, particularly oestrogen, the vaginal epithelial cells secrete increased quantities of glycogen that is metabolised by the lactobacilli into lactic acid. This creates an acid environment unfavourable for the growth of most pathogenic microbes. Because the indigenous vaginal flora varies with age (pre-puberty as well as during and after menopause) and when giving birth, the normal vaginal flora can be colonized by many different microbes during the life time of a woman
  • Sperm
    Male sperm contains spermine, a biochemical factor that acts as a bacteriocide in the vagina after ejaculation.

❑ **The eye**

The natural defence barriers of the eye are as follows

- ❖ Eye infections are effectively controlled by the rinsing action of tears which convey pathogenic microbes into the nasopharynx via the naso-lachrymal duct
- ❖ Tears also contain large quantities of lysozyme which destroy Gram-positive microbes.

5.1.1.2 The elements (phagocytic cells and soluble factors) of the innate immunological defence system

Despite the general effectiveness of various natural protective barriers, pathogens still successfully penetrate the body on many occasions. When this happens, two main defensive strategies of the innate immune system come into play, namely the mechanism of phagocytosis and the destructive effect of soluble chemical factors such as bactericidal enzymes. By killing off the pathogen and therefore preventing disease/infection, the elements of the innate immunological defence response lends thus, via its major elements of soluble factors (lysozyme, complement, acute phase proteins) and cells (phagocytes and natural killer cell), a general resistance to the body. The innate immune system parries/fights the invasion of the infectious agent through phagocytosis, activation of the complement system and other innate processes to kill off the pathogen. The defence processes of the innate immune system may be sufficient to prevent replication and spread of the specific infectious pathogen, thereby preventing the development of a particular communicable infection/disease. When the specific infectious pathogen bypasses and overwhelms the innate immune system and spread through the body, the adaptive physiologic immunological immune system is activated to eliminate the infective pathogen.

Phagocytosis involves the engulfment and killing off pathogens that had gained entry into the body and bonded with the protein of the tissue cells of the body, by specialized cells – the large macrophages and the smaller polymorphonuclear granulocytes (also named polymorphs or neutrophils) (see figure 5.2). Long-living macrophages are present throughout connective tissue, brain tissue, kidney tissue, bone tissue and basement membrane of small blood vessels, with concentrations in the lungs, liver, lymph nodes and spleen to filter off any foreign material. The neutrophils are non-dividing short-lived cells with a segmented nucleus and their cytoplasm contains an array of granules containing soluble chemical factors such as bactericidal enzymes, to kill off the pathogen. Once phagocytosis has had taken place, the soluble factors are activated and released to kill off the specific pathogen. The net result of all the mechanisms and processes of the phagocytic cells and the destructive effects of soluble chemical factors in killing off the infective microbes, is only the prevention of disease/infection as the "humoral"/natural resistance of the innate immune system is not enhanced by repeated contact with microbes and no memory cells to the specific pathogen are produced by the innate immune system.

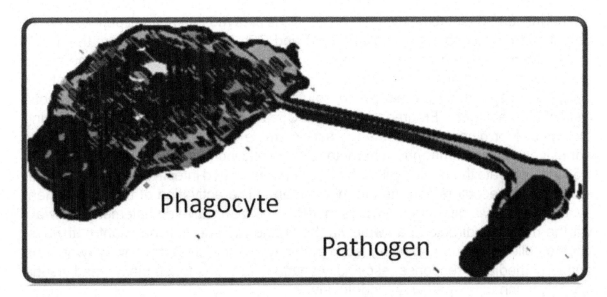

Figure 5.2　Schematic presentation of a macrophage phagocytising a pathogen

Phagocytosis only occurs after the pathogen had attached itself to the surface epithelial cells of the host's body tissue and bonded with the proteins of the cells. As soon as the phagocyte has attached itself to the surface of the pathogen, receptors on the surface on the phagocyte recognizes the repeating molecular patterns on the pathogen. The phagocyte, through its receptors, is then stimulated by the attached pathogen to initiate the ingestion phase as the actin-myosin contractile system of the phagocyte is activated whereby the phagocyte send arms of cytoplasm around the pathogen until it is completely enclosed within a vacuole. Shortly afterwards, the cytoplasmic granules fuse with the phagosome and discharge their contents around the incarcerated microbe. The internalized pathogen is now killed off by an array of killing mechanisms. The internalization and killing off of the pathogen can only happen if the pathogen and phagocyte are physically close to one another.

Although many pathogens produce chemical substances to directionally attract leukocytes, this mechanism/process of "chemotaxis" is a very weak signalling system. To defend the body as quickly as possible, the body has developed a complex mechanism to mobilize phagocytes from afar and target them onto the pathogen – the complement system comprising of a complex series of proteins, collectively named the "complement". The complement system is a multi-component-triggered enzyme cascade (a cascade phenomenon in which the product of the one reaction is the enzymes catalyst of the next) and is activated by the presence of certain molecules on the surface of the specific pathogen (activation via the alternative complement pathway). The most abundant complement (complement components are designated by the "C" followed by a number) in normal plasma, C3 splits into inactive cleavage products C3a (a chemotactic factor) and C3b by a convertase enzyme formed by its own cleavage product C3b and factor B and then stabilizes against breakdown through association with the microbial surface caused by factors H and I. Simultaneously, fragment C3b when formed, becomes covalently linked to the pathogen. The next abundant component to be cleaved is C5. C5 is cleaved into a small peptide C5a (a potent chemotactic factor for polymorphs) and C5b (a residual fragment that binds to the surface of the pathogen). When becoming membrane bound, fragment C5b assembles the terminal components C6, C7, C8 and C9 into a membrane attack complex that is freely permeable to solutes (soluble factors) leading to osmotic lysis of the pathogen. Fragments C3a and C5a as such, acts on mast cells causing the release of other mediators such as histamine whereby capillary permeability, adhesiveness and neutrophils chemotaxis is greatly increased. Fragments C3a and C5a also activate the neutrophils to bind to the C3b-coated infective pathogen by their surface C3b-receptors and then to ingest them. The activation of the complement system occurs via different pathways, namely, the alternative complement pathway; via the mast cell-directed pathway, via the fibrinolytic and anticoagulant pathways, via the collectin mannan-binding lectin pathway; via the classic pathway (when the antibody-mediated response, especially antibody IgA, has taken place); and via the lipopolysaccharides-pathway (endotoxins).

When the complement synergizes with the phagocytic cells, the influx of polymorphs and the increase in vascular permeability constitute the potent antimicrobial acute inflammatory response. The acute inflammatory response is a local non-specific self-limiting reaction lasting 8 to 10 days and occurs in an identical manner regardless of the trigger agent. The local acute inflammatory response starts within seconds after local cell injury or local cell invasion or local cell death and acts by effectively focusing the phagocytic cells onto complement-coated microbial pathogen-targets which are then engulfed by the phagocytes. The local acute inflammatory response is characterized by capillary dilatation (erythema), exudation of plasma proteins and fluid due to hydrostatic and osmotic pressure changes (oedema), and the accumulation of neutrophils. Activation of the local acute inflammatory response also takes place through the mast cell-directed pathway because of the stimulation of macrophages by certain bacterial toxins. This immunological reaction together with the action of C5a as well as by the action of phagocytosis of C3b coated bacteria, greatly enhance the mobilization of phagocytes. As macrophages now secrete other potent mediators of acute inflammation, for example, cytotoxic molecules such as reactive oxygen metabolites, the activation of the local acute inflammatory response is reinforced. The local acute inflammatory response and the rate of phagocytosis are also greatly enhanced and prolonged by the activation of the complement system via the fibrinolytic and anticoagulant pathways, the collectin mannan-binding lectin pathway; the classic pathway (when the antibody-mediated response, especially antibody IgA, has taken place); and the lipopolysaccharides-pathway (endotoxins). On the other hand, the systemic inflammatory response is an abnormal host reaction/ response characterized by general inflammation in organs remote from the primary/ initial cell injury/cell invasion/cell death.

Simultaneously with the activation of the complement, certain proteins in the plasma (such as the mannose-binding protein and C-reactive protein – the "acute phase proteins") increase dramatically in concentration in response to early 'alarm' mediators, such as the cytokines interleukin-1, interleukin-6 and tumour necrosis factor, that are released as a result of infection or tissue injury. As acute phase protein reactants have defensive roles to fulfill, they use pattern recognition receptors to bind to the molecular patterns on the pathogen, generating defensive effector functions at the same time. Also helping with the defense against the invading pathogen, are the different mechanisms of many other extracellular antimicrobial factors. The extracellular microbial agent lysozyme, that operate at short range within the phagocytic cells and which also appear in various body fluids in sufficient concentrations, for example, has a direct inhibitory effect on the infecting pathogen. Similarly, lactoferrin appears in the blood in sufficient concentration to complex iron depriving microbes of this important growth factor.

When body cells are infected with a virus, the body cells synthesize and secrete interferon (a family of broad spectrum antiviral molecules such as the different alpha interferon [IFNα] produced by leukocytes, the different beta interferon [IFNβ] produced by fibroblasts and all cell types, and interferon-gamma [INFγ] produced by T-lymphocytes) which bind to receptors on nearby uninfected cells. The bound interferon exert their antiviral effect by facilitating the synthesis of two new enzymes which interferes with the machinery used by the virus for its own replication while setting up a cordon of infection-resistant cells around the site of the virus infection, thus restraining its spread. Interferon *per se*, plays an important role in the recovery of viral infection/disease rather than the prevention of viral infections. Because viruses have to penetrate the body cells of an infected host in order to subvert the cells' replicative machinery towards viral replication, the body has evolved Natural Killer cells to kill off the specific virus before it has had a chance to reproduce. Natural Killer cells, large granular lymphocytes, are cytotoxic cells that attach themselves by lectin-like receptors to structures on the surface of the virally infected cells and allow them to be differentiated from normal cells. When attachment had taken place, the Natural Killer cell is activated to release its extra-cellular granular content into the space between the target and effector cells. The granular content include perforin molecules that are inserted into the membrane of the virally infected cells and polymerize to form annular membrane pores that permits entry of another granular protein, granzyme B, resulting in the death of the virally infected cells by apoptosis (programmed cell death) - a process mediated by a cascade of proteolytic enzymes, termed caspases, which terminates with the ultimate fragmentation of the DNA of the pathogen by a Ca-dependant endonuclease. Another mode of cytotoxicity is the direct "burning" of the surface of the viral infected cell by the respiratory oxygen bursts that is turned on by the activated macrophages involved by means of a stream of reactive oxygen intermediaries that are produced at the macrophage's membrane. The net end result is the death of the virally infected cell because of damage to the cell's membrane.

Because phagocytes are too small to physically engulf large parasites such as helminths (worms), the body has evolved a more appropriate form of defence by killing through another extracellular form carried out by eosinophils. Eosinophils, polymorphonuclear relatives of the neutrophils, contain distinctive cytoplasmic granules and a characteristic ultra-structural appearance. A major basic protein is contained in the core of the granule while the matrix contains an eosinophilia cationic protein, a peroxidase and a perforin-like molecule. Eosinophils have surface receptors for C3b complement and when activated, generate copious amounts of active oxygen metabolites. As many helminths activate the complement via the alternative pathway, although resistant to C9 attack, their (the helminths) coating with C3b allows adherence to the eosinophils through their C3b-surface receptors. The eosinophils, once activated, launch their extracellular ammunition which includes the release of major basic proteins and cationic protein to damage the helminths' membrane; "chemical burning" by the oxygen metabolites; and "leaky pore"-formation by the perforin – the net result leading to the death of the macro-parasite.

5.1.2 The adaptive physiologic immunological defence mechanism – the specific immunologic memory response

Although primary contact with a specific antigen activates both the innate and the adaptive immune systems, the adaptive immune system is only activated when an infectious pathogen bypasses and overwhelms the innate immune system and spreads through the body or is encountered a second time (see figure 5.3). As infectious pathogens frequently find ways around the innate defences of the body, the lymphocyte-based adaptive immune system provides defences that are "tailor-made" to each individual variant of the different species of microbes, namely, T-lymphocytes that differentiate in T-helper cells [T_H-cells] and cytotoxic T-cells [T_C-cells] and B-immunocytes that mediate antibody (immunoglobulin molecules) – a soluble factor. Antibody specifically binds to antigens (proteins) on the foreign/infective pathogen, followed by a secondary binding to other cells or molecules of the innate immune system such as phagocytes and complement. T-lymphocytes, the second main component of the adaptive immune response, produce cytokines (the hormones of the adaptive immune system) that induce the activation of macrophages; help with antibody production and direct their cytotoxic action on infected intracellular target cells (viruses and other intracellular microbes). Although it takes time for the adaptive immune system to reach it maximum efficiency, the antibody and T-lymphocytes generally eliminates the infective pathogen, allowing recovery from the infection/ disease. The adaptive/specific physiologic immunological response as such greatly strengthens the innate physiologic resistance/immunity of the body as the adaptive physiologic immunological response forms specific immunologic memory cells to the specific infectious agent during the response. Thus, the adaptive physiologic resistance (acquired immunity) protects the body against a subsequent infection by the same specific infectious pathogen as the body has developed an immunological antibody-mediated and cell-mediated resistance with memory to the specific infectious agent. Because the specific memory of the infectious pathogen is imprinted on the adaptive immune system, the particularly/specifically effective response comes into play with remarkable speed and a faster and stronger immunological response is elicited when a subsequent infection by the same pathogen occurs. Therefore, the adaptive immune response is a homeostatic mechanism that protects the body against any subsequent invasion of a specific infectious pathogen.

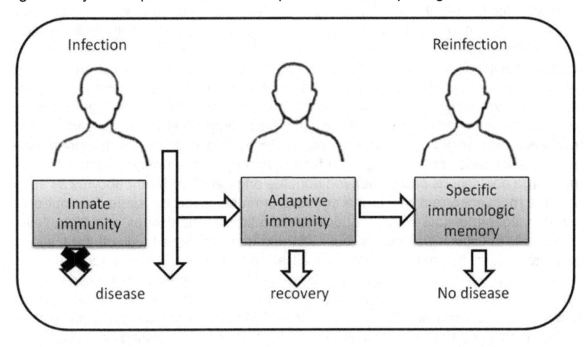

Figure 5.3   Schematic presentation of the integration or symbiosis of the innate and adaptive immune systems.

The adaptive immune response is generated by lymphocytes which are derived from stem cells differentiating within the germinal centres of the primary lymphoid organs (bone marrow and thymus).   From the bone marrow and thymus, the lymphocytes colonize the secondary lymphoid tissue such as the lymph nodes, spleen, and mucosa-associated lymphoid tissues. The lymph nodes are concerned with responses to antigens/pathogens that are carried into them from the body tissue, while the spleen is primarily concerned with antigens that reach the spleen from the bloodstream.   Communication between these lymphoid tissues and rest of the body is maintained by a pool of re-circulating lymphocytes which pass from the blood into the lymph nodes, spleen and other tissues and then back to the blood by the major lymphatic channels such as the thoracic duct.   This circulating of lymphocytes between the tissues, the bloodstream and the lymph nodes enables antigen-sensitive cells, namely, T-lymphocytes (mediating cytokines) and B-immunocytes (mediating antibody) to seek out the antigen/pathogen and to be recruited to sites where the acute inflammatory response is taking place.   In addition, un-encapsulated aggregates of lymphoid tissues, the "mucosa-associated lymphoid tissue" (MALT), lie in the mucosal surface where they respond to antigens from the environment, particularly the heavy bacterial load in the intestine, by producing IgA-antibody for mucosal secretions.   The lymphocytes which constitute the un-encapsulated aggregates of lymphoid tissues and the "mucosa-associated lymphoid tissue" system re-circulate between these mucosal tissues using specialized homing receptors.

The lymphocytes involved in the adaptive immune response are the T-lymphocytes and the B-lymphocytes. Both the T-lymphocytes and the B-lymphocytes are derived from stem cells (S-cells) differentiating within the germinal centres of the primary lymphoid organ, namely, the bone marrow in long bones, from where the differentiated stem cells are disseminated to either the thymus gland to mediate T-lymphocytes or to certain other lymphoid organs that mediate B-lymphocytes, after which cell proliferation by means of clonally expansion takes place. A small number of T-lymphocytes are potently activated by the antigens of intracellular pathogens (when the T-lymphocytes recognize and bind to molecules of the major histocompatibility complex and peptide that were derived from the intracellular pathogen) to clonally expand/proliferate under the influence of soluble growth factors and cytokines (immune hormones) to form large populations of cells derived from the original. The T-lymphocytes as such play the most important role in the adaptive immune response since they not only act as antigen-monitors when continuously scrutinizing the tissues on cellular level for specific infectious pathogens, but also help macrophages to kill off intracellular parasites within the macrophage as well as inhibiting intracellular replication of viruses. The B-lymphocytes are also stimulated for cloning by certain antigens that combine/bind through their components to only those B-lymphocytes whose surface receptors are complementary to the shape of these specific antigens, as well as by other antigens that are polyclonal activators for the stimulating and cloning of B-lymphocytes without the need for intervention by T-lymphocytes. Thus, under the influence of cytokines, soluble growth factors and intercellular communication factors, B-lymphocytes proliferate clonally to form large populations of cells derived from the original. Because the B-lymphocytes are programmed to mediate only antibody (IgA, IgD, IgE, IgG , and IgM) with the same specificity as it surface receptor, the antibody produced by B-lymphocytes are antigen-specific and can only be directed against the epitope on the antigen recognised by the B-lymphocyte surface receptor. A fraction of the clonally expanded population of both the B-lymphocytes and T-lymphocytes differentiate into resting memory cells with specificity (for example, memory cells with specificity for the measles-virus will not afford protection against an unrelated virus such as the mumps-virus).

The adaptive physiologic immunological response, as such, complex three processes, namely,

❖ the ability of the body to recognise an antigen (the specific infectious agent)
❖ the ability of the body (after recognition of the antigen) to produce specific antibody which are capable of destroying the specific infectious agent
❖ the ability to produce dormant long-living memory cells with specificity that retains their function to divide and re-activate should the same specific infectious agent gains entry into the body again.

As soon as an infectious agent gains entry into the body by penetrating the non-specific defence barriers of the body, the body recognises the specific infectious agent as an antigen. The innate immune system is immediately activated to kill off the infective pathogen through phagocytosis by phagocytes, extracellular killing by natural killer cells, and the activation and synergizing of the complement system, acute phase proteins and other factors. Should the body not succeed in killing off the infectious agent at this stage, the adaptive immune system is activated to eliminate the infective pathogen to allow recovery to take place. When the infective pathogen overwhelms the innate immune system, the infectious agent does not only destroy the tissue cells, but simultaneously penetrates the circulatory system to spread through the rest of the body (see figure 5.4).

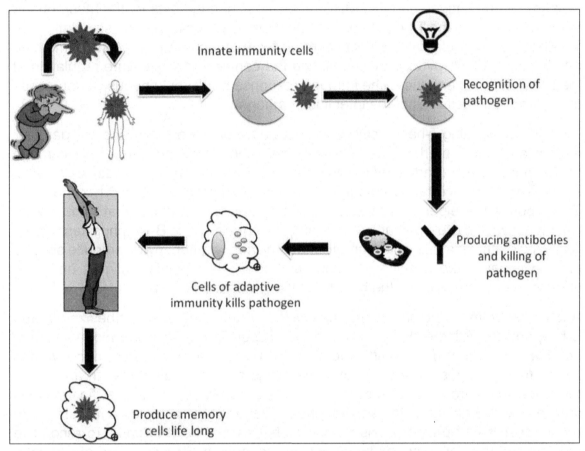

Figure 5.4   Schematic presentation of the immune response by the adaptive immune system

Immediately after the innate immune system is activated, the lymphocytes, in particular the T-lymphocytes, summon the phagocytes, the monocytes, neutrophils and the macrophages to the infected tissue cells. Both the phagocytes and the proteins in reticulo-endothelial cells now secrete several chemical substances, namely, histamine and lymphokines which bring about specific haemodynamic changes to ensure that large numbers of defenders of the innate immune system (phagocytes, macrophages and lymphocytes) reach the infected tissue cells. These chemical substances also enhance the enzyme actions of the macrophages.

Apart from the secretion of these chemical substances, the macrophages also phagocytise and process the infectious agent. After processing, the macrophages reflect in the grooves of the protein-like molecules that form the major histocompatibility complex (MHC) of the macrophages, parts of the assimilated proteins of the infectious pathogen. The protein-like molecules of the major histocompatibility complex then indicate whether the infectious pathogen is friend or foe. As soon as the protein of the infectious pathogen is reflected on the MHC of the macrophages, the macrophages move from the body tissue to the lymph glands where the T-helper cells (T_H1 and T_H2) are always present. When a macrophage and a compatible T-helper cell (T_H-cells) meet, the antigen-carrying MHC molecule is handed over by the macrophage to the receptors on the T-helper cell. Interleuken-1, a specific protein stimulating the T-helper cells to proliferate, is now secreted by the macrophage. At the same time Interleuken-1 elicits pyrexia by stimulating the centre for temperature regulation of the body. Pyrexia enhances the immune response and simultaneously suppresses the proliferating activities of the infectious pathogen.

The fast proliferating T-helper cells now secrete lymphokines which include gamma-inferon and other interleukins. These lymphokines stimulate further proliferation of the phagocytes (particularly macrophages) and the reticulo-endothelial cells. At the same time certain T-helper cells attach themselves to the B-lymphocytes. These bonded T-helper cells secrete specific chemical substances that stimulate the B-lymphocytes to grow fast and proliferate. The proliferating B-lymphocytes quickly grow into mature plasma cells, namely immunocytes. Immunocytes produce specific antibody against the specific infectious pathogen (the specific antigen) and then release these antibody into the blood and the lymphatic system.

Antibodies or immunoglobulin are specialized proteins that are synthesized by the B-lymphocytes with the ability to recognise the specific infectious pathogen and then bond with it so that the specific infectious pathogen can be easier phagocytosed by the macrophages. The antibody molecule is of a multivalent design and multi-functional in nature as it possesses different sites specialized for specific functions such as the recognition of the antigen, the activation of the complement system and the inducement of phagocytosis by macrophages and polymorphs. To recognize the antigen, the antibody has two identical recognition sites made up of a unique amino acid sequence for recognition of the antigen specificities/specifications and a shape that is complementary to the surface of the foreign antigen as to enable the antibody to bind to the specific pathogen/antigen. Instantaneous recognition by the amino acid sequence in the complementary-determining regions occurs the moment the recognition sites (or complementary determining regions) of the antibody has made the first complementary contact with the antigen. Activating of the complement system immediately follows recognition whereby the antibody coats the antigen with the adaptor antibody molecules, namely, antibody IgA or IgD or IgE or Ig or IgM - antibody molecules with the same specificity as its surface receptor. As soon as coating of the infective pathogen with several adaptor antibody molecules had taken place, fixating/complexing/bonding of the complement adaptor antibody molecules happens enabling the antibody to bind with varying degrees of strength to the specific pathogen/antigen. Fixating/complexing/bonding is immediately followed up with inducing of phagocytosis via the classical complement pathway causing the killing off or inactivation of the antigen by macrophages and polymorphs. As such, antibody or immunoglobulin (Ig) helps to destroy the specific infectious agent or inactivate it by

- complexing/binding with the antigen whereby the resulting complex activates the first component of the complement C1. This sets the classical pathway in motion whereby the activation of the enzyme cascade of the complement system is triggered. When antibody IgE complex with microbial antigens, a signal to the interior of the mast cells is transduce (the surface receptors of IgE are cross-linked to specific receptors on the surface of mast cells), signalling the mast cells to release their mediators whereby vascular permeability is increased and polymorph chemotaxis is induced

- neutralising its toxic properties by blocking microbial reactions such as attachment, uptake of nutrients, cell damaging

- making it more vulnerable to phagocytosis when the backbone portions of certain antibody molecules in the antigen-antibody–complex bind to specialized backbone receptors on the surface of the phagocytic cells. When there is more than one antibody in the antigen-antibody–complex, these receptors are cross-linked as to induce the phagocytic cells to put out arms of cytoplasm which enclose the complex in a phagocytic vacuole

- causing it to precipitate through lysis and opsonisation when antibody and complement act together whereby the rate of phagocytosis is thousand-fold enhances

- causing it to agglutinate by the physically attachment of antibody to the antigen(s) and coating of the antigen with several adaptor antibody molecules that then induces complement fixation and phagocytosis.

While the before mentioned process takes place, certain T-helper cells start forming T-killer cells. The T-killer cells bond with the infected tissue cells as the infected tissue cells also reflect tiny particles of the specific infectious agent's protein on their outer cell walls. The T-killer cells destroy the outer cell wall of the infected tissue cells with perforin (a protein-like substance) resulting in the leaking out of the content of the pathogen-cell, causing the infected tissue cells to die off. To ensure that the infected tissue cells die off completely, the T-killer cells release a chemical substance, which stimulates the infected tissue cells to phagocytise their own DNA as well as the DNA of the specific infectious agent. As soon as the specific infectious pathogen has been killed off in this manner, the immune response is inhibited under the influence of the T-suppressor cells [T_S-cells]. The immune cycle is completed when memory cells with specificity have been formed. The immune reaction now settles down. To avoid reaction against the body's own components, the immune system have developed tolerance mechanisms to prevent immunological self-reactivity through eliminating auto-reactive self molecules by some form of clonally deletion, making auto-reactive self molecules anergic (prevent maturation) early in their cell life, or silencing (inactivating) them by T-regulatory cells [T_R-cells] in later life.

While the immune response is still active, a fraction of the clonally expanded population of both the T-lymphocytes and B-lymphocytes differentiate into resting memory cells with specificity that circulates in the bloodstream and the lymphatic system for years to come. These dormant memory cells are more capable of recognizing the specific pathogen and are more readily stimulated and activated by the specific infectious agent should it again gains entry into the body. After recognition, a stronger and faster specific physiologic immunological response is activated against the specific infectious agent, resulting in an attack on and killing off of the specific infective pathogen. Specialised memory cells of the formed antibody are also present in the body's mucous membranes, saliva and tears, in order to protect the body against any further entry of the specific infectious pathogen. It takes a healthy immune system (immune competent immune system) between three and six weeks to complete the immune response. The body is now immune to the specific infective pathogen. Should subsequent exposure to the same specific infectious agent occur, reactivation or a secondary reaction take place and a faster, stronger and more lasting immune response is elicited.

Two types of physiological immunological reactions are mediated by the adaptive immune system, namely the antibody-mediated reaction and the cell-mediated reaction. The antibody-mediated and cell-mediated reactions take place simultaneously and complement each other.

- ❖ **Antibody-mediated immune reaction**
  The antibody-mediated immune reaction results in the circulating of immunocytes that mediate antibody or immunoglobulin (soluble factors) that were formed by the body in reaction to the entry of a specific pathogen into the body. The memory cells with specificity of the antibody are present in the blood and the lymph and circulate in the body for life. The circulating immunoglobulin is subdivided into five main groups, namely IgA, IgE, IgG, IgM and IgO. Each of these main groups has a specific structure with a specific function. IgG forms approximately 75% of the total number of immunoglobulin in the body and protects it against bacteria, viruses and toxins. The memory cells **are able to cross** the placenta barrier.

- ❖ **Cell-mediated immune reaction**
  During the immune response some infectious agents do not stimulate the body to an antibody-mediated immune reaction, but stimulate the immune system to mediate/produce T-lymphocytes with lymphocytic properties. These sensitised T-lymphocytes do not secrete antibody, but reject the specific infectious pathogen by making direct contact with the specific pathogen and destroying its cell. Although the sensitised T-lymphocytes originate simultaneously with the antibody, they function without the support of the immunoglobulin. These sensitised T-lymphocytes also produce memory cells with specificity but the latter (the memory cells) **cannot** cross the placenta barrier.

5.1.3 Eliciting of the adaptive immune response by a communicable disease or through vaccination

The body of any individual who had contracted and recovered from a specific communicable disease (excluded those communicable infections that elicit no immunity with memory), has naturally and actively elicited the antibody-mediated and/or cell-mediated physiological immunological reactions and this immune response with memory is permanent and last lifelong. When a person is vaccinated, an active-artificially immune response is elicited, though the person does not necessarily manifest the specific signs or symptoms of the disease. After vaccination, the immune status of the body is initially high but diminishes with time (after 5 to 12 years the artificial actively-acquired immunological response has diminished more or less all together). As a consequence of this diminished immune status, the individual becomes susceptible and can then contract the disease again (although in a lighter form). When the person now recovers from the disease, his/her body has naturally and actively elicited the antibody-mediated and/or cell-mediated immune reaction, which then last for life. (Booster doses are no longer needed.) Should the vaccinated person want to maintain a high immune status, he/she should have booster doses (for the purpose of further stimulation of the immune system by the specific attenuated living or non-living infectious agent or its toxoid).

Note

A large group of communicable diseases, such as all sexually transmitted infections, some zoonotic infections and all parasitaemia caused by helminths, do not elicit an immune response with memory in the body at all. These diseases can be contracted more than once and the person will manifest the specific clinical picture of the particular disease every time (regardless the severity of the disease).

5.1.4 Infections in the immuno-defected or immuno-deficient or immuno-compromised host

Immuno-compromised hosts are individuals who have one or more defects in their body's natural defences against microbial invaders. Consequently, they are more liable to suffer from severe and life-threatening infections. The numbers of immuno-compromised persons are increasing due to modern medicine and treatment modalities such as organ transplantations, new and improved chemotherapies, etc. Persons can become immuno-compromised in many different ways and the immunodeficiency can take a variety of forms. Immunodeficiency can be classified into two main groups, namely, defects (accidental or intentional) in the body's defence mechanisms (innate and adaptive) and deficiencies in the adaptive immune response. Immunodeficiency can further be sub-classified as 'primary' or 'secondary'. Primary immunodeficiency is inherited or occurs by exposure in uteri to environmental factors or by other unknown mechanisms and varies in severity depending upon the type of defect. Secondary or acquired immunodeficiency is due to an underlying disease state or occurs as a result of treatment of a disease.

The primary defects of the innate immunity include congenital defects in phagocytic cells or complement synthesis and as such confer susceptibility to infection. Secondary defects of the innate defences include disruption of the body's mechanical non-specific protective barriers to infection, for example, damage sustained in the continuity of the skin with poor vascularised tissue near the body surface provide a relatively defenceless site for microbes to colonize and invade when burns, traumatic injury and major surgery occur. Foreign bodies in the body alter the local non-specific host responses and provide surfaces that microbes can colonize more readily than normal equivalents. The causes of secondary adaptive immuno-deficiency include malnutrition, infections, neoplasia, splenectomy and certain medical treatments, for example, Cortisone drugs, radiotherapy for cancer.

Immuno-compromised individuals can become infected not only with any pathogen able to infect non-compromised persons, but also with opportunist pathogens, namely, microbes that are incapable of causing disease in a healthy person, but able to infect immuno-compromised individuals when their immune defences are lowered, often with fatal consequences. The different types of immune defects predispose the host to different infections with different pathogens, depending upon the critical mechanisms of the immune systems operating in the defence against each specific infectious pathogen. Infections of the host with deficient innate immunity due to physical factors, for example, burn wounds, are mostly aerobic and facultative anaerobic bacteria and fungi. In traumatic injury and surgical wound infections, *Staphylococcus aureus* is the most important cause of infection as well as in catheter-associated infections. *Staphylococcus epidermidis* is the cause of infections of plastic devices in situ. Infections also occur if the clearance mechanisms of the body are compromised, for example, damage of the ciliary escalator in the respiratory tract predisposes the lungs to invasion. The underlying immunodeficiency state determines the nature and severity of infections associated with secondary adaptive immunodeficiency and in some cases, infection is the first/prime presenting clinical feature in an individual with an immunological deficit. Bacteria (Gram-positive and Gram-negative), fungi, parasites and viruses are opportunistic pathogens in neutropenic individuals and organ transplant recipients. Individuals suffering from AIDS are often infected concomitantly with multiple pathogens. Most of the pathogens involved are intracellular microbes that require an intact cell-mediated immune response for effective defence. As the immunodeficiency deepens, pathogens that are usually controlled by cell-mediated immunity reactivate to cause disseminated infections not seen in immunological healthy/competent individuals. Effective antimicrobial therapy is often difficult to achieve in immuno-compromised individuals because of the absence of a functional immune response, even when the pathogen is susceptible to the drug in situ.

5.1.5　Factors that alter the body's defence mechanisms

Several factors alter (enhance or compromise/impair) the normal defence mechanisms of the body. These factors must always be considered in order to optimally promote and maintain the person's health and physiologic resistance/immunity (humoral/innate and specific/adaptive).

5.1.5.1　Factors situated in the environment

* **The growing of food** in terms of agrobiodiversity, traditional crops and food provision is not the only purpose of agriculture (though being the most important supplier of food and essential nutrients as well as a source of income and employment and an engine of growth) but at a deeper level it encompasses the growing of healthy, well-nourished individuals, families and communities as well as the prevention of diseases. Whatever happens in the agricultural sector has far reaching and long lasting implications for the health and nutrition

of all individuals, families and communities. As such, when economic and related crisis exist the local, national and global food supply system comes under pressure leading to a local, regional, national and/or global food crisis. Not only does the prize of food increase but food and nutritional security can be drastically reduced leading to a decline in diet quality, diet quantity, and diet variety. These shocks lead to nutritional insults (malnutrition and hidden hunger [micro-nutrient deficiencies]) that have a negative effect on all persons affected, especially infants and children, with effects that can last through generations.

* **Climate changes**, namely, changes in the characteristics such as temperature, humidity, rainfall, wind, and severe weather events together with all consequences in a specific region, as such influence not only the world food supply negatively (in quantity and in quality [both energy and nutrients] as well as in dietary variety) but also has implications for the sustainability and security of the global food supply as changes have to be made in agricultural, animal husbandry, and aquatic (fishery) practices. Furthermore, millions of individuals are displaced as a direct result of these changes in global weather patterns and the compliant changes in agricultural, animal husbandry and aquatic practices lead to poverty and a food crisis (a small to no food supply at all). And in so far that health, food, and water are intimately linked to nutritional well-being, climate changes have direct and indirect influence on the well-being of all humans - especially on displaced or impoverished individuals - as humans start to suffer from hunger as well as hidden hunger (vitamin-mineral deficiencies) that may be felt for decades. (Hidden hunger is largely invisible to human senses as it is often only detected through the presence of its effects or symptoms because hidden huger impairs the physiological immunity of individuals, reduces work productivity or school performance as well as slowing down the cognitive development and growth of the individual. An impaired physiological immunity leads to an increase in bodily infections and other medical diseases which in turn induce nutrient losses because of a reduced appetite as well as furthering the vulnerability of children, mothers and women in general).

* **All agricultural practices**, all animal husbandry practices and all fishery practices directly affect the sustainability of the food supply system globally or of a specific country or a specific region in as much that the diet quality, diet quantity and diet variety of the populations of the world or of the specific country or of the specific region can decline or be improved. The implementation globally of biofortification and climatic resilient food products in agricultural-based programmes during plant breeding to prevent micro-nutrient malnutrition as well as the food-fortification programmes in the food industry to prevent protein-energy-malnutrition (PEM) and micro-nutrient malnutrition can improve and enhance the health of the populations of the world/country/region.

* **The planting of homestead/backyard gardens and the use of permaculture watering practices** (using of grey water like bath water and washing water - not toilet water) as well as practicing organic plant breeding (including climatic resilient plant breeding) and bio-friendly aquatic ecological techniques in fish

breeding can ensure the availability of healthy foods (including micronutrient-dense food choices) while protecting the environment. (Note Organically and conventionally produced foods are comparable in nutrient content as the biological differences detected are due to differences in fertilizer use, namely, the use of organic and/or inorganic fertilizers).

* **Food preparation methods** that conserve nutrients such as steaming and/ or baking when preparing raw food must be facilitated in all households to enhance the immunological system of the individual while overcooking and the frying of foods need to be discouraged (occasional frying is however not excluded).

* **Changes in food handling practices** such as deep-freezing, fast-foods and inadequate cooking allow bacteria and toxins to enter the body.

* **Any factor in the environment**, regardless being physical, biological, psycho-emotional socio-cultural, economical, technological, industrial, agricultural, legal, political etc., that negatively effects the health status of individuals, greatly impairs or compromises the immune systems (innate and adaptive) of the affected individuals while enhancing the chances of contracting communicable diseases.

* **Tourism and modern transport systems** can spread diseases easily and quickly from one continent to another or from one region to another or from one person to another person/group of persons. Examples are the outbreak of Avian Influenza in Asia and Swine Influenza in Mexico that was carried to Africa by individuals who were exposed to the specific virus in the specific country and then travelled by air to South Africa.

* **Civil unrest and guerrilla wars** lead to the displacement of thousands of individuals from their natural homes and environment and their placement in refugee camps. The stresses they experience not only compromise the immunological resistance of these individuals, but being crowded together in circumstances such as poor environmental hygienic conditions, facilitate the rapid spread of communicable diseases.

* **Poverty**, whether in rural or urban areas, is directly linked to poor nutrition and health problems throughout the lifespan, resulting in the impairment of the immune system of an individual and a higher chance to contract communicable diseases. Furthermore, girls and female adults who are poor and are also poorly nourished often fail to develop properly - a state that impairs foetal development when they become mothers and whereby the cycle of ill health is perpetuated for generations to come.

* Although the **causes of death** in industrialized countries have changed to cancer, ischemic heart disease and cerebral vascular incidents, affluent individuals, because of their sedimentary lifestyle, overeating and changed food habits, increasingly suffer from vitamin and mineral deficiency syndromes as an excess of calories does not imply adequate nutrition on macro-nutrient and micro-nutrient level. Thus, because a strong relationship exists between nutritional deprivation (macro- and micro-nutrient) and poor health, the

immunological defence system of many affluent individuals is compromised whereby they become more vulnerable to contract communicable diseases.

* **Importation of goods** between countries causes vectors to be spread from one region to another; for instance, the import of rethreaded tyres to South Africa brought the mosquito, the vector for yellow fever, into the country.

* **Droughts** followed by high rainfall in areas where malaria has a high incidence, cause a proliferation of all mosquito populations (including the vector for malaria). The normal preventive and control measures may become insufficient with the result that the incidence rate of malaria increases drastically.

* **Immigration** - an increase in immigrants (particularly illegal immigrants) can be a reason for the spread of communicable diseases between regions, for example, Tuberculosis.

* The **exploration of unknown/uninhabitable regions and tourism** to these areas such as the tropical and subtropical forests of Africa and South America exposes people to unknown pathogenic microbes, for example, the Ebola virus (a virus of unknown origin). When infected persons from these areas come into contact with other individuals, epidemics quickly develop.

* Because there exist **an integrated relationship between parasitic infection and malnutrition** (in macro- and micro-nutrients), parasitic infections (particularly soil transmitted helminthic infections) in children, adults and the elderly must be prevented as the normal development, the functioning of the immune system, and the life performance of parasitized individuals are significantly negatively affected.

5.1.5.2   Factors related to the host

The factors related to the host can be divided in factors influencing the immune systems (innate and adaptive) and factors influencing the natural defence barriers.

5.1.5.2.1   Factors that enhance or impair the immune system (innate and adaptive) of an individual

❖ **Age**
Infants and young children are more susceptible than adults to communicable diseases because of the immaturity of their immunological system (innate and adaptive) which negatively influence the ability of the lymphoid system to react to infectious agents. Due to the presence of maternally–derived antibody, the effectiveness of some vaccines is reduced when infants younger than three (3) month is vaccinated. The introduction of antigens from the vaccines into the developing immune system of an infant may also have profound effects beyond the induction of a specific immunity, for example, BCG vaccination which induces T_H1 T-cell-immunity, may affect the T_H1 and T_H2 cytokine balance which may make the infant prone to other diseases. When many different types of vaccines are simultaneously administered, overloading of the infant's or young child's immune system may takes place, resulting in a sub-optimal level of immunity to a specific antigen. Because the immune system of all premature (preterm) infants (regardless of being a medically stable preterm baby or a baby of low birth weight or a baby with a birth weight less than

2000g) is very immature, their immune system is not always able to induce an immunity response to a specific antigen administered by vaccination.

The activity of the immune system of an **elderly person** usually slows down, causing the general physiological resistance of the body to become compromised. Age-related changes detrimental to the immune system include changes in the indigenous microbiotical population of the intestinal mucosa, involution of the thymus gland, poor response to evolving pathogens and newly encountered antigens as well as an increased in auto-immunity diseases and inflammation. Regarding the innate immune system, when aging, the functionality of macrophage chemotaxis, phagocytosis, cytokine production and the bone marrow population of stem/virgin cells are compromised. In general, the ability of the macrophages to fight infection becomes impaired and there is deregulation of the molecules the macrophages produce while the production of prostaglandin E_2 (an inflammatory molecule that suppress T-cell function) increases in aged individuals. Other age-related changes that simultaneously take place involve the neutrophils (neutrophils phagocytosis as well as the production of hydrogen peroxide and superoxide become impaired), the eosinophils, the mast cells and the Natural Killer cells. The age-related changes in the skin affect the macrophages that are part of the defence barrier of the skin, in as much that the function of the macrophages is altered leading to increased colonization of bacteria and yeast on the skin and on mucosal surfaces. Wound repair is also affected because of delayed macrophage infiltration and function. As this age-related changes cause delayed symptom manifestation and diagnosis of infection, disease is exacerbated. Although the number of peripheral B-cells and secreted immunoglobulin levels stay constant with aging, the production of naïve/ virgin B-cell lymphocytes is impaired together with less affinity of antibodies to antigen and a higher production of auto-antibodies – all resulting in a physiological state of reduced responsiveness to newly encountered antigens. The immune senescence of the adaptive immune system also affects the T-cells as the production of naïve/virgin T-cell lymphocytes is impaired due to the thymic involution that is taking place while the number of memory T-cells increases. This imbalance leads to a decreased response to new antigens. Additionally, the number and function of CD4 T-helper cells decline while the CD8 cytotoxic effector lymphocytes have a reduced intensity in their response with less production of interferon-gamma during viral infections. In general, the age-associated immunological changes predispose the elderly individual to a higher incidence of communicable infections. In addition, the passage of especially viral antigens through an elderly host can result in several mutations of the virus with increased virulence, leading to a higher susceptibility to infection. If the elderly person also suffers from malnutrition (especially hidden hunger/micro-nutrient malnutrition and protein-energy-malnutrition) the consequences of communicable infections such as nutrient mal-absorption, nutrient and energy store loss and reduced appetite can become life threatening leading to death.

❖ **Nutrition** - Because we are what we eat, good nutrition (in both macro-nutrients [proteins, carbohydrate, fats and fibre] and micro-nutrients [vitamins and minerals]) enhances the general physiological resistance of an individual. Malnutrition in its many forms (whether being apparently well-fed, or under-fed [malnourished], or over-fed [obesity] or suffering from hidden hunger [micro-nutrient malnutrition]) renders the person more susceptible to infections. Consumption of a low protein diet impairs the immune system while a high consumption of folate lowers the absorption of minerals. The consumption of food of low nutritional quality leads to a higher incidence of communicable disease as well as obesity. Vitamin A-deficiency leads to small epithelial lacerations which facilitate the entry of pathogenic microbes into the body. A deficiency in Biotin (a B-group vitamin) and vitamin C increase the body's susceptibility to infections. Deficiency in vitamin C and Zinc correlates with an impaired ability of immune cells to produce interferon-gamma. A deficiency in vitamin D plays a role in the deregulation of the immune response. Vitamin E-deficiency increases upper respiratory tract infections such as the common cold and pneumonia. A deficiency in Zinc leads to a weak immunological response of both the innate and the adaptive immune systems as the zinc deficiency leads to the atrophy of the thymus gland. Selenium-deficiency result in greater pathogenesis in a malnourished host and this individual could potentially transmit a more severe disease to others. The body's inability to produce interleukin-2 by immune cells correlates with a deficiency in iron (leading to iron deficiency anaemia) whiles a deficiency in iodine results in an impaired health status that negatively influence the immune system.

❖ **Obesity** - Obesity is the product of a poor life style as well as the product of poor food choices. The immune system of an obese person becomes compromised because of a low-grade chronic inflammation state caused by hypoxia in white adipose or fat tissue. This state of low-grade chronic inflammation results in macrophage infiltration of the adipose tissue that leads to increased circulating concentrations of pro-inflammatory molecules which include acute phase proteins (elevated C-reactive proteins), cytokines, adipokines and chemokines as these pro-inflammatory factors are predominantly produced by the enlarged adipocytes and activated macrophages in the adipose tissue and the liver. Glucose intolerance and insulin resistance leading to diabetes and other metabolic syndromes can now directly be induced. Furthermore, these pro-inflammatory factors act also as "alarm signals" for triggering the adipocytes to promote the acute phase inflammation process. Because of the state of the low-grade chronic inflammation in the obese person, the production of hepcidin in the liver is up-regulated (100-fold higher than in the adipocytes) leading to a disturbance in the regulation of iron metabolism by blocking iron absorption and re-utilization. The adipose lipocalin-2 expression is also increased by inflammatory cytokines interleukin-1 and tumour necrosis factor-2 resulting in higher iron requirements in obese persons. An iron-deficiency or iron-anaemia now develops because of elevated transferring receptor concentrations and a state of hypoferremia. A Vitamin D-deficiency is also related to a high body fat index resulting in non-skeletal consequences that play a role in the deregulation of the immune response.

❖ **Chronic degenerative medical diseases** - Persons suffering from chronic degenerative medical conditions such as diabetes mellitus, hypothyroidism and adrenal dysfunction have a compromised physiological resistance against infections. Any chronic illness of the kidneys, liver and gastro-intestinal tract leads to a negative nitrogen balance, which in its turn leads to a diminished physiological resistance as proteins are necessary for producing leucocytes and antibody. Alcoholism and chronic neurological illnesses (due to taking medication over a long period) also compromises the individual's resistance.

❖ **The immune status of persons who were vaccinated** diminishes with the passing of years if no booster doses have been given or if the person was not exposed to the specific infectious pathogen causing the particular disease. Regular booster doses strengthen a person's physiologic resistance to a particular communicable disease. Should the specific living infectious agent or the toxin of the specific infectious pathogen be weakened too much during the process of preparation of the vaccine, it cannot elicit an immune response in the body and the person is then susceptible to that particular disease. Regarding live attenuated vaccines, it sometimes happens that the specific infectious agent does not die off during the preparation process of the vaccine. Consequently, when the specific live infectious agent is administered to the person, the person may become seriously ill. When instructions for the cold chain and the procedures concerning storage, transport, handling, reconstituting, and administering are not executed to the letter, the specific infectious agent in the vaccine can die off. Consequently, no physiological immunological response is elicited although the person has been vaccinated.

❖ **The administering of immune-suppressive chemotherapy** (corticosteroids) suppresses the inflammation reaction as well as the cell-mediated immune response, resulting in the compromising of the immune systems (innate and adaptive) to such an extent that any exposure to pathogens leads to disease (despite previous physiologic resistance having been built up) because the general physiologic resistance of the individual is extremely low. Any disease which suppresses the immune system, such as AIDS, renders the person more susceptible to communicable diseases.

❖ **Certain racial groups** who have been exposed for generations to a particular communicable disease, such as tuberculosis, **develop a natural physiologic resistance** to the infectious pathogen causing the particular disease (excluded are the drug-resistant strains of the specific pathogen).

5.1.5.2.2   Factors that enhance or compromise the natural defence barriers of the body

✓ **Chemo-therapeutic drugs**
- Medicines that dry up the mucous membranes, such as antihistamine, compromise the resistance of the mucous membranes to such an extent that pathogenic microbes quickly gain entry into the body
- The intestinal flora plays an important role in the protection against infections and the normal defence actions of the immune system (innate and adaptive). Oral antibiotics/anti-microbial drugs destroy the intestinal flora to the extent that fungi, such as Candida Albicans, gain the upper hand and cause a fungal infection in the intestinal tract. It is therefore necessary to take preparations, such as Probiotics, when oral antimicrobial drugs have been prescribed or to eat yogurt containing live culture
- The taking of supplementation of Probiotics helps to maintain not only the health of the intestinal flora but also maintains the immunological balance of all mucosal sites in the body as well as protecting these sites against invasion by pathogens. Probiotics also helps with the restoration of the impaired innate immunity of the mucosal epithelium.

✓ **Stress** (anxiety and tension) **as well as tiredness** have an adverse influence on the autonomous and endocrine functions of the body and diminish the general physiological resistance of the body.

✓ **Clamminess/moistness of the skin** leads to vasoconstriction, which, in its turn, diminishes the resistance of the skin.

✓ **A sudden hypothermia resulting in a low body temperature**. In any situation where a sudden decrease of the body temperature occurs, vasoconstriction is caused which diminishes the general physiological resistance of the body. The mucous membranes of the airways are also negatively influenced, with the result that viruses and pneumococci gain entry into the body through the mucous membranes.

✓ **Hormonal functions.** In women, a normal level of oestrogen leads to an enhanced physiological resistance against vaginal infections. During pregnancy, cell-mediated immunity is suppressed with the result that pregnant women are more susceptible to certain infections, such as poliomyelitis and influenza.

✓ **Altered behaviour** of individuals, especially sexual habits such as promiscuity, leads to an increase in sexually transmitted infections (STI's).

5.1.5.3   Factors related to the pathogenic microbe

✠ Whenever **mutation** of the pathogenic microbe takes place, the body is no longer able to recognise the new strain of the specific pathogen. Activation of the memory cells can thus not take place any more. Consequently the person becomes ill

✠ Whenever the **antigenic virulence** of the specific pathogen changes, the body is not always able to withstand the infection, despite the physiologic resistance that has been built up. The person thus becomes ill

✠ Increased **viral pathogenicity** takes place when certain mineral deficiencies, such as a deficiency in Selenium, are present in the host as such deficiencies induce permanent changes in the viral genome inducing it to increase its virulence

✠ **The combined effects of age-related immunological impairment and the presence of both macro- and micro-nutrient deviancies** in the elderly not only put the aged at high risks for virulent infections but simultaneously pose a health problem for all age groups by contributing to the spread of more virulent viral species as the compromised immune response in the elderly increases the viral virulence by causing mutations in the infecting viruses

✠ The **routine use of antimicrobial medication/antibiotics** in medical treatment can lead to the emergence of antibiotic-resistant microbes/bacteria. The **abuse and over-use of vaccination** as well as antimicrobial drug interventions also lead to the mutation of infective microbes and the development of new strains of a specific pathogen (most of the time more virulent)

✠ **Changes in food production** with intensive animal husbandry practices under antibiotic protection also leads to the development of drug-resistant bacteria/microbes

✠ **Drug-resistance** (mono-drug resistance, multi-drug resistance, extensively-drug resistance, and complete-drug resistance) shown by many pathogens against chemotherapeutic interventions resulted in a situation where communicable diseases are not always treated successfully or cannot be treated at all (complete drug resistance). Certain pathogenic microbes elicit no immune response at all and the person becomes ill with every exposure

✠ **All human hosts have no immunity to any pathogen that has a natural animal reservoir such as**
  ➢ marine/sea vertebrate mammals (whales) or land vertebrate mammals (whether domesticated [pets], or farming [cattle, sheep, etc] or exotic [wild])
  ➢ rodents like rats and mice
  ➢ arthropods like insects, lice, mosquitoes, fleas, spiders, etc.
  ➢ reptiles
  ➢ birds (whether wild/exotic, or domesticated, or farming [poultry])

5.2   IMMUNITY

Immunity is the highly developed physiologic resistance with memory of the body against the influence and effects of any infectious pathogen (such as viruses, parasites, fungi, protozoa, bacteria and rickettsiae) after it had gained entry into the body. This highly developed physiologic resistance (immunological response) is the result of the antibody-mediated and cell-mediated immunological reactions with memory to the specific infectious pathogen that had caused the particular communicable disease. The level of the physiologic resistance or immune status varies from one person to another while immunity as such varies between males and females as well as between races.

Immunity is classified as natural (genetic-based and species) and acquired (permanent or semi-permanent) immunity. The nature of the immunity is closely associated with the antibody-mediated or cell-mediated immune reactions with memory.

5.2.1 Natural and acquired immunity

Natural immunity is divided in innate and species immunity while acquired immunity is divided in actively-acquired and passively-acquired immunity. Both actively-acquired and passively-acquired immunity may be acquired naturally or artificially (see fig. 5.5).

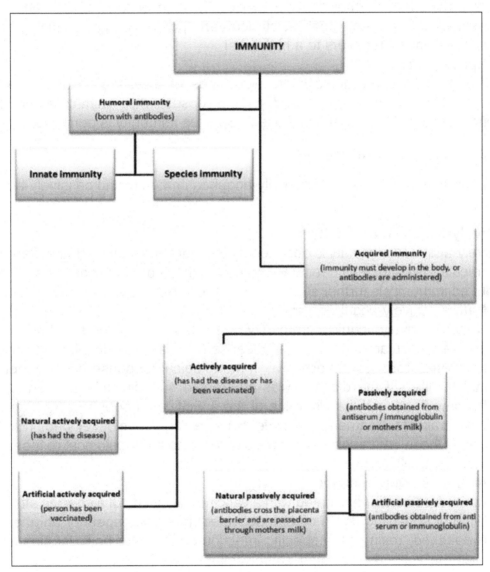

Figure 5.5 Schematic representation of the categorisation of immunity

5.2.1.1   Natural immunity

Natural or humoral immunity is determined by an individual's genetic material and is the innate ability of the body to physiologically resist the influence and effects of any pathogenic microbe. The genetic material also ensures that different species are subjected to its own types of diseases.

Natural immunity is divided into
  ❖ Innate (genetically determined) immunity
    The immunity (innate and adaptive) a person is born with is genetically determined, is permanent and can be on high or low levels. The body's high level of physiological resistance can spontaneously diminish and then spontaneously recovers to a high level
  ❖ Species immunity
    Every species are liable to its own kinds of diseases. Humans are not susceptible to most animal and avian diseases, while animals and birds are not susceptible to human diseases. Species immunity is permanent.

5.2.1.2   Acquired immunity

Acquired immunity is divided into actively-acquired immunity and passively-acquired immunity.

❑ **Actively-acquired immunity**
  Actively-acquired immunity is obtained by the individual having had/suffered from a particular disease or by been vaccinated against a particular disease. Actively-acquired immunity is further subdivided as being naturally or artificially acquired.
  ❖ Natural actively-acquired immunity
    Natural actively-acquired immunity is elicited when a person had suffered from a particular communicable disease (clinically or sub-clinically) and has recovered from it. The adaptive immunological response is permanent and last for life. If the disease was contracted sub-clinically, the person may become ill again if the virulence of the specific pathogen is very high or if a new strain of the same specific infectious pathogen has developed. (Excluded are all those communicable diseases where no immunological response with memory is elicited).
  ❖ Artificial actively-acquired immunity
    When a person is vaccinated with a vaccine consisting of a specific attenuated living or non-living (killed off or inactivated) infectious agent or an attenuated (weakened) toxin of the specific infectious agent, the body is stimulated to elicit the antibody-mediated and/or cell-mediated immune response against the specific infectious agent. Artificial actively-acquired immunity is semi-permanent. Regular booster doses are required to keep the body's level of immunity high (see fig. 5.6) as artificial actively-acquired immunity diminishes with the passing of time (the diminishing process starts about 5 years after receiving the vaccine and after 12 years no physiological resistance exist anymore if booster doses have not been received).

❑ Passively-acquired immunity (passive immunity)

Passively-acquired immunity is classified as being acquired by natural or artificial means. Because antibody cross the placental barrier during the gestation period and are present in the breast milk when breastfeeding, all infants acquire natural passively-acquired immunity. Artificial passively-acquired immunity is acquired when an antiserum or antitoxin is administered to a person who is already suffering from a particular communicable disease.

❖ Natural passively-acquired immunity

Natural passively-acquired immunity is acquired when the memory cells of the immunocytes developed during the antibody-mediated immunological reaction, cross the placenta barrier and start to circulate in the blood and lymph system of the foetus. Natural passively-acquired immunity is temporary because it lasts for only about three months after birth. The unborn foetus receives only the specific antibody to the particular communicable diseases the mother has had herself or against which she was vaccinated (and her artificial actively-acquired immunity has not yet diminished). Breastfed babies also obtain memory cells of the immunocytes developed during the antibody-mediated immunological reaction through their mothers' milk. The infant only receives the specific antibody to the particular communicable diseases the mother has had herself or against which she was vaccinated (and her artificial actively-acquired immunity has not yet diminished). Natural passively-acquired immunity only lasts as long as the infant is breastfed.

❖ Artificial passively-acquired immunity

Artificial passively-acquired immunity is acquired through the injection of an antiserum or antitoxin that contains the antibody already. An antiserum is obtained from horses or humans (see fig. 5.6) and it affords artificial passively-acquired immunity because the body does not produce any antibody itself. Artificial passively-acquired immunity is temporary as the body begins to excrete the antibody after two or three weeks.

Please note: As soon as the body starts to produce its own immunoglobulin during the antibody-mediated immunological reaction, the person develops natural actively-acquired immunity

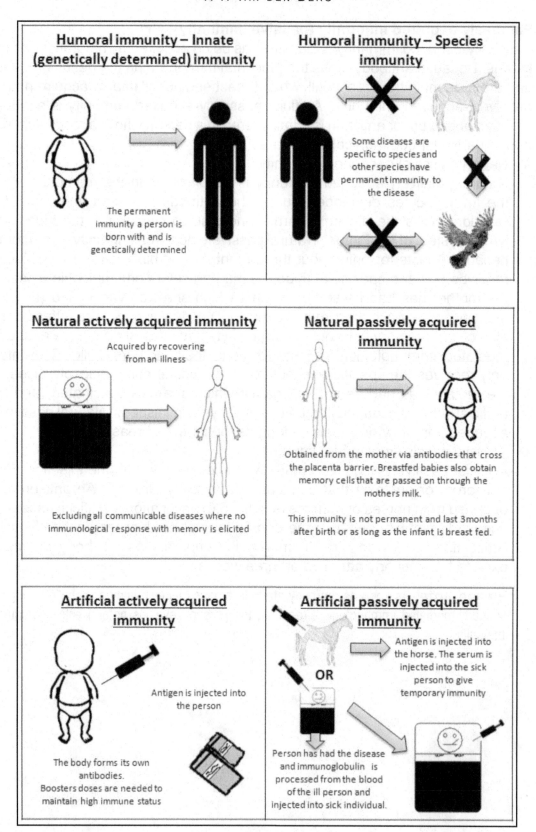

Figure 5.6 Schematic representation of natural and acquired immunity (actively and passively)

5.2.2   Immune status (level of immunity)

The immune status of an individual refers to the level of physiologic immunological resistance the person possesses against a specific infectious pathogen. When a person has mediated his/her own antibody against a specific infectious agent, he/she usually has a high, life-long immune level against that specific infectious agent. When a person has been vaccinated, his/her immune status is high at first, but gradually diminishes (within 5 to 12 years) unless he/she receives booster doses or is exposed to the causative infectious pathogen. A high immune status can be maintained if the individual is given booster doses at regular intervals to enhance his/her antibody-mediated and/or cell-mediated immunity.

5.3.   KEY NOTES

❑ The body possesses several defence mechanisms to prevent pathogenic microbes from gaining entry into the body and causing infection.

❑ The innate immune defences consist of formidable barriers to prevent entry of pathogens and second-line defending by phagocytes and soluble factors. Whenever heredity or acquired deficiency in any of these functions occurs, colonization of the body by normally non-pathogenic microbes takes place and opportunistic infections develop.

❑ The adaptive immune system provides the body with a powerful series of effector mechanisms which augment the actions and processes of the innate immune defences. The lymphocyte–mediated responses, namely, antibody produced by B-lymphocytes and T-cell-mediated responses are extremely effective against both intracellular and extracellular pathogens. The soluble antibody mediated by B-lymphocytes not only effectively neutralizes bacterial toxin, but by interacting with complement, mast cells and polymorphs, produces the acute inflammatory response which is effective against extracellular bacteria and also provide clearance of extracellular bacteria from the blood. Furthermore, the IgE-mediated acute inflammatory response and the secreted IgA defend the mucosal surfaces against extracellular infections. The T-lymphocytes, on the other hand, produce T-helper cells [T_H-cells] and cytotoxic T-cells [T_C-cells] that are directed to intracellular infective microbes. The specialized receptor on the T-cell recognizes the infected cell as a target and the T_H-cell or T_C-cell then binds to the surface major histocompatibility complex molecule (the marker of the infected cell) and peptide derived from the intracellular pathogen. The T-cell-mediated response either triggers the release of macrophage activating factors (interferon gamma) or the secretion of cytokine phenotypes and lymphokines to kill off the pathogen.

❑ A fraction of the clonally expanded population of both the B-lymphocytes and T-lymphocytes differentiates into resting memory cells that are readily stimulated by a given dose of a specific antigen. A secondary antibody and T-cell immune response is elicited that are bigger, brisker and stronger than the primary response. This magnified response forms the principle for vaccination.

❑ It is extremely important to enhance the defence mechanisms of the innate and adaptive immune defences of the body in order to prevent the person falling ill.

❑ When a specific infectious pathogen overpowers the defence mechanisms, the particular communicable disease develops and the person manifests the general and specific clinical signs and symptoms.

❑ Immunity is the highly developed *physiologic resistance with memory* of the body against the influence and effects of any infectious pathogen (whether viruses, parasites, fungi, protozoa, bacteria and rickettsiae) after it had gained entry into the body. This highly developed physiologic resistance (immunological response) is the result of the antibody-mediated and cell-mediated immunological reactions with memory to the specific infectious pathogen that has caused the particular communicable disease. The level of the physiologic resistance or immune status varies from one person to another while immunity as such varies between males and females as well as between races. Immunity is classified in natural (genetic-based and species) and acquired (permanent/semi-permanent) immunity. The nature of the immunity is closely associated with the antibody-mediated or cell-mediated immune reactions with memory.

Chapter 6

VACCINATION

Priming the adaptive immune system

The principle underlying vaccination is based on the fact that, by inducing a primarily "primed state" of the adaptive immune system to the antigen(s) of a specific pathogen, the first infection induces a rapid and effective secondary immune response. Vaccination therefore represents an artificial stimulant/primer of the adaptive immune system as the vaccine induces the adaptive immune system to actively produce antibody-mediated and/or cell-mediated immunity with memory. Vaccination depends on the ability of lymphocytes, both B- and T-cells, to respond to specific antigens and to develop memory cells. Vaccination thus elicits artificial actively-acquired immunity with memory against the specific pathogen that the individual was vaccinated against. The immune response reaches its peak immunological response within 6 weeks after the vaccine had been administered.

6.1   WHY PRIMING THE IMMUNE SYSTEM

The main aim of vaccination is to block the transmission from the infected host (human or animal) to another uninfected human host, to protect the individual against symptoms or pathology, and to eradicate a particular communicable disease. The public health benefits of vaccination lie in the facts that
> (1) an individual is protected against a particular communicable disease, and
> (2) different vaccines can eradicate different communicable diseases if the average age for vaccination is lower than the average age of infection and there is strict adherence to the two stage vaccination programme.

The two–stage vaccination programme entails vaccination at a young age (before 1-2 years) to reduce transmission efficiency, followed by booster dosage(s) at 3-5 years of age to block transmission via the creation of very high levels of herd-immunity – that is a high proportion of the population being immune to the particular disease. By generating herd-immunity through vaccination, the unvaccinated individual who is highly susceptible also benefits because, by reducing the incidence of infection/ disease, a situation is created where there are fewer infected individuals who are able to transmit infection to those still susceptible.

Although political endorsement underwrites the vaccination of all inhabitants of the RSA, vaccination is legally **not compulsory** (it has been since 1987 **voluntary**), except when administered as a chemo-prophylactic measure in the event of an epidemic/pandemic outbreak, when it can become compulsory by law. When travelling to certain countries, proof of vaccination against certain communicable diseases (as specified by the laws of the specific country of entry) is compulsory for the traveller.

Note

ACCORDING TO THE CONSTITUTION OF THE RSA, THE BILL OF HUMAN RIGHTS, AND THE PATIENTS' RIGHTS CHARTER, ALL INDIVIDUALS HAVE THE RIGHT TO REFUSE TO BE VACCINANATED, OR WHEN CONSENTING TO VACCINATION, THE INDIVIDUAL'S WRITTEN CONSENT MUST BE OBTAINED, OR IN AN EMERGENCY, THEIR VERBAL CONSENT (VERBAL CONSENT MUST BE RECORED AS SUCH). **THE ONLY EXCEPTION IS WHEN AN EPIDEMIC/ PANDEMIC HAS BROKEN OUT AND VACCINATION BECOMES COMPULSARY BY LAW AS A CONTROL MEASURE**

THE PARENTS - BOTH OR SINGLE (BIOLOGICAL AND FOSTERING) AND/OR MOTHERS AND/ OR PREGNANT WOMEN AND/OR LEGAL GARDIAN(S) HAS THE RIGHT TO REFUSE TO HAVE THEIR INFANT(S) VACCINATED, WHILE THE PREGNANT WOMEN HAS THE RIGHT TO REFUSE VACCINATION FOR HERSELF DURING THE ANTENATAL, INTRA-PARTUM AND POSTNATAL PERIOD. NO PRESSURE MAY BE PUT ON PARENTS/MOTHERS/PREGNANT WOMEN TO HAVE THEIR CHILD VACCINATED, NOR MAY HEALTHCARE PROVIDERS DISCRIMINATE AGAINST THE MOTHER AND CHILD ON THE BASIS OF THE DECISION OF PARENTS/MOTHERS/PREGNANT WOMEN. BASED ON THE DECISION OF PARENTS (BIOLOGICAL AND FOSTER) /MOTHERS/ LEGAL GARDIAN(S), NO VACCINES MAY BE ADMINISTERED TO ANY INFANT/CHILD AFTER BIRTH (WETHER IN THE LABOUR WARD/NURSERY/CLINIC/PEADIATRIC CARE UNIT) WITHOUT WRITTEN CONSENT OF THE PARENTS OR MOTHERS OR LEGAL GAURDIAN(S) OR FOSTER PARENTS. The National Department of Health respects the decision of parents/guardian(s)/foster parent(s)/mothers not to have their child vaccinated. The decision of the biological/adopted parents/legal guardian(s)/foster parent(s)/single mothers or fathers must, however, be recorded on the child's "Road to Health Card" and healthcare providers may not discriminate against the child and/or parents (biological and foster)/mothers/legal guardian(s) on the grounds thereof. Also note that vaccination of the child may be done under the Children's Act, Act 38 of 2005, without the written or verbal consent of parents/single mothers or fathers/guardians/foster parents when it is in the best interest of the child to be immunized. Counselling of the parents/mothers/guardians/foster parents prior to instituting the Children's Act, Act 38 of 2005, must have taken place

Adults as employees in sensitive occupations do have the right under the Constitution of the RSA and the Bill of Human Rights to conscientiously object to compulsory vaccination. THEY MUST INFORM THEIR EMPLOYER IN WRITING THERETO

6.2 ETHICAL AND CULTURAL CHALLENGES OR ISSUES SURROUNDING VACCINATION

The use of prophylactic interventions to prevent communicable disease is traditionally justified in terms of the best interest of the individual (child and adult) and public health benefits. Routine vaccination prevents the transmission of communicable diseases and is considered as a legitimate prophylactic medical programme by the healthcare professions and endorsed by the National Department of Health. Vaccination programmes, *per se*, have in fact yielded the most significant changes for the better in the health of children and travellers. Public health benefits of vaccination lies the foundation for the control and eradication of communicable diseases – when 90 to 95% of a population is vaccinated against a particular communicable disease, the disease does not spread in the population from person to person (not even in unvaccinated individuals) and might be eradicated because the population have satisfactory herd-immunity and is then practically immune to the particular communicable disease. In spite of the benefits of vaccination, various ethical and cultural controversies/dilemmas surround vaccination today, especially the vaccination of children (including adolescents).

6.2.1   Ethical Issues

Moral principals provide values as a general guide for actions and decision-taking. Values underlie the perspectives from which individuals/families/communities attempt to resolve the controversy of what is right and what is wrong. And because of the strong relationship that exists between values and decision-making, ethical dilemmas arise. An ethical dilemma is a conflict between two or more equally desirable (or undesirable) courses of action in a given situation. The conflict arises when strongly held values that underlie the potential choices are incompatible with each other. When faced with an ethical dilemma, a person engages in moral reasoning to choose the best course of action. Different perspectives based on specific values exist and are used as guide for a person's decision making and actions, for example, stoicism [value of caring]; rational paternalism; collectivism and utilitarianism [value of beneficence for the greatest number of persons]; individualism [values of liberty and self-reliance]; existentialism; libertarianism; rights-based ethics; consequentiality perspectives; etc. In the healthcare setting there exists a clash between the perspectives of the healthcare user and the perspectives of the healthcare providers who see themselves as the gatekeeper of the health of the user - for example,
*__the user__ (individualism [values of liberty and self-reliance], libertarianism [value of individual freedom] and consequentiality/situational perspectives) *versus* __the provider__ (collectivism and utilitarianism [value of beneficence for the greatest number of persons], and stoicism [value of caring]); or
*__the provider__ (collectivism and utilitarianism [value of beneficence for the greatest number of persons], stoicism [value of caring] and rational paternalism [value of the decision maker knows what is best for the beneficiary of the action]) *versus* __the user__ (individualism [values of liberty and self-reliance], libertarianism [value of individual freedom] and rights-based ethics of self-determination).

Although vaccination programmes are ethically and scientifically defensible as it helps society safe-guarding their herd-immunity while optimizing its members' capabilities, vaccination as a preventive intervention on the other hand, interferes with the rights and autonomy of healthy individuals – especially the child. Parents as proxies for their children are legally given the authority to make decisions for a child – but they find themselves in a controversial ethical dilemma situation - must their child be vaccinated or must their child not be vaccinated? Reasons for these ethical controversies/dilemmas are embedded in the following

❑ No vaccine is 100% safe and the risk always exists that the side-effects of the specific vaccine might harm or injure the vaccinee

❑ Vaccine production and delivery processes may not meet the required standard with the result that the vaccine does not induce a satisfactory level of immunity, or when the needle-injection-system in vaccination is used, the vaccinee may contract other infections

❑ Vaccinating of infants younger than three (3) month reduces the effectiveness of some vaccines due to the presence of maternally–derived antibody. The introduction of antigens from the vaccines into the developing immune system of an infant may also have profound effects beyond the induction of a specific immunity, for example, BCG vaccination which induces T_H1 T-cell-immunity, may affect the T_H1/T_H2 cytokine balance which may make the infant more prone to other diseases

❑ By administering many different types of vaccines simultaneously, overloading of the vaccinee's immune system (especially the immune system of infants and young children) may takes place, resulting in a sub-optimal level of immunity to a specific antigen

❑ Compulsory vaccination of children deprives parents of their parental right to make autonomous decisions regarding child rearing and healthcare practices

❑ As artificial actively-acquired immunity elicited by vaccination diminishes with time, a vaccinated child can contract the particular disease later in life, and far more adults die from or are disabled by the complications of vaccine-prevented diseases than children

❑ A wide variety of animals, animal tissues, primary cells or cell lines derived from animals are used in determining the quality of the seed materials as well as in the in-process-control-tests of product quality. Hence, the use of animals and animal products as indicators of the possibly efficacy of vaccines, is therefore questionable

❑ The overused of vaccines for purposes other than the prevention of a particular communicable disease (for example, giving polio vaccine to treat cold blisters), leads to the continuous mutation of new more virulent strains by an specific pathogen – rendering vaccination thus ineffectively while heightening the risk of the vaccinee to contract the particular disease in spite of being vaccinated. The same applies for the overuse of vaccines for the normal vaccination of individuals (for example, vaccinating an individual with the same vaccine after every exposure)

❑ Certain ethnic/religious/cultural groups object to vaccination based on religious reasons

❑ High parental anxiety regarding the administrating of many different types of vaccines simultaneously, leads to the refusal of parents to have their child/children vaccinated

❑ The disadvantages of present injury is more compelling and influential than the benefits of the absence of disease to be expected throughout a future time

❏ Occupational specific vaccination (for example, Hepatitis B-vaccine and Hepatitis A-vaccine) is now routinely administered to infants

❏ Alleged associations between vaccination and diseases, such as autism, intestinal abnormalities and encephalitis, may result in parents refusing to have their child/ children vaccinated

❏ Mistrust and conflict between society and the healthcare profession is exacerbated more and more as the public wants a greater say in their own healthcare decisions, while communication difficulties between professional healthcare givers and lay persons are getting further and further away from being resolved. In the search for new vaccines, the healthcare profession has lost sight that some diseases are controllable equally well by other means, such as traditional preventive healthcare practices (which the healthcare profession sometimes fiercely demolishes as unscientifically and outdated). By only informing the public of the 'so-called' benefits of vaccination and vaccines without explaining the side-effects of vaccine-induced/vaccine-associated diseases, healthcare users feel they are exploited because they are not enabled by healthcare practitioners to make informed decisions regarding their own healthcare

❏ The way in which "Informed Consent" is acquired, leaves many healthcare users feeling that they are coerced by healthcare professionals to give consent

❏ Exploitation and distortion in goal expectation between preventive healthcare and the social context wherein the vaccinee lives is increasing. To increase herd-immunity in the population, the new immunogenic vaccines (high potency vaccines) provide better protection, but the vaccines may be less safe which lead to more cases of vaccine-associated/vaccine-induced diseases.

6.2.2 Cultural and Social issues

Culture has both direct and indirect effects on a person's health. Direct effects stem from specific culturally prescribed practices related to health (prescribed practices to prevent illness and promote health); to disease (prescribed practices to restore health when disease occur); to food and diet (particular dietary practices that contribute to personal and group nutritional status) and to life-events (rituals to be followed in life-events such as pregnancy, birth, child rearing, death). Indirect effects result from the cultural definitions of health and disease, the acceptability of healthcare programmes and of professional healthcare providers, and cultural influences on compliance with suggested health and/or healthcare regimens for diseases.

❏ The cultural definition of health and disease determines which types of health conditions are considered worthy of attention and which conditions are likely to be disregarded. In general, people tend to disregard any type of condition that is not defined as disease (or health) in their own culture. This cultural propensity can lead to serious health consequences, such as not complying with the vaccination programme

❏ Cultural factors, such as religious faith, determine the acceptability of healthcare programmes. For example, when the belief in healing is based on faith in God, scientific medicine will be eschewed and vaccination programmes viewed as inimical to beliefs. If healthcare providers are seen as wicked/lower-class persons/unprofessional and non-caring/ignorant herbalists etc. by healthcare users, healthcare providers/practitioners will have little opportunity to influence the health of the healthcare users for the better

❑ Cultural factors very often determine whether healthcare users will comply with recommendations when they do seek professional help. When the recommendations of healthcare providers are too far removed from accepted cultural practices in a given situation, the healthcare user is unlikely to comply with those recommendations. For example, if the healthcare provider insists that the infant <u>must be vaccinated at the age of 6 weeks</u> without taking the cultural child rearing practices of early childhood in consideration, the mother may not comply when she and her newborn infant are protected from outsiders for a few months after delivery (sometimes up to 4 months)

❑ Cultural-specific healthcare practices regarding life-events, such as birth (antenatal, delivery, and postnatal) and early childhood rearing practices as well as traditional preventive healthcare practices, also influence the compliance with the childhood vaccination programme. In some cultures, mothers are not allowed to leave the protective area where she lives for a period of time after birth and only intimate friends and family members may visit her and her infant there. This practice protects the baby from being exposed to virulent pathogens in the environment while his/her immune system develops to maturity. At the same time, the period of seclusion helps the mother to regain her strength and bond with her infant

❑ Healthcare users take healthcare decisions based on the family's interest, religious convictions and socio-cultural customs (for example, it is morally irresponsible to make a healthy person sick regardless the health benefits gained by vaccination) and not on public health benefits

❑ Other cultural factors of importance include attitudes and beliefs regarding preventive and promotive healthcare practices (traditional and biomedical); individual versus group goals; modes of authority and decision making; attitude toward change; the character of the relationship with the larger society, and the occurrence of epidemics of significant communicable diseases. Cultures that emphasize family and community goals frequently vest authority and decision-making power in elders rather than individuals. For example, the mother is sometimes not allowed to take any healthcare decisions regarding the newborn infant as it is the prerogative of the paternal grandmother (the mother of the father) to do so. When the new mother and infant stays with her own mother during the postnatal period (3-4 months after delivery), the maternal grandmother may make all healthcare decisions for the mother relating to the newborn infant

❑ Because traditional or folk healthcare providers reinforce the value system of the healthcare user, the influence they excerpt on any healthcare programme (for example, vaccination programme) must never be underestimated or underrated

❑ Political interference with and suspension of vaccination programmes leads to outbreaks and the spread of a specific communicable disease(s) in disease-free zones and countries

❑ Civil unrest and guerrilla wars lead to the displacement of thousands of individuals from their natural homes and environment and their placement in refugee camps resulting in the fact that vaccination programmes are suspended or not followed by the refugees in refugee camps across national borders.

Lastly, not only must healthcare providers be knowledgeable about the ethical and cultural controversies and dilemmas surrounding vaccination, but they **must reconcile** scientifically sound healthcare practices with ethical decision-taking and cultural practices/attitudes/beliefs etc. to the satisfaction of both parties. For example, vaccination can be delayed for a few weeks until mother and child has fulfilled the cultural rituals/practices regarding delivery and the postpartum period. By not being paternalistic and by giving all information necessary to take an informed healthcare decision, healthcare practitioners can resolve many ethical dilemmas. By working hand-in-hand with traditional healthcare practitioners and figures of authorities (for example, grandmothers), healthcare practitioners can achieve the aims of preventive healthcare through vaccination programmes. Through cultural brokering, bridging and accommodation, healthcare providers can influence healthcare users for the better.

6.3 DESCRIPTION OF CONCEPTS

6.3.1 Vaccination

Vaccination/immunization is a procedure whereby a vaccine (vaccination inoculant) is administered to an individual in order to stimulate/prime the adaptive immune system with memory to the antigens of a specific pathogen so that a first infection induces/mounts a rapid and effective secondary response leading to prevention of the particular communicable disease. Vaccination, *per se*, is not a modern medical practice. Even before it was put into writing for the first time during the eleventh century, traditional medical practitioners in China primed the immune system of the body by blowing pulverized smallpox scabs into the nasal mucosa of healthy persons. These individuals then contracted a sub-clinical form of smallpox and were immune for a number of years, even in the midst of epidemics of the serious form of smallpox. From the early eighteen century to the beginning of the nineteen century, doctors in America rubbed smallpox pus into wounds or skin pricks made in the skin of healthy healthcare users to protect them (the vaccinee) against smallpox. Edward Jenner inoculated persons with cowpox for the first time in 1796 in order to protect them against smallpox. In 1880 Louis Pasteur prepared a vaccine against cholera, using chickens infected with cholera. Pasteur later also developed a vaccine for human usage against rabies, prepared from the brains of rabid sheep and cattle. With Pasteur's work as basis, medical science has succeeded during the 20th century in preparing vaccines in large quantities by using specific non-living (killed-off) bacteria or attenuated (live) viruses in the vaccine in order to elicit a specific antigen-antibody response with memory. Today, with new recombinant DNA technology and genetically engineered vaccine preparation, the early tedious method of preparing vaccines by using egg embryos has changed drastically as vaccines can now be produced on a large scale in a very short period of time in large vaccine bio-barrels (these bio-barrels are manufactured as result of new metallurgic technology and processes).

Although vaccination elicits artificial actively-acquired immunity with memory against the specific pathogen that the individual was vaccinated against, the artificial actively-acquired immunity begins to diminish as time passes if no booster dosages are administered and after about 12 years no immunological protection exists. The individual can now contract the specific infection/disease and become seriously ill or manifest an atypical form of the disease. The older the individual becomes before he/she contracts "the so-called children's diseases such as Measles, German measles, Chickenpox, Mumps", the more serious ill the person becomes. Because of the expanded vaccination programme for infants and young children, many "so-called children's diseases" is now becoming diseases of adolescents and young adults with serious sequelae. Vaccination *en mass* of especially the older child, can therefore have the following indirect effects, namely, (1) individuals acquire infections/diseases that may leave them with more serious sequelae now at an older average age than before vaccination; and (2) when the risk of disease associated with infection increases with age, a programme of vaccination at levels below that required to block transmission, can have perverse effects (for example, although all levels of Measles vaccination coverage reduce the incidence of encephalitis from Measles, a low vaccination rate of Measles increases the overall incidence of serious disease when suffering from Mumps and Rubella).

6.3.2   Vaccines (immunizing inoculants)

A vaccine is a suspension of a specific non-living (killed-off), or of a living attenuated pathogen (with reduced virulence), or of the attenuated toxin (with reduced virulence) of a specific infectious pathogen in a normal saline solution or glycerine. The vaccine contains some (or at least one) of the protective antigens of the pathogen. When the vaccine is injected into or given orally to the individual, the specific infectious agent is not virulent enough to cause the infection, but the attenuated/killed-off pathogen or toxoid or genetically engineered substance acts as immune response stimulant by priming/stimulating the body's physiological adaptive immunological response to mediate antibody and/or T-immunity with memory.

Different types of vaccines are in use today, each having its merits and drawbacks. A specific vaccine contains one of the following
   (1) a specific pathogen/a combination of different pathogens with artificially reduced virulence ("attenuated"), OR
   (2) microbes with natural reduced virulence for man, OR
   (3) killed-off microbes, OR
   (4) sub-cellular fragments.
Vaccines can be pure (containing only the specific antigen) or monovalent/multivalent (containing one or more biotype(s)/strain(s) of the same pathogen) or combined (containing two or more different pathogens in a single/same suspension).

❑ **Living vaccines** are preparations that contain a living/a live attenuated pathogen, for example, measles vaccine. The living pathogen is not virulent enough to cause the infection, but an antigen-antibody reaction is induced leading to antibody-mediated and/or cell-mediated immunological response. Live attenuated vaccines make up the bulk of successful viral vaccines. Living vaccines induce a strong and a long lasting immune response with memory. The use of living vaccines is contra-indicated in immuno-compromised individuals.

❑ **Non-living vaccines** are a group of vaccines containing the killed-off (dead) or "inactivated" infectious agent, for example, typhoid or whole-cellular pertussis vaccines. Upon administering of the vaccine, the killed-off pathogen still causes an antigen-antibody response. Non-living vaccines have the advantage of non-infectivity and are therefore relative safe, but have the disadvantage of generally lower immunogenicity with the consequent need of several dosages. Non-living vaccines induce a more weak and short-term immune response than the living vaccines.

❑ **Toxoids** are vaccines that contain bacterial toxins that have been inactivated (usually by formaldehyde) and are thus no longer toxic, but can still induce specific protective antibody-mediated and T-cell-mediated immunity with memory.

❑ **Sub-cellular fractions** are used as vaccines when protective immunity is directed against a particular part of the pathogen. Examples of vaccines that are sub-cellular fractions are: acellular pertussis, polysaccharide capsules of pneumococci; haemophilus and meningococci; the surface coat of the hepatitis B-virus that is produced by recombinant DNA technology; and the fragmented virus or purified surface antigens of influenza virus vaccines.

❑ **DNA vaccines** are produced by recombinant DNA technology, when a specific gene is cloned into a yeast vector to produce large amounts of the anti-genetic protein. DNA vaccines are used more and more today, as recombinant DNA vaccines are safe and can be produced on a large scale.

❑ **Genetically engineered vaccines** are vaccines that are produced from cloned genes with gene coding insertion. A variety of virus and bacteria are used as vectors. The expression vector, complete with the inserted gene(s), forms the vaccine itself. When injected, the expression vector proliferates sufficiently to release an immunizing amount of the foreign protein, but without inducing the disease itself. Gene cloning and peptide synthesis can produce immunogenic peptides that can also be used as vaccines.

❑ **Combination vaccines** consist of a combination of different live attenuated or non-living/inactivated pathogens in one specific vaccine preparation. A combination vaccine targets multiple pathogenic microbes (for example, *Corynebacterium diphtheria; Bordetella pertussis* (whooping cough); *Clostridium tetani* [tetanus]; *Poliomyelitis-virus* [inactivated virus]; *Hepatitis B-virus* and *Haemophilus influenzae type B virus*) in a single vaccine injection. Combination vaccines provide a higher level of immunity as the risk of error in the preparation and administering of the separate vaccines is minimised. Hence, a combination vaccine is an alternative to the administering of multiple separate vaccines for example, four separate vaccines. Although the administering of combination vaccines has more or less the same favourable safety and efficacy as when separate vaccines are administered, overloading of the vaccinee's immune system (especially of the immune system of infants and young children) may takes place, resulting in a sub-optimal level of immunity to a specific antigen. Combination vaccines help to alleviate parents worry about the number of vaccines their babies receive during a single visit, and because the stress associated with multiple injections is removed, parents might change their attitude to vaccination whereby failure to complete the infants'/children's vaccination schedules on time might be addressed.

The ideal vaccine must be effective, safe, stable and of low cost. To be effective the vaccine must not only induce an adequate immune response, but the response must also be of the right type, for example, a purely antibody-mediated response is of no benefit against an intracellular infection such as tuberculosis where cell-mediated immunity is required and vice versa. The duration of the primary adaptive immunity response is of utmost importance – for short-term protection of individuals, for example, travellers, the primary adaptive immune response may be perfectly adequate and memory cells may not be strictly necessary. On the other hand, for the protection of individuals against exposure sometime in the future, the inducement of immunologic memory is essential. All vaccines must also undergo rigorous safety testing that requires extensive quality control and animal trials before trials and usage in man. All vaccine compounds destined to remain on the shelf for long periods must be stable. Maintaining of the "cold chain" from production to administering is imperative - especially critical in living attenuated vaccines. Lastly, the cost of a vaccine must not be so high that it is out of reach of the ordinary population or the health system of the country.

It must always be kept in mind that a vaccine may at times elicit not only an immune response, but also the disease/infection itself. This occurs because the specific killed-off/non-living or live attenuated infectious agent was not sufficiently "killed off"/inactivated or "the virulence was insufficiently attenuated" (was not reduced properly or enough)" during the process of preparation. When during the process of preparation, the pathogen or toxin is attenuated or inactivated to the extent that it cannot elicit an immune response, the "immunized/vaccinated" person will contract the particular communicable disease and the severity of the disease will be similar to that of a non-vaccinated person. When the pathogen was not "properly killed off" during the process of preparation, the still living/live pathogen with all its virulent factors is administered to the individual, resulting in the individual becoming ill from the disease/infection he/she was vaccinated against. The severity/seriousness of the disease/infection can varies from sub-clinical to mild to severe to fatal.

6.3.3   Adjuvants

Adjuvants are substances that enhance the consequent immune response when administered simultaneously with the antigen. The adjuvant must be safe, convenient and effective. For example, aluminium salts is an adjuvant that forms a repository of antigen within in the tissue and is used in vaccines such as DTP (diphtheria-tetanus-pertussis) vaccine while BCG (Bacillus Calmette-Guérin) vaccine is used as an adjuvant for other vaccines. Other materials that possess adjuvanticity are mycobacterium and other bacterial derivatives, cytokines, and dendrite cells. In Conjugate Hib-vaccine (*Haemophilus influenzae type B*), tetanus toxoid or diphtheria toxoid is used to conjugate with the capsular polysaccharides of *Haemophilus influenzae* to improve the immunogeniticity of the vaccine. BCG vaccine is also used as either vector for cloned genes of other pathogenic microbes, or as adjuvant in different vaccines.

6.3.4   Herd-immunity

Herd immunity is the raising of the overall level of immunity in a population to a point at which there are insufficient susceptible individuals to maintain effective transmission. A high herd immunity (the vaccination level of the population is 80-86% or higher) interrupts the transmission cycle from infected person-to-susceptible person whereby the susceptible individuals become protected, resulting in the pathogen dying out because it cannot reproduces

6.3.5   Cross-immunity

Cross-immunity occurs when immunity to one infectious agent also confers immunity to a related agent. Cross-immunity can either be passive or active. BCG vaccine induces limited immunity to tuberculosis and cross-immunity to the related mycobacterium Leprae causing leprosy. Polio drops are sometimes given to treat cold blisters, although this practice is not encourage as the shed polio-virus reverse back to the wild type which can cause outbreaks of epidemics.

6.3.6   The cold chain

The cold chain refers to the process whereby the vaccines are kept cold from the moment of production, throughout periods of storage and transportation, during reconstitution and up to the point of administering. Most vaccines have to be stored in a refrigerator between 2–8°C or in a freezer. These vaccines must be transported on ice or in a cool bag, and they must not be warmed or allowed to warm up before the administering.

To maintain the cold chain, adherence to the following principles is of utmost importance

- ✠ **Only one person must be responsible** for the transportation, storage and administering of vaccine
- ✠ **No food or drink may be stored in the refrigerator** in which vaccines are stored
- ✠ **Do not keep too large a stock** of vaccines in the healthcare delivery setting. Leave space around and between each tray to allow the cold air to move around
- ✠ **Do not let DTP-HIV, DTP(a)-IPV-Hib, PCV, RV, DTP, Td, HBV, Hib and TT touch the evaporator plate at the back of the fridge as they may freeze. DO NOT FREEZE THESE VACCINES AND DO NOT USE WHEN BEEN**

FROZEN! (Note – All vaccines and diluents with a "T" in their name are sensitive to freezing as well as the Rotavirus vaccine and the pneumococcal conjugated vaccine)

✠ **Defrosted OPV should not be kept in the freezer or allowed to freeze again**

✠ **A Dial thermometer (not a minimum-maximum thermometer) or the cold chain monitor has to be hung vertically** in the centre of the refrigerator and the temperature monitored twice daily. Should the recorded temperature rise beyond the safety limits, consider the following

* Is there a power failure? Is the refrigerator plugged into the power socket? Is the gas cylinder empty? Is there enough paraffin available to power the refrigerator?
* Does the door close properly and tightly? Is the door opened too often? Was the door of the refrigerator left open?
* Is the refrigerator overloaded?
* Should the refrigerator be defrosted?

6.4 ADMINISTERING OF VACCINES

When a healthcare consumer reports for vaccination, the healthcare provider must **perform the following steps before the vaccine may be administered at all**

* **Assessing the health status of the healthcare user** that consists of
  ◈ Taking the health history of the present and previous vaccination status of the healthcare user and hypersensitivity to any vaccines administered
  ◈ Doing a clinical (physical) examination on the individual to rule out any present infections/diseases/ailments
* **Selecting the correct vaccine**, taking into account the findings of the assessment and the healthcare user's age
* **Administering the vaccine** correctly according to dosage, procedure and route
* **Providing information** regarding the specific vaccine.

6.4.1 Assessing the health status of the healthcare user

The healthcare assessment consists of taking the history of the healthcare user and doing a physical examination.

* **Taking the health history of the healthcare user**
  The main reason for taking the health history of the healthcare user is to be able to identify contra-indication to the administering of a specific vaccine. Contra-indications for routine vaccination/vaccination are set out in table 6.1.

Table 6.1   DATA TO BE OBTAINED WHEN TAKING A HEALTH HISTORY

❑ **Contact details of the healthcare user**
❑ **Age of the healthcare user**
  • Medically stable preterm and low birth weight infants can receive the full dosages of vaccines at the chronological age consistent with the immunisation schedule recommended for full-term infants. Infants with birth weight less than 2000g may require modification of the timing of certain vaccines
  • The pertussis toxoid ($P_{[w]}$) is not to be administered after the age of two years
  • In high risk cases, such as babies who became seriously ill after receiving $DTP_{(w)}$ or $DTP_{(a)}$, the pertussis toxoid must not be administered at all. When the child is older than one year old, only DT vaccine must be administer – as single dosage vaccine or as a combination vaccine
❑ **Family history** – especially drug allergy; convulsions (petit mal and/or grand mal); bleeding disorders; asthma; hay fever; any inherited and genetic diseases
❑ **Vaccines previously received and any adverse event experienced**
❑ **History of hypersensitivity**
  • Physiological responses manifested after the administering of vaccines received previously, for example, fever of 40°C or higher within 48 hours of vaccination not due to another identifiable cause; persistent inconsolable crying for 3 hours or longer within 48 hours after being vaccinated; febrile or non-febrile convulsions occurring within 3 days of vaccination; or collapse or shock-like state (hypotonic-hypo-responsive episodes) within 48 hours of vaccination
  • Substances to which the user is allergic (for example, albumin and drugs such as neomycin)
  • Allergic reactions experienced such as hay fever, rash, asthma, anaphylactic shock, drug allergy
❑ **Drugs taken at present** – the list should be as complete as possible as to eliminate the possibility of contra-indications. For example, cortisone preparations and immuno-suppressants are contra-indicated for the administering of certain vaccines such as the measles and MMR vaccines
❑ **Present illness/ailments** - for example, any serious febrile disease, gastritis, pyrexia, coryza, eczema, and skin lesions
❑ **Prior diseases suffered from**
  • Communicable diseases - only those for which vaccines are available
  • Diseases that are contra-indicated for the administering of certain vaccines such as epilepsy, convulsions, hypogammaglobulinaemia, leukaemia, Hodgkin's disease, untreated tuberculosis or any other serious disease
❑ **Pregnancy** is a contra-indicated for the administering of any vaccine containing attenuated living viruses

✳ Performing a physical examination

A physical examination **must** be performed before vaccination. Particular attention must be paid to the healthcare user's nutritional status, general health status, and whether any signs of diseases (in particular tuberculosis) are present. Should the individual's physical condition justify it, vaccination can be postponed to a later date, or the individual has to be referred to a medical practitioner for further management.

6.4.2 Selecting the correct vaccine

Specific vaccines are administered to healthcare users for different reasons. Infants and children are vaccinated to prime the child's adaptive immunity system against certain communicable diseases; travellers are vaccinated to protects his/her health against diseases endemic to the country of entry; while employees in sensitive occupations who are more exposed to pathogens causing communicable diseases, need specific protection against specific communicable diseases.

✱ Travellers

Vaccines should be administered according to the endemic communicable diseases prevailing in the country of entry or in accordance with the compulsory vaccination(s) required by the country of entry. Travel clinics <u>must issue</u> **certification as to the vaccinations received** by the individual travellers and the certification has to be presented on request by these travellers upon entering the foreign country. Only medical practitioners certified by the National Department of Health may administer the necessary vaccines.

✱ Employees in sensitive occupations

- ☑ Compulsory vaccination of employees in sensitive occupations such as the healthcare professions, police service, environmental health services, military services (especially in field units) etc. is of utmost importance
- ☑ An employee <u>wishing to raise conscientious objections to being vaccinated must inform the employer of this in writing</u>. When the employee does contract the disease(s) he/she would otherwise have been vaccinated against, the employer can be exempted of responsibility.

✱ Adults (adolescents, adults and the elderly)

<u>Meningococcal, influenza and pneumococcal vaccines</u>

- ☑ Adults may be voluntary vaccinated against influenza, pneumococcal and meningococcal infections. Meningococcal vaccination may become mandatory as a chemoprophylaxis measure for both children and adults during an outbreak of meningococcal meningitis.

<u>Influenza vaccine (Trivalent inactivated influenza vaccine or live attenuated influenza vaccine)</u>

- ☑ Influenza vaccination does not induce a good long-lasting immunity - a good long-lasting immunity is also not induced even after recovery from infection in healthy persons. This is due to the ability of the virus to mutate (antigenic drift and shift) and/or due to the phenomenon of "original antigenic sin" - a strange tendency of the adaptive immunological responses to be dominated by the already mediated antibody against the strain first encountered when the individual's adaptive immunological responses react to the different strains of the pathogen

☑ Although influenza is such an important cause of morbidity and mortality, as yet the range of vaccines in use is only partially effective, pending on the development of something better. The most widely used influenza vaccines are formalin-killed off or β-propiolactone-killed off viral vaccines that contain two subtypes of influenza A and one of influenza B as well as the prevalent/anticipated hemagglutinin (H) and neuraminidase (N)

☑ Influenza vaccine is offered to members of high-risk groups such as healthcare practitioners, the elderly, persons suffering from chronic illnesses such as chronic respiratory illnesses, cardiac or renal diseases, anaemia, diabetes mellitus and immunodeficiency

☑ Regular re-vaccination in subsequent years is necessary to maintain antibody levels. Vaccination with the same or a different strain, however, does not give a further boost of titre

☑ Influenza vaccine may also be given to children.

Live attenuated Varicella-Zoster-virus (VZV) vaccine

☑ The heat-inactivated preparation of the live attenuated childhood preparation of the VZV-vaccine helps to prevent re-activation of the virus in persons suffering from cancer who receive haemopoietic cell transplants.

Pneumococcal vaccines

☑ Pneumococcal vaccines are prepared from bacterial cultures and contain polysaccharide antigens from different serotypes of the Streptococcus pneumoniae

☑ The pneumococcal vaccine is offered to members of high-risk groups such as healthcare practitioners, the elderly, and individuals suffering from chronic illnesses such as chronic respiratory illnesses, cardiac or renal diseases, anaemia, diabetes mellitus and immunodeficiency. Pneumococcal vaccine induce antibody in 80% of healthy adults

☑ The response to the vaccine is generally poor in children younger than 2 years, because the IgG2 class of antibody which predominate the response to carbohydrate antigens, develops later in life (older than 2 years) and the polysaccharide antigens behave as T-independent antigens. Vaccines containing conjugation to a protein carrier shows an improve response as it allows the T-cells to participate. The 7-valent pneumococcal conjugate vaccine (PCT$_7$) which protects against pneumococcal pneumonia caused by Streptococcus Pneumoniae helps to decrease hospitalisations resulting from pneumonia. The 7-valent pneumococcal conjugate vaccine (PCT$_7$) is recommended for all infants aged between 2 and 23 months as well as for children aged 24 to 59 months who are at increased risk for pneumococcal infections.

Tetanus Toxoid vaccine (TT vaccine)

☑ Tetanus Toxoid (TT) vaccine must be administered to all pregnant women according to protocol, to prime the foetal adaptive immune system against

Neonatal Tetanus. This strategy also includes the provision of clean delivery services for all birthing mothers and health information about the proper care of the umbilicus of the neonate, as well as the vaccination of the infant(s) through the Expanded programme on Immunisation: South Africa (EPI programme)

☑ Tetanus Toxoid (TT) vaccine must also be administered when tetanus-prone lacerations and injuries were sustained (unless there is proof that Tetanus Toxoid (TT) vaccine was administered in the proceeding 5 years)

☑ Tetanus Toxoid (TT) vaccine must also be administered as a booster series every 10 years

☑ Tetanus Toxoid and reduced amount of Diphtheria (Td) can be used in adolescents and adults for primary vaccination and post-exposure prophylaxis following a tetanus-prone wound when a booster for diphtheria is also needed.

Note

In older children, adolescents, adults and the elderly, any other infection(s) (for example, Malaria etc.) notably interfere with the normal response to vaccines (especially to pneumococcal and meningococcal vaccines)

* ### Children (infants, toddlers and older children)

☑ For the primary series vaccination of infants and children up to the age of 12 years, vaccines should be administered according to the recommended Expanded vaccination/immunization schedule for the public sector or the private sector (see table 6.2A, 6.2B and 6.2C)

☑ In cases where the recommended vaccination schedule was not followed, the catch-up vaccination schedule has to be adapted according to the age of the child and vaccines already received (see table 6.3)

☑ Always take into consideration all contra-indications and act accordingly with regard to the healthcare interventions to be followed (see table 6.4)

☑ Only those vaccines set out in the Expanded programme on Immunisation (table 6.2A and 6.2B) as prescribed by the National Department of Health are supplied free of charge by the National Department of Health when administered in public hospitals and in primary healthcare clinics

☑ When vaccination is administered at mother-and-child/well-baby clinics in private hospitals or at any private medical or nursing practice, the vaccination is not free of charge as payment is asked for the procedure done and vaccine administered. Vaccines (either single dosages vaccines or combination vaccines) are to be purchased privately and administered at the required age, for example, the MMR vaccine (for Morbilli [Measles], epidemic parotitis [Mumps] and Rubella [German measles]); Varicella-Zoster vaccine; Human Rotavirus vaccine and others. These vaccines can be also be purchased from a pharmacy by the parents/guardians/foster-parents and brought to a primary health clinic for administering. The vaccine should be kept cold in a cool bag during transportation. The parents of minor children have to give their written permission for the administering of the vaccine at all public healthcare clinics.

Table 6.2A THE EXPANDED PROGRAMME ON IMMUNIZATION[1] [EPI-SA SCHEDULE] FOR CHILDHOOD VACCINATION WITH PENTAVALENT VACCINES

AGE OF CHILD	VACCINE	BODY SITE FOR ADMINISTERING[1]
At birth	BCG[2] OPV (trivalent oral polio vaccine) {0 dosage}	BCG – Intradermal upper right arm Polio – drops per mouth
6 to 8 weeks	OPV {1st dosage} RV[3] Rotavirus vaccine {1st} $DTP_{[a]}$–IPV-Hib {1st} (diphtheria, tetanus, pertussis acellular[4], inactivated polio vaccine[5], and Hib-vaccine[6]) Hepatitis-B {1st]} (Hep-B) PCV {1st} pneumococcal Vaccine[7]	Polio drops – per mouth Rotavirus Liquid - per mouth Intramuscularly - left thigh Intramuscularly - right thigh Intramuscularly – right thigh
10 to 12 weeks	$DTP_{[a]}$–IPV-Hib {2sd dosage} Hepatitis-B {2sd} (Hep-B)	Intramuscularly - left thigh Intramuscularly - right thigh
14 to 16 weeks	RV {2sd dosage} $DTP_{[a]}$– IPV-Hib {3rd dosage} Hepatitis-B {3rd} (Hep-B) PCV {2sd dosage}	Rotavirus Liquid – per mouth Intramuscularly - left thigh Intramuscularly - right thigh Intramuscularly - right thigh
9 months	Measles[8] {1st dosage} PCV {3rd dosage}	Intramuscularly - right thigh Intramuscularly - right thigh
18 months	$DTP_{[a]}$– IPV-Hib {4th dosage} Measles {2sd dosage}	Intramuscularly - left arm Intramuscularly - right arm
6 years	Td[9]	Intramuscularly - left arm
12 years	Td	Intramuscularly - left arm

Table 6.2B THE EXPANDED PROGRAMME ON IMMUNIZATION 1 [EPI-SA SCHEDULE] FOR CHILDHOOD VACCINATION WITHOUT PENTAVALENT VACCINES

AGE OF CHILD	VACCINE	BODY SITE FOR ADMINISTERING[1]
At birth	BCG[2] OPV[5] (trivalent oral polio vaccine) {0 dosage}	BCG – Intradermal upper right arm Polio – drops per mouth
6 weeks	OPV [1st dosage] RV[3] Rotavirus vaccine {1st} DTP-Hib {1st} (diphtheria, tetanus, pertussis acellular/pertussis whole-cell[4], and Hib-vaccine[6]) Hepatitis-B {1st}(Hep-B) PCV {1st} pneumococcal vaccine[7]	Polio drops – per mouth Rotavirus Liquid - per mouth Intramuscularly - left thigh Intramuscularly - right thigh Intramuscularly – right thigh
10 weeks	OPV {2sd dosage} DTP-Hib {2sd dosage} Hepatitis-B {2sd} (Hep-B)	Polio drops – per mouth Intramuscularly - left thigh Intramuscularly - right thigh
14 weeks	OPV {3rd dosage} RV {2sd dosage} DTP-Hib {3rd dosage} Hepatitis-B {3rd} (Hep-B) PCV {2sd}	Polio drops – per mouth Rotavirus Liquid – per mouth Intramuscularly - left thigh Intramuscularly- right thigh Intramuscularly - right thigh
9 months	Measles[8] {1st dosage} PCV {3rd dosage}	Intramuscularly - left thigh Intramuscularly - right thigh
18 months	OPV {4th dosage} DTP-Hib {4th dosage} Measles {2sd dosage}	Polio drops – per mouth Intramuscularly - left arm Intramuscularly - right arm
6 years	OPV {5th dosage} Td[9]	Polio drops – per mouth Intramuscularly - left arm
12 years	Td	Intramuscularly - left arm

[1] **The prescribed injection sites as indicated** in the Expanded EPI-SA Schedule for Childhood Vaccination (table 6.2A) **must be followed** for the sake of reporting the slight possibility of Severe Adverse Events following Immunisation (AEFI). When the child's immunisation chart (called the "Road to Health") is not available at the time of the reaction, the information obtained from the parent/grandparent/ foster parent/caregiver regarding the body site used for the vaccination, will give an indication of which vaccine could have been administered, possibly implicating the vaccine having caused the AEFI. (Important The reaction must be correlated

with the specific vaccine pamphlet insert before the conclusion is drawn that the vaccine caused the reaction).

2   **BCG vaccine** must be repeated after 6 weeks or later, when any uncertainty exists whether the infant has been vaccinated, or when the growth lesions are not visible.

3   The **Rotavirus vaccine must only be given orally** (never be administered intramuscularly). **The first dosage must not be administered after the age of 14 weeks or any dosage after the age of 24 weeks.**

4   **Pertussis whole-cell (P[w])** contains the inactivated Bordetella pertussis-endotoxin in suspension, while the **Pertussis Acellular (P[a]/P[ac]/acP/aP)** contains purified pertussis toxoid and antigen component (filamentous haemagglutinin). Both P[w] and P[a] act as immuno-stimulant to prime the infant's immune system to produce antibody-mediated immunity against whooping cough. Neither the P[w] nor the P[a] is available as a single dosage vaccine - both come only in combination with other vaccine pathogens, such as diphtheria and tetanus as a combination/valente vaccine. The DTP[a] pentavalent combination vaccine is deemed safe to be given up to the age of 12 years. The DTP[w] combination vaccine is not used any longer at public healthcare institutions in the RSA. (Note When DTP[a] is not available, DTP[w] must still be used taking in consideration the age of the child and all other contra-indications for Pertussis whole-cellular [P[w]]. Pertussis whole-cellular [P[w]] is deemed not save for children older than 2 years). The DTP[a] pentavalent vaccine is provided free of charged by public healthcare facilities or be bought voluntarily and administered to infants at the required ages in the private sector.

5   The **Polio vaccine** can be given at any age either orally (TOPV, namely, the trivalent oral vaccine) or intramuscularly (the inactivated polio vaccine [IPV]). Preferably, the oral vaccine (OPV trivalent/TOPV) must be given to infants under the age of 6 weeks. From the age of 6 weeks, inactivated polio vaccine containing inactivated type 1, 2 and 3 Poliovirus D antigen may be administered intramuscularly either as single dosage vaccine or as a combination vaccine with DTP[a], or alternatively with DTP[a]-Hib. IPV and OPV can be used as substitute for one another. Only IPV must be used when an outbreak of poliomyelitis occurs (when stock of IPV runs out start using TOPV).

6   **Hib vaccine** - Haemophilus influenza type B combination vaccine is administered in combination with DTP[a] and IPV to babies from the age of 6 weeks. Three (3) dosages at intervals of four weeks are administered. It is essential that all children under the age of 5 years be vaccinated before they attend or will be attending crèches/pre-primary schools/play groups/day care centres. Private medical practitioners and private well-baby clinics also administer Hib vaccine as a single dosage vaccine or the combination vaccine DTP[a]-Hib or DTP[a]-IPV-Hib.

7   The **Pneumococcal Conjugated Vaccine** (PCV7) protects the infant or child against pneumococcal pneumonia caused by *Streptococcus Pneumoniae.* The 7-valent pneumococcal conjugate vaccine (PCV7) is administered to all infants aged from the age of six (6) weeks up to the age of 18 months as well as to older toddlers 24 to 59 months who are at increased risk for pneumococcal infections

or whose vaccination where not completed. The Pneumococcal Conjugate Vaccine-7 valente is available free of charge at public health facilities.

8 The **Measles vaccine** should preferably not be administered to babies younger than 9 months. Should an epidemic outbreak occur, however, the vaccine can be administered to babies 6 months and older. In these cases booster dosages have to be administered at the age of 9 and 18 months.

9 The **Td-vaccine** contains Tetanus Toxoid and reduced diphtheria toxoid. It is used as a booster series vaccine as well as a primary series vaccine; for post-exposure prophylaxis vaccine following a tetanus-prone wound (if a booster diphtheria is also needed); and for active protection against tetanus and diphtheria from **6 years of age and older** (adolescents and adults). **This vaccine CANNOT be used to vaccinate children younger than 6 years of age.**

Table 6.2C THE COMPLETE VACCINATION SCHEDULE FOLLOWED IN THE PRIVATE SECTOR

AGE	VACCINE*	BODY SITE FOR ADMINISTERING[1]
At birth	BCG OPV(trivalent oral polio vaccine)	BCG – Intradermal upper right arm Polio – drops per mouth
6 to 8 weeks	RV(Rotavirus vaccine) DTP$_{(a)}$–IPV-Hib(diphtheria, tetanus, pertussis acellular, inactivated polio vaccine, and Hib) Hepatitis-B (Hep-B) Conjugated Pneumococcal Vaccine	Rotavirus Liquid - per mouth Intramuscular - left thigh Intramuscular - right thigh Intramuscular – right thigh
10 to 12 weeks	DTP$_{(a)}$–IPV-Hib Hepatitis-B (Hep-B)	Intramuscular - left thigh Intramuscular - right thigh
14 to 16 weeks	RV DTP$_{(a)}$– IPV-Hib Hepatitis-B (Hep-B) Conjugated Pneumococcal vaccine	Rotavirus Liquid – per mouth Intramuscular - left thigh Intramuscular - right thigh Intramuscular - right thigh
9 months	Measles[1]	Intramuscular – left thigh
12 months	Hepatitis A (Hep-A) paediatric Varicella Vaccine (chicken pox) Conjugated Pneumococcal vaccine	Intramuscular – right thigh Intramuscular – left thigh Intramuscular – right thigh
15 to 18 months	MMR (measles, mumps and Rubella)	Intramuscular - right thigh
18 months	DTP$_{(a)}$– IPV-Hib Hepatitis A (Hep-A) booster	Intramuscular - left arm Intramuscular - right arm

6 years	Td or DTP(a) and inactivated Polio (IPV) (Give Boosters every 10 years thereafter)	Intramuscular - left arm
	MMR	Intramuscular –right arm
12 years	Td or DTP(a) and inactivated Polio (IPV) when missed at 6 years	Intramuscular - left arm
	MMR (when missed at 6 years)	Intramuscular – right arm

*   The same guidelines/information stated under the Expanded EPI-SA Schedule for Childhood Vaccination for the different vaccines indicated in the "Complete Vaccination Schedule" followed in the private sector are applicable to the vaccines

[1]   Although the private sector may not exactly follow the prescribed injection sites that have to be followed in the public sector, it is suggested that the private sector does follow the prescribed injection site as followed in the public sector for the sake of reporting the slight possibility of severe adverse events following immunisation (AEFI). When the child's immunisation/vaccination chart (Called the "Road to Health") is not available at the time of the reaction, the information obtained from the parent/grandparent/foster parent/caregiver regarding the body site used for the vaccination, will give an indication of which vaccine could have been administered, possibly implicating the vaccine having caused the AEFI. (**NB**. The reaction must be correlated with the specific vaccine pamphlet insert before the conclusion is drawn that the vaccine caused the reaction).

Primary series and Booster series using the Expanded or the Complete vaccination schedule

- **Administering of the different vaccines during the same session can be done safely BUT THE ADMINISTERING MUST BE IN SEPERATE INJECTION SITES**
- **Care must be taken <u>not to</u> administer vaccines intravenously or that the needle enters a blood vessel. <u>No vaccine must be injected intradermally</u>**
- **Vaccines must be administered with caution to individuals with thrombocytopenia or a bleeding disorder since bleeding may occur following an intramuscular injection**
- **No drug interaction occurs between vaccines and anti-retroviral drugs**
- **Check the "Road to Heath Chart" on every visit to the healthcare establishment (even when visiting for minor ailments) for missed vaccination dosages. If in doubt whether the child was vaccinated or not, repeat that dosage (extra dosages are not harmful)**
- **Routine vaccination can be done in paediatric units when the child is hospitalized for long periods. When admitted to paediatric units the "Road to Heath Chart" must be checked for missed vaccination dosages. If in doubt whether the child was vaccinated or not, repeat that dosage (extra dosages are not harmful)**

CATCH-UP VACCINATION SCHEDULE

The catch-up vaccination schedules are used for infants and children (up to the age of 12 years) who were never vaccinated or whose vaccination was not completed (partly vaccinated). For these infants and children, an individualized catch-up vaccinated schedule must be drawn up (see table 6.3) based on the **age of the child AND vaccines already received**. The **age** of the infant or child must be taken in account because certain vaccines, such as the Rotavirus vaccine and the measles vaccine, may not be administered after a specific age. A full vaccination history needs to be taken as to ascertain the primary series vaccine(s) that was/were already been administered when the **vaccination** of the infant or child **was not completed** (partly vaccinated), or if the **child was never vaccinated before**. The catch-up schedule must be adjusted accordingly to complete the necessary vaccination as booster series or the primary series vaccination must then be administered to the child.

Table 6.3 CATCH-UP VACCINATION SCHEDULE FOR INFANTS AND CHILDREN WHO WERE NOT VACCINATED OR WHOSE VACCINATION WAS NOT COMPLETED

Infants between 6 weeks and 6 months of age
BCG vaccine* - when in doubt
Rotavirus (RV) vaccine - 2 dosages 4-6 weeks apart before the age of 24 weeks
DTP[a]-IPV-Hib vaccine, or alternatively DT [Diphtheria-tetanus toxoid] and IPV and Hib as single dosage vaccines, or alternatively the combination vaccines of DTP[a]-IPV and Hib. Primary series - 3 dosages 4 weeks apart. Booster series - 1 dosage at 18 months of age
Conjugated Pneumococcal Vaccine. Primary series - 3 dosages 4 weeks apart. Booster series - 1 dosage at 12-15 months
Hep-B vaccine. Primary series - 3 dosages 4 weeks apart
All booster series dosages are to be administered according to the normal recommended time intervals of 4 weeks between administering until the recommended dosages of the specific vaccine have been given

Infants between 6 months to 12 months of age
BCG vaccine* - when in doubt
DTP[a]-IPV-Hib vaccine, or alternatively DT [Diphtheria-tetanus toxoid] or alternatively TT [tetanus toxoid] as well as IPV and Hib as single dosage vaccines. Primary series - 3 dosages 4 weeks apart. Booster series - 1 dosage at 18 months of age
Measles vaccine Primary series - 1 dosage after 9 months of age as a single dosage vaccine. Booster series - 1 dosage MMR at the age 15 to 18 months or alternatively 1 dosage measles vaccine at the age of 18 months as a single dosage vaccine
Conjugated Pneumococcal Vaccine Primary series - 2 dosages 4 weeks apart. Booster series - 1 dosage after 12 months of age and at least 2 months after the 2sd dosage
Hep-B vaccine Primary series - 3 dosages 4 weeks apart
All booster series dosages are to be administered according to the normal recommended time intervals of 4 weeks between administering until the recommended dosages of the specific vaccine have been given

Infants between 12 months to 24 months
<u>BCG vaccine</u>* - when in doubt <u>DTP[a]-IPV-Hib vaccine,</u> or alternatively <u>DT</u> [Diphtheria-tetanus toxoid] or alternatively <u>TT</u> [tetanus toxoid] as well as <u>IPV</u> and <u>Hib</u> as single dosage vaccines, or alternatively the combination vaccines of <u>DTP[a]-IPV and Hib</u>. Primary series - 3 dosages 4 weeks apart. Booster series - 1 dosage 6 months later <u>Measles vaccine</u> When younger than 17 Months - Primary series: 1 dosage measles vaccine as a single dosage vaccine, or alternatively 1 dosage MMR vaccine. Booster series -1 dosage measles vaccine as a single dosage vaccine, or alternatively 1 dosage MMR vaccine 4 weeks later or at the age of 18 months. Children older than 17 months must be given the primary dosage and booster dosage 4 weeks apart <u>Conjugated Pneumococcal Vaccine</u> Primary series - 2 dosages 2 months apart <u>Hep-B vaccine</u> Primary series - 3 dosages 4 weeks apart <u>Hep-A vaccine</u> - **can be given voluntary.** Primary series - 1 dosage. Booster series - 1 dosage 6-12 months later All booster series dosages are to be administered according to the normal recommended time intervals of 4 weeks between administering until the recommended dosages of the specific vaccine have been given

Children 24 months to 12 years of age
<u>DT</u> [Diphtheria-tetanus toxoid] <u>and IPV</u> (or TOPV [Tri-valente oral polio drops]) as single dosage vaccines, or alternatively <u>TT</u> [tetanus toxoid] <u>and IPV</u> (or TOPV) as single dosage vaccines at the same time. Primary series - 3 dosages 4 weeks apart. Booster series - 1 dosage 6 months later <u>Measles vaccine</u> Primary series - 1 dosage measles vaccine as a single dosage vaccine, or alternatively 1 dosage MMR vaccine. Booster series - 1 dosage measles vaccine as a single dosage vaccine or alternatively 1 dosage MMR vaccine at the age of 4-5 years or at the age of 11-12 years <u>Conjugated Pneumococcal Vaccine</u> Primary series - 1 dosage before the age of 5 years <u>Hep-B vaccine</u> Primary series - 3 dosages 4 weeks apart up to the age of 5 years <u>Hep-A vaccine</u> - **can be given voluntary**. Primary series - 1 dosage. Booster series - 1 dosage 6-12 months later <u>Td and IPV vaccines or only Td vaccine</u> – 1 dosage at the age of 6 years and 12 years All outstanding booster series dosages are to be administered according to the normal recommended time intervals of 4 weeks between administering. **Do not, when the child is older than 24 months**, administer any vaccine that contains Pertussis (whole-cell such as DTP[w]-IPV-vaccine, or the combination vaccines of Hib like DTP[w]-IPV and Hib, or DTP[w]-Hib and IPV).

Children who had received DT at 5 years of age
Children who received DT at 5 years of age **MUST NOT receive Td at the age of 6 years.** A dosage of Td must be given at 12 years of age

Children who did not received DT at 5 years of age
Children who did not received DT at 5 years **MUST** wait until they are 6 years old. The child must then receive 1 dosage of Td vaccine at the age of 6 years and 12 years. **BCG*** can be administered to children older than one (1) year who have never received BCG. When there is the slightest suspicion that the child may suffer from tuberculosis, the tuberculin skin test has to be done first. On the grounds of the result, BCG will be administered or treatment will be started Children younger than 8 years of age who have not been previously vaccinated should receive a second dose of Haemophilus influenza type B (Hib) after 4 weeks

Table 6.4 CONTRA-INDICATIONS FOR ROUTINE VACCINATION OF CHILDREN

Contra-indication	Vaccine	Rationale	Healthcare interventions
Acute diseases associated with pyrexia, or a chronic debilitating diseases, or a body temperature of 38,5°C or higher	All	The natural defence mechanisms of the body are compromised	Explain the reason for postponing the vaccination to the healthcare user or parents, and arrange a follow-up visit as soon as possible. In the case of a chronic disease, discuss the matter with the healthcare user's doctor before vaccination
Gastroenteritis	Living attenuated polio virus vaccine (oral polio vaccine only) and Human rotavirus vaccine	Vaccination can impede the colonisation of the virus in the intestinal tract. Colonisation is essential to elicit the immune reaction	When child is younger than 8 weeks of age, explain the reason for postponing the vaccination to the parents/ care giver/mother, and arrange a follow-up visit as soon as possible. When child is older than 8 weeks old, intramuscular polio vaccine (IPV) can be given instead of OPV. When Human rotavirus vaccine cannot be given, postpone until later date, but do not postpone until infant is older than 24 weeks of age
• **Immunological diseases** • **Malignancies,** for example, leukaemia, lymphoma • **AIDS**[1] • **Immunotherapy** (steroids, radiation)	BCG All living vaccines (such as measles, mumps, rubella and poliomyelitis)	Serious reactions to vaccination can occur as these diseases suppress/ compromise the immune system	Emphasise the necessity of preventing exposure to childhood communicable diseases Discuss the matter with the attending physician
Recently received "Artificial-passively-acquired immunity" via antitoxin, or antiserum or gamma-globulin that was administered **(within the previous six weeks)**	Measles, mumps and rubella viruses	The presence of artificial passively-acquired immunity prevents the formation of antibody in response to the vaccine	Enquire (during history-taking) about recent blood transfusions or injections of gamma-globulin or administering of immunoglobulin or an antiserum or antitoxin. If the reply is affirmative, wait six (6) weeks before vaccination

Known allergic/ hyper-sensitivity reactions to substances in vaccines for example, egg protein and drugs such as neomycin, streptomycin, and polymycin B, as well as substances such as thiomersal (an organic-mercuric compound) and glutaraldehyde	Living virus vaccines cultivated in embryos of chickens and treated with neomycin and/or other microbial drugs and/ or substances used in the production of the vaccine	Substances present in the vaccine will cause a hyper-sensitivity reaction in the vaccinee	Check the manufacturer's product information for specific contra-indications and include in the history taking of the healthcare user, ask questions regarding specific allergies and allergic reactions to a previous dosage of a specific vaccine. Do not administer the specific vaccine
• **History of diseases of the central nervous system** • **Side-effects of hyper-pyrexia, drowsiness or convulsions after DTP(a) or DTP(a)-IPV-Hib or DTP(a)-IPV vaccination**	Pertussis vaccine	The risk of a severe neurological reaction to the pertussis vaccine is considerably increased	Take a thorough neurological history, including information regarding epilepsy, convulsions, syncope, tremors, muscular spasms and specific side-effects of DTP(a) vaccination. Refer the client to a medical practitioner for vaccination if necessary. **Diphtheria–Tetanus-Pertussis** must not be given to any individual suffering from epilepsy that is not controlled. Give TT (tetanus toxoid) if younger than 6 years or Td when older than 6 years
Pregnancy	All living viral vaccines and pneumococcal vaccine except polio and tetanus toxoid vaccines	Potential risk to foetus, especially rubella virus	Take a thorough history of all female healthcare users (married or unmarried) in their fertile years regarding being pregnant at present or possible conception within the following two months. When the female user is pregnant, **NO vaccination must be done** (with the exception of polio and tetanus toxoid vaccines)

Severe reaction (collapse, encephalopathy, or non-febrile convulsions) after the first dose	DTP[a]-Hib or DTP[a] or DTP[a]-IPV-Hib, or DTP[a]-IPV	Indication of an allergic reaction that may trigger a similar event when vaccinated again with same vaccine	Give TT (tetanus toxoid) according to age or Td when older than 6 years of age. Administer a separate dosage of Hib and IPV

[1] All HIV-exposed children as well as HIV-infected children who have not developed AIDS must be vaccinated as they need more protection than children that are not HIV-infected

Please note

* **VACCINATION IS NOT COMPULSORY according to regulation R2438 of 30 October 1987,** promulgated under The Health Act, Act 63 of 1977, (Government Gazette No. 11014 of 30 October 1987). As children have a right to protection against Vaccine Preventable Diseases, it now becomes necessarily for all healthcare providers to motivate and encourage all parents/guardians/single mothers or fathers/foster-parents to have their children vaccinated[1]. Every opportunity should be used to vaccinate children or have their vaccination completed, for instance in paediatric wards of hospitals, paediatric outpatient departments, baby clinics and primary healthcare clinics (public and private), and school health services

* **When parents/guardians do not want their child to be vaccinated, it must be recorded as such.** However, under the Children's Act, No 38 of 2005, any child can be vaccinated without the written or verbal consent of the parents/ guardians/single mothers or fathers/foster parents when it is in the best interests of the child to receive immunization (infant's right to receive protection against specific communicable diseases)[1]. Also, when the health of the population of the RSA or any part of the population may be affected by a medical condition against which the population can be vaccinated, the Director-General of Health may, by means of notification in the Government Gazette demarcate an area referred to in the notice for compulsory vaccination of all inhabitants or of a specific group or category of inhabitants, as referred to in the notice, of such a demarcated area

* There exists close collaboration between the National Department of Health and the National Department of Education in the implementation of all revised policies in respect of compulsory and voluntary vaccination as well as school entry and school exit requirements

* Always bear in mind that, although most of the vaccines are designed to protect the infants/children against particular communicable diseases at a very young age and vaccination is carried out as early as possible, the following are **always applicable when vaccinating infants**
  + **The presence of maternally-derived antibody reduces the effectiveness of some vaccines. These vaccines must only be given after the age of 3 month or later**

✚ Live attenuated vaccines can cause severe disease in immunodeficiency states which may not be diagnosed immediately after birth

✚ If the disease is mainly a risk to the elderly (for example, pneumococcal pneumonia) vaccination must be given at a later age

✚ The overuse of vaccines during the early childhood by vaccinating the child over and over again and again with the same specific vaccine after every exposure, may lead to the mutation of new, more virulent strains of the specific pathogen, leaving the individual susceptible to the more virulent pathogen that may cause a more serious disease

✚ As artificial actively-acquired immunity elicited by vaccination decreases with time, "childhood communicable diseases" now becomes diseases of adolescence and young adults - a vaccinated child now contracts the particular disease later in life and because adolescents and adults become more seriously ill than children, more adolescents and adults die from or are disabled by the complications of vaccine-prevented diseases than children

✚ The practice of administering paracetemol or other anti-pyretic preparations to infants one hour before vaccination and then one hour after vaccination followed by four hourly dosises for up to 72 to 96 hours to prevent pyrexia (fever) and a feeling of sickness, suppresses the immune system to such an extent that the adaptive immune system cannot elicit the normal antigen-antibody response. The result of this suppressed immune reaction is that the "immunized/vaccinated" infant will contract the particular communicable disease and the severity of the disease will be similar to that of a non-vaccinated person as no immunologic memory could be induced. A moderate temperature/fever up to 38°C can be well tolerated because a raised body temperature, as a natural body mechanism, is a necessity to enhance the activity level of the immune system of the infant, for example, the complement activation, lymphocyte proliferation and the synthesis of proteins such as antibody and cytokines. At the same times heat sensitive pathogens are killed off.

[1]Please note that subject to Section 132 under the Children's Act, Act 38 of 2005, consent to vaccination can be given by the defined classes of officials/individuals who are accorded with the legal right to give consent on behalf of the child for medical procedures.

Please note
The following is applicable to all situations of vaccination
⊙ All children who are Symptomatic HIV-infective or who suffer from the AIDS syndrome have to be vaccinated according to the vaccination schedule WITH THE EXCEPTION OF BCG, RV (Rotavirus vaccine), and Measles which are NOT TO BE GIVEN

⊙ During epidemics or in special vaccination situations all the different vaccines can be safely administered simultaneously

⊙ There is no danger of transmission of HIV or virus hepatitis B or any other disease transmissible by blood, when a new and unused sterile needle and syringe are used every

time for each individual injection in different injection sites. (When multiple dosage vaccine vials are used, retractable needles can be used to prevent blood borne transmission of infectious agents from person to person). The aseptic technique has to be used during administering of all vaccines and all sharp objects have to be safely disposed of. The skin must be cleaned with water and cotton wool

⊙ **UNDER NO CIRCUMSTANCES MAY SINGLE DOSAGES OF DIFFERENT VACCINES BE MIXED IN THE SAME SYRINGE OR BE INJECTED INTO THE SAME INJECTION SITE WHEN ADMINISTERING**

- ☑ **THE SAME THIGH OR ARM MAY BE USED, BUT DIFFENT AND SEPARATE INJECTION SITES FOR ADMINISTERING**
- ☑ **TWO OR MORE NEW AND UNUSED SEPARATE SYRINGES HAVE TO BE USED IN WHICH TO RECONSTITUTE THE DIFFERENT VACCINES BEFORE ADMINISTERING. USE THE SAME NEEDLE FOR DRAWING UP AND INJECTING THE VACCINE - "ONE NEEDLE, ONE SYRINGE"**
- ☑ **ALWAYS USE DIFFERENT INJECTION SITES FOR DIFFERENT VACCINES**
- ☑ **ALSO REMEMBER THAT DILUENTS ARE NOT INTERCHANGEABLE AS DIFFERENT VACCINES HAVE DIFFERNT DILUENTS. Always use the diluent from the same manufacturer as the vaccine**

⊙ Should other vaccines than those provided by the National Department of Health, such as combination vaccines or single dosage vaccines, be used for the vaccination of a child, the parent(s)/guardian(s)/foster parent(s) have to purchase the vaccine and transport it in a cool bag to the public primary healthcare clinic for administering (this does not apply in the case of private practices and private clinics). Excluded are those specific vaccines for travelling that have to be administered at a travel clinic and be certified

⊙ Only living trivalent oral polio vaccine is used for the priming of the immune system of children under the age of 6 weeks. From 6 weeks and older the inactivated polio vaccine that is administered intramuscularly is used. When an epidemic breaks out, the inactivated polio vaccine should be administered as it prevents the attenuated living polio-virus in the oral vaccine to revert back to the wild type while simultaneously increasing its virulence because the oral attenuated virus is shed in faecal stools. The inactivated polio vaccine is always given intramuscularly

⊙ Considering all contra-indications, only the most serious contra-indications (such as pregnancy and outspoken allergic reactions) are taken into account when a person has to be vaccinated. Low hyperpyrexia (below 39^0C), gastritis and skin conditions, are not considered serious contra-indications for vaccination. The final decision regarding the vaccinating of the individual is based on the findings of the health assessment done (the history taking and the physical examination). Should it be decided not to have the individual vaccinated, the necessary steps have to be taken, namely, referring the individual to a medical practitioner or to provide the person with a future date for vaccination

⊙ Do not vaccinate a sick child when the parent(s)/guardian/foster parent objects – rather encourage the parent/guardian/mother/foster parent to bring the child for vaccination as soon as the child has recovered

⊙ All premature or underweight infants should be vaccinated at the same age as other babies – do not postpone vaccination of these children

⊙ When a child is eligible for more than one type of vaccine, the vaccines can all be given safely during the same session, as long as different injection sites are used

⊙ All vaccines can be administered concurrently with antibiotics and anti-retroviral drugs

⊙ When in doubt whether a child has had a certain dose or not, give that dose – extra doses are not harmful

⊙ **Never miss a change to vaccinate - never turn a child away if vaccination is due**

6.4.3   Administering of the vaccine

The process of administering, storage, transportation and reconstitution of each specific vaccine will be discussed in detail in section 6.5.

<u>Please note:</u>

According to the Expanded Programme of Vaccination, when vaccines are used, the **<u>following steps must always be adhered to in respect to single and multiple dosages and/or any other administering</u>**

■ **Read all vaccine vial monitors (VVMs) carefully before use**. A VVM is a tiny dot on the vial which is sensitive to heat. The cumulative effect of heat and the duration of time cause the dot to change colour, and this indicates that the vaccine is no longer safe to use (See figure 6.1)

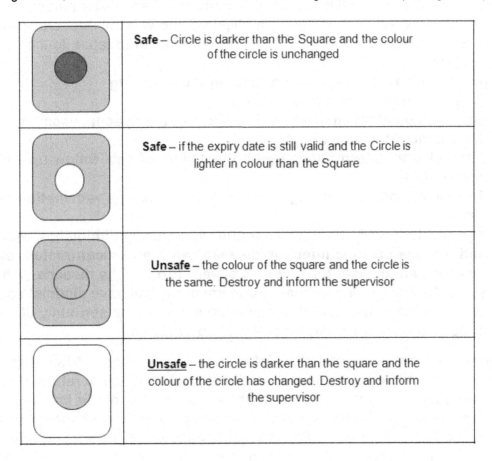

Figure 6.1 Interpretation of vaccine vial monitors (VVMs)

■ **Opened vials of DTP, TT, Td and Hepatitis B vaccine may be re-used** for a maximum of 30 days, provided the opened vials are kept cold at all times and are not taken from the premises

■ **If opened vials are to be re-used, this has to be done before the expiry date, the vials had been stored at 0–8⁰C, the vaccine vial septum had not been submerged in water, the inner** circle of the vaccine VVM is lighter than the outer square, and the aseptic technique was used to withdraw all dosages. If any of the aforementioned conditions were neglected, all vials must be immediately destroyed. Always take careful note of the colour of the VVMS.

■ All opened vials of reconstituted Measles and BCG vaccines MUST be destroyed after SIX (6) hours and at the end of each vaccination session. NO VIAL MAY BE USED AGAIN. Should vaccination campaigns take longer than six hours, new vaccine vials must be opened for use

■ All opened oral polio vials can be used as long as the VVM has not reached the discard point

■ Reconstituted DTP-Hib vials must be discarded after 7 days

■ Reconstituted Rotavirus vaccine must be discarded after 24 hours

■ Complete the necessary records by always labelling vaccine vials with the date and time when opened or reconstituted.

6.4.4 Information to be provided to healthcare users in respect to vaccination, vaccines and side-effects

It is imperative that the healthcare user, parents/guardians/foster-parents be well-informed about the vaccination and side-effects of the vaccine after administering. Not only will this reassure them, it will also motivate them to return to the clinic for follow-up visits.

Information must always be given regarding the following
- **Type of and purpose of the vaccine**
- **Immunological reaction and side-effects of the specific vaccine**
- **Treatment of the side-effects**
- **Date of and information about the value of the follow-up visit (if appropriate)**
- **The importance of keeping of the healthcare user's vaccination record safely**
- **The fact that artificial actively-acquired immunity diminishes with time and that the specific infection/disease can then be contracted, even if it is then an atypical form or less severe form of the disease. After 12 years the artificial actively-acquired immunity will have diminished more or less all together, and the individual can become seriously ill. When booster dosages are required, it must be received.**

Antipyretic drugs must be administered very sensibly. When the body temperature is lowered to a point under the critical body temperature of 36,5⁰C, the immunological response (the innate and adaptive physiologic immunological responses) <u>cannot be activated</u> **and maintained to induce phagocytosis and antibody-mediated and T-cell-mediated reactions to kill off the specific infectious agent.** A low to moderated elevated body temperature (37,5⁰C to 38,5⁰C) can be well tolerated by most individuals. When the ill person can tolerate a higher elevated temperature and <u>there are no indications of complications developing</u> (especially cerebral and neurological complications) the natural course of the vaccination can be followed. Drugs containing acetylsalicylic or salicylic acids/acetylsalicylate/salicylate/ASA (for example, Aspirin, Disprin, Grandpa powders etc.) <u>must never be given to children under the age of 16 years</u> as it can cause Reye's disease of the liver. These drugs must also not be given to children who have received any vaccine(s) containing living attenuated viruses. **A body temperature rising to 40,5ºC and higher within 48 hours after vaccination is a trigger event of a medical incident that needs medical attention, as the hyperpyrexia can be accompanied by vomiting and restlessness leading to febrile convulsions. Such adverse reaction must be medical treated and has to be reported according to law.**

The specific information regarding each specific vaccine which must be given to healthcare users, parents/guardians/foster parents and care takers, is discussed in detail in section 6.5.

6.5 VACCINES

Each of the respective vaccines is discussed under the following headings
✠ Available preparations
✠ Storage, transportation, handling and reconstituting
✠ Contra-indications
✠ Administering
✠ Health information to be given to the healthcare user

6.5.1 BCG (BACILLUS CALMETTE-GUÉRIN) VACCINE

The BCG vaccine, a living vaccine, contains freeze-dried live, attenuated pathogens prepared from a special strain of *Mycobacterium bovis*. BCG vaccination elicits cell-mediated immunity against infection of drug-susceptible *Mycobacterium tuberculosis humanis* only.

✠ **Storage, transportation, handling and reconstitution**
  ✳ The vaccine has to be stored in a refrigerator at 2-8ºC and **must not be frozen, since freezing and thawing will destroy the live attenuated pathogen**
  ✳ The vaccine should be **kept on ice in a cool bag during transit**
  ✳ **The vaccine is extremely sensitive to heat and light, including neon light**
  ✳ If the vaccine is correctly stored, it **remains effective for two years after production**
  ✳ The **diluent must be stored in a cool place**
  ✳ **Reconstitution** of the vaccine is done as follows
    • Reconstitute the vaccine according to the **manufacturer's instructions**
    • **Do not reconstitute the vaccine in bright light**
    • **Keep vial in a cool, dark, dry place. When not in use, store in cool, dark, dry place**
    • After being reconstituted, the **vials must be covered immediately after use and replaced** into a dark container that does not let light in or through
    • **Reconstituted vaccine must be destroyed after six (6) hours**
    • **Do not expose reconstituted vaccine to heat - DO NOT hold it in the hands for any period of time, or handle it under or near neon lights or other electrical appliances.** Keep it cold at all times

✠ **Contra-indications**

The BCG vaccine is **not administered to children who**

⅄ **are being treated with cortisone**

⅄ **are on immuno-suppressant treatment**

⅄ **suffer of immune system deficiencies**

⅄ **have just stopped taking INH (24 hours must have elapsed before BCG-vaccine can be administered)**

⅄ **are taking anti-tuberculosis drugs for active tuberculosis**

⅄ **are symptomatic HIV-infective or suffer from AIDS syndrome**

⅄ **are HIV-exposed and may be infected and/or seriously sick – Do PCR after 6 weeks and give BCG if results are negative. (Healthy HIV-exposed infants can be vaccinated)**

⅄ **have recently had measles** (two months must elapsed before BCG-vaccine can be administered)

⅄ **are older than 12 months**

⅄ **are new-borns whose mothers are receiving anti-tuberculosis drugs – put new-born on TB prophylaxis and follow up with BCG later**

<u>Please note</u>

✴ <u>Asymptomatic HIV-infected children can be given childhood vaccines as normal</u>

✴ <u>In missed opportunities, BCG and measles can be given on the same day BUT different vaccination sites must be used</u>

✠ **Administering**

◈ **Age of vaccination**

BCG vaccination must preferably be **done before the age of 6 months or as soon as possible after birth. Should the vaccination be unsuccessful (for example, no scar, or growing inoculation marks) the child has to be vaccinated once more.**

◈ **Procedure for vaccination**

Use the **multiple puncture vaccination apparatus** when vaccinating

☑ **Clean the right upper arm with water** when it is very dirty. Do not clean with chemical substances, such as ether, alcohol and/or other germicides, as it destroys the BCG vaccine

☑ Draw the vaccine up in a syringe, remove the needle and place a drop of vaccine immediately above the implant of the deltoid muscle. **Spread it with the narrow, un-grooved edge of the collar so that it covers a surface of about 2 cm**

☑ Hold the **cylinder at a right angle to the area spread with the vaccine** with the needles pointing downwards

☑ Push the **cylinder down until the edges of the collar touch the skin**

☑ Lift the cylinder, **rotate slightly and push down a second time.** Repeat the process a third time. (In this way 27 punctures are made in the skin right through the layer of vaccine)

Please note

Eighteen punctures are sufficient for the vaccination of infants. Make these by rotating the cylinder once only

◈ When vaccination campaigns are undertaken away from the service centre at places where an autoclave is not available, the following **method of sterilizing and/or cleaning the vaccination apparatus is recommended**

♦ Submerge the needle end of the apparatus in a full strength solution of any germicidal solution for ten minutes and rinse thoroughly under clean running water before use

♦ If no solution is available, scrub the needle end of the apparatus with soap and water and rinse well under clean running water

PLEASE NOTE

<u>Under NO circumstances must BCG vaccine be administered intradermally into the M. Deltoid using an injection needle.</u> When injected intradermally, a sterile abscess will form at the site of the injection within 2 to 4 months that needs to be drained surgically - scar tissue can leave a lesion. <u>NO IMMUNOLOGICAL RESPONSE</u> is mediated and the child can contract drug-susceptible Tuberculosis from a very early age on wards. Sterile abscesses are seen as an Adverse events/reactions following immunization or vaccination **(Injection site abscess formation following vaccination-AEFI)** and as such must be reported by law

✠ **Health information to be given to healthcare users**

✳ The aim of vaccination, namely, to **prime the infant's adaptive immune system against drug-susceptible tuberculosis by acting as immuno-stimulant in the eliciting of cell-mediated immunity**

✳ The **inoculation/vaccinated area must be kept out of direct sunlight for four hours on the day of administering**

✳ The **inoculation/vaccinated area may be washed with soap and water**

✳ The **inoculation marks begins to grow three to six weeks after vaccination (sometimes sooner).** The marks may grow for three or four months and then gradually disappear. They may, however, remain visible for months, or even years. The growth of the inoculation marks is no cause for concern

✳ **The inoculation marks must not be pricked, scratched or covered**

✳ **A month has to pass before measles vaccine or MMR vaccine may be administered.**

Please note BCG vaccine prevents severe forms of drug-susceptible TB in children but is less effective in preventing pulmonary TB in adults, irrespective of the level of drug resistance of the strain.

6.5.2   POLIO VACCINE (ORAL AND INJECTABLE)

Attenuated oral trivalent polio-vaccine, a living vaccine (TOPV), contains the attenuated living poliomyelitis-virus as a mixture of biotypes 1, 2 and 3 of the poliomyelitis strain. The monovalent oral polio vaccine (MOPV) is a vaccine which contains only the attenuated live/living polio-virus biotype 1 of the poliomyelitis virus strain. The monovalent oral polio vaccine is only used in certain circumstances, for example, during an outbreak of an epidemic caused by polio-virus biotype 1.

Attenuated oral Polio-vaccine (OPV) not only elicits a general antibody-mediated reaction, but also an intestinal-mucosal immunity that affords protection when the polio-virus gains entry into the body again. When the prescribed schedule of administering is followed, the trivalent polio vaccine affords total protection against all three biotypes. The attenuated living virus, when administered as an oral vaccine, does not regain its virulence when shed/excreted from the body (it is shed in the stools). It can, however, improve the general immunity of a population by spreading in the community and competing with the virus of the wild type.

When the inactivated polio vaccine **PV[i]** or **IPV** or **P[i]** is administered intramuscularly, the above does not occur as the pathogenesis of polio does not occur in the gut and the virus cannot be shed in the stools. By administering the inactivated polio vaccine intramuscularly as single dosage vaccine or in a combination vaccine from the age of 6 weeks, the general immunity of the population is enhanced while the risk of epidemics is minimized. During outbreaks of epidemics of poliomyelitis, the administering of inactivated polio vaccine helps to control the epidemic.

✠ **Available preparations**
- ➧ Monovalent oral polio drops given orally **(MOPV)**
- ➧ Trivalent oral polio drops given orally **(TOPV or OPV)**
- ➧ Inactivated type 1, 2 and 3 Poliovirus D antigen polio vaccine administered intra-muscularly **(IPV or P[i] or PV[i])**
- ➧ Purified Diphtheria toxoid-tetanus toxoid-pertussis toxoid (P[a]-filamentous haemagglutinin)-inactivated type 1, 2 and 3 Poliovirus D antigen-Haemophilus influenzae type B-vaccine administered intra-muscularly **(DTP[a]-IPV-Hib)**
- ➧ Purified Diphtheria toxoid-tetanus toxoid-Pertussis toxoid (acellular-filamentous haemagglutinin)-Inactivated type 1, 2 and 3 Poliovirus D antigen vaccine administered intra-muscularly **(DTP[a]-IPV)**

✠ **Storage, transportation, handling and reconstitution**
- ✻ The oral polio vaccine must be **stored frozen** and must not repeatedly be frozen and thawed
- ✻ **After thawing**, the oral polio vaccine must be **kept in a refrigerator at 2-8⁰C** (preferably 4⁰C) or in a cool bag for only a limited time period.
- ✻ Always **keep VVMs in mind**
- ✻ The **cold chain must be maintained** from the moment of production until administering to the healthcare user. This requires that the oral polio vaccine be packed directly onto ice after administering, between administering and during transportation. Since the vaccine is a live virus, **interruption of the cold chain will inactivate it.** The maintaining of the cold chain is of extreme importance in extremely hot or remote areas as to maintain the potency of the live attenuated oral vaccine

* Oral polio vaccine is **sensitive to heat and neon light**. It must therefore never be exposed to direct sunlight or be placed under neon lights
* **ONLY** <u>bright yellow or straw-coloured oral polio vaccine</u> **is suitable for use**
* **Turbid oral polio vaccine** is unsuitable for use and **must be destroyed**
* A **sterile needle** must be used to **puncture the vial of the oral polio vaccine**
* The inactivated polio vaccine (as single dosage vaccine or as part of a combination vaccine) must be kept cold at 2 - 8°C and administered cold intramuscularly

✠ **Contra-indications**

⅄ Oral polio vaccine should **not be administered during a serious illness or in chronic illnesses,** such as leukaemia or Hodgkin's disease or when suffering from AIDS

⅄ In case **of diarrhoea or gastro-enteritis, the oral vaccine may be administered, but a further dosage should be given** four weeks later. Inactivated polio vaccine (IPV) can be given intramuscularly instead when the child is older than 2 months old

✠ **Administering**

◈ Two drops of trivalent oral Polio (TOPV) vaccine are given to all children under the age of 6 weeks

☑ **Preparation**

No special preparation is necessary. Infants and toddlers can be fed before and after administering – withholding of food is therefore unnecessary either before or after administering

☑ **Administering**

* The **first dosage** of trivalent oral polio (OPV) vaccine is given at birth and at the age of 6 weeks where after the combined **DTP[a]-IPV-Hib vaccine is used**
* The **recommended number of drops (2-3) are dropped directly from the container of the oral polio vaccine into the mouth** of the child
* Should the **oral polio vaccine be vomited, the dosage must be repeated immediately**
* **Trivalent oral polio vaccine can be administered simultaneously with the vaccines of BCG, DTP(a), Hep-B**

☑ **Premature babies can also be given trivalent oral polio vaccine. Older children or adults, who have never been vaccinated with oral polio vaccine, are given three dosages of the trivalent oral polio vaccine or three dosage of the IPV vaccine administered intramuscularly at intervals of four to six (4-6) weeks**

◈ Three drops of trivalent oral polio vaccine or three intramuscular IPV vaccine are administered four to six (4-6) weeks apart to

☑ **immigrants** up to 40 years of age

☑ **susceptible contacts** who have been exposed to the disease

☑ **high risk groups** as preventative chemo-prophylaxis when an outbreak of poliomyelitis occurs

◈ Inactivated polio vaccine (as single dosage vaccine or in combination vaccines) is administered intramuscularly to infants and children to prime the infant's/child's immune system (primary series) as well as to travellers and/or local community members as preventive chemo-prophylaxis when an outbreak of poliomyelitis occurs in a specific country or geographical area. Inactivated polio vaccine is highly immunogenic while carrying no risk of vaccine-associated paralytic poliomyelitis (VAPP); and is not contra-indicated in immune-compromised individuals. As the pathogenesis of polio does not occur in the gut with inactivated polio vaccine, the risk of an outbreak due to circulating vaccine-derived poliovirus (cVDPV) is reduced because the polio-virus is not excreted in the stools with the result that the polio-virus cannot revert back to a more virulent form nor attach itself to the wild type of the disease. Inactivated polio-virus vaccine (IPV) and attenuated oral polio-virus vaccine (OPV) can be used as alternatives to each other in priming the infant's adaptive immune system against the poliomyelitis virus or as booster dosages

✠ **Health information to be given to healthcare users**
After administering the vaccine, the healthcare provider must provide the parent/guardian/foster-parent or healthcare user with the following information

✳ The aim of primary vaccination, namely, to **prime the infant's adaptive immune system against poliomyelitis by acting as immuno-stimulant in the eliciting of antibody-mediated immunity.** When given later in life, it acts as a booster for the adaptive immune system, if previously vaccinated

✳ When the infant/child **vomits** the oral polio vaccine, he/she has to receive the polio vaccine once more

✳ The infant/child may **be fed as usual**

✳ The infant/child **will not become ill** as a result of the oral polio vaccine

✳ **After the combined DTP[a]-IPV-Hib vaccine has been administered, the vaccinee should remain under medical supervision for 30 minutes**

Warning
As inactivated polio vaccine (IPV) has to be injected intramuscularly, it must be administered with caution to individuals suffering from thrombocytopenia or a bleeding disorder.

Please note
The practice of treating fever blisters with oral polio vaccine is not recommended.

6.5.3 HUMAN ROTAVIRUS VACCINE

The Human Rotavirus vaccine, a living vaccine, is a lyophilized vaccine containing the live heterogonous attenuated *human rotavirus*. **The Human Rotavirus vaccine gives only effective protection against any severe rotavirus gastro-enteritis** – it does not protect against gastro-enteritis due to other pathogens than the rotavirus.

The Human Rotavirus-vaccine is provided free of charge by the National Department of Health or be purchased from a pharmacy or a medical practitioner and will be administered by the staff of a public healthcare clinic after permission has been given in writing by the parents/guardians/foster-parents. When administered by private healthcare practitioners in private practices or in private well-baby clinics, a fee will be charged for the procedure done and the vaccine administered.

✠ **Available preparations**
➤ Rotavirus vaccine containing the human rotavirus GIP[8] and non-GI serotypes {such as G2P[8], G3P[8], G4P[8] and G9P[8]}
➤ Pentavalent rotavirus vaccine containing the human-bovine (WC3) reassortant rotavirus G1,G2,G3 G4 and P1

✠ **Storage, transportation and handling of the vaccine**
✳ The **vaccine (both lyophilized vaccine and liquid diluent)** must be **stored between +2^{0}C and +8^{0}C in a refrigerator**
✳ The **vaccine must not be frozen and must be protected from light** (sunlight as well as electrical light/neon light)
✳ After **reconstitution the vaccine must be administered immediately or kept in the refrigerator (+2^{0}C to +8^{0}C) for not longer than 24 hours.** When used again, the syringe containing the reconstituted vaccine must be **again** visually inspected and shaken before the vaccine is administered **orally**
✳ If **not used within 24 hours, the vaccine MUST be discarded**
✳ The **cold chain must be maintained** from the time of production until administering to the healthcare user. This requires that the vaccine be transported cold. When a cool bag is used, the time period is limited. As the vaccine contains a living virus, interruption of the cold chain will inactivate the virus
✳ The lyophilized vaccine is a whitish cake or powder in the glass vial, while the diluent is a turbid liquid with a slow-settling deposit and colourless supernatant in a glass pre-filled syringe with a plunger stopper. **In the event of foreign particulate matter and/or abnormal physical appearance, the vaccine must be immediately discarded**
✳ **Disposed of unused vaccine and waste material** in accordance with local requirement
✳ **Both the vaccine and diluent must be inspected visually before and after reconstitution** for any foreign particular matter and abnormal physical appearance prior to administering. A white deposit and clear supernatant is to be observed upon storage of the diluent and the content of the syringe should be visually inspected before and after shaking. **In event of foreign particulate matter and/or abnormal physical appearance the vaccine must be immediately discarded**

✠ **Contra-indications**
⅄ Infants with **known hypersensitivity after previous administering** of the vaccine or any component thereof

215

⅄ Infants who have **known or suspected immunodeficiency**

⅄ Infants with any **history of chronic gastro-intestinal disease** including any uncorrected congenital malformation of the gastro-intestinal tract

⅄ **Do not** administer the **first dosage when the child is younger than 6 weeks of age**

⅄ **Do not** administer the **first dosage when the child is older than 14 weeks of age**

⅄ **Do not** administer **any dosage when the child is older than 24 weeks of age**

⅄ **Do not administer when the child suffers from AIDS or are HIV-infected**

Please note

* The human rotavirus vaccine can be given to asymptomatic human immunodeficiency virus infected infants (asymptomatic HIV+ infants)

* Vaccination with the human rotavirus vaccine must be postponed in infants suffering from severe acute febrile illness, diarrhoea and vomiting

* The presence of a minor infection is, however, not a contra-indication for vaccination

* The human rotavirus vaccine <u>must not be administered after the age of 24 weeks</u>

* <u>When the infant vomits or spits out or regurgitates the vaccine, DO NOT repeat the dosage</u>

■ **Administering**

◇ The Human Rotavirus vaccine **is <u>administered orally</u> and only to infants** between the ages of 6 weeks and 24 weeks

◇ The **first dosage** should be given before the infant is 14 weeks old, and the **second dosage** when the infant is not older than 24 weeks of age

◇ The interval between dosages **should not be less than 4 weeks,** for example, the first dosage when 10 weeks old and the second dosage when 14 weeks old

◇ Human Rotavirus vaccine can be **given concomitantly** with the following vaccine (monovalent or in combination): **purified diphtheria toxoid-tetanus toxoid, purified diphtheria toxoid-tetanus toxoid-acellular pertussis toxoid** vaccine (DTP[a]); **Haemophilus influenzae type B (Hib)** vaccine; **inactivated polio vaccine (IPV)** vaccine, **hepatitis B** vaccine **and pneumococcal** vaccine

WARNING - DO NOT INJECT THE HUMAN ROTAVIRUS VACCINE – IT MUST BE GIVEN ORALLY

◇ To administer the vaccine - Position the infant seated in a reclining position and administer the entire content of the syringe (1ml) **orally** into the mouth of the infant (on the inside of the cheek)

◇ <u>**DO NOT repeat the dosage when the infant vomits/spits out/regurgitate the vaccine**</u>

Please note

* The Human Rotavirus vaccine **is not** intended for use in adults

* THE HUMAN ROTAVIRUS VACCINE SHALL UNDER NO CIRCUMSTANCES BE INJECTED – IT IS AN ORAL VACCINE TO BE GIVEN PER MOUTH

* Repeat dosage **is not** indicated when the infant should spit out, regurgitate or vomit during or after the administering of the vaccine.
* **No restriction** exists on the infant's consumption of food or liquid, including breast-milk before or after vaccination
* Vaccination **must be preceded** by a review of the medical history (especially with regards to previous vaccination and the occurrence of undesirable events) and a clinical examination
* **The two-week (2 weeks) interval between giving Trivalent Oral Polio Vaccine (TOPV) and giving the Rotavirus vaccine must be respected - or give in accordance to the Expanded Programme on Immunisation – (EPI (SA) Revised Childhood Immunisation Schedule**

⨯ Health information to be given to healthcare users

After administering the vaccine, the healthcare practitioner must provide the parent/guardian/foster-parent or healthcare user with the following information

* The aim of vaccination, namely, to **prime the infant's adaptive immune system against rotavirus gastro-enteritis by acting as immuno-stimulant in the eliciting of protective intestinal-mucosal viral-antigen immunity**
* **Side-effects**

Various side-effects may occur after the administering of the human rotavirus vaccine

General side-effects	Rare side-effects
➤ Irritability	➤ Constipation
➤ Crying	➤ Upper respiratory tract infection
➤ Sleep disorder	➤ Hoarseness
➤ Somnolence	➤ Rhinorrhoea
➤ Loss of appetite	➤ Gastro-enteritis
➤ Diarrhoea	➤ Dermatitis
➤ Vomiting	➤ Rash
➤ Flatulence	➤ Muscle cramps
➤ Abdominal pain	
➤ Regurgitation of food	

* **Treatment of side-effects**

Symptomatic and supportive
* Other information to be communicated regarding the administering of human-rotavirus vaccine
    * ➤ The protective immune response may not be elicited in all vaccinees
    * ➤ The vaccine does not protect against gastro-enteritis due to other pathogens than the rotavirus
    * ➤ Two-week (2 weeks) interval between the administering of Trivalent Oral Polio Vaccine (TOPV) and Rotavirus vaccine must be respected or given as required by the Expanded Immunisation Programme (EPI-SA)
    * ➤ **No restriction** exists on the infant's consumption of food or liquid, including breast-milk before or after vaccination.

6.5.4 DIPHTHERIA VACCINE (PURE AND IN COMBINATION)

Diphtheria vaccine, a toxoid vaccine, is prepared from the endotoxin of the diphtheria bacillus and is absorbed in an aluminium phosphate gel. The diphtheria vaccine is obtainable as a pure diphtheria vaccine or as a reduced amount of diphtheria toxoid vaccine combined with toxoid of specific inactivated pathogens or in a combination vaccine with specific different live attenuated pathogens.

✠ **Available preparations**
  ➔ Absorbed pure diphtheria toxoid vaccine - **Diph PTAP**
  ➔ Absorbed diphtheria toxoid-tetanus toxoid vaccine - **Diphtet (DT)**
  ➔ Purified diphtheria toxoid-tetanus toxoid-pertussis toxoid (acellular-filamentous haemagglutinin) vaccine – **DTP[a]**
  ➔ Purified diphtheria toxoid-tetanus toxoid-pertussis toxoid (acellular-filamentous haemagglutinin)-Haemophilus influenzae type B-vaccine – **DTP[a]-Hib**
  ➔ Purified diphtheria toxoid-tetanus toxoid-pertussis toxoid (acellular-filamentous haemagglutinin)-Inactivated type 1, 2, and 3 poliovirus D antigen-Haemophilus influenzae type B-vaccine – **DTP[a]-IPV-Hib**
  ➔ Purified diphtheria toxoid-tetanus toxoid-pertussis toxoid (acellular-filamentous haemagglutinin)-Inactivated type 1, 2, and 3 poliovirus D antigen vaccine – **DTP[a]-IPV**
  ➔ Purified diphtheria toxoid-tetanus toxoid containing 2 IU of purified diphtheria toxoid and 20 IU of purified tetanus toxoid - **Td**

Warning
✱ **All absorbed vaccines must be injected intramuscularly and must not be frozen**
✱ **All vaccines that have to be injected intramuscularly, must be administered with caution to individuals suffering from thrombocytopenia or a bleeding disorder**
✱ **Td-vaccine must never be administered intravascular and the needle must never penetrate a blood vessel. To reduce the risk of hypersensitivity reactions, avoid administering the Td-vaccine to persons having received full primary vaccination course and a booster dose the previous 5 years. Because immuno-suppressive therapy or immuno-deficiency may induce a diminished antibody response to active vaccination, vaccination must be delayed until the end of treatment or after the protection level of the person has been checked. In cases of chronic immuno-depression such as HIV-infection, vaccination is recommended when the underlying pathogenesis allows the induction of an antibody response, even if limited**

✠ **Storage, transportation, handling and reconstituting**
  ✳ All diphtheria vaccines must be **stored in a cool place at a temperature of 2-8⁰C**
  ✳ The vaccines **must not be frozen**. Freezing causes irreversible changes in the phosphate gel and bacterial growth in vaccines containing diphtheria endotoxin

(forming of flakes). This may lead to unequal dosages and sometimes to the formation of cysts and abscesses at the injection site

✳ Although the **vaccine is fairly stable, it must be kept cold during transportation** and must not be exposed to direct sunlight

✳ **Always take note of VVMs and expiry date**

✠ **Contra-indications**

The following are **contra-indications to the administering of all diphtheria vaccines - single or combined or combination dosages. When there is any doubt, consult a medical practitioner before proceeding with vaccination**

⅄ **Any serious illness**

⅄ **Hyper-pyrexia of 40,5°C and higher**

⅄ **A history of neurological disorders, for example, epilepsy**

⅄ **Convulsions/epilepsy that are/is not controlled**

⅄ **Allergies or a previous violent reaction to vaccination**

⅄ **Encephalopathy of unknown aetiology occurring within 7 days following previous vaccination with a vaccine containing pertussis (whole-cellular or acellular)**

⅄ **Babies older than 24 months must not receive any vaccine containing Pertussis**

When **Td** is used the following contra-indications must be adhered to

⅄ **Hypersensitivity to any ingredients, especially thiomersal - an organic-mercuric compound**

⅄ **Acute infectious disease, except in the presence of a potentially lethal risk such as a tetanus-prone wound**

⅄ **Evolving immunological disorders**

⅄ **History of severe reaction to previous dosage**

⅄ **Not to be administered to children younger than 6 years of age**

✠ **Administering**

◈ The **choice of vaccine depends on the age and vaccination history** of the healthcare user (child/adult)

◈ Before injecting the inactivated combination vaccine, all combination vaccines must be shaken well to obtain a homogenous whitish-turbid suspension

Vaccinating with diphtheria vaccine	
Preparation of all available diphtheria vaccines for administering •	• All vaccines must be examined before use and vials with absorbed vaccine must be shaken well before use. This should result in the contents forming a milky white but smooth suspension. **Should the contents not meet these requirements, especially if there is flocculation, the vaccine must not be administered. This also applies if the VVMs do not indicate safe conditions.** Vaccines that are unsuitable for use must be sealed and marked with full particulars, including the batch number. • Only one dosage must be drawn up in the syringe immediately before being administered. When multiple dosage vials are used, they have to be shaken well before each withdrawal of vaccine. The vial has to be kept cool at all times. All procedures have to be executed under sterile conditions • Lightly massage the injection area after administering
Infants between the ages of 6 weeks and 2 years	
Vaccine administering procedure **DTP[a]** or alternatively **DTP[a]-Hib** or alternatively **DTP[a]-IPV** or alternatively **DTP[a]-IPV-Hib**	<u>DTP[a]</u> or alternatively <u>**DTP[a]-Hib**</u> or alternatively <u>**DTP[a]-IPV-Hib**</u> or alternatively <u>**DTP[a]-IPV**</u> • Three (3) intramuscular injections of 0.5 ml vaccine are given alternately on the antero-lateral aspect of the left thigh (NOT the buttocks of babies under one [1] year of age) or left deltoid muscle region (infants of I year and older) at four (4) weeks intervals. Record must be kept of which thigh was injected, namely, the left thigh • The fourth dosage of 0.5 ml vaccine is administered 18 months after the abovementioned primary series course was administered. The fourth dosage is given in the left deltoid muscle (left upper arm) when the child is older than one (1) year

Infants who are older than nine (9) months but younger than two (2) years and who have never been vaccinated or whose vaccination was not completed, should receive **DTP[a]-IPV-Hib vaccine** and **Measles**, or alternatively dosages of **IPV (or TOPV)** and **DTP[a]-Hib**, or alternatively **DTP[a] and Hib**, or alternatively **DT and Hib**, or alternatively **DTP[a]-IPV** as single dosages or as combination dosages. Intervals of four (4) weeks are to be maintained until the necessary number of vaccination dosages has been administered. Booster series dosages are given at the recommended age or when the child is once again brought to the health establishment

Note

→ When, after the administering of **DTP[a]** (as a single dosage or as in a combination vaccine), an infant should have convulsions or any other severe reaction (i.e. reaction within 3 hours which renders the infant very ill) **NO FURTHER** dosages of pertussis must be administered

→ Single dosages of DTP[a], **or** Hib, **or** IPV **MAY NEVER** be mixed in the same syringe or be injected into the same area of administering

➔ Children older than two (2) years **may develop encephalitis if they are given the whole cellular pertussis (P[w]) portion of the vaccine. The acellular pertussis (P[a]) portion is deemed safe to be administered up to the age of 12 years although it is advisable not to administer it to any child older than 24 months**

Children between the ages of 2 and 5 years

Vaccine administering procedure **Diphtet-DT** or alternatively **DTP[a]-IPV** or alternatively **DTP[a]**	**Diphtet-DT** or alternatively **DTP[a]-IPV** or alternatively **DTP[a]** Administering is done at 4 weeks intervals for 4 dosages. One intramuscular booster dosage of 0,5 ml vaccine is administered when the child is 4-5 years old

When the child has never been vaccinated or has only been partially vaccinated, it must be ensured that the child receives the necessary five (5) dosages. Intervals of four (4) weeks are maintained between dosages

Please note
Diphtet-DT can be administered simultaneously with single dosages of Hep-B, IPV (or TOPV) and measles. Further administering of Diphtet-DT, IPV (or OPV), and measles are then given with normal time intervals of 4 weeks. The TT vaccine together with the single dosages of Hep-B, IPV (or OPV) and measles can be given in the place of Diphtet-DT vaccine or the combined vaccine TDP(a)-IPV and measles can be given in place of Diphtet-DT vaccine

Children between 6 and 12 years

Children between 6 and 12 years must receive booster dosages of Td-vaccine at the age of 6 years and 12 years.

Please note
Td can be administered simultaneously with Hep-B, TOP or IPV and measles. When Td is used as the primary series vaccination, the necessary subsequent dosages are then given at the normal time intervals of 4 weeks. Do not administer Td to children younger than 6 years of age

All persons older than 12 years of age

Since children over the age of 12 years as well as adults show severe reactions to vaccination, an individual should not be vaccinated until an assessment of his/her immune status has been done first. This is done by means of a Schick test or by means of an antibody count. Should vaccination be indicated, only the absorbed pure diphtheria vaccine (Diph PTAP) **or** the combined vaccine DT is used. The prescribed dosages are administered every four weeks

When Td-vaccine is used as routine booster, one (1) injection of 0.5 ml is administer intramuscular in the M. Deltoid or deep sub-cutaneous. When used as primary vaccination 3 dosages of 0.5ml is administered at 4 weekly intervals

Please note

* If any of the combination vaccines have been administered (for example, the absorbed diphtheria-tetanus-pertussis (acellular)-haemophilus influenzae type B-vaccine, (DTP$_{[a]}$-Hib) or the DTP$_{[a]}$-IPV-Hib or the DTP$_{[a]}$-IPV vaccine, the vaccinee should remain under medical supervision for 30 minutes after vaccination

* The different vaccines containing diphtheria can be administered simultaneously with other paediatric vaccines as long as the different vaccines are administered in separate sites. It can also be given in any temporal relationship with any other vaccine

* The administering of all other combination vaccines must be done according to the manufacturer's instruction. Most of these vaccines are privately available and must be bought before administering from private healthcare providers

Health information to be given to healthcare users

To ensure that the infant/child is successfully cared for at home, the healthcare practitioner must provide the parents/ guardians/foster-parents or the healthcare user with the following information

* The aim of vaccination, namely, to **prime the infant's adaptive immune system against diphtheria** or alternatively **diphtheria, tetanus, whooping cough** or alternatively **diphtheria, tetanus, whooping cough, poliomyelitis and haemophilus type B influenza by acting as immuno-stimulant in the eliciting of antibody-mediated immunity**

* The injection site **may be washed** with soap and water

* The injection site **may be rubbed** to relieve discomfort

* When the site is **red and swollen and painful, local heat** can be applied and an analgesic given (not aspirin or disprin)

* Other side-effects that can start within an hour after vaccination and last up to 2 days, are - headache; irritability; eating and drinking less than usually; sleeping more than usual/drowsiness; crying, restlessness

* Should the child **develop pyrexia (higher than 39^{0}C)**, Panado syrup or another antipyretic may be given 4-hourly according to age. Antipyretics may not be given for longer than 48 hours as pyrexia stimulates the adaptive antibody-antigen immune response. (Children younger than 16 years must not be given any drug containing aspirin or disprin.) When pyrexia persists for longer than 72 hour, <u>a medical practitioner must be consulted</u>

* The healthcare user may **feel ill for a day or two**. This may occur after the first, second or third injection. Sometimes the individual feels ill after every dosage

* It is important to keep the **appointment for the follow-up visit**

* **Children may suffer an atypical attack of pertussis/whooping cough years later** when they come into contact with the pertussis-bacteria due to the fact that natural artificially-acquired immunity disappears with time

* When the **individual has a severe reaction (temperature [40.5^{0}C and higher); general collapse; or shock-like state [hypotonic or hypo-responsive episode]; bronchospasm or laryngeal oedema; persistent, inconsolable crying; or convulsions) within 3 to 48 hours after receiving the injection, a medical practitioner (doctor or nurse) must be consulted.**

The reaction must be reported before the following dosage is administered. (**The pertussis component of the vaccine must not be administered any further in this case**)

✳ Side-effects of Td-vaccine include both local and systemic side-effects
Local reactions such as pain, redness, indurations and swelling can occur within 24 hours, as well as aseptic abscesses (rare condition). The severity and incidence of local reactions is influenced by the site, route and mode of administering as well as the number of previous vaccinations.
Systemic reactions that can occur are transient fever (associated or not to a local reaction); lymph-adenopathy; and an immediate hypersensitivity reaction (pruritis, urticaria, swelling, malaise, hypotension, shivering, myalgia, arthralgia and headache). These reactions may occur more likely in hyper-immunized persons, mainly after too frequent booster dosages. Neurological disorders are extremely rare

Warning: As this vaccine has to be injected, it must be administered with caution to individuals suffering from thrombocytopenia or a bleeding disorder.

6.5.5 HAEMOPHILUS INFLUENZA TYPE B VACCINE (HIB VACCINE)

The single dosage Hib vaccine, a capsular polysaccharide vaccine, is prepared from the capsule of the *Haemophilus influenzae type B-virus* and then bonded to the tetanus protein of the detoxified tetanus toxoid to form a conjugate. The carrier protein does not elicited immunity against tetanus. Nor does the Hib vaccine afford immunity against other pathogens that cause meningitis or infections that are caused by other pathogens.

✠ **Preparation available**
➜ Several preparations as a single dosage are available. Most of these are second, third or fourth generation polysaccharides Haemophilus influenza type B vaccine which is bonded as conjugate to the tetanus protein (PRP-T). The diluent contains 0,5ml of 0.4% NaCl solution, while the vaccine itself contains 10µg of the polysaccharide in the conjugate
➜ Combination vaccines
✓ Purified diphtheria toxoid-tetanus toxoid-pertussis toxoid ($P_{[a]}$)-Haemophilus influenzae type B-vaccine **$DTP_{[a]}$-Hib**
✓ Purified diphtheria toxoid-tetanus toxoid-pertussis toxoid ($P_{[a]}$-filamentous haemagglutinin)-Inactivated type 1, 2 and 3 Poliovirus D antigen-Haemophilus influenzae type B-vaccine **$DTP_{[a]}$-IPV-Hib**

Warning
As the single and combined dosage vaccine has to be injected intramuscularly, it must be administered with caution to individuals suffering from thrombocytopenia or a bleeding disorder. The vaccine must then be given subcutaneously.

✠ **Storage, transportation, handling and reconstitution**

✶ All preparations have to be stored in a refrigerator at 2-8⁰C **and must not be frozen**

✶ It is a very stable vaccine and can be kept in a refrigerator for **two years at the correct temperature**

✶ The single dosage and the combination vaccine has to be **transported and administered cold**

✶ Parents/guardians/foster-parents have to buy the single dosage preparation themselves and take it to the clinic in a cool bag. Permission to administer the vaccine has to be obtained in writing

✶ The singe dosage vaccine is reconstituted by mixing the freeze-dried lyophilisate with the diluent (sodium chloride)

✠ **Contra-indications**

⅄ When a person **suffers from an acute communicable disease or any other illness (acute or chronic)** or hypersensitivity to the ingredients of the vaccine (particularly the tetanus protein), the vaccine should not be administered

⅄ **Pregnant women and mothers breastfeeding** their babies should not be vaccinated

✠ **Administering**

◇ **Primary series vaccination**

☑ Three injections of 0.5 ml vaccine (single dosage vaccine) **or** DTP$_{(a)}$-IPV-Hib vaccine are administered intramuscularly on the area of the left antero-lateral thigh of babies (6 weeks and older) at 4 weeks intervals when 6 weeks, 10 weeks and 14 weeks of age (not less than one month [4 weeks] must be allowed between injections)

☑ The fourth dosage of DTP$_{[a]}$-IPV-Hib must be given at the age of 18 months

☑ When the single dosage vaccine is used, a booster must be given after one year

◇ **Second chance vaccination (Catch-up vaccination)**

☑ If a child has not received the primary vaccination, he/she has to be vaccinated as follows:

• **Infants 6–12 months** - Two injections of the single dosage vaccine **or** alternatively the combination vaccines DTP$_{[a]}$-Hib or alternatively DTP$_{[a]}$-IPV-HIB are administered in the left antero-lateral thigh with intervals of one or two months, followed by a booster dosage 12 months later

• **Children 1–5 years old** - Only one injection to be given in the left Deltoid muscle

◇ **Preterm and Low Birth Weight infants**

☑ Preterm and Low Birth Weight infants benefit from Hib vaccine from the age of 6 months before the beginning of and during the influenza season. Although the immunogenicity of the vaccine may be decreased, the concentrations achieved usually are protective

Please note

✱ The vaccine **may never be given intravascular**
✱ **After the vaccine has been administered, the vaccinee should remain under medical supervision for 30 minutes**
✱ In individuals suffering from immunodeficiency or receiving immunosuppressive therapy, **an adequate response may not be achieved**

✠ **Health information to be given to healthcare users**
After administering the vaccine, the healthcare practitioner must provide the parent/guardian/foster-parent or healthcare user with the following information
   ✳ The aim of vaccination, namely, to **prime the infant's adaptive immune system against Haemophilus influenza type B by acting as immuno-stimulant by eliciting antibody and memory responses**
   ✳ The injection area **may be painful**
   ✳ The injection area **may be red and swollen – it resolves spontaneously**
   ✳ A fever **may develop (above 38°C) which could last 24-48 hours**
   ✳ **Any analgesic and/or antipyretic remedy may be taken 4-hourly, only if necessary and taken with discretion** as pyrexia is necessary to stimulate the adaptive antigen-antibody reaction. Aspirin or disprin must not be given to children younger than 16 years
   ✳ The injection **area may be washed with soap and water**
   ✳ Children may **feel ill for a day or two – loss of appetite, restlessness, vomiting, diarrhoea and crying**
   ✳ The vaccine **can be safely administered simultaneously with DTP[a] and IPV/OPV and Hep-B.**

6.5.6 HEPATITIS-B VACCINE (HBV/HEP-B)

Hepatitis-B vaccine is produced either as a recombinant DNA yeast cell vaccine that contains the refined surface antigen of the virus **or** as a multi-determinant plasma-derived DNS hepatitis B-virus vaccine that contains the refined surface antigen of the virus.

❑ The recombinant DNA yeast cell vaccine or the genetically-engineered vaccine is produced when the gene of the surface antigen is primed into a yeast vector and prepared as a suspension of the antigen and absorbed to aluminium hydroxide.

❑ The multi-determinant plasma-derived DNS hepatitis B-virus vaccine consists of a non-living antigenic preparation derived from refined heat-treated plasma of the blood of virus carriers. Apart from the surface antigen, the multi-determinant plasma-derived DNS hepatitis B-virus vaccine also contains pre-S1 molecules and high levels of pre-S2 molecules which are critical in the formation of immunity. Regular safety tests have to be done on the vaccine derived from blood to ensure that it contains no viruses (such as HIV) or any other pathogen.

✠ **Preparations available**
  ➜ The **recombinant DNA yeast cell vaccine** or **genetically-engineered vaccine** consist of an adult dosage containing 20 μg antigen protein per ml and a paediatric dosage containing 10 μg antigen protein per 0,5ml
  ➜ The **plasma-derived DNS virus vaccine** is seldom used today as antibody levels start to fall after 1–2 years and booster dosages are necessary

<u>Warning</u>
<u>**As this vaccine has to be injected intramuscularly, it must be administered with caution to individuals suffering from thrombocytopenia or a bleeding disorder**</u>

✠ **Storage, transportation, handling and reconstitution**
  ✳ Hepatitis-B vaccine must be transported cold and be stored at 2-8°C. **IT MUST NOT BE FROZEN**
  ✳ **During storage, a fine, white sediment may be formed with a clear, colourless top layer**
  ✳ The vaccine **may not be used after its expiry date**

✠ **Contra-indications**
  ⅄ **Hypersensitivity** for any component of the vaccine
  ⅄ **Serious febrile infections**
  ⅄ **Pregnancy** - it is not known what the effect of the antigen is on the development of a foetus – pregnant women therefore **must not be vaccinated**. Should there be any doubt, consult with a medical practitioner

✠ **Administering**
  ◈ The **particular vaccine to be used depends on the age and vaccination history** of the person concerned.

Vaccinating with hepatitis-B virus vaccine	
Target population	New-born babies; persons in endemic areas; healthcare personnel; healthcare users who frequently need blood transfusions or concentrates of coagulation factors; personnel and residents of institutions; persons subjected to increased risk owing to their sexual habits; illegal abusers of drugs which are injected; persons exposed to hepatitis B-virus by reason of their life-style; persons exposed by reason of their career, such as policemen, firemen, army personnel and healthcare providers
Preparation of vaccine (paediatric as well as adult type)	The vaccine has to be examined for flocculation. **WHEN FLOCCULATION APPEARS, THE VACCINE MAY NOT BE USED.** Shake the vial well before use. <u>Administer intramuscularly</u>. **THE VACCINE MAY NEVER BE ADMINISTERED INTRAVENOUSLY, NOR IN THE M. GLUTEUS OR IN THE SKIN.** In highly exceptional cases, such as persons with tendencies towards severe bleeding (for example, haemophilia), the vaccine may be administered subcutaneously

	All children younger than 10 years of age
Vaccine	<u>Hepatitis-B vaccine - 10 µg antigen in 0,5 ml suspension (paediatric type)</u> • A dosage of 10 µg antigen protein in 0,5 ml suspension is administered intramuscularly on the anterior-lateral right thigh from the age of six weeks. Intervals of four (4) weeks are maintained until three (3) dosages have been administered • When the child is <u>older than one year</u>, the following policy may be followed - a first dosage given on a chosen date, a second dosage one month later and the third dosage six months from the date of the first dosage • <u>A booster dosage will be necessary after a number of years</u> for both groups of children
	Children older than 10 years of age and adults
Vaccine	<u>Hepatitis-B vaccine - 20 µg antigen in 1 ml suspension (adult)</u> • A <u>dosage of 20 µg antigen in 1 ml suspension</u> is administered intramuscularly in the M. Deltoid. Primary vaccination is done as follows First dosage - on a chosen date Second dosage - one month later Third dosage - 6 months from the date of the first dosage Booster dosage - a number of years later

➜ **Cases where quick protection is needed** (for example, contacts of carriers, vaccination of travellers)
   ☑ Administer three injections intramuscularly every four weeks
➜ **Cases where exposure had occurred**
   ☑ Administer hepatitis-B vaccine simultaneously with hepatitis-B immunoglobulin
<u>**Please note:**</u> *The vaccine **MUST NOT BE ADMINISTERED IN THE SAME INJECTION SITE** as the immunoglobulin
*Preterm and Low Birth Weight infants weighing less than 2000 gram may require modification of the timing of Hep-B immunoprophylaxis depending on maternal hepatitis B surface antigen. Although the immunogenicity of the vaccine may be decreased, the concentrations achieved usually are protective

✠ **Health information to be given to healthcare users**
After administering the vaccine, the healthcare provider must provide the parent/ guardian/foster-parent or healthcare user with the following information
   ✳ The aim of vaccination, namely, to **prime the infant's adaptive immune system against hepatitis B infection by acting as immuno-stimulant**
   ✳ The injection area **may be washed** with soap and water
   ✳ If the injection **area is painfully red and swollen, local heat** can be applied
   ✳ Should **headache and/or pyrexia (higher than 39⁰C) develops, an antipyretic may be taken** every 6 hours until pyrexia can be tolerated. The reaction will lessen after two days. <u>NB</u> **Antipyretics must be taken with caution as pyrexia stimulates the adaptive antibody-antigen reaction**

* Should an adult **develop dizziness, he/she should not drive a vehicle and be alerted that occupational accidents can happen.** It is advisable for the person to stay at home. Dizziness should clear up within a day or two
* **Nausea can be avoided by having small helpings of food often during the day** and avoiding all types of food which will increase nausea. The nausea also clears up within a couple of days. Ginger can be taken for nausea
* If the individual **is tired, taking short rest periods throughout** the day is advisable

Warning
*Owing to the long incubation period of hepatitis-B infection, the possibility exists that an undiagnosed infection may already be present when vaccination takes place. In such a case **the vaccine cannot prevent** the disease
*Babies born to mothers known to be hepatitis surface antigen positive are given hepatitis B-immunoglobulin.

6.5.7 PNEUMOCOCCAL CONJUGATED VACCINE (PCV)

The pneumococcal conjugated vaccine contains a sterile solution of saccharides of the capsular antigen of *Streptococcus pneumoniae* serotype 4, 6B, 14, 18C, 19F, and 23F individually conjugated to diphtheria CRM_{197} protein. It also contains aluminium phosphate as an adjuvant.

Each 0,5 ml dose is formulated to contain 2µg of saccharides for serotype 4, 9V, 14, 28C, 19F, and 23F, and 4µg of serotype 6B per dosage (16µg total saccharides) and approximately 20µg of CRM_{197} carrier protein. The conjugated pneumococcal vaccine is indicated for active vaccination of infants and children from 6 weeks until 9 years of age against invasive disease, pneumonia and otitis media caused by *Streptococcus pneumoniae* serotype 4, 6B, 14, 18C and 23F.

* **Storage, transportation and handling of the vaccine**
  * The conjugated pneumococcal vaccine must be **stored in a refrigerator at 2-8⁰C and must not be frozen**
  * **Discard if the vaccine has been frozen**

* **Contra-indications**
  * **Hypersensitivity to any component** of the vaccine, including diphtheria toxoid
  * The **vial stopper contains dry natural rubber** that may cause **hypersensitivity reactions** when handled by or when the product is injected into persons with **known or possible latex sensitivity**
  * The **safety and effectiveness** of the conjugated pneumococcal vaccine **in children younger the age of 6 weeks and older than 10 years have not been established**
  * The vaccine should **NOT be administered to infants and children with thrombocytopenia or any coagulation disorder**
  * The vaccine is **NOT RECOMMENDED FOR USE IN ADULTS**

⅄ **Safety in pregnancy** (it is not known whether foetal harm will be caused) **and lactation** (it is not known whether vaccine antigens or antibodies are excreted in human milk) **has not been established**

⅄ **It has not been established whether the vaccine can affect reproductive capability**

⅄ **Under no circumstances must the vaccine be administered intravenously**

<u>Please note</u>
- The conjugated pneumococcal vaccine may be administered simultaneously with other paediatric vaccines in accordance with the recommended immunisation/ vaccination schedules as long as different injection sites are used
- In healthy subjects, the presence of a minor infection such as a mild respiratory infection with or without low-grade fever, however, is not a contra-indication for vaccination
- When suffering from acute febrile illness, the administering of the vaccine MUST BE POSTPONED
- The conjugated pneumococcal vaccine may be administered in any temporal relationship with oral polio vaccine (OPV) or inactivated polio vaccine (IPV); hepatitis-B vaccine; DTP[a] or DTP[a]-IPV-Hib or DTP[a]-Hib vaccine; *Haemophilus influenza* type B vaccine (Hib); measles or MMR vaccine; and varicella-zoster-virus vaccine. DIFFERENT INJECTION SITES MUST BE USED when vaccinating concurrently with the different vaccines
- The use of the conjugated pneumococcal vaccine does not replace the use of 23-valent pneumococcal polysaccharide vaccine in children older than or equal to 24 months of age with conditions such as sickle cell disease, asplenia, HIV infection, chronic illness, or who are immune-compromised, placing them at higher risk for invasive disease due to *Streptococcal pneumoniae*
- The different injectable vaccines MUST always be administered in different injection sites
- Although some antibody response to diphtheria toxin may occur, vaccination with the conjugated pneumococcal vaccine does not substitute for the routine diphtheria vaccination

- **Administering**
  - ◈ The conjugated pneumococcal vaccine **<u>must only be administered intramuscularly</u>** – <u>never administer intravenously</u>. Care must be taken to avoid injecting the vaccine into or near nerves and blood vessels. The preferred injection sites are the antero-lateral aspect of the right thigh in infants or the deltoid muscle of the right upper arm in older children. The vaccine **must not be injected in the gluteus muscle**
  - ◈ Since the conjugated pneumococcal vaccine is a suspension containing an adjuvant, the vaccine container (vial or pre-filled syringe) must be shaken vigorously immediately prior to administering as to obtain a uniform suspension. **The contents of the container must be administered immediately after being drawn up into a syringe.** The vaccine should not be used if it cannot be re-stored to a white suspension

◈ After shaking, the vaccine must have a homogeneous white suspension appearance. The vaccine **must be inspected visually for particulate matter and discolouration prior to administration.** The vaccine **must be discarded if particulate matter or discolouration is found**

◈ The conjugated pneumococcal vaccine is administered as follows
*<u>Infant primary series vaccination</u> - 3 dosages of 0,5 ml vaccine beginning at the age of 2 months of age (or at 6 weeks of age). An interval of 4-8 weeks should be respected between dosages. The fourth dosages must be administered in the second year of life – 12 to 15 months
*<u>Unvaccinated infants from 7 to 11 months</u> - 2 dosages approximately one (1) month apart followed by a 3rd dosage after 12 months of age. The interval between the second and the third dosages must be at least 2 months
*<u>Unvaccinated children from 12 to 23 months of age</u> - 2 dosages at least 2 months apart
*<u>Children who are 24 months of age and older</u> - only a single dosage

<u>Warning</u>
<u>As this vaccine has to be injected intramuscularly, it must be administered with caution to individuals suffering from thrombocytopenia or a bleeding (coagulation) disorder</u>

<u>Please note</u>
✳ <u>Vaccination of children with impaired immune responsiveness due to the use of immune-suppressive therapy (including radiation, corticosteroids, antimetabolites, alkylation agents, and cytotoxic agents); a genetic defect; HIV infection; or other causes</u>
The vaccine may have a reduced antibody response to active vaccination

✳ <u>Special precautions</u>
Appropriate medical treatment should always be readily available, including adrenaline in case of rare anaphylactic reactions following administering of the vaccine. **<u>For this reason, the vaccinee should remain under medical supervision for 30 minutes after vaccination</u>**

✳ <u>Vaccination of infants and children suffering from thrombocytopenia and any coagulation disorder or who are receiving anticoagulant therapy</u>
The potential benefits of vaccination must clearly outweigh the risk of administering. If the decision is made to administer the vaccine, it must be done with caution

✳ <u>Incompatibilities</u>
<u>The conjugated pneumococcal vaccine must never under any circumstances be mixed with other vaccines in the same syringe</u>

✳ <u>Overdosing</u>
Care must be taken not to overdose with the conjugated pneumococcal vaccine, that is the administering of a higher than the recommended dosages and/or the administering of subsequent dosages closer than recommended to the previous dosage. Although most individuals may be asymptomatic, adverse events can occur

✠ **Health information to be given to healthcare users**

After administering the vaccine, the healthcare practitioner must provide the parent/guardian/foster-parent or healthcare user with the following information

❋ The aim of vaccination, namely, to **prime the infant's adaptive immune system against invasive disease, pneumonia and otitis media caused by** *Streptococcus pneumoniae* **serotype 4, 6B, 14, 18C and 23F**

❋ **Side- effects**

Various side-effects may occur after the administering of the conjugated pneumococcal vaccine

General side-effects	Rare side-effects
➢ Injection site erythema, induration/ swelling (sometimes greater than 2,4 cm), and pain/tenderness that may interfere with movement, ➢ Fever (sometimes higher than 39ºC) ➢ Irritability and crying ➢ Drowsiness ➢ Restless sleep ➢ Diarrhoea ➢ Vomiting ➢ Decreased appetite	➢ Injection site dermatitis, injection site urticaria, injection site pruritis ➢ Skin rash, urticaria or urticaria-like rash ➢ Seizures (including febrile seizures) ➢ Hypotonic or hypo-responsive episode ➢ Lymphadenopathy localized in the region of the injection site ➢ Hypersensitivity reaction including face oedema, dyspnoea bronchospasm, anaphylactic/anaphylactoid reaction including shock ➢ Angio-oedema and erythema multiforme ➢ Apnoea (especially when medical conditions such as a history of apnoea, infection, prematurity, and/ or seizures exist) ➢ Hospitalization because of bronchiolitis (diagnosis of wheezing)

❋ **Treatment of side-effects**

Symptomatic and supportive

❋ **Other information** to be communicated regarding the administering of conjugated pneumococcal vaccine

  ➢ The protective immune response may not be elicited in every vaccinee

  ➢ The vaccine does not protect against other *Streptococcal pneumoniae* serogroups than those included in the vaccine nor other microbes that cause invasive diseases such as bacteraemia, meningitis, pneumonia or otitis media

  ➢ Prophylactic antipyretic medication can be given especially when the conjugated pneumococcal vaccine is administered simultaneously with vaccines containing whole cell pertussis (medication containing salicylate acids, for example, Aspirin, Disprin, Grandpa powders, must not be given at all as it can result in Reye's disease)

> Prophylactic antipyretic medication should be given to children at higher risk for seizures than the general population (medication containing salicylate acids, for example, Aspirin, Disprin, Grandpa powders, must not be given as it can result in Reye's disease).

6.5.8   MEASLES VACCINE

The measles vaccine, a living vaccine, contains the freeze-dried attenuated living *measles-virus* (Schwartz strain).

The Measles vaccine is provided free of charge by the Department of Health and administered by the staff of public healthcare clinics. If administered by private healthcare practitioners in private practices or in private well-baby clinics, a fee is charged for the procedure done and the vaccine administered.

✠ **Storage, transportation, handling and reconstitution**
  ✳ The measles vaccine is **extremely sensitive to light and heat** and must be protected from exposure to sunlight
  ✳ It must always be **stored in a refrigerator at 4-8⁰C**. Freezing will not damage the vaccine
  ✳ It **has a limited life-span**. When stored under optimum conditions, it will last a year from the time of production. After the date of expiry, the vaccine has to be disposed of
  ✳ The **measles vaccine is reconstituted** according to the manufacture's instruction. Dilution of the vaccine in order to save on stock constitutes malpractice
  ✳ The **reconstituted vaccine loses its affectivity very rapidly** and must therefore be used **within one hour of opening**
  ✳ All **opened vials must be destroyed after six (6) hours**
  ✳ **Opened vials may not be re-used**

✠ **Contra-indications**
  There are several contra-indications to the administering of the measles vaccine, namely,
  ⅄ **Children with conditions such as**
    + A serious illness associated with pyrexia
    + Hypogammaglobulinaemia
    + Leukaemia
    + Hodgkin's disease
    + An allergy (particularly to eggs and anti-microbial drugs)
    + Active, untreated tuberculosis
    + Recent exposure to other communicable diseases
    + Symptomatic HIV infection or full blown AIDS
  ⅄ **Treatment with corticosteroids or immunosuppressive drugs**
  ⅄ **Pregnancy** - the vaccine can cause foetal abnormalities

⋏ In cases where artificial passively-acquired immunity was elicited with gamma-globulin, active vaccination with the measles vaccine must be withheld for at least six (6) weeks since the vaccine impairs the antibody reaction

⋏ **Administering of measles vaccine simultaneously with DTP[a] or DTP[a]-IPV-Hib and OPV or IPV polio vaccine is not advisable**

⋏ **The vaccine must be given with caution to persons with a history of allergic diseases or to those with a history or family history of convulsions**

⋏ **All children sick with AIDS or who are HIV-infected – refer for medical opinion**

✠ **Administering**

* The measles vaccine is administered intramuscularly to infants from the age of **nine months up to about four/five (4-5) years old**. Artificial actively-acquired immunity is elicited

* Should there be an **outbreak of measles, the vaccine can be administered to babies from the age of 6 months. A booster dosage is administered at 18 months**

* Children **over the age of two (2) years receive only one (1) dosage of measles vaccine**

* During **health campaigns** the measles vaccine can be **administered to children up to the age of 15 years**
  Please note:
  Older children tend to become very ill after being vaccinated and may sometimes develop a **hypersensitivity reaction** to the measles vaccine

* **MMR can be used as a substitute for measles - administer at 15-18 months**

* In missed opportunities, measles and BCG can be given on the same day BUT separate administrating sites must be used

Vaccinating with and target population for measles vaccine	
Preparation	Ether, alcohol and other germicidal solutions destroy the measles-virus in the vaccine. Therefore, do not use these preparations to clean the skin before vaccination. The healthcare user's skin must be washed with soap and water when it is very dirty. The washed skin must be completely dry before the injection is administered
Administering	The dosage of reconstituted measles vaccine is given as a single intramuscular injection of 0,5 ml vaccine , preferably on the antero-lateral thigh (for babies younger than 12 months) or the upper arm in Deltoid muscle (for children older than 12 months)
TARGET POPULATION	
Infants 6-7 months of age	The measles vaccine is given at this early age only if there is a high incidence of measles among infants under one year of age in a particular community. This is due to the fact that the protection level is very low at this age. A booster dosage must be administered at the age of 18 months

All children over the age of 9 months	A high protection level (more than 95%) is obtained when the measles vaccine is administered after the age of nine months. A booster dosage must be given at the age of 18 months. Children older than two (2) years need only one dosage of the measles vaccine. MMR can be used as a substitute for measles vaccine – to be administered at the age of 15 or 18 months
High risk groups	Children of any age with serious illnesses such as heart disease, cystic fibrosis and tuberculosis must be vaccinated when they are susceptible. All children in institutions are considered high risk individuals and must be vaccinated when they are admitted to the institution, particularly if there is the slightest doubt that the child has not been vaccinated previously, or whether the child had ever contracted measles
Susceptible children	Susceptible children, who have been in contact with measles, should be vaccinated as soon as possible after exposure
Persons who have been vaccinated with BCG	The measles vaccine may not be given until four (4) weeks has expired after BCG was administered, and BCG may not be administered until two (2) months after a person had contracted measles. In missed opportunities, BCG and measles can be given on the same day BUT different vaccination sites must be used
Infected children	Children, who have already been infected, may develop a milder or modified form of the disease if they are vaccinated with gamma-globulin shortly after exposure

Warning
As this vaccine has to be injected intramuscularly, it must be administered with caution to individuals suffering from thrombocytopenia or a bleeding disorder

✠ **Health information to be given to the healthcare users**
 After administering the vaccine, the healthcare practitioner must provide the parent/guardian/foster-parent or healthcare user with the following information
 ✳ The aim of vaccination, namely, to **prime the infant's/child's adaptive immune system against measles by acting as immuno-stimulant in the eliciting of antibody-mediated immunity**
 ✳ **Side-effects**
 Various side-effects may occur after the administering of the measles vaccine
  ➢ The injection site **may become swollen**
  ➢ The injection site **may become red**
  ➢ The child **may develop a temperature of 39°C or higher**, 5-12 days after vaccination
  ➢ A **sore throat and/or cough may develop**
  ➢ A **typical measles rash may appear within 5-12 days after vaccination**
  ➢ The child may feel ill for several days

＊ **Treatment of side-effects**
> ➤ **Panado syrup may be given 4-hourly for a period of up to 72 hours for pyrexia**. Because pyrexia stimulates the adaptive immune response (antibody-mediated immunity), Panado syrup must only **be given when the pyrexia cannot be tolerated or when it stays high (higher than 39^{0}C) for more than 24 hours.** If the temperature does not subside, a healthcare practitioner (nursing practitioner or medical practitioner) must be consulted
> ➤ When the **child becomes seriously ill within 72 hours**, a medical practitioner must be consulted
> ➤ **Heat may be applied** locally to relieve redness and swelling
> ➤ **The rash may be washed with soap and water**, and if it is itchy, an antihistamine cream or calamine lotion can be applied. The rash disappears within three to ten days

＊ **General information**
> ➤ **Transmission of the measles-virus will not occur** despite the manifestation of the disease which develops after vaccination. It is therefore not necessary to isolate the child or kept away from other babies or children
> ➤ **Children may suffer an atypical attack of measles years later** when they come into contact with the measles-virus due to the fact that natural artificially-acquired immunity disappears with time
> ➤ **BCG vaccine may be given one (1) month after** administering of the measles vaccine.
> ➤ The **measles vaccine offers no protection against German measles (Rubella).**

6.5.9 HEPATITIS A VACCINE (HAV/HEP-A)

The hepatitis A-virus vaccine, a non-living vaccine, contains the inactivated *hepatitis A-virus* in suspension and is absorbed onto aluminium hydroxide.

✠ **Preparations available**
> ➜ An adult dosage containing a viral antigen content of not less than 1440 ELISA units of viral antigens (HM 175) per 1.0 ml suspension
> ➜ A paediatric dosage containing a viral antigen content of not less than 720 ELISA units of viral antigens (HM 175) per 0.5 ml suspension

Warning
As the vaccine has to be injected intramuscularly, it must be administered with caution to individuals suffering from thrombocytopenia or a bleeding disorder

✠ **Storage, transportation, handling and reconstitution**
> ＊ Hepatitis A vaccine must be transported cold and be stored at 2-8^{0}C. **IT MAY NOT BE FROZEN**
> ＊ **If the vaccine has been frozen, discard it**

* The **vaccine must be protected from light** (sunlight as well as electrical/neon light)
* **Shake well before use**
* The vaccine **may not be used after its expiry date**

✠ **Contra-indications**
⅄ **Hypersensitivity** for any component of the vaccine
⅄ **Serious febrile infections**

✠ **Administering**
◇ The **particular vaccine to be used depends on the age** of the person concerned

Vaccinating with hepatitis A-virus vaccine	
Target population	New-born babies; persons living in intermediate to high prevalence endemic and urban areas; persons for whom the disease is an occupational hazard, such as healthcare personnel and sanitation workers; healthcare users who frequently need blood transfusions or concentrates of coagulation factors; individuals subjected to increased risk owing to their sexual habits; illegal abusers of drugs which are injected; individuals exposed to hepatitis A-virus by reason of their life-style, such as frequent travellers; individuals for whom there is an increased risk of exposure and transmission by reason of their career, such as policemen, firemen and army personnel; individuals who need prophylactic treatment for protection after an outbreak occurred; contacts of infected individuals; healthcare users suffering from chronic liver disease or who are at risk to develop chronic liver disease; specific population groups known to have a higher incidence of hepatitis A
Preparation of vaccine (paediatric as well as adult type)	The vaccine has to be visually examined for any particulate matter or discolouration prior to administering. **IF FLOCCULATION APPEARS AND/OR DISCOLOURATION IS VISIBLE, THE VACCINE MAY NOT BE USED.** Shake the vial/syringe well before use to obtain a slightly opaque white solution. Discard if the contents of the vial/syringe appear otherwise. Administer intramuscular in the deltoid muscle of older children and adults and in the antero-lateral part of the thigh in young children. **THE VACCINE MAY NEVER BE ADMINISTERED INTRAVENOUSLY, NOR IN THE M. GLUTEUS OR IN THE SKIN**
All children and adolescents from I year up to 16 years of age	
Vaccine	Hepatitis A vaccine: 720 ELISA units in 0,5 ml suspension (paediatric type) • A dosage of 0,5 ml suspension is administered intramuscularly on the anterior-lateral thigh or the M. Deltoid from the age of 1 year as primary series vaccination • A booster series dosage of 0,5 ml suspension is given 6 to 12 months after the primary vaccination

Children older than 16 years of age and adults	
Vaccine	Hepatitis A vaccine: 1440 ELISA units in 1.0 ml suspension • One single dosage of 1.0 ml suspension administered intramuscularly in the M. Deltoid of the vaccinee for the primary series vaccination • A single dosage of 1 ml suspension is given as a booster at any time between 6 to 12 months after the primary series dosage
HIV-infected persons	Sero-positivity is not contra-indicated

Special precautions

* Appropriate medical treatment should always be readily available, including adrenaline in case of rare anaphylactic reactions following administering of the vaccine. **For this reason, the vaccinee should remain under medical supervision for 30 minutes after vaccination**

* The administering of the vaccine must be **postpone in individuals with severe febrile illness**

* The vaccine must only be used **during pregnancy and lactation when clearly needed,** as the effect of the vaccine on foetal development has not been assessed

* In **ill healthcare users on haemodialysis and in subjects with an impaired immune system,** adequate anti-hepatitis A-virus titres may sometimes not be obtained after a single dosage of the vaccine. Such individuals may therefore **require administering of additional dosages of the vaccine**

* As the vaccine is an inactivated vaccine, it can be **administered concomitant with other inactivated vaccines** (typhoid, yellow fever, cholera and tetanus) and interference with the immune response will likely not result

* Concomitant **administering of immunoglobulin does not impact on the protective effect of the vaccine**

* When it is deemed necessary to simultaneously administer other vaccine(s) intramuscularly in the M. Deltoid, the vaccine(s) can be administered concomitantly. **Precaution must be taken that the different vaccines are given with different syringes and at different injection sites**

* **Concomitant vaccination with the recombinant hepatitis B-virus vaccine is satisfactory.** No interference takes place in the respective immune responses to both antigens

* **UNDER NO CIRCUMSTANCES MUST THE VACCINE EVER BE MIXED WITH OTHER VACCINES OR IMMUNOGLOBULINS IN THE SAME SYRINGE**

* **Health information to be given to healthcare users**
  After administering the vaccine, the healthcare practitioner must provide the parent/guardian/foster-parent or healthcare user with the following information
  * The aim of vaccination, namely, to **prime the infant's/child's/adolescent's/ adult's adaptive immune system against hepatitis A-virus infection by**

acting as immuno-stimulant for the production of specific anti-hepatitis A-virus-antibody

* The injection area **may be washed** with soap and water
* If the injection **area is painful, red and swollen, local heat** can be applied
* Should **headache and/or pyrexia (higher than 39ºC) develops, an antipyretic may be taken** every 6 hours until pyrexia can be tolerated. The reaction will lessen after two days. Important: **Antipyretics must be taken with caution as pyrexia stimulates the adaptive antibody-antigen reaction**
* **Nausea and loss of appetite can be avoided by having small helpings of food often during the day** and avoiding all food which will increase nausea. The nausea also clears up within a couple of days
* If the individual **is tired, taking short rest periods throughout** the day is advisable
* Treatment of **other side-effects** such as diarrhoea, myalgia, arthralgia, is symptomatic and supportive

Note

Owing to the fact that the possibility exists that an undiagnosed infection may already be present when vaccination takes place, **the vaccine cannot prevent** the disease.

6.5.10   VARICELLA-ZOSTER-VIRUS VACCINE

The varicella-zoster-virus vaccine against chickenpox, a living vaccine, is a lyophilized preparation of the live attenuated OKA strain of the *Varicella-zoster virus*, obtained by propagation of the virus in MRC_5 human cell culture.

* **Storage, transportation and handling of the vaccine**
  * The varicella-zoster-virus vaccine must be **stored in a refrigerator at 2 to 8ºC and must not be frozen**
  * The **vaccine must be protected from light** (sunlight as well as electrical light)
  * If **not used within 24 hours the vaccine MUST be discarded**
  * The cold chain has to be maintained during transportation
  * **Disposed of unused vaccine and waste material** in accordance with local requirement

* **Contra-indications**
  * Any child with a total lymphocyte count of less than $1200/mm^3$ or presenting other evidence of lack of cellular immune competence
  * Children with **known systemic hypersensitivity to neomycin**, but a history of contact dermatitis to neomycin is not a contra-indication
  * **Pregnancy and breastfeeding**
  * **Sick/ill persons suffering from acute severe febrile illness**
  * In **high-risk ill individuals**, the varicella-zoster-virus vaccine **must be postponed** as it cannot be administered at the same time as other live attenuated vaccines

⅄ Primary or acquired immunodeficiency states - persons with leukaemia, lymphomas, blood dyscrasias, clinically manifested HIV-infection or healthcare users receiving immunosuppressive therapy and drugs.

Note - Vaccination can be considered when individuals are susceptible to varicella, are in haematological remission, and/or treatment has been stopped from one (1) week before and one (1) week after vaccination. A booster dose must be given

Please note

- **In healthy subjects, the presence of minor infection, however, is not a contra-indication for vaccination**
- **Inactivated vaccines may be administered in any temporal relationship to the varicella-zoster-virus vaccine, given that no specific contra-indications have been established**
- **In individuals who have received immunoglobulin or a blood transfusion, <u>VACCINATION MUST BE DELAYED</u> for at least three (3) months because of the likelihood of vaccine failure due to passively-acquired varicella antibody**

✠ **Administering**

◈ The varicella-zoster-virus vaccine **must only be administered subcutaneously** – <u>never administer intradermally or intravenously</u>

◈ The varicella-zoster-virus vaccine is reconstituted by adding the contents of the diluent to the vaccine vial and **the contents of the vial must be administered immediately after reconstitution.** The diluent must be inspected for visible particles – if present, discard the diluent

◈ The varicella-zoster-virus vaccine is administered as follows
*From the **age of 9 months to 12 years** – one dosage of 0.5 ml vaccine subcutaneously
*From 13 years and older – **2 dosages** of 0.5 ml vaccine subcutaneously **with an interval of a minimum of 6 weeks between dosages**
*In high risk individuals **additional dosages** of vaccine might be required

Vaccinating with and target population for varicella-zoster-virus vaccine	
Preparation	Ether, alcohol and other germicidal substances destroy the varicella-zoster-virus in the vaccine. <u>Therefore, do not use these preparations to clean the skin</u> before vaccination. The healthcare user's skin must be washed with soap and water when it is very dirty. The washed skin must be completely dry before the injection is administered
Administering	The dosage of reconstituted varicella-zoster-virus vaccine is given as a single subcutaneous injection of 0.5 ml vaccine, preferably on the thigh (for babies younger than 12 months) or in the Deltoid muscle of the upper arm (for children older than 12 months)

TARGET POPULATION	
Healthy individuals	The varicella-zoster-virus vaccine is administered from the age of 9 months, to healthy infants, children and adolescents for active vaccination against varicella
High-risk individuals and healthy close contacts	The varicella-zoster-virus vaccine is also administered to susceptible high-risk individuals and their susceptible healthy close contacts for active vaccination against varicella
Persons with acute leukaemia	Individuals suffering from leukaemia have been recognized to be at special risk when they contract varicella and should therefore receive the vaccine when they have no history of having suffered from the disease or are found to be sero-negative
Persons with planned organ transplantation	When organ transplantation (for example, kidney transplant) is being considered, vaccination should be carried out a few weeks before the immunosuppressive treatment is administered
Persons suffering from chronic diseases	Individuals suffering from chronic diseases such as metabolic and endocrine disorders, chronic pulmonary and cardiovascular diseases, mucoviscidosis and neuromuscular abnormalities, may also be predisposed to suffer from severe varicella
Healthy close contacts	Susceptible healthy close contacts should be vaccinated in order to reduce the risk of transmission of the virus to high-risk ill individuals. These include parents and siblings of high-risk ill individuals, medical and paramedical personnel, and other individuals who are in close contact with ill healthcare users suffering from varicella or healthcare users classified as high-risk individuals
Sick healthcare users under immunosuppressive treatment	Sick healthcare users under immunosuppressive treatment (including corticosteroid therapy) for malignant solid tumours or for serious chronic diseases (such as chronic renal failure, auto-immune diseases, collagen diseases, severe bronchial asthma) are predisposed to suffer from severe varicella Generally, ill healthcare users are vaccinated when they are in complete haematological remission from the disease. It is advised that the total lymphocyte count should be at least $1200/mm^3$ or no other evidence of lack of cellular immune competence exists

Please note

* **When vaccinating ill healthcare users in the acute phase of leukaemia**
  Maintenance chemotherapy should be withheld one (1) week before and one (1) week after vaccination. Ill healthcare users under radiotherapy should normally not be vaccinated during the treatment phase

* **Special precautions**
  Appropriate medical treatment should always be readily available, including adrenaline in case of rare anaphylactic reactions following administering of the vaccine. **For this reason, the vaccinee should remain under medical supervision for 30 minutes after vaccination**

* The **varicella-zoster-virus vaccine can be administered at the same time as any other vaccine**. Different injectable vaccines should always be administered at different injection sites. Should a **measles-containing vaccine** needed to be given at the same time as the varicella-zoster-virus vaccine, it is recommended that **an interval of at least one (1) month should be respected** since it is recognized that measles vaccination may lead to a short-lived suppression of the cell-mediated immune response. As the varicella-zoster-virus vaccine is highly immunogenic, it must be expected that the **reactogenicity (lower safety/less safe) following co-administering** of the varicella-zoster-virus vaccine and more reactogenic (less safe) vaccines will be determined by the **reactions of the latter**

* <u>Incompatibilities</u>
<u>The varicella-zoster-virus vaccine must never under any circumstances be mixed with other vaccines in the same syringe</u>

* **Health information to be given to the healthcare users**
After administering the vaccine, the healthcare practitioner must provide the parent/guardian/foster-parent or healthcare user with the following information
   * The aim of vaccination, namely, to **prime the individual's adaptive immune system against** the varicella-zoster-virus infection **by acting as immuno-stimulant in the eliciting of antibody-mediated immunity**
   * **Side-effects**
   Various side-effects may occur after the administering of the varicella-zoster-virus vaccine
      ➢ **Reactions at the site of** injection are usually mild
      ➢ **Papular-vesicular eruptions.** These eruptions are generally mild and short-lived
      ➢ **Mild to moderate fever** can appear a few days up to several weeks after vaccination
   * **Treatment of side-effects**
   Symptomatic and supportive
   * Other information to be communicated regarding the administering of varicella-zoster-virus vaccine
      ➢ **Pregnancy should be avoided** for three (3) months after vaccination
      ➢ **An interval of at least one month should be respected between the administering of** a **measles-containing vaccine** and the varicella-zoster-virus vaccine.

6.5.11   MMR VACCINE (MEASLES, MUMPS AND RUBELLA)

MMR vaccine, a living vaccine, is a freeze-dried suspension of attenuated live *measles-, mumps-* and *rubella viruses.*

The MMR-vaccine, as well as the single dosages of German measles vaccine and mumps vaccine are not provided by the Department of Health and must thus be purchased from a pharmacy or a medical practitioner and will be administered free of charge by the staff of a public health clinic after permission has been given in writing by the parents/guardians/foster-parents. A fee will be charged when administered by private healthcare practitioners in private practices or in private well-baby clinics for the procedure done and the vaccine administered.

✠ **Storage, transportation and handling**
   * The vaccine must be **administered as soon as possible after purchase**
   * The **cold chain must be maintained**. Parents must therefore be instructed to transport the vaccine on ice in a cool bag and ensure that it is administered within half an hour of purchase
   * Vaccine **has to be destroyed after if it was opened and not used**, or if the **VVMs are discoloured**, or if **six (6) hours have lapsed since reconstitution**
   * **Do not clean the skin with alcohol, ether or any other germicidal solutions as it destroys the measles virus – wash skin with water and soap when dirty and let completely dry before administering**

✠ **Contra-indications for MMR**
   Several contra-indications exist for the administering of MMR, namely,
   ⅄ <u>**Absolute contra-indication - Pregnancy**</u> **(including the single vaccine dosage of German measles)**
   ⅄ **Post-adolescence**
   ⅄ **Any acute disorder associated with fever**
   ⅄ **Acute respiratory infections**
   ⅄ **Any infectious condition**
   ⅄ **Active tuberculosis**
   ⅄ **Any chronic disease**
   ⅄ **Any immunological abnormality or deficiency**
   ⅄ **Sensitivity to neomycin**
   ⅄ **Allergy – particularly to egg-white**
   ⅄ **Treatment with corticosteroids or immuno-suppressive drugs**
   ⅄ **Any child suffering from AIDS or who are HIV-infected**

Please note:
<u>The vaccination must not be given within 3 months after receiving blood or plasma transfusions or the administering of human immunoglobulin.</u>

✠ **Administering**
   ◈ A **single dosage is given intramuscularly** in the Deltoid muscle. No booster dosage is necessary
   ◈ The vaccine is administered **only after the age of 12 months.** The eliciting of an **adaptive antibody-antigen immune response by MMR vaccine is optimal at the age of 15 months**
   ◈ **MMR vaccine can be administered** to babies of 12 months and older (up to the age of 4-5 years) (preferably at 15 or 18 months old) **whether the measles vaccine had been administered previously or not**
   ◈ If the vaccine had been administered at a much younger age (younger than 12 months) **a booster dosage has to be given at 15 months**

◈ A **single dosage of German measles vaccine is given to young girls, adolescent and adult women of fertility age if they are not pregnant or plan to become pregnant within the next three (3) months**

◈ The **vaccine can be administered to susceptible women** (who have never been vaccinated against rubella or never had the disease and whose serological titre is very low) **during the immediate postpartum period.** (It is advisable to have serological tests done for rubella sensitivity before inoculation is done)

◈ **Four (4) weeks must elapse after BCG vaccination** before MMR or the single dosage of measles vaccine, the single dosage of German measles vaccine, or single dosage of mumps vaccine may be administered

◈ **Single dosage of mumps-virus vaccine can be given to adolescent boys** if they have never had the disease as a child

◈ It is **not recommended that DTP[a] or DTP[a]-IPV-Hib and OPV or IPV** (as combination or single dosage vaccines) **be administered together with MMR vaccine**

<u>Warning</u>
<u>As this vaccine has to be injected intramuscularly, it must be administered with caution to individuals suffering from thrombocytopenia or a bleeding disorder</u>

✠ **Health information to be given to the healthcare users**
After administering the vaccine, the healthcare practitioner must provide the parent/guardian/foster-parent or healthcare user with the following information

✳ The information is the same as that is given for the measles vaccine

✳ The aim of vaccination, namely, to **prime the individual's adaptive immune system against measles, mumps and rubella by acting as immuno-stimulant in the eliciting of antibody-mediated immunity**

✳ Other information to be communicated regarding the administering of MMR vaccine

➤ **Post-pubertal women have to be informed that the rubella vaccine can cause** a general self-limiting arthralgia and/or possibly arthritis 2 to 4 weeks after administering

➤ **Breastfeeding mothers, who had received rubella vaccine, needs not to worry** about the infant receiving the antibody with breast milk

6.5.12 TETANUS TOXOID VACCINE

Tetanus Toxoid vaccine, a toxoid vaccine, is prepared from the toxin of the *Clostridium tetani* bacillus and is obtainable as a pure vaccine (absorbed and non-absorbed) or in combination with other vaccines.

✠ **Available preparations**
➔ Purified non-absorbed Tetanus Toxoid vaccine - **Tetanus toxoid or TT**
➔ Purified absorbed Tetanus Toxoid vaccine - **absorbed tetanus vaccine**
➔ Purified absorbed diphtheria toxoid-tetanus toxoid vaccine - **DT or Diphtet**

- ➜ Purified diphtheria toxoid-tetanus toxoid-pertussis toxoid vaccine (acellular- filamentous haemagglutinin] - DTP[a]
- ➜ Purified diphtheria toxoid-tetanus toxoid-pertussis toxoid (acellular-filamentous haemagglutinin–Haemophilus influenzae type B-vaccine - **DTP[a]–Hib**
- ➜ Purified diphtheria toxoid-tetanus toxoid-pertussis toxoid (acellular-filamentous haemagglutinin)-inactivated type type 1, 2, and 3 poliovirus D antigen vaccine - **DTP[a]–IPV**
- ➜ Purified diphtheria toxoid-tetanus toxoid-pertussis toxoid(acellular-filamentous haemagglutinin)–inactivated type type 1, 2, and 3 poliovirus D antigen-Haemophilus influenzae type B-vaccine - **DTP[a]-IPV-Hib**
- ➜ Purified Tetanus toxoid-Reduced amount of diphtheria vaccine - **Td**
- ➜ Typhoid fever-tetanus toxoid vaccine - **typhoid fever-tetanus vaccine**

Warning
<u>**As this vaccine has to be injected intramuscularly, it must be administered with caution to individuals suffering from thrombocytopenia or a bleeding disorder**</u>

✠ **Storage, transportation, handling and restitution**
- ✳ Tetanus Toxoid vaccine must be **stored in a refrigerator at 2-8⁰C and must not be frozen**
- ✳ Not **only will freezing harm the pure non-absorbed Tetanus Toxoid vaccine, it can also cause the vial to explode**
- ✳ **Freezing of the purified absorbed Tetanus Toxoid vaccine will lead to irreversible changes** in the phosphate gel
- ✳ The cold chain has to be maintained during transportation
- ✳ **Expiry dates and VVMs have to be taken into account** and adhered to

✠ **Contra-indications**
- ⅄ There are **no contra-indications** to the administering of Tetanus Toxoid (TT) vaccine
- ⅄ Do not administer Td to children younger than 6 years.

✠ **Administering**
- ◈ The various preparations of Tetanus Toxoid vaccine are administered intramuscularly as follows
  - ☑ Combination purified Tetanus Toxoid vaccine to infants and children - routinely with DTP[a]-IPV-Hib or other vaccines (as recommended as single dosages vaccines or as combination dosages vaccines) at 6 weeks (1st), 10 weeks (2sd), 14 weeks (3rd), 18 months (4th), and Td (or TT) at school entry 6 yrs (5th) and when leaving primary school 12 yrs (6th)
  - ☑ Typhoid fever-Tetanus Toxoid Vaccine and typhoid fever/paratyphoid fever A and B vaccine are only given under special circumstances, for example, epidemics, persons in sensitive occupations
  - ☑ Purified Tetanus Toxoid (non-absorbed) vaccine or Purified Tetanus Toxoid (absorbed) vaccine are given to
    - ◆ Adults who have not previously been vaccinated

- Women before or during pregnancy to protect the new-born infant against tetanus neonatorum
- Previously vaccinated children and adults to boost their immunity

---

Vaccinating with Tetanus Toxoid (TT) vaccine (excluding DTP[a]-IPV-Hib and other combination vaccines, DT and Td)

Purified Tetanus Toxoid (TT) vaccine, whether non-absorbed or adsorbed, can be used for the primary series vaccination as well as for booster series dosages. The absorbed vaccine, in which the toxoid is absorbed on aluminium phosphate, is undoubtedly the better of the two vaccines for primary series vaccination. Tetanus Toxoid vaccine (absorbed) must be used when vaccination is commenced and can be administered together with tetanus antitoxin

Primary series vaccination (for healthcare users who have not received DTP[a] or alternatively DTP[a]-IPV-Hib or alternatively DT or alternatively DTP[a]-HIB/DTP[w]-Hib or alternatively DTP[a]-IPV

*Tetanus Toxoid (TT) vaccine (non-absorbed)
Three (3) intramuscular injections of 0.5 ml are given with a 4 week interval between the first two dosages and an interval of six months between the second and third dosages. The 4th dosages must be given 1 year later and the 5 dosage 1 year later

*Tetanus Toxoid vaccine (absorbed)
Two (2) intramuscular injections of 0.5 ml vaccine are given with an interval of 4 weeks. A third dosage of 0.5 ml vaccine is recommended 6 months later and is **essential if tetanus antitoxin was given at the time of the first injection**. The 4th and 5th dosage must be given 1 year apart after the 3rd dosage

Booster series Dosages with Tetanus Toxoid
A booster dosage of 0.5 ml vaccine should be given every 10 years, as well as immediately after a tetanus-prone injury (if more than one (1) year has passed since the last vaccination with any of the vaccines containing tetanus toxoid or it can be proved that tetanus toxoid was given during the preceding 5 years)

Women of childbearing age
Five (5) adequately spaced dosages should be given to all women throughout the childbearing age

Pregnant women and breastfeeding mothers
→ Pregnant women (primigravidae and multigravidae) and mothers breastfeeding their babies who have **not** been immunized **before**, should receive three (3) intramuscular injections of 0.5 ml vaccine (depending on the type of vaccine used) over a period of time as follows: the **first vaccination** is administered during the first visit to the health clinic, followed 4 weeks later by the **second vaccination,** and 6 months later for the **third vaccination**. When the pregnant woman goes into labour before receiving the third recommended dosage, the last dosage(s) must be given postnatal. The six-week' postnatal visit, or the first time when the mother brings the infant for his/ her first vaccination visit, is ideal for the mother's 3rd dosage. At the first visit for antenatal care with all subsequent pregnancies, a booster series dosages must be given until 5 dosages have been received

> ➔ <u>Pregnant women (primigravidae and multigravidae) and breastfeeding mothers who have been vaccinated before</u>, should receive booster series dosages until 5 dosages have been received – the first booster dosage to be given at the first visit to the health clinic when pregnant and with all subsequent pregnancies until 5 dosages have been received. (Note that 1 year interval must lapsed between the booster dosages)
>
> ➔ <u>If no record of vaccination exist, or no record exist for antenatal care in previous pregnancies,</u> treat the healthcare user as a pregnant woman who has not been vaccinated before and give three (3) dosages vaccine. At the first visit for antenatal care with all subsequent pregnancies a booster dosages must be given until 5 dosages have been received
>
> ➔ <u>Record all TT dosages administered to the pregnant woman on her permanent "Woman's Health Card"</u> as well as on the antenatal card

✠ **Health information to be given to healthcare users**
After administering the vaccine, the healthcare practitioner must provide the parent/guardian/foster-parent or healthcare user with the following information
* The aim of vaccination, namely, to **prime the healthcare user's adaptive immune system against tetanus by acting as immuno-stimulant in the eliciting of antibody-mediated immunity**
* The injection site **may be painful**
* **Any analgesic may be taken 4-6 hourly for 48 to 72 hours if the body temperature is higher than 39⁰C** (pyrexia stimulates the antigen-antibody reaction). **Aspirin or disprin must not be given to children younger than 16 years**
* The injection site may be washed with soap and water
* The healthcare user **may feel unwell for a few days**
* Should the **healthcare user feel very ill within three to six hours** after administering, **he/she should return to the healthcare facility or immediately consult a medical practitioner.**

6.5.13 TYPHOID FEVER VACCINE

Typhoid fever vaccine, a non-living vaccine, is prepared from killed-off *Salmonella typhi* or *S.paratyphi bacilli*. Typhoid fever vaccine elicits short-term immunity lasting only for a year or two.

✠ **Available preparations**
➔ The **pure typhoid fever vaccine** is prepared from killed-off *Salmonella typhi*. It is preserved in phenol and offers protection against typhoid fever. (This vaccine is not used very often these days)
➔ The **living attenuated typhoid fever vaccine** induces local immunity in the intestines but no immunity to the systemic disease. The vaccine is prepared from the typhoid bacillus (TY21a) and is taken orally (as a tablet to be taken with sodium bicarbonate or in enteric-coated capsules)

➜ The **capsular polysaccharide typhoid fever vaccine** is composed of purified "Vi" (virulence) antigen

➜ The **typhoid fever-and-tetanus vaccine** is an inactivated vaccine, containing killed-off Salmonella typhi and inactivated tetanus toxoid. The vaccine offers protection against typhoid fever and tetanus

➜ The **typhoid fever-cholera vaccine** contains inactivated killed-off *Salmonella typhi* and killed-off *Vibrio Cholerae* offering a short duration protection against typhoid fever and cholera

✠ **Storage, transportation, handling and restitution**

⁎ Typhoid fever vaccine as a single dosage vaccine or as a combination vaccine, must be stored in a **refrigeration at 4 to 8⁰C and must never be frozen**

⁎ It must **not be used after the expiry date** given on the label

✠ **Contra-indications**

⅄ There are **no contra-indications** to vaccination against typhoid fever

✠ **Administering**

◈ **Vaccination against typhoid fever is indicated only in certain circumstances**, examples of which are exposure to a carrier, an outbreak of typhoid fever in a community, or in an institution, or in a group such as a military unit in field conditions. In the latter case typhoid fever-tetanus vaccine is given. The typhoid fever-cholera vaccine is useful for travellers in areas where these diseases are endemic and for sanitation workers exposed to the risk of contracting the diseases

◈ The **vaccine against typhoid fever may be given to all age groups,** but the dosage must be proportionally decreased for children under 10 years old

Vaccinating with purified typhoid fever vaccine and combinations thereof	
Typhoid fever vaccine (TAB) *Children	This vaccine is presently preferred to the other combinations since it causes fewer side-effects The dosage for children under the age of ten years is 0,25 ml vaccine injected subcutaneously. A booster dosage can be given after two years
*Adults	Two dosages of 0,5 ml vaccine each with an interval of two (2) weeks are injected subcutaneously for primary series vaccination
Typhoid fever-tetanus toxoid vaccine *Children	Children under five (5) years of age must be given half a dosage (0,25 ml) vaccine injected subcutaneously. Since most children of this age have already been vaccinated with DTP[a] vaccine (single dosage vaccine or combination vaccines), they must not be given tetanus vaccine unnecessarily

*Adults	Three (3) subcutaneous injections are given for the primary series vaccination with an interval of eight (8) weeks between the first and second dosages and six (6) months prior to the administering of the third dosage. A booster series dosage of typhoid fever vaccine (TAB) may be given two (2) years later, and a booster dosage of Tetanus Toxoid vaccine should be given after ten (10) years
Typhoid fever-cholera vaccine *Children	The above dosage is decreased according to the child's age
*Adults	Adults receive 1ml vaccine subcutaneously, followed by a further 1ml vaccine 7-14 days later
The oral typhoid fever vaccine must be given orally and must be administered according to instructions. The same goes for the health information to be given.	

✠ **Health information to be given to healthcare users**

After administering the vaccine, the healthcare practitioner must provide the parent/guardian/foster-parent or healthcare user with the following information

* The aim of vaccination, namely, to **prime the individual's adaptive immune system against typhoid fever by acting as immuno-stimulant**
* The healthcare user, parent or guardian or foster parent(s) must be warned that a **severe reaction may follow with swelling of the injection site, general symptoms and signs associated with pyrexia, headache and rigor**
* The treatment of this acute reaction includes the application of **local heat to the injection site and arm exercises**
* **Aspirin or disprin must never be given to children younger than 16 years**
* **Antipyretics must only be given when pyrexia is higher than 39°C.** Give only a few dosages (not more than 6) every 4-hourly until temperature has been lowered to 38°C or lower and can be tolerated, as pyrexia is necessarily to stimulate the adaptive antibody-antigen reaction
* **Give health information according to instructions** for orally administered typhoid fever vaccines

Please note

At **present little emphasis is placed on routine vaccination for the prevention of typhoid fever.** The emphasis is rather on the importance of other preventive measures, for instance, good sanitation, safe water supplies and hygienic food handling. When travelling to foreign countries where typhoid fever is an endemic disease, typhoid fever vaccine may become compulsory under the laws of the country of entry.

6.5.14   CHOLERA VACCINE

The cholera vaccine, a non-living vaccine, is a suspension of killed-off *Vibrio cholerae* of the Inaba and El-Tor biotypes.

✠ **Available preparations**
- ➜ **Pure cholera vaccine** containing only heat-killed-off *Vibrio cholerae*
- ➜ **The two new vaccines (living and non-living)** that is given orally. Two doses of the vaccines must be given to induce immunity
- ➜ **Typhoid fever-cholera vaccine**, a combination non-living vaccine, containing killed-off *Salmonella typhi* and killed-off *Vibrio cholerae*

✠ **Storage transportation, handling and reconstitution**
- ✳ The cholera vaccine must be **stored in a refrigerator between 4 to 8⁰C and must not be frozen**
- ✳ It must **not be used after the indicated expiry date**

✠ **Contra-indications**
- ⅄ **A severe reaction to previous vaccination against cholera** is a contra-indication, in which case a medical certificate for the contra-indication must be issued

✠ **Method of administering**
- ◈ **Infants under the age of 6 months** need not be vaccinated
- ◈ For **children 6 months to 1 year**, the first dosage must be decreased to 0,1 ml vaccine. If this does not elicit a reaction, a second dosage of 0,2 ml vaccine is given. For **children over the age of 12 months**, the age of the child determines the dosage of vaccine to be administered
- ◈ **Primary series vaccination** of persons **over the age of 14 years** consists of an initial subcutaneous injection of 0,5 ml cholera vaccine, followed 7 to 14 days later by a second dosage of 1ml vaccine. When exposure is a probability, a booster dosage of 0,5 ml vaccine must be given every six (6) months
- ◈ **International travelling purposes** - One (1) injection of 1ml vaccine is sufficient
- ◈ **The new oral vaccines (living and non-living)** must be given according to instructions as well as the health information to be given

✠ **Health information to be given to healthcare users**
After administering the vaccine, the healthcare practitioner must provide the parent/guardian/foster-parent or healthcare user with the following information
- ✳ The aim of vaccination, namely, to **prime the individual's adaptive immune system against cholera by acting as immuno-stimulant**
- ✳ The information given to the healthcare user is similar to that given for typhoid fever vaccination
- ✳ **Further information to be communicated regarding the administering of cholera vaccine**
  - ➢ An **international certificate of vaccination against cholera is required from time to time** on entering certain countries in Asia, Africa and the Middle East. The certificate is issued by the office of a travel clinic or by private medical practitioners certified to issue such a certificate
  - ➢ No proof of vaccination against cholera is required regarding entry into South Africa

Please note
The most important indication for cholera vaccination is travelling to areas where the disease is endemic or where epidemics occur. But, the effectiveness of vaccination against cholera is questionable. Vaccination may promote a sub-clinical infection and travellers may well become healthy short-term carriers. Furthermore, immunity lasts six months at the most, and the vaccine does not prevent sub-clinical or latent infection. Pure water supplies and sanitation are considered more important than vaccination.

6.6 INTERNATIONAL CERTIFICATION OF VACCINATION AGAINST SPECIFIED DISEASES

An international certificate of vaccination is a requirement for entry into several foreign countries. Each foreign country has its own requirements regarding vaccination, for example, against encephalitis, Yellow fever, etc. Such a certificate of vaccination is issued by the office of private travel clinics or certain private medical practitioners who are certified by the National Department of Health to issue such certificate. Information regarding the specific vaccination required by a specific country is available from these offices. A fee is charged for the procedure done and the vaccine administered.

Please note: The instructions given by the manufacturer must be followed with regard to the different vaccines; their storage, handling, and reconstitution; as well as all contra-indications, administering, side-effects and health information to be communicated to healthcare users regarding to the vaccine administered.

6.7 ADVERSE EVENTS OR REACTIONS FOLLOWING IMMUNIZATION OR VACCINATION (AEFI)

Although vaccines used in South Africa have been proven over many years to be very safe and effective, no vaccination can be declared entirely without risk. Some individuals (babies, children, adolescents, adults and the elderly) do experience adverse reactions (events) after vaccination. These adverse reactions may range from hypersensitivity with mild side-effects to serious illness, namely, anaphylactic shock. Adverse reactions are caused either by an error in the administering of the vaccine, or by sensitivity of an individual to a component within the vaccine that precipitate a reaction to the specific vaccine, or it may be co-incidental or the cause may be unknown. Hence, all vaccinators must be familiar with **true contra-indicators** and **vaccine-specific side-effects** of vaccination/immunization. Vaccine-specific side-effects are usually mild and self limiting and can be treated by the vaccinee self/ parents/relatives. In most instances vaccine-specific side-effects can be prevented or minimised. The adult vaccinee self, or the parents/relatives of a child vaccinee must thus be informed of the possibility of side-effects and informed how to deal appropriately with such side effects. However, when they are concerned, they have the right to return to the healthcare facility for further help and management. Vaccine-specific side-effects need not to be reported. **On the other hand, <u>any serious side-effect (trigger event of a medical incident) perceived to have been caused by a vaccination/immunization must be immediately treated, reported and investigated</u>**.

The case definition of an adverse event following vaccination/immunisation (AEFI) according to the EPI Disease Surveillance Field Guide (1998:53) is "A medical incident (trigger event) that takes place after immunisation and is perceived to be caused by immunisation." Adverse events following immunisation are classified in local reactions and systemic reactions. **<u>The following AEFI's trigger events must be reported according to law.</u>**

LOCAL REACTIONS

Local reactions may be caused by the volume of the vaccine injected and the following local reactions need not to be reported

- ➢ Immediate pain at the injection site
- ➢ Pain that disappears after a few minutes
- ➢ Tenderness lasting a few hours or sometimes a whole day

The following local reactions, however, **must be reported**

- ✱ **Severe local reactions following vaccination** with swelling further than 5 cm from the injection site or pain, redness and swelling of more than 3 days duration. Frequently, a nodule may develop at the injection site that last several weeks. In rare cases the nodule may become inflamed and turn into an aseptic abscess. **(All abscess formation must be reported)**
- ✱ **All cases of BCG lymphadenitis following vaccination** with regional inflammatory adenitis (simple or latent or suppurative) **occurring in the territory corresponding** to the vaccination site
- ✱ **Injection site abscess formation following vaccination.** Abscesses are severe local reactions with the formation of a fluctuating abscess at or near the injection site. As the abscess can be either suppurative (caused by an un-sterile needle) or aseptic/sterile (caused by a reaction to the vaccine itself), <u>a culture must be taken when the abscess is drained</u>

SYSTEMIC REACTIONS

Although systemic adverse events are rare, they are far more serious and may result in hospitalization. Hypersensitivity with severe anaphylaxis (sometimes followed by death) is the most severe systematic reaction that can occur. Sometimes vaccination is followed by an intense feverish syndrome characterized by headaches, and/or digestive disorders lasting 1-2 days. As long as the pyrexia remains below 40,5°C, this event needs not to be reported

The following systemic reactions, however, **must be reported**

◆ **All cases of hospitalisation thought to be related to immunisation/ vaccination**
Post–immunisation illness is indicated when, according to the history taken of the current illness and the onset of symptoms, hospitalization and treatment are needed within 3 days of vaccination

◆ **Encephalopathy within 7 days of vaccination.** Investigation must be done when any diagnosis of encephalopathy is made in a child who was vaccinated within 7 days prior to the onset of encephalopathy

◆ **Collapse or shock-like state within 48 hours of immunisation/vaccination.** Anaphylaxis may occur either immediately after the first injection of the vaccine (infants and adults) or within six to ten (6-10) hours (delayed reaction occurring particularly in persons previously vaccinated). Persons vaccinated for the first time may also show a delayed reaction

◆ **Fever of 40,5°C within 48 hours of vaccination.** Hyperpyrexia of 40,5°C and higher that is accompanied by vomiting and restlessness may result in febrile convulsions that needs hospitalization and medical treatment

◆ **Seizures/convulsions within three (3) days of vaccination.** Investigation needs to be done in all cases of any seizure/convulsions (febrile or non-febrile) within three (3) days after vaccination

◆ **Any delayed onset of an unusual medical incident thought to be related to vaccination within one month after being immunized**

◆ **All deaths thought to be related to vaccination.** All fatal events following vaccination must be fully investigated. Delictual (relatives of the deceased instigate civil court action) and/or criminal (police investigation followed by criminal court prosecution) and/or professional (code of conduct hearings by professional councils) proceedings may follow

As the post-immunisation period is not defined, death thought to be related to immunisation/vaccination is the most severe AEFI that can occur. Openness and a sympathetic approach (not defensive) much prevail to ensure that the relationship of trust between healthcare providers and the community prevails. All deaths must be reported to the National Department of Health within 24 hours.

All suspected cases of AEFI's must immediately detected, treated and reported by all healthcare providers. Hospitalization, severe unusual medical incident thought to be related to immunization and deaths are considered as "serious" and must be reported within 24 hours to the National Department of Health. Individuals affected by an adverse reaction must be immediately treated at any healthcare facility where the individual presents and, if necessary, referred for specialist treatment. An investigation must follow a reported case of AEFI to determine the cause of the event, to prevent a cluster of events (further AEFI's of the same cause), and to prevent mistrust of the public regarding vaccination programmes. Where necessary, laboratory investigation will be done by the National Control Laboratory in Bloemfontein, for toxicity, sterility, and confirmation that the contents of the vial is in accordance with the label, as well as whether contamination of the specific vaccine had taken place, and whether the vaccine has been frozen.

Any other vaccine-related tests (for example, identifying diluent or adjuvant) will also be done when deemed necessary. A final classification of the cause of the AEFI needs to be made by the Provincial and National EPI managers, taking into consideration the inputs from the Medicines Control Council (MCC), which have a statutory responsibility with regard to the safety, medical efficiency and quality of all medicines, including vaccines, and the manufacturing companies.

To prevent or minimize adverse events, healthcare providers must be knowledgeable and well-trained vaccinators. **Programme-related AEFI's** are medical incidents caused by some error in the transportation, storage, handling, or administrating of a vaccine. The following programme-related AEFI'S that needs to be prevented are

- giving too much vaccine in one dosage
- administering the vaccine in the wrong body site (for example, injecting oral vaccine)
- using un-sterilized needles and syringes
- carelessly handling and use of medical stock and equipment (for example, needles and swabs)
- reconstituting vaccine with the wrong diluent
- using wrong amounts of diluent
- using incorrect amounts of diluent and/or the wrong diluent
- preparing vaccines incorrectly
- substituting drugs for vaccine or diluent
- contaminating the vaccine or diluent
- storing vaccines incorrectly
- ignoring contra-indications (for example, vaccinating a child using the same type of vaccine for which a vaccine-related side effect had previously been reported)
- not discarding vaccine at the end of a vaccination session and using it again during a subsequent session.

A **cluster** of AEFI's events may have been caused by the following possible programme-related errors, when

- ◈ the same healthcare provider has administered all of the suspected vaccinations
- ◈ all vaccinated persons in the same age group in the same geographical area have the same symptoms (for example, during mass vaccination campaigns)
- ◈ all individuals that were vaccinated with the same vaccine batch/lot in the same healthcare facility on the same day experience the same symptoms.

Vaccine–induced AEFI's are a medical incident caused by the reaction of a specific individual to specific vaccine. To a certain extent vaccine-induced AEFI"s can be minimized by taking a **comprehensive medical history** and doing a physical examination **before every vaccination session. Special attention has to be given to**

- ✓ **all medical conditions (acute and chronic) suffering from at present, and all those suffered from in the past (including treatment and outcome)**
- ✓ **allergies (all drugs, vaccines, and food, for example, eggs)**

253

- ✓ **any side effect[s] previously experienced following any form of vaccine administration**
- ✓ **contra-indications for the specific vaccine**
- ✓ **familial history of adverse reaction to drugs and vaccines and other heredity diseases contra-indicated**
- ✓ **current medical treatment and drug taking (including over the counter drugs and herbal medicine).**

<u>**Please Note**</u>

A vaccine-related adverse reaction <u>can never and will never</u> be completely prevented regardless the most comprehensively medical history taken and correct procedures followed. All healthcare providers must thus be well-trained in cardio-pulmonary resuscitation (CPR) and the management of a hypersensitivity reaction.

Co-incidental AEFI's are medical incidents that would have occurred whether the individual had received a vaccination prior to the incident or not – the AEFI happen co-incidentally at the same time as the vaccination. Co-incidental AEFI's are very difficult to prevent or minimize as co-incidental AEFI's are wholly unrelated in any way to vaccinations or vaccines that were administrated except for the time that they had occurred. If the same event is diagnosed in persons who were not been vaccinated, it can be said that a co-incidental AEFI medical incident has occurred.

6.8 HYPERSENSITIVITY REACTION (ANAPHYLACTIC SHOCK) – THE MOST SERIOUS ADVERSE REACTION

A hypersensitivity reaction is a severe systemic allergic reaction to a specific antigen, characterized by multisystem involvement of the skin, respiratory system, cardio-vascular system, neurological system, urinary system and gastro-intestinal tract. The severe antibody-antigen response leads to decreased tissue perfusion and initiation of the general shock response. <u>**Anaphylactic shock as result of a hypersensitivity reaction is life threatening**</u>. Hypersensitivity reactions/anaphylactic reactions are either IgE-mediated or non-IgE-mediated response.

6.8.1 Pathophysiology of a hypersensitivity reaction

When an antigen gains entry into the body, an immunoglobulin (antibody), namely, an IgE-immunoglobulin specific to the antigen, is formed during the antibody-mediated antibody-antigen response. When the antigen-specific IgE-immunoglobulin has been formed, the IgE- and IgG-immunoglobulin conjugate with surface receptors of mast cells in connective tissue surrounding the blood vessels and the basophiles in the blood itself – the primary immune response. The result is that the conjugated IgE-immunoglobulin accumulates in the respiratory and gastro-intestinal tracts, the intravascular system and in the skin. The activation of the biochemical mediators, when released locally and systemically, causes increased mucous membrane secretions, increased capillary permeability and leakage, and remarkably reduces the smooth muscle tone not only in blood vessels (vasodilatation) but also in the bronchioles. Together, all these substances result in shock due to the dilatation of the blood vessels, hyper-permeability of the small blood vessels, spasm of the walls of hollow organs and increased secretion of mucous membranes. The enhanced venous permeability causes a reduction in the circulating blood volume with diminished pressure, as well as an accumulation of fluid outside the blood vessels. (See Figure 6.2 and Table 6.5 for a schematic representation of the antigen-antibody reaction and the effect of biochemical mediators on the body). When the same antigen again gains entry into the body, the preformed IgE-immunoglobulin reacts with it and a secondary immune response occurs. This reaction triggers the release of biochemical mediators from the mast cells and basophiles that then initiates the cascade of events that precipitates anaphylactic shock.

Some anaphylactic reactions are non-IgE-mediated responses as it occurs in the absence of the activation of the IgE-immunoglobulin. These responses occur as a result of direct activation of the mast cells to release biochemical mediators. The direct activation of mast cells is triggered by antibody-mediated mediators such as the complement system and the coagulation-fibrinolytic system. Biochemical mediators can also be released as a direct or indirect response to drugs that then leads to an anaphylactic reaction.

Please note
Many anaphylactic shock reactions, however, occur without a documented prior exposure

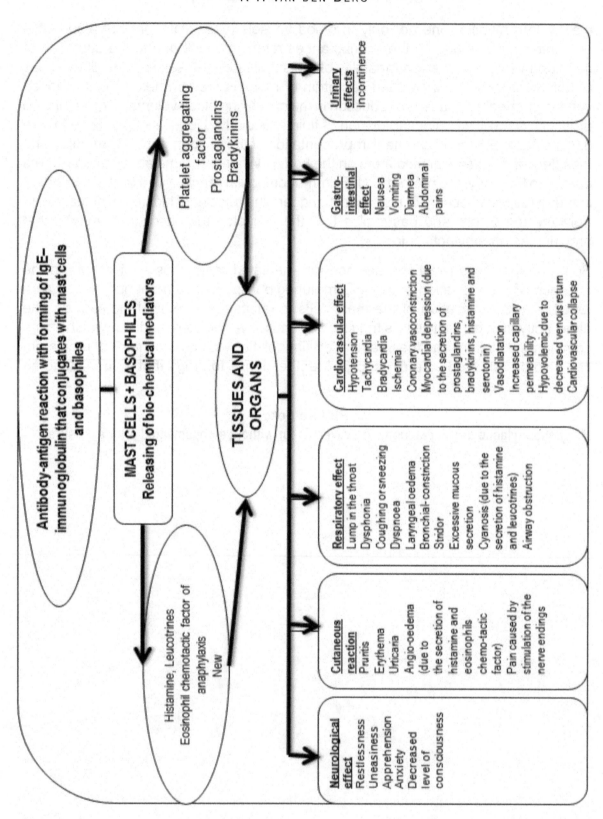

Figure 6.2 Depiction of the antigen-antibody reaction and the physiological functions of the mediators that are released

Table 6.5 TABULATION OF THE PHYSIOLOGICAL REACTION OF THE BIOCHEMICAL REACTIVE MEDIATORS ON THE TISSUES OF THE BODY

Biochemical reactive mediators	Physiological reaction
Bradykinins	Sweat and saliva secretion increases Bronchial constriction occurs Systemic vasodilatation takes place Vascular permeability increases
Eosinophil chemotactic factor	Cellular infiltration takes place
Histamine	Vascular secretions increase Pulmonary secretions increase Urticaria develops Bronchial constriction takes place General vasodilatation takes place Altered myocardial function occurs Dysrhythmia occurs Altered coronary blood flow takes place
Leucotrines (slow-acting substances of anaphylaxis)	Bronchial constriction of the small airways occurs Neutrophil chemotaxis increases Vascular constriction increases Vascular permeability increases Wheal and flare reaction develops Promote plasma leakage with increased leukocyte adhesion to vascular endothelium
Platelet aggregating factor released by mast cells, basophiles, macrophages, neutrophils, platelets and damaged endothelium	Platelet coagulation aggregation and detachment increases Coronary blood flow decreases because of vasodilatation Vascular permeability and bronchial constriction increases Dysrhythmia occurs Negative isotropic effect on the heart occurs Neutrophil adhesion increases
Prostaglandin released by arachidonic acid metabolites	Pulmonary hypertension takes place Lung secretions increase The effect of histamine and permeability increases Vasoconstriction occurs Platelet activation and aggregation take place

6.8.2　Aetiology of a hypersensitivity reaction

Any antigen capable of activating IgE-immunoglobulin can be a trigger for anaphylaxis - a life threatening hypersensitivity reaction that may suddenly occur in the following circumstances

❖ When administering vaccines, particularly those containing albumin such as vaccines against rabies, yellow fever and pertussis

❖ When administering a antiserum or an antitoxin, for instance, diphtheria antitoxin, tetanus antitoxin and snake-bite antiserum

❖ When taking an extensive course of drugs and antimicrobial drugs (antibiotics) such as penicillin, streptomycin, aspirin, insulin and pethidine

❖ After being bitten by a snake or being sting by an insect or bee (venoms)

❖ When contact occurs with chemicals such as chrome, nickel sulphate, and turpentine, or environmental agents

❖ When eating food such as meat, fish, eggs, nuts and seeds etc. as well as food additives

❖ When a drug, serum, or vaccine is given to an individual with allergic disorders such as asthma, hay fever, eczema, urticaria, or to individuals who have developed skin reactions to drugs or antibiotics, or to individuals who have previously developed a severe reaction after having an antiserum or vaccine administered to them.

6.8.3 Clinical manifestation of a hypersensitivity reaction

The nature and onset of a hypersensitivity reaction depend on
- ✠ the route by which the antigen gained entry into the body
- ✠ the quantity of antigen absorbed
- ✠ the absorption rate
- ✠ the degree of hypersensitivity the individual has already developed.

6.8.3.1 The severity of the hypersensitivity reaction

The shorter the interval between exposure and reaction, the more likely the reaction is to be severe

- **Sudden severe and life threatening hypersensitivity reaction (anaphylactic shock)**. The signs and symptoms of an acute systemic reaction appear within seconds/minutes after the antigen has gained entry into the body. The signs and symptoms develop very rapidly and death may ensue within minutes
- **Delayed hypersensitivity reaction**. This hypersensitivity reaction develops more slowly than the immediate reaction (6 to 10 hours later).

6.8.3.2 Clinical manifestation

A variety of clinical manifestations occur depending on the extent of the body systems involvement. The signs and symptoms are the same for both of the hypersensitivity reactions mentioned above. Anaphylaxis must be considered when responses from **two or more body systems** (cutaneous, respiratory, cardiovascular, neurological or gastro-intestinal) are noted.

Please note - the cardiovascular and respiratory systems may not always be involved

✱ **Prodromal signs**
   ▪ vague complaints of discomfort

- intense anxiety
- headache
- paraesthesia (pins and needles in the limbs)
- pain in muscles and joints
- dyspnoea
- lacrimation
- excessive perspiration
- a flushed face

✱ **Signs and symptoms of a hypersensitivity reaction**
- **Skin** - pruritis, pallor, urticaria, angio-oedema of the eyelids, lips and tongue, and a cold, clammy skin
- **Respiratory system** - the person experiences a "lump in the throat" and hoarseness, coughing and sneezing, dyspnoea and stridor occur. The uvula, vocal cords and posterior pharynx may become oedematous and abnormal lung sounds and protracted expirations can be heard on auscultation. Fatal laryngeal oedema and bronchial spasm develop
- **Cardiovascular system** - cardiovascular collapse takes place because the plasma volume is reduced due to dilatation of the blood vessels and the extravasation of intravascular fluid into the extracellular spaces. Hypotension, tachycardia, bradycardia and ischemia with myocardial suppression set in. Cardiac arrest follows
- **Gastro-intestinal system** - nausea, abdominal cramps, severe vomiting and severe diarrhoea
- **Metabolic abnormalities** - raised serum histamine levels, metabolic acidosis and a reduction of blood clotting factors
- **Level of consciousness** - anxiety, restlessness, may become stuporous or unconscious and convulsions may occur.

The duration of the signs and symptoms varies. Urticaria and angio-oedema may clear up quickly or may last for days or weeks. **Moderate systemic signs and symptoms** such as nausea and pruritis may last for a few hours, but may continue for longer than 24 hour. **Severe systemic signs and symptoms** such as hypotension and laryngeal oedema may last for days, although they usually clear up when treatment commences.

Individuals can deteriorate over a brief period of time ($\frac{1}{4} \rightarrow \frac{1}{2} \rightarrow 3$ hours) with progressive development of stridor, dysphonia or aphonia, laryngeal oedema, massive lingual swelling, facial and neck swelling and hypoxia. The airway obstruction together with the severe cardiovascular collapse leads to death within minutes.

6.8.4   Treatment of a hypersensitivity reaction

The management of a hypersensitivity reaction includes early recognition, anticipation of deterioration, and aggressive support of the airway, oxidation, ventilation and circulation. The goal of treatment is to remove the offending antigen, reverse the effects of the biochemical mediators and promote adequate tissue perfusion by supporting of the airway, breathing and circulation.

Note

Since the development of a hypersensitivity reaction may be extremely rapid and often has fatal consequences, emergency treatment must be started immediately

Every clinic or service where vaccines or where drugs are administered, must be equipped with an emergency tray for immediate use. The emergency tray must be checked DAILY before vaccination commences and the COMPLETENESS and EXPIRY DATES of drugs must also be checked

Furthermore, all healthcare providers must ensure that their knowledge of and cardiopulmonary resuscitation skills (CPR) are up to date

Emergency tray requirements

Drugs
Adrenaline (1:1000) 1 ml ampoules
Corticosteroids – betamethasone (Betnasol 40 mg/ml) or hydrocortisone (Solu-Cortef 100 mg in 2 ml H_2O)
Antihistamine

Equipment
Disposable sterile syringes (2 ml) and needles
Airways – large, medium and small
Tongue spatula
Tongue forceps
Bowl, gauze swabs, Savlon and kidney basin
Adhesive plaster
Container for disposal of sharp instruments

Emergency treatment by healthcare providers of a hypersensitivity reaction in healthcare users

Immediate emergency treatment

✱ **Give a subcutaneous injection of Epinephrine 1:1000 or Adrenaline 1:1000** according to the following schedule

Healthcare user's age	Dosage
New-born to 2 months	0,1 ml
3–4 months	0,1–0,2 ml
1–2 years	0,2–0,3 ml
3–4 years	0,3–0,4 ml
5–6 years	0,4 ml
7–11 years	0,5 ml
12–15 years	0,8 ml
16 years and adults	1 ml

Please note
Adrenaline must always be given SLOWLY and SUBCUTANEOUSLY, except if the person show early signs of a systematic reaction (hypotension, airway swelling or difficult breathing) or is severely shocked, in which case it is given intramuscularly. Do not remove the needle after the first injection. MAKE SURE THAT THE NEEDLE HAS NOT BEEN INSERTED INTO A VEIN

◈ When the person shows no improvement after the first injection, another injection of adrenaline 1:1000 injection 0,3 – 0,5 mg may be administered after 15 to 20 minutes. Hereafter adrenaline may only be given four (4) hourly if necessary. **Adrenaline may only be given three times at the most since it can cause cardiac arrest**

◈ Administer intravenous epinephrine 1:1000 only if the anaphylaxis does not clear up or if immediate severe life threatening manifestations appear. Give epinephrine (1:1000) 0,1 mg slowly over 5 minutes (dilute epinephrine to 1:1000 before infusion)

Note An intravenous infusion at a rate of 1 to 4 µg/mm may prevent the need to repeat epinephrine injections frequently

✳ **Monitor the person closely**

◈ Monitor for tachycardia, hypertension, dyspnoea and dysrhythmia while adrenaline 1:1000 is being administered. Monitoring is critical because fatal over-dosage of epinephrine can occur

◈ Stop administering of epinephrine 1:1000 as soon as any of these abovementioned signs appear

◈ The rest of the dosage of adrenaline 1:1000 may only be given when the signs have cleared up

Note **Adrenaline may NOT be given if the signs do not improve**

✳ **Consolidate the person's respiratory status**

◈ Ensure an open airway by moving the mandible forward, putting the head in extension and inserting an airway into the mouth while pulling the tongue forward. Intubation must be done when hoarseness, lingual oedema, stridor and oro-pharyngeal swelling are manifested

◈ Always keep the person's head and shoulder higher than the chest, with the legs elevated and the trunk flat

◈ When respiration cease and the pulse weaken, apply aggressive mouth-to-mouth respiration and external cardiac massage over a prolonged period of time. Administer simultaneously massive volume replacement (4 to 8 litres) of isotonic crystalloid (for example, normal saline) intravenous fluid therapy as quickly as possible

◈ When the person is in full cardiac arrest, give 1–3 mg adrenaline intravenously for 3 minutes, then 3–5 mg adrenaline intravenously for 3 minutes, and then 4–10 µg/ml per infusion

◈ Administer oxygen at high flow rates

✱ **Measure vital signs every 5 to 15 minutes for 4 hours**
  ◈ When tachycardia and hypotension occur, let the individual lie flat and elevate his/her legs to ensure venous return

✱ **Call a medical practitioner**
  ◈ Remain with the person until the medical practitioner has taken over
  ◈ When a medical practitioner cannot be reached, transport the person to the nearest hospital after his/her condition has improved

✱ **Administer high dosage of corticosteroid (intravenously or intra-muscularly) AND an antihistamine (intra-muscularly) very slowly**
  ◈ **(i) Corticosteroid (intravenous or intramuscular), namely, Betnasol or Solu-Cortef**

Betamethasone, for example, **Betnasol 4 mg/ml**		OR	Hydrocortisone for example, **Solu-Cortef 100 mg in 1 ml sterile water**	
Client's age	Dosage		Client's age	Dosage
0-2 years	0,25 ml		0-2 years	0,5 ml
2-12 years	0,25-0,75 ml		2-12 years	0,5-1,5 ml
16 years and older	1 ml		16 years and older	1-2 ml

AND

  ◈ **(ii) Antihistamine such as Anthisan or Phenergan to be given intramuscularly**

Healthcare user's age	Dosage
0-2 years	0,5 ml
2-12 years	0,5-1,5 ml
6 years and older	2 ml

✱ **Commence an intravenous infusion** of normal saline or Ringer's lactate to raise the blood pressure. A rapid infusion of 1–2 litres or even 4 litres may be needed initially

✱ **Observe the person for signs of hypervolumia** such as
  ◈ Adventitious lung sounds, lung murmurs, dyspnoea, coughs, frothy sputum and congestion of the jugular vein, as well as bronchial spasm, respiratory obstruction, tachycardia and hypertension
  ◈ Monitor urinary output (30 ml per hour is normal)

✱ **Monitor the person's condition for 24 hours or longer** after his condition has improved

✱ **Write a report of the events in red** on the chart of the healthcare user

✱ **Inform the person that he/she may not**
  ◈ take any vasodilators since they may cause a drop in his/her blood pressure

> ◈ drink any alcohol
> ◈ take a hot bath
> ◈ take any medication whatsoever without the permission of his/her medical practitioner

Please note

Some persons (up to 20%) show a biphasic response with symptoms recurring within 1 to 8 hours (even as long as 36 hours) despite an intervening asymptomatic period

6.8.5 Measures to prevent a hypersensitivity reaction

A hypersensitivity reaction is life-threatening and can be prevented by determining the healthcare user's history of sensitivity to certain substances and by carrying out a sensitivity test on the healthcare user

✱ **History taking for sensitivity**
  ◈ Always ascertain whether any medication (i.e. penicillin) or the vaccine to be given, had been administered to the healthcare user before, and whether any drug or vaccine caused a sensitivity reaction within 48 hours after administering
  ◈ **When the healthcare user reports a previous reaction to either of the above mentioned substances (drugs or vaccine), it must not be given (not even as a sensitivity test)**
  ◈ Before any vaccine is administered, ascertain whether the healthcare user is prone to allergic reactions such as asthma, eczema, nettle rash, urticaria, egg-white allergy, or an allergy to any component of the vaccine
  ◈ When the healthcare user shows a tendency to allergic reactions, a sensitivity test may be done to determine whether a reaction to the vaccine or preparation will occur. However, always consult the medical practitioner of the healthcare user first

✱ **Sensitivity test to be done**
  ◈ Do the skin test using a tuberculin or other small syringe and a fine needle. Inject 0,2 ml of the vaccine (diluted 1:10) intra-dermal on the inside of the forearm
  ◈ **Hypersensitive individuals will develop a characteristic wheal and flare at the injection site within a few minutes.** This is a raised pale area surrounded by redness. The reaction disappears within 20 minutes to one (1) hour. **The vaccine is NOT TO BE ADMINISTERED when the skin test is positive**

6.8.6 Recording of and information to be provided regarding a hypersensitivity reaction

Any hypersensitivity reaction to any drug or vaccine, or a reaction to a skin test, must be charted in **large red letters on the medical chart of the healthcare user**

◈ The **following information MUST BE SPECIFICALLY BROUGHT TO THE HEALTHCARE USER'S ATTENTION**
  - ➢ **He/she will be provided with a card** containing the information that has been recorded on his/her medical chart. Instruct the person **to show this card** whenever he/she requires medical attention and treatment
  - ➢ **The value of wearing a Medic-Alert disc/bracelet or a SOS disc/bracelet. Encourage the healthcare user to wear the disc/bracelet 24 hours per day, every day, year in, and year out.**

6.9   KEY NOTES

- ❑ In view of the serious complications which may arise when a person, especially a young child or the elderly, suffers from a communicable disease such as measles or influenza, it is necessary that individuals (especially infants, children, elderly, and travellers) be vaccinated against certain diseases as recommended.
- ❑ Vaccination aims to prime the adaptive immune system with memory to the antigens of a specific pathogen so that a first infection induces a secondary response.
- ❑ Vaccines contain either live attenuated pathogens, or killed-off whole pathogens, or sub-cellular fractions or antigens produced by artificially gene cloning or chemical synthesis. Live attenuated vaccines are more effective than the other types, but carry the risk that they may revert to virulence or induce disease in immuno-compromised individuals.
- ❑ It is the responsibility of all healthcare providers to encourage parents/guardians/ foster-parents to have their children vaccinated as vaccination is not compulsory (voluntary). By doing so, epidemics and the complications of certain communicable diseases may be prevented.
- ❑ Childhood diseases are now becoming diseases of adolescence and young adults - a vaccinated child now contracts the particular disease later in life and because adolescents and adults become more seriously ill than children, more adolescents and adults die from or are disabled by the complications of vaccine-prevented diseases than children.
- ❑ Travellers may require certain compulsory vaccinations against specific communicable diseases prevalent or endemic in the country of entry.
- ❑ Employees in sensitive occupations (for example, healthcare profession, police and environmental health workers) must be encouraged to abide to compulsory vaccinations as required.
- ❑ **Healthcare providers must always bear in mind that vaccination can lead to a hypersensitivity and anaphylactic shock reaction. For this reason, all healthcare providers must be well prepared and able to recognize the signs and symptoms of hypersensitivity and anaphylactic shock reaction, and execute the necessary emergency treatment, including cardio-pulmonary-resuscitation.**

Chapter 7

THE GENERAL PATHOGENESIS AND NON-SPECIFIC CLINICAL MANIFESTATION OF COMMUNICABLE INFECTIONS

Every infection is a race between the capacities of the pathogen to multiply, spread and cause infection and the ability of the host to control and finally terminate the infection. A 24-hour delay before an important host response comes into operation, gives a decisive advantage to a rapidly multiplying pathogen – causing enough damage in the host to cause disease while the pathogenic microbe gets the opportunity to be shed from the body in larger amounts or for an extra day or two. As humans are host to normal commensally microbial flora as well as infectious pathogens, the host's surfaces, skin and mucosa, must be intact and the systemic defences, innate and adaptive immune systems, must be competent to prevent infection. When this state of *balanced pathogenicity* between host and pathogens is disrupted, disease/ infection arises.

All communicable diseases run a natural course with five distinctive stages, each of which is recognisable from the general and specific pathogenesis and reaction between the body tissue[s] and the infectious agent, as well as from the manner in which the signs and symptoms are clinically manifested (see figure 7.1)

- ❑ The **first stage** is that of pre-pathogenesis. By this stage, the person has already been exposed to the infectious pathogen. Based on the body's innate and adaptive physiological immune systems, the person may become ill or may not. When the person becomes ill, the non-specific and specific characteristic signs and symptoms will then be clinically manifested
- ❑ The **second stage** is that of pathogenesis (disease mediated by pathogens) which can be divided into four sub-stages, namely
  - ❖ **Early pathogenesis** - During this stage the person is already infected (as the disease has been contracted) although the clinical signs and symptoms (general/non-specific and typical/specific) of the particular disease are not yet manifested. The individual appears to be healthy. This stage correlates with the incubation period and can last from a few hours to a number of days. The individual can already transmit the particular disease to other persons.

❖ **Prodromal stage (pre-clinical stage)** (early non-specific discernible signs) - The signs and symptoms which appear during this stage are not typical of the disease. The individual manifests the signs and symptoms of a general systemic illness (such as pyrexia) and already feels ill. Sometimes a prodromal rash may appear. This stage lasts until the characteristic-specific/typical signs and symptoms of the disease are manifested. During this period the infected person continues to transmit the particular disease to other persons

❖ **Characteristic-specific clinical manifestation/clinical picture (clinical stage)** - This starts with the appearance of the characteristic-specific signs and symptoms of the particular disease. The clinical picture lasts as long as the clinical signs and symptoms are visible. The ill individual continues to transmit the disease to other persons. (Note that some communicable diseases can only be transmitted as long as pyrexia is present. In other cases the disease is transmissible until the ill individual has fully recovered)

❖ **Recovering stage (stage of resolution)** - During this stage the ill individual recovers and the characteristic clinical signs and symptoms disappear. When the ill individual has recovered, he/she is immune to the specific communicable disease when immunity with memory was mediated. When no immunity with memory has been elicited, the individual may contract the specific communicable disease once again. After recovering from certain specific communicable diseases a carrier state may develops.

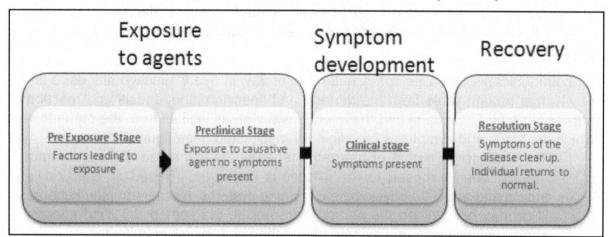

Figure 7.1 Schematic presentation of the pathogenesis of an infection

Pathogens that successfully penetrate the body's natural defence barriers have adapted and evolved strategies to evade the immune responses. These strategies enable the infectious agents to stay in the body long enough to complete their replication, spread, infection and shedding to fresh hosts. The clinical manifestation or signs and symptoms of infection are produced by the infective pathogen or by the host's immune system. Many successful infectious agents multiply in the epithelial cells at the site of entry on the body surface but do not spread to deeper structures or through the body. Local spread takes place readily on the body surface and fluid-covered mucosal surfaces with the result that large areas of the body surface can be involved within a few days with shedding to the exterior. In contrast, infective pathogens that spread systemically through the body via lymph and blood, invade the various tissues stepwise before reaching the final site of replication and shedding to the exterior.

The clinical picture of any particular communicable disease can be divided in two stages, namely, (1) non-specific or general signs and symptoms and (2) characteristic-specific clinical signs and symptoms of the disease itself. The non-specific signs and symptoms develop during the stage of pre-pathogenesis after exposure had taken place and the early stage of pathogenesis when the pathogen attaches and establishes itself in the host cells, multiplies, spreads and sheds from the body to be transmitted to new hosts. As soon as the host manifests the characteristic (specific) signs and symptoms of the particular infection, the disease can be diagnosed as such. Resolution follows and the ill person recovers.

Note

In this chapter, only the **general pathogenesis underlying** all communicable diseases and the NON-SPECIFIC OR GENERAL CLINICAL PICTURE WHICH IS MANIFESTED IN ALL COMMUNICABLE DISEASES are discussed.

Also note that the general pathogenesis and non-specific clinical picture must always be read in conjunction with the specific pathogenesis and the characteristic-specific clinical picture of the particular communicable disease as fully described in THEME IV of the book

7.1 THE GENERAL PATHOGENESIS IN THE NATURAL COURSE OF A SURFACE AND SYSTEMIC INFECTION

The human host can be considered as a series of body surfaces serving as sites for microbial infection and shedding, namely the mouth and the respiratory tract, the mouth and the alimentary tract, the eye, the skin and the urinary-genital tract. To establish themselves on or in the host, the infective pathogens must either attach themselves to the outer body surface or penetrate one of the inner body surfaces. The skin as outer surface forms a horny, dry, relatively impermeable outer layer to protect and isolate the body. Where there are more intimate contact and exchange with the outside world, the alimentary, respiratory and urinary-genital tracts - where food is absorbed, gases exchanged and urine and sexual products are released - the surface lining consist of one or more layers of living cells. In the eye the transparent layer of living cells is replaced by the conjunctiva. Well-developed cleansing and defense mechanisms are present at all these body surfaces. However, successful infectious pathogens possess efficient mechanisms to attach themselves to and to transverse these body surfaces. Once attachment has taken place, the successful pathogen must survive the defense mechanisms of the host, then multiply/replicate itself, spread through and infect body cells after which it must exit from the body to be transmitted to fresh hosts. As soon as the defense mechanisms of the body have successfully defended the body by killing off the infective pathogen, resolution of the infection takes place and the ill person recovers. When recovery does not take place, a persistent chronic infection follows.

7.1.1 Entry and attachment – the stage of pre–pathogenesis after exposure had taken place

Microbes possess specific molecules on their bodies to attach to receptor molecules on host cells either at the body surface (viruses and bacteria) or in the tissues (viruses). The receptor molecules on the host cells, of which there are many, have specific functions to perform in the life of the cell, over and above to bind with the specific infective pathogen. Very occasionally the receptor molecule is present only in certain cells which are then uniquely susceptible to infection, for example, the CD4 molecule for the *HIV-virus* and the C3d receptor for the *Epstein-Barr virus*. In these cases, the receptor molecule determines the virus tropism and accounts for the distinctive pattern of infection. Thus, the receptor molecules on the body cells of the host are critical determinants of the body cells' susceptibility at the body surface and in all the tissues. After binding to the susceptible cell, the infective pathogen multiplies at the surface, for example, *Mycoplasma or Bordetella pertussis*, or enters the cell and infects it, for example, *viruses*.

Infective pathogens invade the body through different sites/portals of entry, namely, the skin, the conjunctiva, the respiratory tract, gastro-intestinal tract, the urinary-genital tract and the oropharynx.

⇨ **Skin**

Infective pathogens on the skin, other than residents of the normal flora, are inactivated by fatty acids, substances secreted by sebaceous and other glands, keratinocytes, and material produced by the normal flora. Bacterial pathogens enter the skin via hair follicles or sebaceous glands to cause sties and boils, or via teat canals to cause mastitis. Fungi (dermatophytes) infect the non-living keratinous structures (stratum cornea, nails, hair) produced by the skin. (The infection is established as long as the downward growth of the dermatophytes into the keratin exceeds the rate of shedding of the keratinous product. When the latter is very slow, as in the nails, the infection becomes chronic). Wounds, abrasions (even microscopic small) and burns are also portals of entry for especially virulent microbes, such as streptococci, Leptospira and *Hepatitis B-virus,* present at the site. Microbes, such as Leptospira and the larvae of Ancylostoma and Schistosoma (helminths), are able to traverse the unbroken skin via their own mechanisms.

Biting arthropods such as mosquitoes, ticks, fleas, and sand flies penetrate the skin during feeding and then introduce infectious agents into the body. The arthropod transmits the pathogen as an essential part of the lifecycle of the microbe; or mechanical via contaminated mouthparts without the pathogen multiplying in the arthropod; or the pathogen multiplies in the arthropod and appears in the saliva or faeces of the arthropod and is then transmitted (injected in, defecated on or scratched into the byte wound) during a blood feed.

⇨ **Conjunctiva**

The eye is kept clean by the continuous flushing action of tears aided by the windscreen viper action of the eyelids every few seconds. Infective pathogens (such as Chlamydia or gonococci) that infect the normal conjunctiva possess effective and efficient attachment mechanisms. Non-specialist microbes establish themselves in the conjunctiva when damage to the eyelid occurs, or there is a decrease in the lachrymal gland secretion, or there is interference with the local defenses. Contaminated hands and fingers often carry infectious material (for example, *Chlamydia trachomatis* that causes trachoma) to the conjunctiva.

⇨ **Respiratory tract**

Efficient cleansing mechanisms in the respiratory tract deal with the constantly inhaled suspended particles (smoke, dust) and airborne microbes. The inhaled microbes are entrapped in the respiratory mucus and carried by ciliary action to the back of the throat and are then swallowed. The microbes that invade the normal healthy respiratory tract have developed specific mechanisms to avoid this fate by either interfering with the cleansing mechanisms (by attaching firmly through adhesion molecules to the surfaces of cells forming the muco-ciliary sheet and/or inhibit the ciliary activity) or avoid destruction by alveolar macrophages (by avoiding phagocytosis or by avoiding destruction after phagocytosis had taken place, for example, *Mycobacterium tuberculosis humanis*). When damage to the alveolar macrophages occurs after inhaling toxic particles or certain dust, the susceptibility of the cells of the muco-ciliary sheet is greatly enhanced.

⇨ **Gastro–intestinal tract**

Apart from the general flow of the intestinal contents, no particular cleansing mechanisms exist in the alimentary tract. Under normal circumstances, the multiplication of the commensal flora of the intestinal tract is counterbalanced by their continuous passage to the exterior with the rest of the intestinal content. Infectious pathogens, on the other hand, must attach themselves by specific binding mechanisms to the intestinal epithelial cells and then avoid being carried straight down the alimentary tract to be excreted with the rest of the intestinal contents. The fact that pathogens such as the Shigella infect largely the colon or the Rotaviruses and Salmonellae the small bowel, indicates the presence of specific receptor molecules on the mucosal cells in these sections of the alimentary tract. These infective pathogens are also capable of surviving in the presence of acid, mucus, enzymes and bile by counteracting their defense mechanisms. The final pathogenicity of infective pathogens which penetrate the intestinal epithelium depends upon

- subsequent multiplication and spread
- toxin production
- cell damage
- the inflammatory and immune responses.

Microbial exotoxins, endotoxins and proteins are also absorbed from the intestine on a small scale. The intestinal lumen can, apart from taking up large molecules, also take up particles the size of viruses especially in certain sites where Peyer's

269

patches occur (isolated collections of lymphoid tissue lying immediately below the intestinal epithelium consisting of highly specialized mucus-cells. The mucus-cells take up particles and foreign proteins and deliver them to underlying immune cells with which they are intimately associated by cytoplasmic processes).

Crude mechanical devices are used by parasitic protozoa and worms for attachment in the intestines. Some worms such as *Giardia lamblia,* have specific molecules for adhesion to the microvillus of epithelial cells, but also possess its own microvillus sucking disks. Hookworms attach themselves to the intestinal mucosa by means of a large mouth capsule containing hooked teeth or cutting plates. Other worms, such as the Ascaris, maintain their position by "bracing themselves against peristalsis", while tapeworms adhere closely to the mucus covering the intestinal wall. The anterior hooks and sucker disks play a relatively minor role for the larger worms. Some worms, such as the Trichinella and Trichuris, actively penetrate the mucosa as adults or traverse the gut wall to enter deeper tissues.

⇨ **Urinary-genital tract**
The regular flushing action of urine is the major urethral defense and urine in the bladder is normally sterile. The wall of the bladder possesses intrinsic defense mechanisms that include a protective layer of mucus, the ability to stimulate/activate the acute inflammatory response, and the secretion of antibody and immune cells. The urinary-genital tract is a continuum resulting in the easy spread of microbes from one part of the tract to another. The urinary tract is nearly always invaded from the exterior via the urethra and the invading pathogens must first and foremost avoid being washed out during urination. Successful invaders have therefore developed special attachment mechanisms, such as the parasite-directed endocytosis whereby the pathogen binds with the urethral cell and then induce the cell to engulf it (the pathogen). The foreskin also enhances transmission in the sense that sexually transmitted pathogens often remain in the moist area beneath the foreskin after detumescence (when semen has been shed), giving the pathogens more opportunity to invade. Because the sexual anatomy of women is a major determinant of infection, intestinal bacteria (mainly *Escherichia coli or E.coli*) are common invaders of the urinary tract of women.

The vagina has no cleansing defense mechanisms and the repeated introductions of a contaminated and sometimes pathogen-bearing foreign object, the penis during coitus, makes the vagina particular vulnerable to infection, at the same time forming the basis for sexually transmitted diseases. During the reproductive life of women, the vagina is protected by additional defenses such as the vaginal pH of about 5.0 which inhibits colonization by all microbes except lactobacilli, certain streptococci and diptheroids. These defenses, however, diminishes with age and in the absence of estrogens the vagina becomes more vulnerable to infection.

⇨ **Oropharynx**
The flushing action of saliva is a natural cleansing mechanism aided by the masticator and other movements of the tongue, cheeks and lips. Material borne

backwards from the nasopharynx is firmly wiped against the pharynx by the tongue during swallowing, resulting in an opportunity for microbes to enter the body at this site. Factors that reduce mucosal resistance leading to the overgrowth of bacteria are, for example, gum infections caused by vitamin C deficiency; while Candida invasion is promoted by the changed resident flora after taking broad-spectrum antimicrobial drugs, as well as the salivary flow that decreases between meals and during dehydration. Many infective pathogens possess attaching mechanisms to attach themselves firmly to mucosal and tooth surfaces.

7.1.2 Defending of the body once penetration by invading pathogens has taken place – the commencement of the process of pathogenesis

As soon as a pathogen had penetrated a specific natural defense barrier of the body - either the skin or the respiratory tract or the alimentary tract or the urinary-genital tract - and has attached itself to the receptor cells of the body, the innate and the adaptive immunological defense systems are activated to defend the body against invasion of the body by the pathogen. When activated, the innate immunological defense system together with its backup mechanisms comes rapidly into play to defend the body as it offers the main resistance to microbial pathogens within the first minutes, hours or days of an infection. Although the defense mechanisms of the innate immunological system does not enable antibody as the adaptive immune system does, the defense mechanisms of the innate immune system are vital to the survival of the host due to the considerable specificity of the innate immune system to be able to discriminate not only between pathogens and self but as well as between classes of pathogens, and to mediate the acute inflammatory response. The adaptive immune system, on the other hand, comes only into play after a lapse of days or weeks when specific recognition of the antigens by lymphocyte T-cells and B-cells is enabled and immunity is elicited. The antibody mediated by immunocytes are of utmost importance in combating infections by extracellular pathogens, particularly pyogenic bacteria, while the T-cell-mediated immunity controls intracellular infections by bacteria, viruses, fungi and protozoa.

* **The innate immune system**
  ◈ **Phagocytes** - Phagocytes (macrophages in tissues and monocytes in blood) recognize invading pathogens and then engulf, kill off and digest it as first defense against parasitism. (See chapter 5 for the description of phagocytosis). Phagocytes kill off the pathogens using either an oxidative or a non-oxidative mechanism. Anaerobic pathogens are killed off by to a burst of oxygen consumption (respiratory burst) by the phagocytes accompanied by the activation of microbiocidal reactive oxygen intermediaries, such as super-oxide ions, hydrogen peroxide and free hydroxyl radicals that are extremely toxic to the pathogens because they damage the microbial cell membrane as well as its DNA and proteins while altering the pH to acidity. Cytotoxic lipids prolong the activity of the microbiocidal reactive oxygen intermediaries when interaction between microbiocidal reactive oxygen intermediaries and

serum lipoproteins take place to form stable lipid peroxides. Non-oxidative killing off involves the use of the phagocyte's cytotoxic granules, namely, myeloperoxidase; acid hydrolyses; cathepsins G, B, and D; defensins; cationic proteins; and lysozyme. Activated macrophages secrete nitric oxide that is also cytotoxic to a variety of cells, such as viruses and helminths

◇ **Natural Killer cells** - The activation of Natural Killer cells are a rapid but less specific means of controlling viral and other intracellular infections. Natural Killer cells differentiate from the common lymphoid progenitor generating B- and T-lymphocytes and mature in the bone marrow, lymph node, spleen, tonsils, and thymus from where it enters into the circulation. The activation of Natural Killer cells is determent by the balance of inhibitory and activating receptor stimulation which plays important function roles that include self tolerance and the sustaining of the cell activity of the Natural Killer cells as well as responding to interferon's or macrophage-derived cytokines. Natural Killer cells provide an early source of cytokines and chemokines during infection until activation of and proliferation of antigen-specific T-cells takes place. Natural Killer cells also provide an important source of interferon-gamma during the first days of an infection. The cytokine production of Natural Killer cells is induced by monokines which in turn is induced by macrophages in response to microbial components. Natural Killer cells, by producing cytolytic/ cytotoxic granules and perforin, also act as cytotoxic effector cells mediating cytolytic apoptosis of host cells when these cells are infected with viruses and bacteria and cell lysis of the virus or bacterium as Natural Killer cells secrete antimicrobial agents. Natural Killer cells also play a role in the adaptive immune response because of their ability to readily adjust to the immediate environment and mediating antigen-specific immunological memory. Persons deficient in Natural Killer cells are highly susceptible to early phases of herpes virus infection

◇ **Complement** - The activation of the complement system induces the acute inflammatory response while chemotaxis, phagocytosis and vascular permeability are enhanced. Activation of the complement system occurs via the alternative complement pathway; via the mast cell-directed pathway, via the fibrinolytic and anticoagulant pathways, via the collectin mannan-binding lectin pathway or lectin-complement pathway; via the classic pathway (when the antibody-mediated response, especially antibody IgA, has taken place); and via the lipopolysaccharides-pathway (endotoxins). In this way the acute inflammatory response and the rate of phagocytosis are greatly enhanced and prolonged

◇ **Acute phase proteins** - Acute phase proteins, such as lectins (also called collectins), ficolins, C-reactive proteins, complement factors, ferritin, ceruloplasmin, serum amyloid A and haptoglobin, are antimicrobial reactins that destroy or inhibit the growth of microbes and are produced by liver cells within 24 hours in response to cytokines, particularly interleukin-6, with subsequent activation of both complement and phagocytosis. Because acute phase proteins are produced in increasing amounts early in infection, they also act as opsonins and as antiproteases, over and above, as antimicrobial agent. Acute phase proteins also play an immuno-modulator role, and are also involved in the fibrinolytic and anticoagulant pathways in the activation of the complement system. Collectins are specific acute phase proteins that consist of (A) a collagen-like domain, namely, a set of pattern-recognition receptors for recognition of the specific class of the micro-organism when binding to the conserved pathogen-associated molecular patterns of the microbe and (B) a carbohydrate-recognition domain, namely, receptors for recognition of oligosaccharide/carbohydrate (sugar, glucose, mannose) molecules/ structures or lipids expressed on viral, bacterial (gram-positive and gram-negative), parasites, mycobacterial and fungal surfaces membranes. When binding to the oligosaccharides/carbohydrates on the membrane takes place, activation of the complement cascade via the lectin-complement pathway is induced as well as the enhancement of phagocytosis by macrophages. The mannose-binding lectin/mannan-binding lectin, a specific soluble C-type lectin, activates the complement cascade in an antibody-independent way through the mannose-binding lectin pathway/mannan-binding pathway when binding takes place of the carbohydrate recognition heads/domains on the mannose-binding lectin to specifically arranged cell-surface sugar/mannose residues expressed on the pathogen

◈ **Other extracellular antimicrobial factors** - Many other extracellular microbial agents/factors such as lysozyme that operate at short range within the phagocytic cells and which also appear in various body fluids in sufficient concentrations have direct inhibitory effects on the infecting pathogen. Similarly, lactoferrin appears in the blood in sufficient concentration to complex iron and deprive bacteria of this important growth factor

◈ **Pattern recognition surface receptors** - Many complement components are acute phase proteins and those that play a role in the protection against infection are termed "pattern recognition receptors" (such as the mannose-binding lectin and lipopolysaccharides binding protein) as they reduce pathogenesis by binding with toxic bacterial products. Another family of surface receptors, the Toll-like receptors on macrophages and other cells, bind with conserved microbial molecules such as endotoxin, bacterial DNA, double-stranded RNA and bacterial flagellum. Pattern recognition receptors recognize the repeated structures of pathogens followed by the release of pro-inflammatory cytokines such as interleukin-1 and interleukin-7. Signaling through the Toll-like receptors also leads to the increased expression of major histocompatibility complex (MHC) molecules and of co-stimulatory molecules, whereby the antigen presentation is enhanced, together with the stimulation of T-helper cells (T_H1)

◇ **Elevated body temperature (Fever)** - A raised body temperature almost invariably accompanies infection when cytokines, such as interleukin-1 or interleukin-6, are released. Fever, an abnormal elevation of the body temperature, is a protective response of the host and is produced in response to an exogenous pyrogen such as the endotoxin in the cell walls of Gram-negative pathogens, and/or the endogenous pyrogen such as interleukin-1 released by phagocytic cells. The homeostatic mechanisms of the body maintain a constant body temperature with daily fluctuations not exceeding 1-1.5°C (circadian temperature rhythm) and individuals vary in their body temperature – as low as 36°C to as high as 38°C. When feverish, the oral temperature is higher than 37.6°C while the rectal temperature is higher than 38°C. Fever, *per se*, enhances the activity level of the immune systems of the host, for example, the activation of the complement, the proliferation of lymphocyte and the synthesis of proteins such as antibody and cytokines. At the same time heat sensitive pathogens are killed off

A fever can be continuous or intermittent – when continuous fever occurs the body temperature is elevated over the whole 24-hour period and swing less than 1°C, (for example, in typhoid and typhus fever), while when an intermittent fever occurs, the body temperature is elevated above the normal throughout the 24-hour period but swings more than 1°C during that time (as in pyogenic infections, abscesses, and tuberculosis). Always bear in mind that significant infection(s) may be present in the absence of fever, as in serious ill neonates, in the elderly, in persons suffering from uremia, in persons taking corticosteroids, and in persons continuously taking antipyretic drugs. Other signs and symptoms of infection have now to be sought

◇ **Cytokines** - Cytokines are a family of non-antigen-specific molecules with diverse activities that are involved in cell-to-cell communication. Cytokines contribute to the control of infection as well as to the development of pathology. The beneficial effects of cytokines are directly and indirectly attributed to their induction of some antimicrobial processes through producing interferon within 24 hours after infection had taken place. An antiviral state is also induced resulting in the inhibition of viral RNA translation and hence protein synthesis. Unlike cytotoxic T-cells, interferon does not damage the cells when inducing the antiviral state. Cytokines are also active against a wide range of pathogens such as rickettsiae, mycobacterium and protozoa. Certain cytokines such as TNFα, on the other hand, enhance the replication of certain viruses, such as the *HIV-virus* in T-cells, and also contribute to the pathogenesis of malaria.

✳ **The adaptive immune system**
  ❖ **Antibody-mediated immunity**
    The primarily function of the antibody molecule is to bind specifically to antigens (proteins) on the foreign/infective pathogen. This binding is followed by secondary binding to other cells or molecules of the immune system such

as phagocytes and complement. The effectiveness of the antibody response is influenced by the following features

→ *Speed, amount and duration*
Because of the cell interactions involved and the need for proliferation of a small number of specific precursor lymphocytes to first take place, the primary antibody response takes dangerously slow in reaching protective levels. Thus, a race exists between bacterial multiplication and antibody production, with one side winning dramatically. The rate of replication (doubling time of viruses and bacteria lasting from one hour to days to weeks) plays an important role in this race in the sense that, when the incubation period is only a few hours/days (for example, rhinoviruses, rotaviruses, cholera), the antibody response is too slow to affect the initial outcome. In these instances, the rapidly produced cytokines, such as interferon, are of far more importance in combating the infection. Because the antibody response continues as long as the antigen is present in the body, (although down regulating occurs in prolonged responses in an effort to limit immuno-pathology), lifelong immunity results from either regular boosting by viruses and other bacteria still circulating in the community, or from the non-specific stimulation of memory B-cells and T-cells by cytokines during responses to other antigens (bystander activation)

→ *Affinity*
Antigen-binding affinity is determined by the germ-line antibody pool and the somatic mutation in individual B-lymphocytes – both being under genetic control. A high antigen-binding affinity renders the antibody more useful, while a tendency towards a low affinity antibody predisposes the individual to immune complex diseases

→ *Antibody classes and iso-types (sub-classes)*
The different backbone portions of the antibody molecule are responsible for most of the differentiations in the functioning of the different classes of antibody. By switching from one portion to another portion while preserving the same recognition portion, the immune system is allowed to 'try out' effector mechanisms against the pathogenic invader. This flexibility is not total because T-cell-independent antigens only induce IgM antibody, while T-cells are required to make the switch between IgG, IgA, and IgE. The IgG–responses alternated between IgG1 (anti-protein for viruses); IgG2 (anti-polysaccharide for bacteria); IgG3 (viruses); and IgG4 together with IgE for helminths. IgA on the other hand, is mainly induced by antigens that reach the digestive tract, as IgA is the only type of antibody that can function in this protease-rich intestinal environment. The preferences of the antibody to adhere to specific antigens are greatly regulated by the T-cells and cytokines

➔ *Blocking and neutralizing effects of antibody*

The mechanism of mere binding to a microbial surface by antibody molecules, results in the physical interference with the receptor interaction whereby the entry of the pathogen into the cell is blocked and the binding of a toxin to its host receptor is prevented. This mechanism of binding is sufficient to protect the host as the blocking of attachment and entry is effective against all viral, bacterial and protozoan pathogens that use specific attachment sites. The exception is those pathogens that parasitize the macrophage (for example, the virus of Dengue fever) where the presence of a low concentration of IgG actually enhances the infection by promoting the attachment to the back bone receptors. The interference with the essential surface components of the pathogen, particular if the surface components are enzymes or transport molecules is a more subtle blocking effect of antibody

➔ *Immobilization and agglutination*

The large pentameric IgM, an immunoglobulin antibody of the same size as the smaller viruses and larger than the thickness of a bacterial flagellum, is able to considerably restrict the activities of motile microbes through physical attachment of the antibody to the pathogen. The multivalent design of the antibody molecule enables it to link (agglutinate) two or more pathogens together. Once clumped, most pathogens are probably rapidly phagocytosed, although clumps of still motile trypanosomes can be seen in blood in the presence of enough serum antibodies

➔ *Lysis*

Lysis (suicide of the cell) of bacteria in the presence of complement provides a convenient reason for the presence of antibody. As such, lysis plays a major protective role in only a restricted range of infections caused by some viruses and Neisseria

➔ *Opsonization*

Opsonization/opsonisation is the process whereby pathogens are coated with the substance opsonin marking the pathogen out for phagocytosis (ingestion and destruction). After binding of opsonin to the cell membrane of the pathogen had taken place, phagocytes are attracted to the pathogen. Opsonization is the most important overall function of the antibody molecule by which it directs the binding of the CH2 and CH3 regions of the immunoglobulin to receptors on the cell membrane of the pathogen and whereby it, via the classical complement pathway, activates the complement allowing C3b to bind to its receptor on the phagocytic cells. When antibody and complement act together, the rate of phagocytosis is increased up to a thousand-fold. The effectiveness of opsonization also depends on the phagocytic cell being capable of finishing off (killing off) the indigested pathogen.

Effective opsonization *per se*, cannot take place with pathogens that inhibit or avoid the normal intracellular killing processes, such as the mycobacterium

- *Antibody-dependant cellular/cell-mediated cytotoxicity*
  As phagocytosis of macro-parasites such as helminths, is not possible, several types of cells (conventional phagocytes, eosinophils and platelet) make contact with the parasite through antibody and backbone receptors and inflict damage extracellular

Note

The presence of antibody by no means denotes a protective role under all circumstances. Antibody may be directed against irrelevant or non-critical microbial antigens or the infection may be of a type that it is not controlled by antibody, such as intracellular infections caused by *Mycobacterium tuberculosis, Salmonella typhoid, Herpes–virus*. The precise way in which antibody protects against infection is, in the majority of cases, still unknown

- **Cell-mediated immunity**
  T-cells, the second main component of the adaptive immune response, act not only by producing cytokines that induce the activation of macrophages, but also help with antibody production as well as by directing their cytotoxic action on infected intracellular target cells (viruses and other intracellular bacteria). Before acting, T-cells need to recognize or "see" by its receptor, being the combination of the specific peptide and the major histocompatibility complex molecule. The cytotoxic T-lymphocytes (CD8-positive T-cells) not only recognized the pathogen via involving an antigenic fragment that becomes associated with a specific major histocompatibility complex molecule, but also kill off the infected cell by inserting perforin into the cell which causes leaks in the cell and by inducing apoptosis. Although the lysis of the infected cell does not always kill off the intracellular pathogen, the cell lysis releases the microbe from its hideaway – leading thus to phagocytosis and killing off by a more highly activated macrophage. The cytotoxicity of T-cells can also be mediated by CD4-T-cells and by $\gamma\delta$-T-cells.

Note

In the early stages of infection, the adaptive immune system, however, seems to appear somewhat very ineffective. Since the lymphocytes are only programmed to recognize the shapes of antigenic epitopes, they cannot distinguish between virulent pathogens and harmless microbes, nor can they "know" which type of immune reaction (antibody-mediated or cell-mediated) will be the most effective. Thus, it is likely that the majority of responses in any individual infection will be irrelevant to recovery, and the detection of antibody, cytokines or cytotoxic T-cells is no proof that the responses are doing what they should do. Often, one mechanism/response is responsible for recovery while another is responsible for resistance to re-infection (for example, cytotoxic T-cells and interferon in recovery and antibody in prevention of a second attack). In some infections, notably those by protozoa and helminths, there is still controversy as to which of the numerous responses that can be detected are useful, harmful or neutral

7.1.3 Survival of the pathogen and inducing an infection/disease in the host – the incubation and prodromal period

To survive as human parasites, microbes have developed survival strategies to host defenses, so as to replicate and spread in the body of the host. Parasite survival strategies take on as many forms as there are pathogens, but can be classified as (1) strategies to evade natural non-adaptive defenses, and (2) strategies to evade adaptive defenses, grounded in the immune component that is to be evaded and the selected means to achieve it. As a result, the pathogen is able to undergo a lengthy time period of growth and spread during the incubation period before being shed and transmitted to the next host, for example, as in hepatitis B-virus infection and in tuberculosis. Shedding of the microbe for just a few extra days after clinically recovery, gives more extensive transmission in the community – a worthwhile result for the pathogen.

❖ Strategies to evade natural non-adaptive defenses (innate defense mechanisms
   The strategies to evade natural non-adaptive defenses include the following
   ◈ killing off the phagocyte by antiphagocyte devices
   ◈ inhibiting the phagocyte by eluding contact or gaining protection against intracellular death allowing the pathogen to survive within the phagocyte
   ◈ interfering with the ciliary action of the cleansing mechanism
   ◈ interfering with the activation of the complement via the alternative pathway by preventing the insertion of the C5, C6 and C7 complex, or inhibiting complement activation, or enhancing the coating with non-complement fixing antibody such as IgA to avoid lysis
   ◈ producing its own powerful iron-binding protein molecules to overcome the limited availability of host's iron-binding protein such as transferrin for metabolism
   ◈ blocking alpha and beta interferon which are formed by the host's cells within 24 hours after infection, by producing molecules that block the action of interferon in cells or by being a poor inducer of interferon. Interferon gamma, an essential part of the adaptive immune response, is also affected.

❖ Strategies to evade adaptive defenses
   The strategies to evade adaptive defenses include the following
   ➤ By causing a rapid "hit-and-run" infection whereby the pathogen invades, multiplies and is shed within a few days before the adaptive immune defenses have had time to come into action. Infection of the body surfaces fall into this category.
   ➤ Concealment of antigens to elude the lymphocytes is another principal strategy. This is done by remaining inside the cell without the pathogen's antigen being displayed on the surface – the pathogen therefore cannot be recognized by specific antibody and T-cells. Persistent latent viruses, such as the *Herpes simplex-virus* in sensory cells behave in this way although when

reactivation occurs, re-exposure and boosting of the immune defenses is inevitable. Several viruses, such as the *HIV-virus* and corona viruses conceal themselves within macrophages and display their proteins "secretly" on the walls of intracellular vacuoles instead of at the cell surface and then replicate by budding into these vacuoles. When adeno-viral proteins (E19) combine with the major histocompatibility complex molecules, passage of the virus to the cell surface is prevented resulting in the non-recognition of the infected cell by the cytotoxic T-cells.

Another form of concealment is the colonizing of privileged sites such as the skin and the intestinal lumen, together with those sites that shed directly into external secretions, for example, the central nervous system; joints; testes; and placenta, where they (the microbe) are effectively out of the reach of circulating lymphocytes. The site, however, loses it privilege as soon the inflammatory response is induced and lymphocytes, monocytes and antibody are rapidly delivered to the site. The DNA of the host is the most privileged site to colonize (as done by retroviruses) and through reverse transcriptase the retroviral RNA becomes integrated into the DNA of the host cell. Once integrated and as long as no cell damage takes place and no viral products are expressed on the cell surface where it can be recognized by immune defenses, the virus enjoys total anonymity. Lastly, additional privileged sites can be created by infective pathogens themselves. A good example of antigen concealment in their own created privileged sites, are the hydatid cysts that develops in the liver, lungs and brain around growing colonies of the tapeworm, *Echinococcus granulosis* - in this way ensuring the survival of the worms even when the blood contains protective levels of antibody.

Mimicry or mimicking the host antigens is another form of concealment because the body is not able to recognize self/own antigens as foreign. Pathogens, such as the *group A beta-hemolytic streptococci* cross-reacts with human myocardium and antigen concealment can be obtained for a short period. (This cross-reaction underlies the development of rheumatic heart disease as the body mediate antibody against the cross-reacting determinant meromyosin). Mimicry, however, does not prevent the host from inducing an antimicrobial and auto-immune response. Certain microbes, one of which is the blood fluke Schistosoma (a type of worm), conceals themselves with a complete surface coat of host molecules such as host blood group glycolipids, host major histocompatibility complex molecules, and host immunoglobulin from the plasma, resulting in the virtually invisibility of the flukes to lymphocytes. By producing and displaying back bone-receptors on their surface, certain viruses and bacteria take up immunoglobulin whereby they are enabled to bind to immunoglobulin molecules of all specificities in an immunologically useless upside-down position - thus preventing the access of specific antibody or T-cells to the pathogen or the infected cell.

An alternative strategy used by pathogens is the induction of tolerization (*not eliciting* an immune response)

- in an infection during early embryonic life before the development of the immune system, antigens present such as the *rubella-virus*, *cytomegalovirus*, and *Treponema pallidum* [syphilis], are regarded as "self" (although the fetus does eventually produce IgM antibody later in life). And because T-cell-mediated responses also are seriously impaired, tolerance results

- by producing large quantities of microbial antigen or antigen-antibody complexes that circulate in the blood, immune tolerance to that specific antigen is induced
- by exploiting genetically "gaps" in the host's immune system, such as when the host makes a poor immune response to certain peptides
- by upsetting the balanced between antibody and T$_H$1 and T$_H$2 responses, the pathogen promotes its own survival because of ineffective T-cell responses.

➢ <u>Antigenic variation</u>

Antigenic variation occurs during the course of an infection in a given individual and during the spread of the pathogen through the host community. Antigenic variation is common when microbes pass through the host community as microbial survival is enhanced by long-living humans who are re-infected multiple times during their lifetime. Antigenic variation also commonly occurs in infections limited to the respiratory and intestinal epithelial where the incubation period is less than one (1) week, as the pathogen can infect, multiply and be shed before a significant secondary adaptive immune response is mediated. In systemic infections such as mumps, measles and typhoid fever, the incubation period is longer and the adaptive immune response has more opportunity to come into action and control the infection by the antigenic variant (strain) of the pathogen. At molecular level, antigenic variation takes place through mutation, recombination and gene switching. When an pathogen <u>mutates</u>, repeated mutations or "antigenic drift" in the gene coding machinery of the microbe occur, causing small antigenic changes that are sufficient to reduce the effectiveness of B-cell and T-cell memory build up in response to earlier infections. Mutations affecting the epitopes recognized by cytotoxic T-cells are the source of "escape mutants". During <u>recombination</u> a more extensive and sudden alterations in antigens take place when two different microbes exchange genetic material (genetic shift) with the result that a complete new strain of one of the two pathogens emerges. A classic example of genetic shift is the sudden recombining of strains of the *human influenza A-virus* with strains of the avian virus H5N1, resulting in a completely new strain of influenza A-virus brandishing a new hemagglutinin or neuraminidase of avian origin. This new human influenza A-virus gives rise to an influenza pandemic in humans, as the present world population has not previously experienced the new virus (for example, the influenza pandemic of 1918 and the threatening Bird flu and H1N1 [swine flu] pandemic of the 21st century). Note that mutations have already occurred in the avian influenza A-virus envelope as the antigenicity of the H5-surface antigen and H7-surface antigen had changed and a new antigenicity of H5- and H7-surface antigens have been isolated in the mucous of the throats of dogs that may result in dogs becoming a vector for the *avian influenza A-virus H5N1*. Mutations have also occurred in the swine influenza A-virus envelope as the antigenicity of the H1-surface antigen had changed to a new strain formed consisting of swine, avian and human antigens. Some microbe, such as the trypanosome, is able to switch genes as it carries genes for about 1000 quite distinct surface molecules (known as variant–specific glycoproteins) which cover almost the entire surface and are immunodominant. A sequence of unrelated infections at approximately weekly intervals results, as the trypanosome is able to switch from using one gene to using another. The gene switching enables the trypanosome to persist in the host while the immune system of the host constantly tries to catch up with the switching. The antibody response may trigger the trypanosome to gene switching. Gene switching may also occur in relapsing persistent infections, such as relapsing fever and brucellosis

➢ Immuno-suppression

Many viral infections cause a general temporary immuno-suppression in the infected host, giving the virus enough time to replicate, spread and to be shed before being eliminated. A lasting general immuno-suppression, on the other hand, results in detrimental effects as the host becomes more susceptible to other infections that cause damages (sometimes extensively) in the host. When immuno-suppressed, the host shows a depressed/compromised immune response not only to the antigens of the infecting pathogen (antigen-specific suppression), but also to antigens of unrelated other pathogens.

Immuno-suppression by microbes often involves the infection of the immune cells such as

- the T-cells (by *the HIV-virus, measles virus*)
- the B-cells (by the *Epstein-Barr-virus*)
- the macrophages (by *the HIV-virus*)
- the dendrite cells (by the *HIV-virus*)

The end result of this infection is impaired cell functioning, because cell division is blocked, the release of interleukin-2 or other cytokines are blocked, or the death of the cell is caused. The toxins released by pathogens act as powerful immuno-modulators as they are potent T-cell mitogens (super-antigens) acting as polyclonal activators of T-cells thereby upsetting the delicate balance of immune regulation, killing off T-cells and other immune cells, and diverging T-cells of all specificities into immunologically unproductive activity. Other successful pathogens interfere with the signaling between immune cells as well as with the signaling between the molecules of the essential components of the host defense (such as cytokines, chemokines, the major histocompatibility complex, the apoptotic and complement receptors) and with the signaling of the cytotoxic T-cell recognition – the net result is the suppression of the activation of the immune system. Some successful pathogens do not interfere with the development of the adaptive immune response but actively interfere with the local expression of the immune response in tissues. Microbes such as *Neisseria gonorrhoeae, Streptococcus pneumoniae* and strains of *Haemophilus influenzae* liberate a protease that cleaves IgA antibody while protein A from virulent staphylococci inhibits the phagocytosis of antibody-coated bacteria.

Certain viruses, such as the herpes-viruses and *Zoster-Varicella-virus*, code for molecules that act as backbone portion-receptors for IgG, while streptococci produce backbone portion-receptor for IgA.

It must always be taken in account that certain pathogens are able to remain (persist) in the host for many years, often for life. Persistence is worthwhile for the pathogen as shedding occurs during the persistence. Persistent pathogens fall into two categories, namely, (1) those that are shed more or less continuously, such as the *Epstein-Barr-virus* into the saliva; *Hepatitis B-virus* in blood; and eggs in faeces in various helminthic infections; and (2) those that are shed intermittently, such as *Herpes simplex-virus*, *polyoma-viruses*, *typhoid bacilli*, *Mycobacterium tuberculosis humanis* (tuberculosis bacilli) and malaria parasites. All persistent infections represent a failure of host defenses, as the defenses are designed to control microbial growth and spread and to eliminate the microbe/pathogen from the body. Pathogens, such *as Hepatitis B-virus* in the blood and the schistosoma in the blood vessels of the bladder/alimentary tract, persist in the body in a flagrantly defiant infectious form, while adenoviruses in the tonsils and adenoids persist in a form with low or partial infectivity

Viruses are particular good at thwarting immune defenses on the grounds of the following reasons
  * Viruses often invade tissues and cells "silently" as they do not form toxins in the way bacteria do. As long as the virus does not cause extensive cell destruction, and this sometimes does not happen for several weeks after infection has had occurred, there is no sign of illness until the onset of immune and inflammatory responses, for example, infection with *Hepatitis B-virus* infection
  * Viruses such as the *rubella virus*, *wart viruses* and *Hepatitis B-virus* can infect cells for long periods without adverse effects on cell viability

Based on the intimate molecular relationship that exists between the virus and the infected cell, latent virus infections can persist in the body in a completely non-infectious form. In virus latency, the virus, although present in the host cells, does not produce any antigens or infectious material, but as soon as reactivation occurs, production of antigens or infectious material starts. When viral activity in the infected cell is resumed, latent infections become patent (stage A of virus reactivation). Stage B of virus reactivation is the infecting of other cells, replication, spreading and shedding. Stage B of reactivation can be controlled by the immune system without symptom formation, but when not controlled because of a poor lymphocyte response, reactivation may progress to cause clinical disease.

7.1.4   The end result of the host-pathogen-battle Disease as manifested in the characteristic-specific clinical manifestation of the particular communicable infection

As soon as the state of "balanced pathogenicity" between host and pathogen is disrupted, disease/infection arises. The particular disease that arises is either a surface infection or a systemic infection. A variety of factors, among others temperature and site of budding, determine whether an infection is a surface infection or a systemic infection. Temperature-sensitive pathogens are restricted to certain surface body sites as they can only multiply/replicate efficient at a specific body temperature. Certain viruses are also restricted to the surfaces of the body as they can only bud there. Pathogens that fail to multiply and spread at the site of initial infection or portal of entry (the body surface) are obliged to spread systemically. For example, the *measles virus* replicates next to nothing at the initial site of infection, but after spreading systemically, large numbers of the measles virus are delivered back to the same surface [respiratory surface] where the virus replicate and sheds to the exterior. Other pathogens, for example, the *mumps virus and hepatitis A-virus*, must also spread systemically as they are committed to infection by one route only (mumps-virus via the respiratory route and hepatitis A-virus via the alimentary route), while major replication and shedding occurs at another site (the mumps-virus in the salivary glands and the hepatitis A-virus in the liver).

Essential to any surface infection is the rapid replication of the pathogen - a doubling rate of replication/multiplication of every 20 minutes to a few hours. "Hit-and-run" surface infections need to replicate/multiply rapidly and to be shed in large numbers. Local spread takes place readily on a fluid-covered mucosal surface and is often aided by the ciliary action of the respiratory tract, while movement of fluid spreads the infection to more distant areas on the surface as in the gastro-intestinal tract. In the upper respiratory tract, high winds, such as sneezing or coughing, can splatter the infectious agent onto new areas of mucosa or into the openings of sinuses or the middle ear resulting in sinusitis or otitis media, while the downward trickle of mucous during sleep seeds the pathogen into the lower respiratory tract. As a result, large areas of the body surface can be involved within a few days with shedding to the exterior. Infections restricted to the body surfaces, for example, the common cold, have a very short incubation period. Only the innate immunological response is mediated as there is not enough time to activate the adaptive immunological system. To control the infection, the body relies on non-adaptive responses such as phagocytosis, interferon, and Natural Killer cells. Hence, re-infections occur most of the time.

When a pathogen divides every few days, a systemic infection/disease evolves slowly with a long incubation period. A systemic infection invades the body tissues in a stepwise way, from the site/portal of entry to the lymph and then to the blood. By multiplying locally or in lymph nodes and by evading phagocytosis, a great deal of inflammation is caused by the pathogen. In the early stages of infection, the lymph flow is increased but eventually when enough inflammation and tissue damage had taken place in the lymph node itself, the flow of lymph ceases. Viruses and intracellular pathogens, in contrast, silently and asymptomatically invade the lymph and blood during the incubation period by infecting the monocytes and lymphocytes without initially damaging them. Once in the bloodstream, the fate of the microbes depends on whether they are free circulating pathogens or associated with circulating cells, namely,

◇ when free circulating and in small numbers, the pathogens are usually quickly filtered out and destroyed by macrophages lining the liver and spleen sinusoids. A transient bacteraemia may develop, giving the bacteria the opportunity to localize in less well-defined sites, such as the heart and growing end of long bones

◇ when present in circulating cells such as the monocytes and lymphocytes, the monocytes and lymphocytes protect the pathogens from the host defences and carry them around in the body, from where the pathogens localize and invade body structures and organs - for example, malaria protozoa enters the erythrocytes; some viruses invade the platelets; some pathogens spread to adjacent hepatic cells in the liver (such as the *measles virus*); while others re-invade the blood (like the *Salmonella typhi* and *hepatitis virus*).

When the uptake of pathogens by the reticulo-endothelial system is not complete within a very short time or if large numbers of pathogens are in the blood, localization elsewhere in the vascular system takes place. Each circulating pathogen <u>invades a specific target organ</u> due to

◇ the presence of specific receptors for that particular infectious pathogen on the vascular endothelium of the target organ, or

◇ the accumulation of the particular circulating pathogen in sites where there is local inflammation as the blood flow there is slow and the endothelium in the inflamed vessels is sticky, or

◇ suitability of the specific pathogen to colonize and replicate in that particular organ only, regardless of the random localization of the pathogen throughout the body After localization and invasion of the specific organ, the pathogen replicates and is then shed from the body to the exterior if the organ has a surface with access to the outer world, or if not, the pathogen is shed directly back into the bloodstream or shed via the lymphatic system into the bloodstream.

Other mechanisms of spread through the body are via the nerves, via the cerebrospinal fluid and via other routes. Certain viruses such as the *Poliomyelitis-virus*, *Rabies-virus*, *Herpes simplex-virus*, and *Varicella-zoster-virus* as well as tetanus toxin, spreads via the axons of peripheral nerves from peripheral parts of the body to the central nerves system and vice versa. Few, if any, host defences are in a position to control this type of viral spread once nerves are invaded. These pathogens, once localized in the nervous system, are not shed to the exterior after multiplying in the meninges or spinal cord. Viruses and bacteria in the nasopharynx are spread to the central nervous system via the blood or via the olfactory nerve with axons terminating in the olfactory mucosa (for example, free living amoeba in fresh water pools causing meningo-encephalitis in swimmers). Pathogens that have crossed the blood-cerebro-spinal barrier spread rapidly in the cerebrospinal fluid spaces infecting ependymal and meningeal cells. Pathogens such as bacteria spread easily from one visceral organ to another resulting in peritonitis if the omentum is injured or diseased (the peritoneal cavity is lined by macrophages and also contains an antimicrobial armoury consisting of the omentum, lymphocytes, macrophages and mast cells). When the chest cavity is injured or diseased, pathogens spread easily, leading to lung infections or pleurisy.

An infection/a disease are fundamentally determined by genetic factors situated in both the host and in the pathogen. Some of the genetic determinants in the pathogen that influence the spread and replication are pathogenicity (mutation may lead to a reduced/increased/changed ability of the pathogenic microbe to cause infection) and the gene coding for virulence of the pathogen that are involved during different stages of pathogenesis (virulence factors such as adhesion, penetration into cells, anti-phagocytic activity, production of toxins and interaction with the immune system, are coded by different genes and gene products). The genetic determinants in the host are the genetic constitution of the host and the influence the brain wields on the immune response. The ability of a pathogen to infect and cause disease in a host is influenced by the genetic constitution of the given individual in so far that susceptibility to infection depends on the immune responses the individual mediate. A poor response to a given infection leads to increased susceptibility to infection/disease, whereas an immune response that is too vigorous, leads to immuno-pathological diseases. The brain, acting via the hypothalamus, pituitary and adrenal cortex, influence the immune responses in so far that, when a shortage or an excess of glucocorticoids (a hormone that has powerful actions on immune cells and is needed for resistance to infection and trauma) exists, the shortage or the excess results in an increased susceptibility to infection. The brain, the endocrine and the immune systems also use the same molecular messengers – cytokines, peptide hormones and neural-transmitters; while neural cells have receptors for interferon and interleukins; and the thymic lymphocytes produce prolactin and growth hormones (the immune-neuron-endocrine crosstalk – the basis of the influence of the brain on immunity and infectious disease). Other host factors that influence the susceptibility of a given individual to infectious diseases are pregnancy (hepatitis viruses, urinary infections); malnutrition (*measles virus*); age (respiratory infections, re-activation of the *Varicella-zoster-virus*, *Epstein-Barr-virus* infection); atmospheric pollution (silicoses, raised sulphur dioxide levels); foreign bodies (necrotic bone fragments and tissue); hormones and stress.

7.1.5 The resolution of the infection – the recovery stage

After being ill for days, weeks or even months, the ill persons recovers from the particular communicable disease. The adaptive immune responses mediated by antibody and T-cells, are responsible for the recovery from the infection, although these mechanisms take days to weeks to reach peak efficiency. In common viral infections, cell-mediated immunity is responsible for recovery from infection and antibody for the maintenance of immunity. In some cases, the ill person is subsequently immune to the disease, while in other cases he/she can be infected again and then becomes ill again (for example, sexually transmitted infections). When a person recovers, it can fairly be stated that the lymphocytes of the adaptive (specific) physiological-immunological response have been activated because

- the existence of signs and symptoms of infection implies that the natural defenses barriers had been penetrated by a specific pathogen and the innate immunological defense mechanisms that acts rapidly, did not succeed to eliminate the pathogen
- a period of days or weeks is typical of the time period that the adaptive immune mechanisms take to reach their maximum peak levels of efficiency

- subsequent immunity is a sign of the immunological memory exclusive to lymphocytes that are able to specifically recognize antigens and to proliferate into clones and survive as memory cells, thereby protecting and allowing the host to progressively adapt to infectious pathogens in the environment. The older an individual is, the better he/she is to adapt to the environment – until old age begins to weaken the individual's immune system

The reason for an individual's failure to recover from an infection is not easy to pinpoint. When the infection is one from which most individuals recover (for example, Measles, Mumps) or from which humans do not suffer at all (for example, Pneumocystitis), an immunological deficiency must be considered. When infections are rapidly fatal in normal individuals (for example, Lassa fever, Bird flu), these infections are frequently those to which the human immune system has not been exposed before, since the infections are normally maintained in animals (zoonotic diseases) and only accidentally infect human beings. When the infection runs a prolonged course without being eliminated or when the host (the ill person) dies, the pathogen can be considered extremely successful due to one or more survival strategies.

7.2 THE NON-SPECIFIC LOCAL AND SYSTEMIC CLINICAL MANIFESTATION OF AN INFECTION

The signs and symptoms (non-specific and characteristic-specific clinical manifestation) of infection or disease are produced by either the specific pathogen or by the host's immune responses. Signs and symptoms that appear rapidly after acquisition of an infection are usually due to the direct action of the invading pathogen or its secretions. Bacteria provoke most of their acute effects (signs) by causing tissue injury and/or releasing toxins while virulent bacteria, such as staphylococci, can inhibit the acute inflammatory response to some extent. Viruses in cells, on the other hand, cause metabolic "shut down" or lysis of the cells. Also, pathogens do not always produce the same disease/infection in all infected individuals. The biological response gradient causes a spectrum that range from asymptomatic to mild to serious to fatal leading to the death of the infected individual.

In reaction to the invasion of the body by pathogens, the innate defence mechanism of the body mediates the acute inflammatory response propagating inflammation - locally at the portal of entry on the body surface or systemically when internal organs are infected. As expression of the innate immunological system, the acute inflammatory response is a non-specific stereotyped complex biological response of short duration that is usually induced within minutes or hours after invasion of body cells by pathogens had occurred or cell damage had taken place and ceases upon removal of the harmful or injurious stimulus. The classical signs of acute inflammation are heat, pain, redness, swelling and loss of function. Because the innate and the adaptive immune systems always act in close synergy/integration with one another, the adaptive immune responses are also activated when the acute inflammatory response is mediated on contact with the invading pathogen. In chronic and persistent infectious diseases, however, the pathological changes are often secondary to the activation of the immunological mechanisms that are normally thought of as only protective as both the innate and the adaptive immune systems can mediate these pathological changes - the tissue damage mediated by the adaptive immune responses always cause "immuno-pathology".

7.2.1 Non-specific signs and symptoms produced by pathogens

The signs and symptoms elicited by infective pathogens can be classified according the pathology induced at the local site of entry and the systemic pathology induced by the activity of the secretions produced by the pathogen (see figure 7.2 - The local and systemic inflammatory reaction).

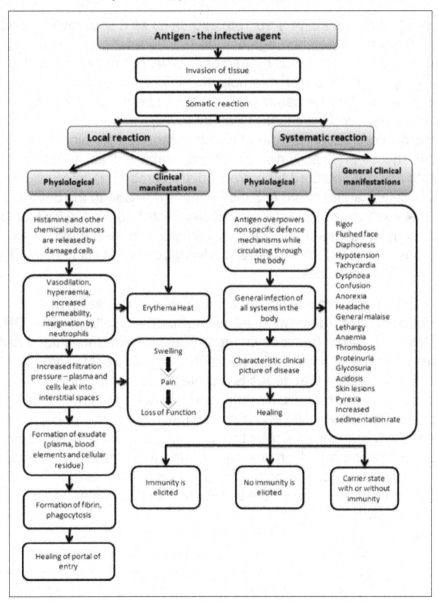

Figure 7.2 Schematic representation of the course of the acute inflammatory response and the accompanying clinical manifestations

The tissue damage directly caused by the pathogen is the result of cell rupture, organ blockage or pressure effects. Many viruses, some intracellular bacteria and protozoa multiply in the cells and usually spread by rupturing the cells. Other pathogens, such as certain viruses and bacteria, do not spread this way but remain latent in the body - for example, *Herpes simplex-virus* and *Varicella-zoster-virus* in nerve ganglia and *Mycobacterium tuberculosis humanis* {TB} in macrophages - while certain viruses will bud from a cell without disrupting it. The type of cell that has been infected may also help with the survival of the pathogen, for example, *Human immunodeficiency-virus* (HIV-virus) lysis T-cells but persists (remains alive) in macrophages. Blockage of normal hollow viscera (for example, worms); blockage of lung alveoli by dense growth (for example, Pneumocystis); and the mechanical pressure effects of large cysts (for example, Hydatid) are other direct effects.

Many bacterial pathogens actively secrete exotoxins as it strategy for entry into and spread in the body or as defence against the host's defences. Most exotoxins are proteins and are often coded not by bacterial DNA but in plasmids (for example, *Escherichia coli*) or phages (for example, *clostridia botulinum* causing botulism, *Corynebacterium diphtheriae* causing diphtheria, *streptococcus pyogenes (group A β-haemolytic streptococcus* causing Scarlet fever). In some cases the exotoxins consist of two or more subunits, one of which is required for binding and entry into the cell, while the other[s] activates or inhibits some cellular function. The most powerful exotoxins are secreted by extracellular microbes as intracellular microbes that multiply in cells, cannot afford to cause serious damage to the cells at a too early stage. Thus, exotoxins secreted by intracellular microbes tend to be less prominent and of lower concentrations in intracellular infections, for example, *Mycobacterium tuberculosis humanis* (TB); *Chlamydia* and *Mycoplasma*, resulting in the dysfunction of immune and phagocytic cells.

The mode of action of exotoxins and its consequences are as follows
   ❖ by producing enzymes, such as hyaluronidase, collagenase, DNase, and streptokinase, which break down the tissues or the intracellular substances of the cells of the host, allowing the infection to spread freely. Some staphylococci release a coagulase that deposits a protective layer of fibrin onto and around the host cells – thus localizing them and promoting their survival
   ❖ by producing haemolysins such as lecithinase or phospholipase that enzymatically damages the membrane of host cells or by inserting pore-forming molecules into the cell which destroy the integrity of the cell. Both staphylococci and streptococci produce pore-forming toxins while pseudomonads release haemolysins. (Please take note that many other cells than red blood cells can be affected by haemolysins)
   ❖ by entering the host cell and actively alter some of the metabolic machinery, for example, toxin of diphtheria and cholera. These toxins characteristically have two subunits A and B. The subunit-A is the active component while the subunit-B is the binding component that is needed to interact with receptors on the surface of the cell membrane. When binding occurs the subunit-A or

the whole toxin-receptor complex is taken into the cell by endocytosis and the subunit-A becomes active

❖ by blocking the protein synthesis of host cells. For example, the diphtheria toxin is synthesized as a single polypeptide that is partially cleaved. When the subunit-B binds with the receptors of the target cell, the entire toxin-receptor complex is internalized. The subunit-A now splits off and enter the cytosol where it inactivates the transfer of amino acids transferring RNA to the polypeptide chain during the translation of mRNA by ribosome. This inactivation effectively blocks the protein synthesis of the cell

❖ by preventing the regulatory mechanism of a cell to turn off production, resulting in massive loss of water. The subunit-A of the exotoxins of *Vibrio cholerae*, *Escherichia coli*, *Salmonellae typhoid and para-typhoid*, and *Bordetella pertussis* is cleaved into fragments A1 and A2 and held together by disulfide bonds. After endocytosis has taken place the two fragments separate from one another. The A1-fragment then ribosylates one of the regulatory molecules involved in the production of cyclic adenosine monophosphate resulting in the inability of the cell to turn off production. The increased levels of cyclic adenosine monophosphate in the cell change the sodium-chloride (Na^+)-(Cl^-) flux across the cell membrane leading to a massive outflow of water and electrolytes from the cell. In the intestinal tract profuse diarrhoea is caused while in pertussis a watery sputum is coughed up

❖ by interfering with the synaptic transmission of neurotransmitter release. The subunit-A exotoxin of *Clostridia tetanus* (the subunit-B binds with ganglioside receptors on nerve cells) is carried by axonal transport from the point of production to the central nervous system where it interferes with the synaptic transmission of the inhibitory neurones by blocking neurotransmitter release. This allows the excitatory transmitter to continuously stimulate the motor neurones causing spastic paralysis. The exotoxin of *clostridia botulinum* enters the body via the intestinal tract, escapes digestion and then crosses the gut wall from where it is transported to peripheral nerve endings. At the neuron-muscular junction, it blocks the release of acetylcholine, preventing the muscle to contract – resulting in flaccid paralysis.

Endotoxins, on the other hand, are typically lipopolysaccharides and are integral parts of the microbial cell wall of most Gram-negative bacteria and are normally released only when the cell dies. Endotoxins are compose of a lipid portion inserted in the cell wall which is responsible for much of the toxic activity; a conserved core polysaccharide and a highly variable O-polysaccharide that is responsible for the serologic diversity of certain microbes such as Salmonellae and Shigellae. Microbial endotoxins activate the immune system and induce cytokines (especially interleukin-1), causing a bewildering variety of biological effects such as fever, hypotension and vascular collapse, disseminated intravascular coagulation leading to thrombosis, hypoglycaemia and bacterial septicaemia (septic shock). Endotoxin bacterial septicaemia (septic shock) is usually associated with the systemic spread of Gram-negative microbes in the body although exotoxins such as the pyrogenic (erythrogenic) exotoxins that are released by streptococcal bacteria can also cause bacterial septicaemia (septic shock)

7.2.1.1 Clinical signs and symptoms manifested at the local portal of entry

As already described, the acute inflammatory response propagating inflammation is mediated by the innate defence mechanism of the body in reaction to the invasion of the body by pathogens - locally at the portal of entry on the body surface or systemically when internal organs are infected. The acute inflammatory response, as expression of the non-specific innate immunological system, is from its very nature a stereotyped complex biological response of short duration that is mediated within minutes or hours after invasion of body cells by pathogens had occurred or cell damage had taken place and ceases upon removal of the harmful or injurious stimulus. As such, the acute inflammatory response is an essential, tightly regulated and controlled innate protective mechanism of local response to invasion by microbes or to local tissue damages. During the acute inflammatory response a lethal micro-environment is created by the increased movement of plasma and leukocytes (especially granulocytes) from the blood into the injured/infected tissues as to localize and kill off the specific pathogen and to initiate the healing process. The acute inflammatory response always propagates inflammation because inflammation is part of the complex biological response of vascular tissues to any harmful stimuli such as invading pathogens or damaged cells. Acute inflammation, *per se*, is the stereotyped initial biochemical and cellular response that only occurs in vascularised tissue when cell injury or cell invasion or cell death is caused by any harmful stimulus (such as microbial pathogens) and is as such not a synonym for infection. Acute inflammation is not only propagated locally at the portal of entry but also systemically when internal body organs are involved and is mediated by a cascade of biomedical events that furthers and matures the acute inflammatory response which involve the vascular system, the immune system and various cells within the injured/infected tissue self. The cardinal signs of acute inflammation on the body surface are redness (rubor); heat (calor); swelling (tumor); pain (dolor), and loss of function (function laesa), whereas the acute inflammation of internal organs may not result in the full set of cardinal signs (for example, pain can only be felt where the appropriate sensory nerve endings exist in the inflamed area). Note that prolonged inflammation (also known as chronic inflammation), on the other hand, leads to a progressive shift in the type of cells present in the site of inflammation mediating a host of diseases and is characterized by simultaneous destruction and healing of the tissue from the inflammatory process.

In summary it can be said that the process of capillary dilatation, extravasation of plasma proteins and fluid due to hydrostatic and osmotic pressure changes and the accumulation of neutrophils is collectively termed the "acute inflammatory response". The acute inflammatory response is an important innate protection mechanism of the host as vascular permeability is vital for the rapid mobilization of cells such as neutrophils and serum components like complement and antibody. Inflammation, as such, is therefore intrinsically a healthy sign as it is part of the complex biological response of vascular tissue to kill off pathogens so that healing can take place (see figure 7.3). The acute inflammatory response results in a highly effective way of directing and focusing phagocytic cells onto complement-coated pathogenic targets. The local inflammation at the portal/site of entry is manifested as **pain, heat, swelling and loss of function** due to the mediating of haemo-dynamic and cellular changes, phagocytosis and the formation of the inflammatory exudate. Systemic inflammation on the other hand, affects all the organs of the body and manifests as a general infection characterised by pyrexia, heightened metabolic functioning, haematological and cardiovascular changes, and impairment of renal, liver and brain functions. (See Theme IV for the full description of the specific clinical manifestation of specific communicable diseases).

The physiological course of the acute inflammatory response can be divided in different phases, namely, activation of the acute inflammatory response (reaction to invasion), vascular phase, exudative phase, and resolution. Furthermore, the acute inflammatory response requires constant stimulation to be sustained because inflammatory mediators have short half lives and are quickly degraded in tissue. Hence, the acute inflammatory response ceases once the invading pathogen has been killed off. Also, the working/actions/mediations of the inflammatory mediators are responsible for the clinical signs of inflammation, namely, **redness and heat** due to <u>vasodilation and its resulting increased blood flow</u>. The increased permeability of the blood vessels induces an <u>exudation (leakage) of plasma proteins and fluid</u> into the tissue which manifests itself as **swelling**. Some <u>released mediators such as bradykinin</u> increases sensitivity to **pain** while the **loss of function** can be <u>attributed to a neurological reflex to pain</u>.

- ❖ **Activation of the acute inflammatory response (reaction to invasion)**
  In response to the invasion of body cells by pathogens, the acute inflammatory response is initiated by specific cells present in all body tissues such as resident macrophages, dendritic cells, histiocytes, Kupffer cells and mastocytes. Because these cells present with pattern recognition receptors on their surfaces, they are able to recognize pathogens as foreign to the host molecules/cells. Following this recognition, these cells immediately become activated and start to release cell-derived inflammatory mediators such as Interleukin-1 and Interleukin-6 and lysosomal products whereby the processes and course of the acute inflammatory response is set in motion.

- ❖ **Vascular phase**
  In response to the cell-derived inflammatory mediators, vascular and haemodynamic changes take place whereby the capillary hydrostatic pressure increases; blood vessels in the vicinity of the tissue(s) infiltrated by the pathogen, temporary constrict and then dilate and become leaky/permeable allowing plasma to escape into the tissue inducing the colloid osmotic pressure to increase in the extra vascular space while blood cells are retained in the vessels. Due to the initial transient process of arteriolar constriction, blood stasis follows (although the blood vessels stay dilated) leading to an increased blood

viscosity because of the increase in the concentration of cells within the blood. As soon as vasodilation occurs, first at the arteriole level and then progressively at the capillary level, blood cells begin to flow in the plasmatic zone near the vessel wall rather than in the axial stream, allowing plasma fluid to escape. Simultaneously, the mediators up-regulate certain molecules such as the intracellular adhesion molecule-1 and the endothelial cell leukocyte adhesion molecule-1, to bind to specific complementary molecules on the polymorphs, especially the neutrophils, thereby encouraging them to stick (adhere) to the walls of the capillaries (the process of pavementing and adhesion) whereby the action of "margination" is initiated. (Note that normal flowing blood prevent margination of cells due to the shearing force of the flowing blood along the periphery of the blood vessels [plasmatic zone] resulting in the moving of cells in the blood into the middle of the vessel [axial stream]).

❖ The Exudative phase

The extravasation of fluid and plasma components to the site of the infection is allowed through the actions of the vascular permeability mediators which have mediated the transitory permeability of capillaries by modifying the intercellular forces between the endothelial cells of the vessel wall. The exudation (escape) of fluid into the tissue constitutes the fluid exudate consisting of a high protein-rich content. The proteins present include immunoglobulin to kill off the invading pathogen; preformed plasma proteins to mediate the enzymatic/acellular biochemical cascade systems; white blood cells, namely, leukocytes to form a cellular barrier against and phagocytise the invading pathogen; and coagulation factors such as fibrogen to form a fibrin deposition on contact with the extra vascular tissues. A considerable turnover of the inflammatory exudate occurs constantly as it is drained away by the local lymphatic channels and replaced by new exudate. Both the terminal lymphatics (blind-ended endothelium-lined tubes present in most tissues) and the collecting lymphatics (which have valves) dilate as to drain away the oedema fluid of the inflammatory exudate by propelling the lymph passively, aided by the contraction of neighbouring muscles, to the lymph nodes. Because of the ability of the lymphatics to carry large molecules and particulate matter, large proteins and antigens are carried to the regional lymph nodes for recognition by lymphocytes and the mediation of the adaptive immune response.

The fluid exudate presents with two important components that further mediates the acute inflammatory response, namely, the plasma component and the cellular component. The **plasma component** contains four enzymatic/acellular biochemical cascade systems consisting of preformed plasma proteins - the plasma complement, the kinins, the coagulation factors and the fibrinolytic system - which are inter-related and act in unison to further initiate and propagate the acute inflammatory response. The activation of the complement cascade takes place as to, together with the activity of the complement proteins, kill off the invading pathogen through promoting opsonization, chemotaxis and agglutination. Activation of the complement cascade with the consequent cleaving (splitting) of very large numbers of C3 complement molecules into C3a and C3b fragments results in the production of large numbers of C3b-fragments. As these C3b-fragments are produced in the vicinity of the microbial membrane, the C3b-fragment binds covalently to the surface membrane of the pathogen. Simultaneously, the C3b-fragments act as opsonins by making the particles they coat more susceptible to engulfment by the phagocytic cells. The C3b-fragment, together with the C3 convertase, acts now on the next component in the sequence, C5, to produce the C5a-fragment which, together with the C3a-fragment that stimulates histamine release by mast cells, directly affects the mast-cells to cause their degranulation. Consequently, mediators of vascular permeability and chemotactic factors for polymorphs, especially granulocytes, are released by the mast cells. As polymorphs have a well-defined receptor for C3b-fragments on their surface, the opsonised pathogen adheres very firmly to the surface of these newly arrived polymorphonuclear leucocytes. The kinin system mediates proteins such as bradykinin that are capable of sustaining vasodilation and other physical inflammatory effects like pain. The activation of the coagulation cascade (clotting cascade) results in the discharging of coagulation factors such as thrombin that cleaves the soluble plasma protein fibrinogen to produce insoluble fibrin, into the immediate area forming a protective protein fibrin mesh over the site of entry. In this way the damaged area is occluded, thus preventing the spread of toxic substances to the rest of the body. While acting in opposition to the coagulation system as to counterbalance clotting, the fibrinolytic system generates several other inflammatory mediators such as plasmin as to lysis fibrin into degradation products (break down fibrin clots), cleave complement protein C3 and activate Factor XII (Hageman Factor) which mediates the activation of the kinin system, the fibrinolytic system and the coagulation system.

The **cellular component** involves the leukocytes, mainly neutrophils, which normally reside in the blood to form the first line of cellular defence against the invasion of the specific pathogen. The cell-derived and plasma-derived inflammatory mediators attract these phagocytic white blood cells such as granulocytes and neutrophils to the infected area which extravasate into the extracellular space and accumulate at the portal of entry. The recruitment of leukocytes is receptor-mediated in venules and small veins whereby the leukocytes (including neutrophil and eosiophil polymorphs as well as macrophages) localize at the endothelial cell surface bonding firmly to immunoglobulin ligands that were mediated by cytokines (margination). Chemokine/chemotactic factors/endogenous chemical mediators such as lysosomal compounds, prostaglandins, leucotrines, serotonin and lymphokines, provide a chemical gradient for the transmigration of the adhered/marginated leukocytes, via the process of diapedesis (hydrostatic pressure forcing the leukocytes out), through the walls of the venules and small veins, into the tissues and then move the leukocytes, via chemotaxis, towards the source of inflammation resulting in large quantities of neutrophils moving to the site of invasion and amassing there. Some leukocytes act as phagocytes ingesting bacteria, viruses and cellular debris and other as granulocytes releasing enzymatic granules that damage the pathogenic invader while simultaneously releasing inflammatory mediators to aid in inflammation. Because the invading pathogen was opsonised by immunoglobulin or the complement components (C3b which has opsonising properties), the pathogen adheres firmly to the surface of the neutrophils resulting in phagocytosis of the pathogen by the polymorphonuclear leucocytes. Being a highly specialised cell, the neutrophil polymorph contains microbiocidal agents such as hydrogen peroxide (oxygen-dependent mechanism) and lysozyme (oxygen-independent mechanism) mediating the intracellular killing off of the pathogen.

Blood monocytes also arrive at the site of infection and transform into macrophages when transmigrating from the blood vessel. On transformation into macrophages, the cells become metabolically active, motile and phagocytic. Because the macrophages appear late in the acute inflammatory response, they play a lesser role in phagocytosis compared with that of the neutrophil polymorphs and are usually responsible for clearing away tissue debris and damaged cells. Both the macrophages and the neutrophils can discharge their lysosomal enzymes, via exocytosis, into the extracellular fluid or release their entire cell content when the cell (macrophage or neutrophil) dies. Releasing of these enzymes assists in the digesting of the inflammatory exudate. In this way the macrophages attempt to localise the invasion by the pathogen by forming a cellular barrier against the migration of the infectious agent to the lymph.

The classification of the inflammatory exudate that is formed by the plasma and blood cells which have extravasate from the intravascular compartment, the chemical substances (products) released by the damaged cells are as follows

➢ A clear serous exudate with a high protein count is formed in the early stages of the inflammatory reaction and consists mainly of fluid with a few cells and fibrin. As the inflammatory process continues, the serous exudates changes to a creamy white fluid containing cellular debris

➢ When the exudate contain a great deal of fibrinogen, a fibrinogenous exudate is formed

➢ A purulent/suppurative exudate (pus) forms a thick fluid consisting of leucocytes, living and dead (killed off) pathogens, dead tissue, fluid and elements of blood. In tissue an abscess is formed locally when the pus is walled-off by granulation tissue or fibrous tissue. When pus fills a hollow viscus it is called empyema

➢ A catarrhal exudate is formed when hyper-secretion of mucus accompanies the acute inflammation of a mucous membrane

➢ A membranous exudate is formed when a membranous epithelium becomes coated by fibrin, desquamated epithelial cells and inflammatory cells, for example, the grey membrane seen in infection by Corynebacterium diphtheriae

➢ A pseudo membranous exudate is formed when superficial mucosal ulceration with an overlying slough of disrupted mucosa, fibrin, mucus and inflammatory cells occurs

➤ A <u>haemorrhagic exudate</u> is formed when vascular injury or depletion of coagulation factors had occurred. A haemorrhagic exudate is seen in acute pancreatitis due to proteolytic destruction of the vascular walls and in meningococcal septicaemia when disseminated intravascular coagulation has taken place

➤ When high pressure due to oedema lead to vascular occlusion and thrombosis, a <u>necrotising/gangrenous exudate</u> is formed and widespread septic necrosis of the organ occurs. The combination of necrosis and bacterial putrefaction is gangrene.

The accumulation of the inflammatory exudate, in the short term, <u>dilutes the toxin</u> released by the specific infectious agent and be carried away in the lymphatics; <u>allow the entry of antibodies</u> into the extra vascular space when increased vascular permeability takes place as to mediate lysis of the pathogen through participation of complement, phagocytosis by opsonisation and neutralisation of toxins; <u>promotes drug transport</u> by the inflammatory fluid; <u>induces fibrin formation</u> to impede the movement of pathogens by trapping them while facilitating phagocytosis; <u>aids the delivery of nutrients and oxygen to cells</u> by neutrophils which have a high metabolic activity; and <u>helps to stimulate the immune response</u> due to the drainage of the fluid exudate into the lymphatics whereby particulate and soluble antigens reach the local lymph nodes. **But** the accumulation of the inflammatory exudate, in the long term, hampers the exchange of nutrients and oxygen and the removal of waste products from the cells as well as from the blood and because of the increased pressure, the normal functions as well as the normal physiological functioning of cells and tissues are impaired. Enzymes such as collagenase and protease may digest normal tissue leading to their destruction. Sometimes the inflammatory response may be inappropriate as when the provoking environmental antigen poses no threat of infection and the resulting allergic inflammatory response becomes life-threatening.

❖ **The resolution of the acute inflammatory response/the stage of repair and healing**
The outcome/sequelae of the acute inflammation depend upon the type of tissue involved and the amount of tissue destruction which depend in turn upon the nature of the pathogen. Tissues that regenerated over the lifespan, regenerated quickly while tissue that are composed of stable cells which stop regenerating when full growth is attained, take much longer to regenerate. Permanent or fixed cells are unable to regenerate and are always replaced by fibrous tissue. With the passing of time, resolution or healing at the site of entry takes place when complete <u>restoration/regeneration</u> of the normal parenchyma (functional) cells are formed by the affected tissues after an episode of inflammation. Complete regeneration occurs when vascular dilatation had disappeared, the infection had occurred in an organ or tissue which has regenerative capacity while minimal cell death and tissue damage had taken place because of the rapid killing off and phagocytosis of the pathogen with rapid removal of fluid and debris by good local vascular drainage. When regeneration is not possible, because

large amounts of fibrin were formed that cannot be completely removed by the fibrinolytic enzymes together with exudate and debris that could not be removed or discharged while substantial volumes of tissues became necrotic or died, <u>organisation</u> takes place characterized by the growing of new capillaries into the inert inflammatory exudate together with the migration of macrophages into the zone, connective tissue cell (fibroblasts) proliferation, and collagen synthesis resulting in normal tissue replacement by granulation tissue (fibrosis). Only fibrotic cells are laid down by the affected tissue when the injured area is filled by scar tissue. Resolution occurs when the structure and function of damaged tissues have been restored or regenerated. <u>Necrosis</u> (death of the tissue), instead of healing, may occur. When bacteria invade the necrotic tissue, decomposition follows resulting in gangrene. As the innate and immunological defence mechanisms cannot defend the body anymore because none to very little blood reaches the area, surgical debrination has to be done of the injured area before healing can take place. When the pathogen causing the acute inflammation is not removed, the acute inflammation progresses to the chronic stage characterized by the organisation of the tissue as well as a change in the character of the cellular exudate whereby the neutrophil polymorphs are replaced with lymphocytes, plasma cells and macrophages (including sometimes multinucleate giant cells).

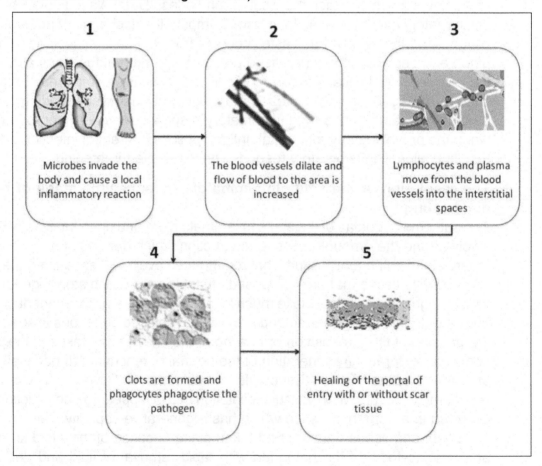

Figure 7.3 Schematic representation of the local inflammatory reaction

7.2.1.2   Clinical signs and symptoms manifested of the systemic inflammatory response

When the local inflammatory response cannot be contained within the restricted environment, the systemic inflammatory response/reaction is elicited because the specific infectious pathogen has invaded the blood and lymph circulation of the body in spite of the local inflammation reaction that had taken place. Unregulated inflammation occurs with uncontrolled coagulation, widespread leakiness of blood vessels with mal-distribution of circulating volume and unbalanced oxygen supply and demand. The endothelial cells are activated throughout the body, resulting in widespread extravasation of fluid into the interstitial compartment and systemic activation of the immune system and coagulation cascade. Substantial extra-vascular fluid accumulation takes place with widespread forming of microthrombi in blood vessels and in the interstitial compartment. The combination of the intravascular coagulation and low circulating volume leads to the decreased perfusion of all vital body organs. All body organs and systems are afflicted and the clinical picture of the systemic inflammation reaction depends on the system/organ being involved. When the systemic inflammatory response cannot be contained, several consequences occur that lead to organ dysfunction, including further excessive activation and production of inflammatory cells and biochemical mediators; direct damaged of the vascular endothelium; the disruption or altered regulation of the acute immune cell functioning; persistent hyper-metabolism; and mal-distribution of circulatory volume to organ systems. Multiple organ dysfunction syndromes develop as result of progressive physiological failure of two or more separate organ systems. The cellular or micro-circulatory dysfunctional events lead to a loss of critical organ function induced by the failure of delivery of oxygen and other substrates and the inability to remove end-products of metabolism. The early impairment of organs is normally manifested in the immuno-regulatory function of reticulo-endothelial organs such as the liver and the gastro-intestinal tract. Moderate to severe inflammatory responses produce systemic manifestations such as hyperthermia (elevated temperature or fever); an increase in white blood cells (leukocytosis); and an increased erythrocyte sedimentation rate.

The non-specific signs and symptoms of the systemic inflammation reaction occur prior to the appearance of the characteristic-specific clinical picture of the relevant communicable disease. (The characteristic-specific signs and symptoms will be discussed under the various diseases – see Theme IV). The following general non-specific signs and symptoms of the systemic inflammation reaction are manifested in all communicable diseases. The infected person feels ill, but it is not yet possible to make a specific diagnosis. A specific diagnosis can only be made when the characteristic-specific clinical signs and symptoms of the particular disease are manifested, after which treatment can commence. Some (or all) of the non-specific signs and symptoms of the systemic inflammation reaction may clear up as soon as the typical (characteristic-specific) clinical picture is manifested. In other cases, the level of severity of the non-specific signs and symptoms may increase to form part of the typical characteristic-specific clinical picture.

The pathogenesis, physiological and general non-specific signs and symptoms of the systemic inflammation response are set out in Table 7.1 and figure 7.4. Please note that because all organ systems of the body are involved, organ-specific signs and symptoms can be manifested.

Table 7.1 THE GENERAL NON-SPECIFIC SYSTEMIC SIGNS AND SYMPTOMS, PATHOGENESIS AND PHYSIOLOGY OF INFLAMMATION CHARACTERISTIC OF ALL ACUTE COMMUNICABLE DISEASES

BODY SYSTEM, OR PART OF BODY	CLINICAL MANIFESTATIONS - SIGNS AND SYMPTOMS
Body as a integrated unit • Onset	Malaise; lethargy; light-headedness; headache; anorexia; pains in joints, body and nerves; inability to concentrate; feeling of discomfort; weakness and lack of motivation, vomiting
• Advanced	Flushed face, dehydration, elevated body temperature (38⁰C and higher), confusion, delirium (at times), weight loss when condition lasts for a period of time and muscle wasting
Temperature regulating-mechanism of the body	Pyrexia/hyperthermia is a pronounced sign and usually reaches its peak in the afternoon and early evening and its lowest level 12 hours later. Rigors are common There may be a distinctive pattern of body temperature changes, which may be of diagnostic importance in some diseases. The different pattern of pyrexia is characterized by either a <u>sustained</u> or a <u>remittent</u> or an <u>intermittent</u> or a <u>recurrent fever</u> <u>Please Note</u>: Not all infected persons have pyrexia. It does not occur in leprosy, cholera or sexually transmitted diseases
Pulmonary-respiratory system	The respiratory rate does not increase dramatically The breath has an acetone-like smell Coughing
Haematological system (Blood)	Leukocytosis, lymphocytosis, anaemia, increased erythrocyte sedimentation rate, thrombosis, haemorrhages, an elevated C-reactive protein (CRP) concentration (>5 mg/L)
Cardiovascular system	• Pulse rate increases (in some medical communicable diseases, the pulse rate is lower than expected {a temperature-pulse-dissociation}, for example, in typhoid, brucellosis, epidemic parotitis and virus meningitis) • Blood pressure does not change unless hypo-volumia or shock is mediated. Hypotension may occur • Septicaemic shock develops which leads to tissue anoxia, metabolic acidosis and oedema. The extremities are cold

Renal system	• Dysuria, urgency and frequency • Proteinuria • Glucosuria • Ketonuria • Pyuria • Oliguria and/or anuria • Haematuria • Polyuria • Increased serum creatinine levels
Gastrointestinal tract, liver and spleen	• Anorexia and intolerance of food • Abdominal tenderness and distension with either a decreased or an increased in bowel sounds • Diarrhoea and bacterial overgrowth in stools • Jaundice • Haemorrhage • Hepato-splenomegaly
Immune system and lymph glands	• The lymph nodes become enlarged and may be tender (lymph-adenitis). In some cases they suppurate • Positive serological tests for antibody
Central nervous system	• Changes in behaviour, such as anxiety, confusion, stupor, delirium • Convulsions • Coma • Increased cerebro-spinal cell counts • Paralysis (flaccid or rigid) • Loss of sensation • Muscle spasms
Cutaneous system (Skin)	Skin lesions occur in some communicable diseases. Skin lesions are superficial growths or patches of skin that do not look the same as/resemble the areas around it (see fig. 7.4). Skin lesions are grouped in primary and secondary lesions. Skin lesions are a hallmark sign of most communicable diseases due to the infection of part of or all the systems of the entire body **Primary lesions** • A **maculae** is a circum-scribed red or brown or white discolouration of the skin. No elevation or depression occurs in the skin and the lesion is less than one centimetre in size. A lesion larger than one centimetre is known as a patch. Maculae associated with communicable diseases are mostly red in colour • A **papulae** is a solid, raised area varying in size, but usually less than one centimetre in diameter. A patch of closely grouped papulae larger than one centimetre is known as a plaque.

Papules and plaques are sometimes rough in texture and can be red, pink, or brown in colour • A **vesicle** is a circum-scribed superficial, elevated/raised lesion containing clear serous fluid and is less than 5 milli-centimetres in diameter. Lesions larger than this is known as bulla or blisters • A **pustule** is a vesicle or a bulla containing pus • **Petechiae** are small areas of blood in or under the skin. If large areas of haemorrhages in the skin occurs, it is called ecchymosis • A **nodule** is a small solid node with distinct edges, developed from connective tissue and palpable under the skin as an elevated lesion • A **wheal** is a well-defined swelling in the skin. The swelling has an even surface with clearly palpable edges. A wheal can be itchy and usually disappears as soon as it has erupted **Secondary lesions** • An **ulcer** is a lesion that involves the loss of the epidermis and part of the dermis. Ulcers may result in acute bacterial infections • A **crust** is a collection of dried cells, serum, blood or pus which dries on the skin and can be either hard or soft • A **scab** is a collection of fibrinogen, which is formed over the primary lesion. Healing takes place under the scab which falls off eventually, usually leaving scars. The scar may disappear after a while or if not, it is permanent. Scars may be limited to the dermis only or reach into the epidermis • A **scar** is discoloured fibrous tissue that permanently replaces normal skin after the destruction of the dermis has taken place. A very thick and raised scar is called a colloid

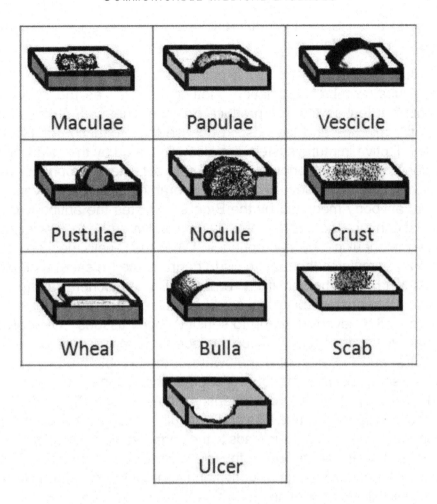

Figure 7.4   Schematic diagrams of primary and secondary skin lesions

7.2.2   Non-specific signs and symptoms produced by the host's immune responses

The pathologic effects of infection cause not only tissue damage directly (as set out in 7.2.1) but also indirectly via the over-activation of the immunological system. Over-activation or prolonged stimulation of either the innate or the adaptive immunological system, or both, can occur, leading to pathological changes with tissue damage inflicted by the immunological system itself. The potent innate immune system has an in-built safety as far as specificity is concerned, because the innate immune system and the adaptive immune system have to evolve in the constant presence of the host's "own/self antigens" to which neither the innate nor the adaptive immune system respond. However, the innate and the adaptive immunological systems are not so well controlled quantitatively, and when over-activity occur, the innate immune system not only damages and kills off the invading pathogen, but also damages "innocent" host tissue. The expression of the innate immunity causes a certain amount of inflammation and if severe, tissue damage follows. The complement and polymorphs are also involved in several tissue-damaging reactions, such as the immune complex disease and the adult respiratory distress syndrome characterized by severe pulmonary oedema.

The endotoxin(s) released by the dying pathogen results in vascular collapse and disseminated intravascular coagulation (clotting) as well as the activation of the polymorphonuclear leukocytes that produce enzymes that can inflict damage in the cells of both the microbe and the host. Because the production of T-cells and the B-cells of the adaptive immune system are also stimulated by the invading pathogen, the B-cells start to mediate antibody while the T-cells activate macrophages that release Interleukin-1 resulting in an elevated body temperature (fever) and eventually tissue damage. The antibody mediated by the B-cells activates the antibody-complement complexes that enhance the enzyme production of polymorphonuclear leukocytes and the releasing of interleukin-1 by macrophages. When the B-cells mediate IgE-antibody, the IgE-antibody stimulates the mast cells to degranulate (release) their biochemical mediators resulting in a hypersensitivity reaction. These biochemical mediators have neurological, cutaneous, respiratory, cardiovascular, gastro-intestinal and urinary effects that can inflict severe damage to sensitive body tissues. Over-production of the T-cells leads to cytotoxicity with tissue damage as the end result. Direct stimulation (via the classical and the alternative pathway) of the complement by toxic amounts of endotoxins also results in bacterial septicaemia shock characterized by a profound drop in the levels of complement components such as C3 and C5, production of large amounts of the fragments C3a and C5a and a simultaneous decrease in the number of polymorphonuclear leukocytes. This leads to the aggregation of the polymorphonuclear leukocytes in and their adherence to the blood vessel wall and their activation to release their toxic molecules, both oxidative and non-oxidative. Tissue damage of the blood vessel wall follows as well as disseminating intravascular coagulation.

Hypersensitivity is the pathological consequence of the excessive or prolonged stimulation of the adaptive immune response. Although the antimicrobial effects of the lymphocyte responses act mainly on the innate immune system, the enhancement of the non-specific effector mechanisms can also enhance the overreaction of the adaptive immune system resulting in hypersensitive reactions. The pathologic tissue-damaging effects of hypersensitivity are termed "immuno-pathologic effects - tissue damage". Hypersensitivity, *per se*, can be divided in four types based on the immunological mechanism underlying the tissue-damaging reaction. Each of the four types of hypersensitivity can be of microbial or non-microbial origin. Microbes of many sorts can mediate a hypersensitivity reaction, and the hypersensitivity reaction of microbial origin includes some of the most serious of these responses. One common feature of the hypersensitivity reaction of microbial origin is that the infection is prolonged with continuous or repeated antigenic stimulation.

* Type-I hypersensitivity
  This type of pathological hypersensitivity is a feature of helminthic/worm infections, especially following the rupture of a hydatid cyst or a tapeworm cyst. Slow leakage of worm antigens ensures that the mast cells are sensitized with specific IgE-antibody and the massive flood of antigens, when ruptured, can

cause acute fatal anaphylaxis with vascular collapse and pulmonary oedema. Even a small amount of antigen used in diagnostic skin tests may have the same effect. Parasitisation with the Ascaris worm also mediates a type-1 hypersensitivity reaction as it is associated with high levels of IgE-antibody. The pathological consequences are mostly respiratory, with eosinophilic infiltrates and asthmatic episodes that correspond to the passage of the parasite migrating through the lungs. The itchy rashes characteristic of helminthic parasitisation when the worms die in the skin, are also a hypersensitivity reaction of this type – for example, the swimmer's rash due to animal or avian schistosomes.

* <u>Type-II hypersensitivity</u>
Type-II hypersensitivity reactions, both the protective and the pathological reactions, are mediated by antibody to the infectious pathogen or by auto-antibody. Antibody-IgG are mostly responsible for mediating type-II hypersensitivity leading to cytotoxicity, either extracellular or intracellular after phagocytosis had taken place. The antibody binds to the cell and, if the complement has been activated, lysis of the cell takes place. The antibody kills the host's cells, as the cells displays the foreign antigens picked up from the pathogen (for example, when red blood cells are infected by the Plasmodium pathogen causing malaria, the antibody to the parasite-derived antigen or the antigen-antibody complex binds to the cell and lysis the cell resulting in haemolytic anaemia). Although the anti-myocardial antibody of group A β-haemolytic streptococcal infections are triggered by the *group A β-haemolytic streptococcal* pathogen, the presence of a same cross-reacting carbohydrate antigen on the bacterium and on the myocardium mediates a cross-reaction between the microbial and the host's own human antigens. This cross-reaction between the microbial and the host's own human antigens result in an auto-antibody hypersensitivity reaction underlying a number of diseases.

Note

Cytotoxicity caused by T-cells is considered a number type-IV hypersensitivity reaction

* <u>Type-III hypersensitivity</u>
Type-III pathological hypersensitivity reaction is mostly triggered by chronic infections such as malaria and chronic glomerulonephritis (acute glomerulonephritis is a serious complication of streptococcal throat infection). When immune complexes are formed, activation of the complement takes place, leading to phagocytosis and removal of the antigen. But when complexes escape removal by the phagocytes of the reticulo-endothelial system, complications set in as the complexes get lodge in the tissues or the blood vessels, resulting in attracting complement and neutrophils. With the release of lysosomal enzymes by the leukocytes, local damage is inflicted in the tissues and blood vessels, which are particularly serious in small blood vessels, especially in the renal glomeruli of the kidneys. The polymorph infiltration leads to alterations in the basement membrane, causing leakage of albumin and even red cells in the urine. When complexes are deposited

over a long period, as in malarial nephropathy, the mesangial cell intrusions and fusion of foot processes cause a more irreversible impairment of the glomerular function of the kidneys.

Note

The prerequisite of a bacterial trigger is not the only role player in this type of hypersensitivity - a poor antibody response in terms of amount and affinity, the particular tendency of the antigen itself to bind to vascular endothelium, or the inhibition of the normal function of the phagocytes, or complement in removing circulating complexes, may also be predisposing factors

* Type-IV hypersensitivity

The type-IV hypersensitivity protective reaction is mostly mediated by cell-mediated immune responses when T-cells and macrophages are activated. Type-IV hypersensitivity invariably causes the destruction of tissues that may be permanent. The cell-mediated response to microbial antigens is responsible for granuloma formation and plays a major role in diseases such as tuberculosis, tuberculoid leprosy, lymphogranuloma inguinale and Toxocara infection. The different patterns of the complex cytokine network in type-IV hypersensitivity responses, determines the tendency of some granulomas to undergo necrosis (for example, caseation in tuberculosis) while others do not (for example, leprosy). The clinical features of schistosomiasis are also produced by cell-mediated immunity. The *Schistosoma Mansoni* (blood fluke) lays eggs in the mesenteric venous system while some become lodged in the small portal vessels in the liver. The strong cell-mediated reactions to the secreted helminthic enzymes lead to granulomatous reactions around each egg and egg destruction – thus sparing the parenchyma of the liver from the toxic effects of the egg enzymes. The coalescent calcified granulomas, however, ultimately cause portal cirrhosis with portal hypertension, oesophageal varicose and haematemesis.

The variety of skin rashes also have an immunological origin as some of the skin rashes are immunological mediated by T-cells. The characteristic skin rash of measles, for example, is absent in children with T-cell deficiency who, instead, develop a fatal systemic disease. This indicates that the typical rash of measles is T-cell-mediated and as such represent some form of successful cell-mediated immunity. When children with T-cell deficiency are vaccinated with live attenuated vaccinia virus, they develop an inexorable spreading skin lesion which is a direct effect of the vaccination and not an immuno-pathological effect. The following common skin rashes/skin conditions are of immunological origin in which an infectious pathogen is involved

- ⇨ **Virus infections**
  - ◈ Maculo-papular rash – measles and rubella
  - ◈ Vesicular rash – chicken pox and shingles, herpes simplex infection
  - ◈ Hepatitis infection - urticaria
- ⇨ **Bacterial infections**
  - ◈ Erythematous rash consisting of papulae – scarlet fever
  - ◈ Disseminated infections and rashes – syphilis
  - ◈ Sparse rose spots – typhoid and enteric fever

◇ Petechiae or maculo-papular lesions – meningitis, spotted fever
◇ Blotchy skin lesions - tuberculoid leprosy
◇ Maculo-papular or hemorrhagic rash – typhus

⇒ **Fungal infections**
◇ Allergic rash – dermatophytoid infection

⇒ **Protozoan infections**
◇ Papules ulcerating to form crusted infectious sores – cutaneous leishmaniasis.

7.3. KEY NOTES

❑ To establish infection in man the host, pathogens must successfully penetrate the body's natural defence barriers and attach themselves to, or pass across, different body surfaces (respiratory, urinal-genital, intestinal and skin).

❑ To enable the pathogens to stay in the body long enough to replicate, spread, infect and be shed so as to be transmitted to fresh hosts, many microbes have developed chemical and/or mechanical mechanisms to evade the actions and processes of the innate and adaptive immune systems.

❑ Many successful pathogens multiply in the epithelial cells at the site/portal of entry into the body surface, but do not spread to deeper structures or through the body. Infective microbes that spread systemically via lymph and blood through the body, invade the various tissues stepwise before reaching the final site of replication and shedding to the exterior.

❑ A local and a systemic inflammation reaction are elicited by all infectious agents. The clinical manifestation or signs and symptoms of infection are produced by the infective pathogen or by the host's immune system.

❑ All communicable diseases run a natural course with five distinctive stadiums, namely, pre-pathogenesis, early pathogenesis, prodromal stage [pre-clinical stage], characteristic-specific clinical manifestation/clinical picture [clinical stage], and recovering stage [stage of resolution]. Each stage is recognisable from the general and specific pathogenesis and reaction between the body tissue[s] and the infectious agent as well as from the manner in which the signs and symptoms are clinically manifested.

❑ The biological context of the host-parasite/infective pathogen-relationship and the dynamics of the immune system in conjunction with the microbial invasion strategies, provide a basis for understanding the cause, symptomology and control of communicable diseases.

Note

The characteristic-specific clinical picture of the relevant communicable disease that is manifested will be discussed in Theme IV. The non-specific systemic signs and symptoms as set out in table 7.1 must always be read together with the characteristic clinical manifestation of the specific disease

Chapter 8

INVASION HAD OCCURRED

The rendering of healthcare to the ill individual grounded in a comprehensive and holistic approach within a familial and community context

Healthcare is embedded in life itself and commissioned by culture and always take place between the healthcare provider and the healthcare user(s). Healthcare is thus both a interpersonal and a cultural phenomenon taking place within an interpersonal context (two unique cultural human beings disclosing themselves to one another in the structures and fellowship of the healthcare user-healthcare provider-relationship), and cultural context (the ethical and professional practice of healthcare is based on and regulated by cultural norms and values, beliefs, ideas, practices, rules and regulations, behaviour, attitudes and traditions). Healthcare *per se*, consist of a science (a comprehensively integrated scientifically-based knowledge) and an art (an ensemble of care and cure activities - activities to fulfil the needs of the healthcare user while helping persons to become self-caring for themselves, their families and the communities they live in). Hence, the aim of the rendering of compassionate, comprehensive, holistic and culturally congruent healthcare to ill persons suffering from a particular communicable disease, their families and their communities, is the self-actualization of all healthcare users (individuals, families, and communities) through **living a meaningful life** (or dying a dignified death) and **becoming self-caring (totally or partially)** by enhancing their well-being.

To support all healthcare users to become self-caring and to actualizes themselves, the rendered healthcare must satisfy the ill person, his/her family and the community wherein they live - that is, the healthcare must be rendered according to the ill person's and his/her family's cultural beliefs, convictions, norms and values, health behaviour and multi-dimensional lifestyle/pattern. Culturally congruent healthcare rendering is a specific mode of healthcare rendering (it can be distinguished but not differentiated from other forms of healthcare rendering) that is meaningful and culturally appropriate and acceptable to and fulfil the healthcare user's expectations. And because culturally congruent healthcare rendering is also an interpersonal and cultural phenomenon, it is grounded in the healthcare brokering process. As such, the science and art of healthcare not only grounds culturally congruent healthcare within its specific points of departure, but the science and art of culturally congruent healthcare supports the science and art of healthcare. The content and context of holistically-culturally congruent healthcare is based on an eclectic approach and when rendering holistically and culturally congruent healthcare to all ill persons, their families and their communities, all biomedical factors as well as all socio-cultural factors must be taken in consideration during the healthcare brokering process - when gathering data, when interventions are designed and implemented and when the outcome(s) is/are evaluated. In support of and supplementary to the healthcare brokering process (that is, the assessment of the health status and needs of the healthcare users, their families and their communities, the diagnosing of their health status [wellness state, illness state and at risk state] and their unique human needs, the designing and implementing of the planned healthcare interventions and the evaluation and recording of the outcomes [self-actualization as human beings]), a cultural assessment must also be conducted, a cultural diagnosis has to be made, culturally appropriate interventions have to be designed and implemented to achieve cultural brokering and cultural bridging and the cultural outcome(s) has/have to be evaluated (healthcare rendering that was/is beneficial and satisfying to all persons served). Because cultures are so diverse, a wide range of activities needed to be planned and rendered to the healthcare user, his/her family and their community to

> maintain cultural care by conserving the healthcare users' values and beliefs and, where necessary, improve it to promote health; or
> provide care that requires cultural accommodation or negotiation as to prevent/minimize cultural shock to both healthcare user and provider by accepting the way different persons do certain activities their own way or to seek explanations when not understood without undermining/condemning the values and beliefs of the healthcare user, his/her family and their community; or
> provide care that requires a re-designing or restructuring of cultural beliefs by identifying those life threatening areas within the tradition and decide together with the healthcare user and his/her family how best these threatening areas can be avoided or replaced with cultural accepted activities beneficial to health.

Based on the fact that in any multicultural environment barriers between healthcare users and healthcare providers do exist and occur frequently, cultural sensitivity for relevance of care must continuously be upheld by all healthcare providers to avoid incongruence brought about by impositions and ethnocentrism. When only biomedical-based healthcare is imposed on healthcare users (taking in account all legislative and other aspects to be complied with in the context of communicable diseases), the healthcare user-healthcare provider-relationship breaks down and healthcare rendering loses its meaning because healthcare rendering then becomes a conglomeration of mechanical procedures carried out on the ill person, on his/

her family and on his/her community. The end result is the disintegration of the personhood of the healthcare users, their families and their communities. Therefore, cultural imposition of the ill person, his/her family and his/her community must be prevented at all cost. Thus, all healthcare providers must be knowledgeable of and skilled in culturally congruent healthcare rendering, cultural brokering and cultural bridging as well as its incorporation into all healthcare plans to meet the health needs of all ill persons, their families and their communities. As compassionate, comprehensive, holistically and culturally congruent healthcare has to be rendered to all individual hosts, their families and their communities, all healthcare practitioners need to be culturally competent in their rendering of healthcare.

Intercultural communication in multicultural environments is a complex undertaking and the role of a liaison interpreter as a cultural broker is invaluable in any intercultural context. But, the provision of an interpreter often solves only the linguistic problem, not the other problems of communication created between the healthcare provider and the healthcare user[s] (healthy, ill, contact, carrier – individual, family, community). These other problems are mostly not simply a matter of language, but problems equally created and compounded by fact that the healthcare provider and the healthcare user[s] is/are separated by a wide gap of authority and power related to class; race and/or culture; gender; and the differential authority-relations between the professional care giver and his/her lay client[s]. Furthermore, all metaphorical and idiomatical language or terminology, as well as dialect, is embedded in the specific language and culture of the healthcare user and as such, can result in major problems for both the interpreter and the healthcare provider (for example, interpretation of the concept "bad blood"). When the healthcare interview is also conducted in a learned medical corpus (in medical jargon or in medical scientific language – even if scientifically correct translated) that is not suited to the healthcare users' educational level or background, many healthcare users have difficulty in understanding and become alienated and lose confidence in the healthcare environment.

The non-verbal aspect of communication (for example, intonation patterns and facial expression and gestures) also tell their own stories and both interpreter, healthcare provider and healthcare user[s] must see and hear as well as act out with one another. Many healthcare users may also add irrelevant material because it lessens their feeling of embarrassment as they feel more comfortable when the attention is not focussed on their medical problem (especially if it is of a personal nature). As health is culturally defined, cultural factors may also come into play (for example, if healthcare users belief that health is directly related to aspects such as the weather, environment, eating habits, plants, and much more), they will add these highly important relevant information – information that may be irrelevant to the healthcare practitioner and/or the interpreter. Some healthcare users have a complete absence of register[1] with regard to certain medical and other subjects. Many female healthcare users have never given names to body parts such as the vagina while both male and female healthcare users may not understand/discuss words such as "single partner", "multiple partners", "sexual intercourse". Because of embarrassment, the healthcare user may provide the wrong information or none at all, or label the healthcare provider as ill-mannered.

To overcome such culturally-based difficulties, language must be seen as an integrated system of culture (language in culture), not language and culture, and interpretation as the reproduction of culture (because culture defines health and disease). Both interpreter and healthcare provider must understand the complex nature of the linguistic activity and the limitations of each practitioner (the healthcare giver and the interpreter) as human beings. The liaison interpreter needs to meet with the healthcare user[s] before the interview, to determine the healthcare user's educational background, language register[1], attitude[s] towards healthcare and other aspects of his/her social background. Healthcare providers must use accessible (plain) medical/ healthcare language and everyday expressions as a way to guarantee linguistic intelligibility for the liaison interpreter and the target language listener[s], namely, the healthcare user(s). The interpreter must also not cut the healthcare user short (nor be prompt by the healthcare provider to do it), but must encourage the user to speak more freely while rendering all seemingly irrelevant information faithfully. Furthermore, the translation must not summarize the information offered by the healthcare user nor must the user's language be polished as nuances may be lost and statements misinterpreted. Because some healthcare users may have learned the meaning of a word in one context and then apply it in other contexts, the healthcare provider and interpreter must make sure that the healthcare user[s] clearly understand what he/she [they] has/have been asked or has/have told the provider. The "Nodding syndrome or Yes syndrome" (nodding or saying yes in agreement out of fear or embarrassment without understanding or insight in what is said) must be prevented, as both the liaison interpreter and healthcare provider represents the healthcare users interests, assess their needs and help them to obtain the best healthcare they are entitled to.

[1] Languages have several registers, for example, specialist, conversational, business, medical, and technical, etc. which is generally defined by the social/intellectual level of the speaker as well as the situation wherein he/she himself/herself finds. As such, the medical register of the healthcare user must be determined and communication must be conducted in that specific register.

The care rendering to ill persons suffering from a communicable medical disease does not differ in principle from the care rendered to any other person suffering from any other medical disorder. What is different though is the additional responsibility of the prevention and control of the spread of the communicable disease. Therefore, the healthcare to be rendered to all ill persons suffering from any particular communicable medical disease consists thus of four components, namely,

- ❖ rendering of individualized, compassionate, comprehensive, holistic and culturally congruent fundamental (supportive and symptomatic) and specific healthcare to the ill person, his/her family and the community they live in
- ❖ administering specific chemotherapeutic drug-therapy and/or other medically prescribed treatment
- ❖ preventing the spread of the disease by taking all necessary preventive measures and isolating (if necessary) the person(s) suffering from the particular communicable medical disease
- ❖ rectifying all risks and hazards in the environment (physical-biological, psychological, socio-cultural, economical, and other milieus) to maintain a healthy living environment.

Persons suffering from communicable medical diseases may be cared for at home or in a hospital, depending on the nature of the particular disease. When the person is cared for at home, healthcare providers do not render the care themselves – they assist the members of the family who care for the individual. This entails continual instruction of the family and continual evaluation of the care rendered in order to timely call in expert help when the course of the disease and the severity of the condition of the ill person demand it. When the ill person is hospitalised, he/she is usually cared for in semi-isolation (for example, taking of enteric precautions) or in full isolation or in a specialised high grade isolation care unit. Thus, to enable healthcare practitioners to care for the ill person at home or in a hospital, they must be well knowledgeable regarding the following

- the interrelatedness of the host, the environment and the specific pathogen (the Epidemiological Triad of Communicable Diseases model)
- the characteristic properties of the specific pathogen (infectious agent/pathogen)
- the portal of entry and exit as well as the intermediaries in the transmission of the specific infectious agent
- the incubation period and the period of communicability (infectivity/transmission)
- the most effective methods of killing off/eliminating the specific infectious agent
- the clinical manifestation and complications of the particular communicable disease
- the way in which specific antimicrobial and other chemotherapeutic drug-therapy changes or influence the clinical picture and course of the disease
- the individualized, comprehensive, holistic and culturally congruent healthcare to be rendered – fundamentally and specifically
- the rehabilitation programmes required by ill persons when recovered
- healthcare interventions to be instated to prevent the re-occurrence of the particular communicable disease
- control interventions to be instated to prevent the spread and further outbreaks of the particular communicable disease
- legislative requirements to be adhered to in the care programme
- the supervision to be instated over all professional practitioners and all non-professional workers participating in the care of ill persons.

Since all healthcare rendering situations are initiated purposefully by healthcare providers because of their responsibility towards healthcare users as the life of the healthcare user is endangered and because healthcare rendering only finds meaning and purpose within the healthcare user-healthcare provider-relationship, the healthcare brokering process (integrated with the cultural brokering and bridging process) are discussed under the following headings

- assessment to be made of the health status and needs of all hosts (individuals, families, communities)
- general fundamental supportive and symptomatic healthcare to be rendered to the ill individual and his/her family at home and in a hospital (excluding high-grade isolation care)
- meeting the unique age-related health needs of children and adults

- the general specific healthcare to be rendered to the ill person and the immunotherapeutic and chemotherapeutic products available for the treatment of communicable diseases.

8.1 THE HEALTHCARE BROKERING PROCESS

The healthcare brokering process is the only scientific clinical decision-making strategy the healthcare provider uses to assess the health status of all host (individuals, families, and communities – healthy, ill, contact, carrier); to identify all risks/hazards in the environments wherein the hosts live, and to identify the causative pathogen. As such, the healthcare brokering process consists of three identifiable phases that merges into one another, namely,

✠ **The data gathering phase** during which an assessment is made of the health status of all hosts as well as the identification of the causative pathogen and all the risks/hazards in the environments. During this phase, a comprehensive assessment is simultaneously made of all the cultural factors that may influence the health of the hosts and the care interventions to be rendered

✠ **The intervention phase** consists of diagnosing the hosts as either healthy, or ill, or carrier, or contact while categorizing all identified health risks in the environments. This is followed by the planning and execution of the healthcare interventions (fundamentally and specifically) when caring for the ill individual and his/her family. Incorporated into the biomedical healthcare interventions, is the cultural diagnosis of all cultural impositions that may negative influence the rendering of the biomedical healthcare and the cultural interventions planned and executed to overcome these impositions. Reconstruction of the environment(s) takes place simultaneously to control the spread of the particular communicable disease and to prevent further outbreaks. The specific interventions aimed at the reconstruction of the environment are done in collaboration with environmental health officers, officials of appropriate governmental departments and non-governmental organizations

✠ **The outcome phase** during which evaluation of the outcome and process is done to confirm whether the projected aims and objectives set for the hosts, environment and disease control and prevention, have been achieved. If non-achievement has occurred, the process is repeated → gathering of data → planning and executing of interventions → evaluation whether aims have been achieved.

8.1.1 The data gathering phase - the assessment of the health status and health needs of all hosts - individuals, their families and the communities they live in

Prior to initiating the required healthcare interventions, it is of utmost importance to assess the health status of all hosts in order to determine the specific and supportive healthcare to be rendered. Using the Epidemiological Triad of Communicable Diseases Model as point of departure in order to render personalized, compassionate, comprehensive, holistic and culturally congruent healthcare (fundamentally and specifically) to all hosts, it is of **utmost importance** that the data gathering phase (assessment) of every host-group (individuals, families, communities), **include** the following four (4) aspects in the assessment process

- assessment of the health status (healthy, ill {including carriers} and at risk {contacts}) and health needs (wellness, high-risk, need-focused [prevailing]) of all hosts (individuals, families, communities - children and adults) as well as identification of all cultural impositions that needs to be brokered/bridged
- identification of all health risks/hazards in the environment (physical, biological, socio-cultural, psychological, economic, and the many others of importance)
- identification of the properties of the specific infectious agent (whether immediately or presumably identifiable)
- establishing a database-line (biomedical and cultural) to guide the decision making process regarding whether the ill person(s) is/are to be cared for at home or in hospital and the healthcare (both the fundamental supportive and the specific care) to be rendered to all hosts within their familial and community context.

The aim of the data gathering process is to establish a database in order to

- ➢ confirm the wellness state or illness state or "at risk" state of all hosts-groups (individuals, families, communities)
- ➢ diagnose all prevailing and high-risk health needs of all ill persons/families/communities to be attended to as well as all cultural impositions to be bridged or changed
- ➢ identify all aspects of the well-being (strengths) of ill persons/families/communities that have to be enhanced and strengthen
- ➢ identify all hazards/risks in the environment (physical-biological, psychological, socio-cultural, economical, and other milieus of importance) that need to be rectified as well as all healthy attributes of the environment that needs to be maintained
- ➢ identify the properties of the specific infectious agent to administer the appropriate medical therapy as well as to prevent and control the spread of the particular disease (including all legislative measures to comply with).

The dimensions included in the database-line of all hosts (individuals, families, communities) must reflect all dimensions of health, (namely, the bio-physical dimension of health, the psychological dimension of health, the socio-cultural dimension of health, the behaviour or lifestyle dimension of health and all healthcare system factors), as well as all the environmental risks/hazardous factors (physical, biological, psychological, socio-cultural, economical, etc.),and all the properties of the identified infectious agent. Furthermore, the data to be collected regarding the health status of all hosts must include

- all subjective data (data reported by all ill persons or significant others and as such cannot be validated by the healthcare practitioner)
- all objective data (data that are observed, described and verified by the healthcare practitioner)
- all historical data (information about the past of all hosts that influence their current health status)

- all current data (data that reflect all present factors [negatively and positively] affecting the health of all hosts).

PLEASE NOTE

The order in which the data gathering/assessment process is described in this book is done solely on the basis of convenience. **In order to prevent the non-assessment of any element in the Epidemiological Triad of Communicable Diseases,** the assessment of the properties of the specific identified infectious agent is discussed first, followed by the assessment of the environment (physical, biological, psychological, socio-cultural, economical, and others). The assessment of the different host-groups are discussed last - first the assessment of the community followed by the assessment of the family. The assessment of the individual host is presented at the end as the specific data gathering base-line is discussed in-depth. BUT**, healthcare providers will found that in the practical healthcare rendering situation, the assessment to be done, is completely reversed from the theoretical presentation in this book. Always remember that the individual person must be assessed first, before the family, the community, the environment and the disease causing agent can be assessed and healthcare interventions designed.** Also take in account that sometimes, after the infectious agent has been identified, a new database has to be compiled through the re-assessment of both the hosts and environment, and the healthcare interventions have to be re-designed as to align it to the identified properties of the specific infectious agent

8.1.1.1 Identifying the properties of the specific infectious agent (pathogen)

To render the necessary fundamental and specific healthcare to all individuals/ families/communities (whether healthy, ill, contact, carrier), and because any particular communicable disease is caused by a specific pathogen, the causative pathogen must be identified by different laboratory tests and investigations. The description of the main properties of all pathogens has already been done in chapter 1. Attention must be specifically given to **the specific properties** of the identified infectious agent as these properties are to be taken as the point of departure in the planning of all fundamental (general supportive and symptomatic) and specific individualized, compassionate, comprehensive, holistic and culturally congruent healthcare plans for individuals, families and communities. Simultaneously, specific healthcare interventions based on the database-line compiled, must be designed/redesigned to eliminate the specific pathogen as well as to prevent and control the spread of the identified communicable disease.

Note

As some of the healthcare interventions are executed in collaboration with environmental health officers and officials of appropriate governmental departments, these interventions are not discussed in detail, but the healthcare practitioner must give his/her cooperation in full

8.1.1.2 Identifying all the healthy attributes of and risks/hazards in the environment

Because environmental hazards lower the resistance of the body making it easier for infectious agents to invade the body, the health of the environment has to be maintained to prevent and control communicable diseases. All attributes of the community (whether healthy or hazardous) needs to be assessed as to plan preventive, promotive and reconstructive interventions to either enhance the health of the environment or to rectify the risks in the environment at the same time. The description of the importance of the environment and risks/hazards in the physical, biological, socio-cultural, psychological, economic and other environments/milieus was given in chapter 1 and 3. As the risks/hazards are of such magnitude and so multi-faceted, the main categories to be assessed, must be aligned to the identified infectious agent causing the particular communicable disease. Based on the database-line compiled, specific interventions must be designed to rectify the identified health risks/hazards in the environment, while at the same time, control the spread of and prevent further outbreaks of the identified communicable disease. Special attention must also be given to aspects such as

- settlement – formal or informal
- safe water supplies
- sanitation system in use - water-borne, pit privy, burying, other
- garbage disposal system used by local authority - burning or burying
- housing - brick, hut, corrugated iron, other and air conduction in homes
- sensitive occupations as well as work environment, contacts and contact material, nature of work which may predispose the individual to come in contact with a communicable disease
- mosquito-proofing of houses, the use of other mosquito repellents
- the presence of biological vectors such as rats and mice and other animals, insects
- sick animals - pets, livestock, wild and exotic animals/birds/reptiles
- chemical and gaseous hazards such as water pollution and air pollution as well as physical, biological, and chemical gases that aid environmental hazards
- urbanization – high density populations contribute to closer contact between persons as well as between people and animals (vectors).

The health environment in the home and the hospital or clinic, including housekeeping, laundry and sanitation, also needs to be regularly assed and monitored as it can become a source of infection and positively enhances the spread of communicable diseases.

Note

As most of these healthcare interventions are executed in collaboration with environmental health officers and officials of appropriate governmental departments, these interventions are not discussed in detail. Healthcare providers must not only identify the risks/hazards in the environment and bring it to the attention of the environmental health officers but also give his/her cooperation in full during the execution of the necessary interventions

8.1.1.3   Confirming the health status of the host-system

The host-system refers to the individual person, his/her family and the community they live in. Thus, the assessment of the health status and health needs of the hosts-system must include the individual (healthy, ill, contact, carrier), his/her family (as individuals and as a group) and the community (as individuals and as a group) wherein he/she lives. The assessment of the individual person must be comprehensive (all subjective data, all objective data, all historical data and all current data) and include all dimensions of health, namely, the bio-physical dimension of health, the psychological dimension of health, the socio-cultural dimension of health, the behaviour or lifestyle dimension of health, and all healthcare system factors. Based on the database-line compiled, a diagnosis of healthy, ill, carrier, contact must be made regarding all individual persons/all individual members of family/all individual members of a group/community and of the family and community as individual units. As the individual person always relates to other persons (as a member of a family, a group and a community), the effects (both direct and indirect) of the family/group/ community on the health and personhood of the individual must also be explored and recorded. Also, based on the database-line compiled, all the fundamental (general supportive and symptomatic) and all the specific healthcare interventions must be designed to render personalized, comprehensive, holistic and culturally congruent healthcare to the individual host (whether healthy, ill, carrier, contact), his/her family and the community wherein they live.

8.1.1.3.1   Confirming the health status of the community as host-unit

As the community as a whole or part of the community or certain groups in the community can contract the particular communicable disease identified, all attributes (healthy and problematic) of the community must be assessed as to plan preventive, promotive and reconstructive interventions to prevent and control the spread of the identified communicable disease. The community wherein the ill individual lives is constituted of all formal and informal groups that are interdependent on one another and whose function it is to meet the collective needs of the group members. Because the ill individual and his/her family are members of a specific community and because the possibility always exists that the community as a system or only specific members of the community can become ill, **the community (as an unit) always forms part of the host system of the ill person and must therefore be meticulously assessed.** The description of the attributes of the community that has to be taken in account has already been given in chapter 1. Attention must be given specifically to the most important characteristics considered necessary. An assessment of all socio-cultural attributes must be done as they may contribute to the infection/disease or may constrain the control of the disease. All those cultural customs and practices that the ill individual and his/her family will follow/adhere to during illness and recovery or death (when the ill person dies) must also be assessed. Furthermore, all traditional healthcare practices/customs to enhance, to maintain and to restore health and wellness should be used as the basis for culturally congruent healthcare rendering.

8.1.1.3.2   Confirming the health status of the family as host-unit

To render all the necessary support to the family, all attributes (healthy and problematic) of the family need to be identified as to plan and execute preventive, promotive and reconstructive interventions for the family as a unit. As such, the ill individual's family (whether monogamous or polygamous) are individuals (infants, children, adults, elderly) living in a nuclear conjugal family/an extended family/a same gender (gay or lesbian) family/a single-parent family/a step family/a cohabiting family/a tribal family (married

315

according to traditional marriage laws)/a communal family (families living in communes) or an inter-racial family. The description of the attributes of the family that has to be taken in account has already been given in chapter 1. As every family is a social system that has its own cultural values, specific functions and structure, and moves through recognizable developmental stages, the family as a unit (as individual members and as a system) has to be assessed. Particular attention must be given to all characteristics of the family as the ill individual reflects his/her family in conceptualization, behaviour, beliefs and rituals. Attention must also be given to a history of illnesses (including communicable diseases) suffered by the family members as well as the health status of other individual family members, friends, and strangers who have had visited the family or to whom visits had been made by the family (families/groups/communities). Sensitive occupations held by individual family members must also be clarified.

8.1.1.3.3 Confirming the health status of the individual as a healthy, ill, contact, carrier host

To plan and to render the correct personalized, comprehensively, empathically, holistically and culturally congruent healthcare to all individual hosts within their familial and community context, the health status of the individual must be assessed and confirmed (either a state of wellness or a state of disease or a state of contact or a state of carrier). The state of health of the individual person, the individual members of the family, and the individual members of the community is determined by the interplay of all the multiple factors of the different dimensions of health – the combined effect influencing the individual person's exposure, susceptibility and response to the infectious agent. The description of the attributes of the individual as person and the dimensions of health that have to be taken in account has already been given in chapter 1. Based on the classification of the health status of the individual (healthy or ill or contact or carrier), culturally congruent preventive, promotive, curative (fundamental and specific) and rehabilitative healthcare interventions that are individualized, comprehensively, empathically and holistically in nature have to planned and executed.

* **Confirming the wellness status of the individual as a healthy host**
  The assessment of the bio-physical dimension of health, the psychological dimension of health, the socio-cultural dimension of health, the behaviour or lifestyle dimension of health, and all healthcare system factors, must confirm the wellness state of the individual person, the individual members of the family and individual members of the community. All healthcare interventions (preventive and promotive) to be planned and implemented must enhance the wellness state of all the individuals (as persons, as members of the family and as members of the community).

* **Confirming the health status of an individual as a contact host**
  The assessment of the bio-physical dimension of health, the psychological dimension of health, the socio-cultural dimension of health, the behaviour or lifestyle dimension of health, and all healthcare system factors, must confirm the "at risk" state of the individual, the family and the community. Depending on the data obtained, contacts must be diagnosed as healthy, immune or

susceptible. All healthcare interventions to be planned and implemented aimed at healthy and immune individual, familial and community contacts must enhance their wellness state. Simultaneously, all susceptible (individuals, families and communities) contacts must be kept under observation, prophylactic treatment must be commenced immediately (when necessary) and quarantine measures must be instated as necessary because they are "at risk" to become ill. As soon as any contact - individuals, family members, community members (regardless whether diagnosed as healthy, immune or susceptible) complain of or present with any prodromal signs and symptoms of the particular identified communicable disease, the person must be **immediately re-diagnosed** as ill (sick). A new database-line must now be compiled and a new individualised, comprehensively, empathically, holistically and culturally congruent healthcare plan, based on the non-specific and characteristic-specific signs and symptoms of the particular identified communicable disease, must be designed and implemented. The spread of the specific disease must also be controlled. All the individuals the ill contact has been in contact with are now regarded as susceptible contacts and the process is repeated.

* **Confirming the health status of an individual as a carrier host**
In all relevant cases and based on the nature of the particular identified communicable disease, such as meningitis, poliomyelitis, diphtheria, typhoid fever and cholera, etc., it must be ascertained whether any carrier(s) has/have been responsible for/contributed to the outbreak of the specific communicable disease. The assessment of the bio-physical dimension of health, (including the necessary laboratory tests) must confirm the carrier state of the individual(s). Depending on the data obtained, carriers must be diagnosed as a healthy or temporary/recovering or permanent/chronic or intermittent carrier. Treatment must be immediately commenced and the carrier(s) must comply with all legislative measures laid down (parents take responsibility for their child/children). Where necessary, long term follow-up of carriers must be done.

* **Confirming the sickness status of an ill/sick individual as an sick host**
The assessment of the bio-physical dimension of health, the psychological dimension of health, the socio-cultural dimension of health, the behaviour or lifestyle dimension of health, and all healthcare system factors, must confirm the sickness state of the individual, and/or family member(s) and/or community member(s). The healthcare assessment of all ill persons suffering from any particular communicable disease to be carried out, must be comprehensive - consisting of all subjective data, objective data, historical data and current data of all biomedical factors and all socio-cultural factors and as such include all dimensions of health, namely, the bio-physical dimension of health, the psychological dimension of health, the socio-cultural dimension of health, the behaviour or lifestyle dimension of health, and all healthcare system factors

In compiling the data base-line, the data base-line must always be based on both the subjective and objective data obtained. All subjective data is collected when a health history is taken while all objective data is collected when a physical examination is done and the necessary specimens collected for diagnostic and special investigations.

❖ **Subjective data to be collected during the compilation of the data base-line health history**

The subjective data to be collected are mostly collected by an interview (structured or semi-structured) to assess the interplay of all the multiple factors influencing the ill person's health. Aspects to be included in the interview schedule are cultural, religious, familial and personal attitudes to and all practices related to health and disease. The information can be supplied by the ill person himself/herself as well as/or by any significant person of the ill person's choice (in case of a child the parent[s], great parent[s], care giver[s] or any other person who has intimate knowledge of the child must be the informant[s]). Because the healthcare practitioner cannot verify the information given, the information must be comprehensive and in detail as to give a broad and in depth picture of the ill person, his /her family and the community he/she lives in. Always keep in mind that the information gathered is directional in the planning of all interventions to care for the ill individual as well as in the control and prevention of further outbreaks of the particular communicable disease.

The health history of the ill person is taken down to collect all subjective data pertaining to the ill individual/person. In this chapter only the subjective data relevant to communicable diseases which demand special attention will be discussed. (Data that must be obtained for a complete health history and physical examination are set out in other literature). The data to be collected during the taking down of the health history is set out in table 8.1. Although the data is set out in such a way that it must be obtained from the ill person himself/herself or significant other person(s), information relating to the family, community and environment can be obtained from other sources. During history taking, data must also be collected, amongst others, to determine whether the ill person must be hospitalised or can be cared for at home (see table 8.3).

It is also important to determine the ill person's immunological (innate and adaptive) resistance as well as the number of infections (general and communicable) he/she has had, and how often these have occurred as well as the presence of other non-communicable diseases. The ill person's vaccination history must also be taken (especially if the ill person is a child or an adolescent or a young adult). Regarding the family's history of illnesses, data referring to communicable diseases that have occurred in the family provide valuable information.

Table 8.1   SUBJECTIVE DATA TO BE COLLECTED DURING THE HISTORY TAKING REGARDING THE ILL PERSON

BIO-GRAPHICAL AND SOCIAL DATA PERTAINING TO THE ILL PERSON

* Surname and first names
* Date of birth and age
* Gender
* Partnership or type of family system living in
* Home address - **physical address** (not postal address)
* Telephone and cell numbers
* Medical fund (check whether certain diseases are covered or not) and/or pension number
* Occupation and income (individual and family)
* General practitioner (family doctor) or usual source of healthcare provider
* Religion
* Cultural grouping or ethnic heritage
* Mother tong language

THE BIOPHYSICAL DIMENSION OF HEALTH

Main complaint
* Reason for visit
* Details concerning the signs and symptoms:
  * <u>Onset</u> Date, nature of onset, precipitating and predisposing factors
  * <u>Characteristics</u> Nature, localization and distribution, intensity or severity (quality), frequency, duration, factors which relieve or intensify signs and symptoms, associated signs or symptoms
  * <u>Course</u> Progress, effect of treatment
  * <u>Effect</u> Daily living and/or work/school, leisure activities

Medical history
* <u>Communicable disease</u>
  All communicable diseases that the person already had contracted
  Knowledge of a communicable disease that has broken out in the vicinity (school, work, friends) or of persons in the area who suffer from a communicable disease
* <u>Tests and investigation done previously and reasons why</u>
  Tuberculin, Schick and Widal tests and other investigations (microscopic and culture) done as well as x-rays taken
* <u>Allergies</u>
  Food, environmental elements, animals, medications, textiles and other substances
* <u>Hospitalisation</u>
  Periods and reasons for admittance
* <u>Vaccination</u>
  A complete history of vaccination is most important when the ill person is a child – less so for older adults. The date of the last tetanus vaccination is particularly important where older

children, adolescents and adults (including the elderly) have been injured. If the ill person has travelled to foreign countries - compulsory vaccinations received for entry into a specific country

✳ Treatment and Medicines
Drugs taken according to a doctor's prescription, the reason for this and the period of treatment. Medicines bought over the counter, such as herbal medicines, homeopathic medicines and the period of time taking it. Medicines prescribed by a sangoma (traditional healthcare practitioner) and the period of use thereof. Religious, magical, cultural practices and scientific treatments adhering to when taking drugs

✳ Chronic disease conditions
A complete history of all diseases suffering from (genetically and other medical conditions). Genetically determined illnesses prevalent in family and community

✳ Age-related conditions (medical and communicable diseases) prevalent in individuals, families and community

✳ Age-composition of family and community in relation to communicable diseases and age-related health concerns

Physiological functioning of the body systems
The general health/abnormal functioning/failure of body organs and systems and body parts

✳ General
*General state of health (for the past month)
*Period of weakness or malaise
*Ability to perform daily activities
*Inability to concentrate
*Anorexia
*Recent significant weight loss
*Lethargy and fatigue
*Pyrexia - highest peak, manner of fluctuation, duration, nature of own treatment
*Attacks of rigor
*Perspiration pattern, night sweats
*Weight
*Growth pattern (for babies and children)

✳ Skin
*Intactness of skin
*Changes in colour, temperature, moistness
*Tendency to bruising, petechiae, ecchymosis, pruritis
*Rash - onset, duration, body part on which rash first appeared, distribution, nature (macular, maculo-papular, vesicular, pustular, haemorrhagic, urticaria), stages of development, colour, swelling, smarting, itchiness, discharge and scab formation

✳ Nails - changes in colour, cyanotic nail bed

✳ Hair - alopecia, change in texture

✳ Face - paralysis, facial distortions and abnormalities

✳ Sensory organs
*Eyes: photophobia, burning, itchiness, pain, redness, discharge, visual disturbances such as blurring
*Ears: tinnitus, vertigo, discharge, earache, ear infections, hearing loss

* Pulmonary-respiratory system
  *Nose and sinuses: rhinitis, epistaxis, nasal catarrh, pain in the infra-orbital area, post-nasal discharge
  *Coughing, *sputum, *stridor, *wheezing *respiratory distress, *orthopnoea, *dyspnoea, *haemoptysis, *chest pain
* Gastro-intestinal system (alimentary system)
  *Mouth: bleeding, exudative lesions, blisters, ulcers, increased or decreased salivation, problem to open and close mouth, halitosis
  *Throat: sore throat, hoarseness, problem with swallowing, feeling of discomfort or swelling in the throat
  *Change in appetite and stools (frequency, composition, amount, consistency, odour and colour), *diarrhoea, *abdominal pain, *colic, *nausea, *vomiting, *constipation *haematemesis, *jaundice, *melaena stools
  *Hepatic system: discomfort/dyspepsia, anorexia, pruritis, alteration in nutritional status, fluid and electrolyte (fluid volume deficit or volume excess), activity intolerance
* Urinary tract and system
  *Dysuria, *urgency, *frequency, *supra-pubic pain, *oliguria, *incontinence, *changes in colour or odour of urine, *haematuria, *purulent discharges
* Genital tract and reproductive system
  *Genital discharges, *genital lesions such as ulcerations and chancres, *changes in menstrual cycle, *sexual history and activities (when necessary), *dispareunia,
* Central and peripheral nervous system
  *Headache associated with stiffness of neck, *pyrexia, *photophobia, *vomiting not associated with food intake, *rash,* convulsions
  *Vertigo, *syncope, *history of black-outs, *behaviour changes, *phobias, *hallucinations, *changes in cognitive ability, *motor and sensory problems, *paraesthesia, *poor coordination, *Sleeping: disturbed sleeping pattern, insomnia, tendency to sleep more than usual
  *Mental status: anxiety, confusion, delirium, stupor, coma, loss of consciousness, changes in level of consciousness, changes in mood and behaviour, changes in communication and speech, aphasia and dysarthria, changes in perception,
  *Changes in sensory status (pain, temperature, touch, mobility and position)
* Muscular-skeleton system
  *Extremities: discolouration, oedema, limited movement, paralysis
  *Muscles: aches, cramps, weakness, *weakening of muscles in face
  *Joints: pain, stiffness, swelling, redness, backaches and pains in the neck
  *Neck: pain, stiffness of neck, limited movement
* Haematopoietic system and Reticulo-endothelial system
  *Tendency to bleeding, *enlarged glands, *enlarged lymph nodes,* liver pain,*haemoglobin and haematocrit, *anaemia, *lymph-oedema
* Cardiovascular system
  *Palpitations, *chest pains, *tiredness, *oedema, *irregular pulse, *tachycardia, *bradycardia, *syncope, *fatigue
* Immunological system
  *Communicable diseases contracted and vaccinations received

*Physiological maturity of the individual's immunological system (premature and newborn infants have an immature immunological system while the immunological system of elderly persons diminishes with age)

*Diseases suffering or suffered from that leads to immunodeficiency

*Recurrent infections and recurrent fevers

*Allergies: food, contrast mediums, pollen, insect stings, medications, other substance

✳ Nutritional status

*Nutritional habits

*Appetite

*Well-nourished

*Under-nourished

*Malnourished

Please note : Malnutrition, on the one hand, helps to reduce the incidence of certain diseases (for example, typhus, malaria) due to a reduction in immuno-pathology while, on the other hand, predisposes the individual to greater severity of many other diseases (for example, measles, meningococcal infection, tuberculosis)

CULTURAL-BASED ATTITUDE TOWARDS ANATOMICAL STRUCTURE AND PHYSIOLOGICAL FUNCTIONING OF THE BODY AND PRESCRIBED CULTURAL AND RELIGIOUS PRACTICES RELATED TO HEALTH AND DISEASE

➤ The ill individual's and family's perception of health and disease (as culturally, familial and personal defined); their acceptance of healthcare programs; as well as cultural, familial and personal influence re compliance with the suggested healthcare regimen(s)

➤ Beliefs regarding the causation of disease and disability and treatment to be rendered

➤ Individual and familial perception of a diagnosis and treatment regime as well as scientific medical diagnosis's prevailing in family and community

➤ Folk designation of physical diseases and folk classification of diseases

➤ Cultural, religious, familial, and personal prescribed practices related to health and disease - preventive practices, promotive practices, curative practices, and rehabilitative practices

➤ Cultural, familial and personal significance attached to certain body parts (for example, head, heart, hands, genitals etc.) as it influence the acceptance of scientific medical procedures such as examination, transfusion, autopsy of the body

➤ Cultural, familial, and personal attitudes to bodily (anatomical and physiological) functions and hygiene practices (cleansing of body, skin-, hair-, and care of teeth)

➤ Cultural, familial, and personal significance of exposure of certain body parts, touching of body parts and who may touch them (opposite sex or same sex), physiological functions in terms of modesty and privacy as well as periods during which individuals are considered ritually unclean

➤ Cultural, familial, and personal attitude and beliefs regarding mental illnesses; occurrence of significant health problems; the importance of individual versus group goals; modes of authority and decision-making; and attitudes towards change and the character of relationships with the larger society

➤ Familial and personal beliefs in folk/traditional medicine and folk diseases (including culture bound syndromes); use of herbal and other traditional treatment and being treated by traditional practitioners

> Primary and secondary preventive healthcare measures taken by the individual, the family and the community
> Potential harmful folk healthcare practices used by individual and family
> Relationship of folk (traditional) and scientific healthcare systems within the family and community and to what extent do family members use both systems, the family's preference for one specific system and system used first by family when ill/sick
> Behaviour expected in one's interaction with others in wellness/disease/disability/death
> Cultural attitudes to age (for example, elderly and children)
> Gender of the ill individual and gender inequities that prevails

PSYCHOLOGICAL DIMENSION OF HEALTH

* Coping skills
* Ability to adapt to change
* Level of emotional maturity
* Self-esteem
* Abilities and strengths
* Coping mechanisms
* Developmental tasks accomplished (functional, interpersonal, psychosocial)
* Levels of stress and anxiety and coping mechanisms
* Emotional support available or lack availability of emotional support
* Attitude to life, health, disease, death and dying
* Cognitive and emotional status
* Emotional status (mood)
* Fears
* Worries (for example, financial, pets, children, housing etc.)
* Reaction to disease (being sick) and caring
* Personal space

CULTURAL ASPECTS OF IMPORTANCE

> Confidant(s) in times of crisis
> Reticence regarding personal matters
> Expectations regarding care to be rendered and care providers
> Importance of familial and personal tokens and cultural totems
> Importance of visitors and contact with the outside world
> Value of children and their socialization
> Kinship ties, family-centeredness and extended family
> Behaviours that are considered aberrant in the family and community
> Social space

SOCIO-CULTURAL DIMENSION OF HEALTH

* Desirable health behaviour
* Desirable illness behaviour
* Desirable role behaviour
* Role behaviour in disease (acute and chronic roles)

* Accepted modes of behaviour
* Cultural, social and personal norms adhering to
* Social networks
* Religious affiliation (including religious practices, religious health practices, religious beliefs re death, dying and burial practices), as well as the emotional aspects of religion - comfort or joy, ritualistic, idealistic (beliefs, dogma), standards of conduct expected of members and integration of religious beliefs and practices to be incorporated in healthcare
* Prevailing social attitude re health, disease (medical and communicable diseases) and disability
* Situational constraints in social milieu

CULTURAL ASPECTS OF IMPORTANCE

➤ Time orientation of individual, family and community, for example, future-orientated persons/families/communities have long-range goals, while present-orientated persons/families/communities do not plan their activities by a clock or calendar but respond to needs as they arise, and past-orientated persons/families/communities dwell in the past (whether something should/could have been done differently)
➤ Interpersonal relationships and commitment to family and social group as well as rules governing these relationships
➤ Gender roles and task-division in the family and community life as well as roles and task-division in health as well as in acute and chronic diseases, disabilities and death
➤ Organizational structure of family life, structure and patterns of residence as well as family ties
➤ Role and status of individual family members
➤ Language and communication (both verbal and non-verbal); the context in which the message is conveyed and contextual considerations; culturally prescribed reticence (openness about personal matters and direct eye contact); courtesy titles (hugs and kisses, handshakes, and/or bows); epithets (word and phrases that are derogatory in nature) and gestures
➤ Cultural, familial, and personal beliefs and values regarding mankind, nature and non-nature, time and life (present, past, and future); activities, interpersonal relationships (for example, competitiveness/non-competitiveness) and material goods
➤ The relative priority given to different values by the individual, the family and the community
➤ Magic and religion – beliefs and attitude, and religious beliefs and practices incorporated in healthcare
➤ Appropriate demeanour in interpersonal relationships – acceptable/unacceptable behaviour and modes of address (formal and informal)
➤ Spatial orientation and use of individual social, interpersonal and personal space
➤ Acceptance of the chronic sick role in the family and community after complications have set in and the ill person does not recover completely
➤ Typical childrearing practices adhered to by the family and community
➤ Social organization regarding support by family members and social-group organization (for example, family visits and presence in care and providing necessary follow-up care after discharge)

BEHAVIOR DIMENSION OF HEALTH AND LIFESTYLE FACTORS

* Employment and sensitive occupations of ill individual and family members as well as the nature of employment and effect of disease on employment. For children the school situation has to considered, infants – day care facilities, toddlers – pre-school facilities, and older children (7-18 yrs) – school facilities as well as the effect of the disease on the education of the child

* Consumption patterns
  * food preferences and consumption patterns of ill individual
  * the use of certain foods as primary and/or secondary preventive measures by ill individual and family
  * specific nutrients (micro and macro) lacking in the diet of ill individual and family
  * nutritional habits of the individual/family/community that enhances or undermines the innate immune system of a person
  * other foodstuffs recently consumed that are not part of the daily diet; when it was purchased and how it was prepared
  * pattern of daily intake of food and composition of meals
  * level of activity
  * appetite
  * facilities for obtaining food, source of water supply, source of milk and use of un-pasteurised/pasteurised milk, purchase of meat (abattoir, butchery or other source)
  * cultural rituals/taboos regarding food
  * methods and practices of food preparation
  * use of alcohol during meals
  * use of nutritional additives (for example, capsules, tablets etc)

* Activities of daily living – personal hygiene, sleeping pattern, relaxation activities, cultural activities, sexual history and practices (including the number of unrelated sexual partners)

* Rest and exercise patterns

* Language (mother tongue)

* Level of educational and economic welfare of individual, family and community

* Using/not using of drugs, making use of injections during drug abuse and/or the sharing of needles and injections

* Patterns of alcohol and tobacco use

* Leisure and other lifestyle factors such as
  * leisure activities (swimming or fishing in infested rivers), outdoor camping, touring of own country, hiking
  * recreational activities and type of materials being used
  * art, cultural and educational activities
  * keeping of pets (dogs, cats, birds and other animals such as mammals [apes], reptiles whether domestic, wild, exotic) and/or farming with any animal/avian/reptile species
  * the individual's sexual behaviour and activities
  * travelling and exploring of foreign territory
    * countries as well as specific areas/scenery visited
    * sanitary facilities and refuse disposal facilities at the places visited

✠ general environmental hygiene of the places visited

✠ sources of food at places visited for example, meat, milk, water, vegetables and fruit

✠ sleeping arrangements for example, camping, hostels

- friendships and family visits received and made

✠ domestic visits to known endemic areas

✠ general visits made and received (± past 4 weeks)

✠ visits to people who were ill during visit

✠ visits received form persons who became ill during the visit

✠ persons visited or guests with children who have never had any communicable diseases or have never been vaccinated/partially vaccinated

✠ the children of the abovementioned persons or guests who attend pre-primary, primary and secondary schools, tertiary educational institutions or are in the army

✠ sanitary facilities and refuse disposal facilities at the places visited

✠ general environmental hygiene at the places visited

✠ pets and/or other animals (domestic, wild, exotic) of persons who were visited or kept by guests

✠ sources of food at places visited, for example, meat, milk, vegetables, fruit, and water

CULTURAL ASPECTS OF IMPORTANCE IN LIFESTYLE BEHAVIOURS

➢ Level of acculturation

➢ Cultural, religious, familial and personal prescribed practices related to lifestyle

➢ Lifestyle regarding diet practices - food preference, therapeutic uses of food, social and religious symbolism of food, methods of preparation, frequency of meals and regularity of consumption patterns, food practices [sharing, eating alone]; fasting; discouragement of foods when ill/dying

➢ Life events – cultural practices during birth (including pregnancy, labour, delivery and postpartum care); cultural practices regarding death and dying (rites, caregivers, afterlife, reincarnation); fears; mourning; clothing and funerals

➢ Whether family members to be informed of approaching death, who should be present at time of death; mode of disposal of body after death; special practices related to grief and mourning; legislation and death practices

➢ Religious customs regarding life and life-events

➢ Level of education

❖ **Objective data to be collected**

Objective data is all data that can be observed, described, and verified as such by the healthcare practitioner. Objective data are collected by a physical/ clinical examination; investigations done such as tests, microscopy and culture studies; sonar, CAT-scans, MRI-scans, X-rays taken; observations made; a review of all medical records and diagnostic reports and through collaboration with multi-professional team members. The healthcare professional must collect the objective data self or refer the ill individual for specialized medical investigations.

To complete the database, a physical examination has to be performed on the ill person and special investigations have to be carried out to obtain the necessary objective data such as the severity of the infection; the overall clinical manifestation of the infection; complications already set in; and the identification of the causative pathogen. The data to be obtained during the physical examination concerns the various systems of the body and general health of the ill person while the investigations to be done, must confirm the preliminary diagnosis. The specific data to be obtained during the physical examination are set out in table 8.2.1 and the investigations to done, is set out in table 8.2.2. (See relevant literature for a complete exposition of the physical examination and investigations to be done for infants, toddlers, children, adolescents, adults, and elderly).

Note

When performing the physical/clinical examination, it is of utmost importance to be knowledgeable of the cultural mind/attitude/character and meaning of the word "privacy". Where there exist a public mind of "privacy" during medical procedures, "privacy means away from other persons but not alone/isolated for long periods of time", for example, during the performance of the examination procedure, family members or friends or even strangers may enter/look into the room/cubicle to see what is happening and chat to the person being examined because there is no need to hide anything from each other. The companions of the ill person may at times even become the main informants and assistants to the healthcare practitioners. The meaning given to spatial orientation by a specific group or culture also plays a role in the interpretation of privacy

In some cultures, male healthcare practitioners may not examine a female healthcare user without the physical presents of a male family member, whether husband, brother, father, or any other male member appointed by the family. Female healthcare user may not, in some cultures, answer any questions without permission granted by the male head of the household (sometimes, the male head member may answer all or part of the questions on behalf of the ill female individual), nor take any decisions regarding the care to be rendered to her. Sometimes, the ill female individual may even refuse to listen to any healthcare practitioner (especially a male practitioner) until such time that medical prescriptions and orders have been explained to the head male family member and he has talked to her and given his permission in person to her to follow the prescriptions. In some cultures women are totally forbidden to be touched by men or men by women

Table 8.2.1 SPECIFIC DATA TO BE OBTAINED BY MEANS OF THE PHYSICAL EXAMINATION THAT MUST BE PERFORMED

BODY SYSTEMS AND BODY PARTS	DATA TO BE OBTAINED DURING THE EXAMINATION
General appearance	General state of health Signs of anxiety or distress Facial expression, skin colour, mood, speech Posture, movements and gait Nutritional status Dress, grooming and personal hygiene Breath and body odour Mental status
Vital signs	Body temperature, pulse, respiration, blood pressure (for example, hypotension with clinical picture of shock)
Head and face	Form of face, ability to use facial muscles Speech - intensity, pitch, speed and articulation
Skin	Skin colour and pigmentation Hydration of skin Skin turgor and elasticity Vascularity and erythema Rash Temperature of skin Texture and thickness Odour
Nails	Hygiene, colour, form, suppleness Skin around nails, change in colour, swelling, tenderness and infective conditions
Hair	Local or total loss of hair Changes in texture and characteristics Hygiene - lice, mites, nits, dandruff
Eyes	Cardinal directions of gaze Colour of conjunctiva and sclera Ocular pressure and ocular movement Pupils - size, form, alikeness, and reaction of pupils to light Discharges Eyelids - ptosis, ectropion, entropion Pupillary reflexes and acuity of vision Lens - transparent or opaque
Ears	Sound changes in auscultation of auricle and mastoid bone External tract - pus, blood or serous discharge Tympanic membrane - otitis media (acute, chronic or serous) Hearing acuity Balance and gait

Nose and sinuses	Discharges and forming of membranes, runny nose Sinuses - tenderness of frontal and maxillary Nostrils - colour, oedema, exudate Nasal obstruction - breathing through mouth while voice has a nasal tone
Mouth and pharynx	Lips - colour, moistness, ulcers, pendulous lip Mouth cavity - fissures, ulcers, chancres Gums - colour, redness, pallor and bleeding Buccal mucosa - Koplik's spots, pallor, bleeding, redness Tongue - coating, redness, whiteness Oropharynx - colour, oedema, forming of membranes, ulcerations, discharges, exudate and elevation of the uvula and soft palate Halitosis or any other odour Tonsils - ulcerations, discharges
Neck	Enlarged lymph nodes - location, characteristics, consistency symmetry, mobility and discomfort on palpation (extending to the entire body) Determination of stiffness of neck Trachea - position
Chest and lungs	Posterior and anterior chest - skin, respiration and form, symmetry of expansion Lungs - resonance - normal, additional and abnormal respiratory sounds Rib retraction during breathing Breathing pattern
Heart and pulse	Heart murmurs, tachycardia, bradycardia, dysrhythmia, skin colour and colour of mucous membranes
Abdomen	Skin temperature, abdominal tenderness, muscle stiffness, enlargement of liver and spleen, increased bowl sounds
Genitals	Ulcers, chancres, painless lesions, Condylomata, discharges, erythema and warts, pubic hair for lice and mites, inspection and palpation of the female external genitalia (including perineum and anus), inspection of the penis and anal-rectal area, palpation of the scrotum Enlargement of lymph nodes
Extremities and back	Muscles spasms, paralysis and curvature
Neurological system	Cerebellar system Motor nervous system - muscle tonus, muscle strength, presence of reflexes and tremors, gait and stance, coordination Sensory nervous system - pain, light touch, vibration and stereognostic perception Cranial nerves and protective reflexes Meningeal irritation Breathing pattern and oxygenation status Thermoregulation Bowel and urinary elimination

Table 8.2.2 SPECIAL INVESTIGATIONS AND TESTS TO BE DONE

The special investigations to be performed are
* non-specific investigations to be done when an infection is suspected but has not yet been confirmed
* collecting of specimens for identification and/or isolation of the pathogenic microbe
* requesting specific diagnostic tests.

Based on the result of these tests, treatment interventions will then be prescribed.

* **NON-SPECIFIC INVESTIGATIONS**

These investigations are done to determine the presence or absence of an inflammatory reaction in the body. Non-specific investigations comprise investigating for signs and symptoms of an infection, rashes, the presence of arthropods, as well as anything that can be seen, heard, felt, tasted and smelled which may be indicative of the presence of an infection. Non-specific investigating is divided into local and systemic indications of an infection.

✠ **LOCAL INDICATORS OF AN INFECTION**

Signs of localized infection such as redness, warmness/heat, swelling, pain, tenderness and loss of function are observed on the limbs, torso, skin, face and mucosa. Sores, eczema, papulae, rashes, vesicles or pustules (not diffused), insect bites and stings, scratches, scabs, eschar, bite-marks from animals, arthropods such as fleas, lice (head, armpits and pubic hair), crawl passages (mites) and chancres may be observed on the skin and body. Discharges (serous, purulent or bloody) from body orifices such as the nose, urethra and vagina, as well as the eyes, can be observed. Coughs, rales and rhonchi can be heard while a runny nose, redness of throat can be seen as an indication of a respiratory tract infection. Objective data related to gastro-intestinal tract infection are vomiting and diarrhoea. Characteristic symptoms of genital-urinary tract infection are frequency, burning and painful micturition, changes in colour or smell/odour of urine. Symptoms of generalized infection are fever, altered mental status, and tachycardia.

✠ **SYSTEMIC INDICATORS OF AN INFECTION**

A systemic infection is suspected based on the following biochemical analysis
> Clear indications of an infection are an increase in leucocytes in the body fluids, as well as in secretions and discharges such as in urine and cerebrospinal fluids; or in secretions from wounds (pus) and in peritoneal fluids
> An increase in leukocytes in the peripheral blood could also be an indication of an infection. For instance, an increase in lymphocytes indicates a virus infection, while an increase in phagocytic cells or neutrophils are an indication of a bacterial infection while an increase in eosinophils indicates a helminthic infection
> An increase in monocytes could be an indication of tuberculosis, brucellosis, syphilis, rickettsiae infections, and protozoan infections
> The rate of erythrocytic sedimentation increases when a mounting infection is present
> Anaemia (low red blood cell count) occurs with chronic infections. Anaemia is unusual in short-term acute infections with the exception of infections caused by pathogens such as the Epstein-Barr virus.
> Albuminuria; glucosuria; oliguria; and the presence of nitrates and leucocytes in the urine are also indicators of the presence of an infection

> An elevated C-reactive protein (CRP) concentration (>5 mg/L) is also an indicator of the presence of an infection. As chronic inflammation is not always revealed by CPR alone, other biomarkers need to be analysed, namely, alpha-1-acid glycoprotein (AGP - a second acute phase protein. With the onset of infection, the CRP increases rapidly before the onset of clinical signs, indicating the incubation phase of the disease. A raised CPR and a raised AGP indicate early convalescence (recently recovered) with the concentration of AGP rising slower (AGP takes 4-5 days to reach plateau concentrations {>1 g/L}). A normal CRP concentration (<5 mg/L) together with an elevated AGP indicates late convalescence as the concentration of AGP remains elevated for longer than the CRP concentration after clinical signs have disappeared. A normal concentration of the CRP and AGP indicates that the individual is healthy
> An elevated Pro-calcitonin blood level is an indication of a bacterial infection
> Hypotension
> Altered mental states such as confusion, convulsions, photophobia, hypersensitivity to noise
> Shock
> Tachycardia or brachycardia

✱ **IDENTIFICATION AND ISOLATION OF THE SPECIFIC INFECTIOUS PATHOGEN (CULTURE STUDIES) AND/OR ANTIBODY ALREADY FORMED (SEROLOGICAL TESTING)**
The identification and isolation of the specific pathogen is based on the collection of various types of specimens from the ill person. Proper collection and handling of laboratory specimens are essential to ensure accurate laboratory results. Cultures must be obtained in a manner that avoids contamination. Correct interpretation of laboratory results is a necessity.
- Specimens collected from the body fluids and body secretions and discharges such as blood, cerebrospinal fluid, urine and sputum. Such specimens are microscopically examined and cultivated in specific cultures for identification and isolation of the pathogen and drug sensitivity for treatment
- Serological testing for antibody can be requested such as precipitation reactions, haemagglutination assays; and the Enzyme-linked Immunosorbent Assay (ELISA)
- A biopsy can be done of the afflicted tissue. Specimens obtained for this purpose are prepared according to various techniques in order to facilitate identification of the specific pathogenic microbe.

✱ **REQUESTING SPECIFIC DIAGNOSTIC TESTS**
Tests such as the Schick, Widal or tuberculin test, Acid Fast Bacilli test can be specially requested. Radiographs (x-rays), ultrasound scans, computed topographical scans (CAT scan), and magnetic resonance imaging scans (MRI scan) can also be requested.

8.1.2 The culturally-holistic healthcare brokering phase

The aim of the culturally congruent and holistic healthcare brokering phase is to help/support the ill individual and his/her family to become self-caring (wholly or partially) leading to their self-actualization as human beings. As the ill individual and his/her family are not passive receivers of care but active participants in the healthcare and cultural brokering process, the healthcare provider must therefore ensure that the ill person actively partakes in his/her own care activities (where possible) while family members become partners of the provider in the brokering process. All healthcare activities must be under taken within the boundaries of all norms and values of the healthcare professions, the specific culture wherein the hosts and provider live and all interpersonal relationships. Comprehensive, compassionate, holistic and culturally congruent healthcare is only meaningful if it takes place within the context of healthcare user-healthcare provider-relationship and is family-centred. The healthcare provider uses himself/herself therapeutically in the healthcare user-healthcare provider-relationship when supporting the ill person and his/her family to become independent, self-caring and actualize themselves through living a meaningful life within their limitations (or supporting the ill person to die a dignified and humane death while supporting his/her family in their crisis situation).

8.1.2.1 Rendering of general fundamental (supportive and symptomatic) and specific individualized, comprehensive, holistic and culturally congruent healthcare to maintain, promote and restore health

The healthcare to be rendered to any individual suffering from a communicable disease/infection consists of both fundamental and specific support/help activities/ healthcare interventions to promote, maintain and restore health.

- The **fundamental interventions** consist of all general supportive and symptomatic healthcare activities to be set (to maintain health and protect health) regardless of the infection/diseases the individual suffers from and are rendered to the individual and his family within their familial, community and cultural context.
- The **specific healthcare activities** (to restore health) are specifically set for the particular communicable disease/infection and include all those specific medical and other professional care activities either to cure the disease; or to alleviate the symptoms of the disease/infection; or to render palliative care until the individual dies; or to prevent complications; or to help the individual to cope with the specific disability/disabilities when complications have set in as well as all those specific control measures set to control the spread of the particular communicable disease/ infection and to prevent further outbreaks of the particular communicable disease.

All fundamental and specific healthcare interventions to be set and rendered, must therefore consist of all primary, secondary and tertiary caring interventions (to maintain health, to protect health and to restore health) appropriate to the ill person's healthcare needs within his/her familial and community context (where possible). The priority given to a particular need of the ill individual is based on the degree to which it threatens the ill person's life/health or the ill person's concern about the particular need or its contribution to other health problems the ill individual experience. As all healthcare interventions can furthermore be classified as either daily living activities or therapeutic healthcare activities, both types of activities must thus also be included in the healthcare plan.

- **Daily living activities** forms part of the daily living of the ill person to maintain life (for example, comfort, safety, food consumption, hygiene, mobility, sleep, relaxation

COMMUNICABLE MEDICAL DISEASES

– all those activities related to the fulfilment of the ill person's daily habits, customs and health behaviour and grounded in the personal and cultural life of the ill person and his/her family). When possible, the ill person must always perform these activities himself/herself or if he/she is unable to do it himself/herself, he/she must be supported by his/her family or by the healthcare provider. As all daily living activities are personal and culturally-based, no need exist to change the execution of any of these activities except if it promotes the spread of the identified communicable disease. When necessary, **cultural brokering and bridging has to be done** to prevent imposition of the ill person and his/her family during the execution of all daily living activities as to meet the wellness needs of the ill person and his/her family.

■ **Therapeutic healthcare activities** (to restore health) are all those specific medical and other professional care activities/interventions set for the particular communicable disease/infection with the objective of either (1) curing the disease; or (2) alleviating the symptoms of the disease/infection; or (3) rendering palliative care until the individual dies; or (4) helping the individual to cope with the specific disability/disabilities when complications have set in, as well as (5) all those specific control measures set to control the spread of the particular communicable disease/infection and to prevent further outbreaks of the particular communicable disease. These activities are to be rendered by the healthcare provider(s) and to be taught to the ill person and/or his/her family to perform by himself/herself/ themselves because he/she/they does/do not have the knowledge, skills and competency to do it himself/herself/themselves.

Grounded on the above, **all** healthcare interventions set for the ill individual **must therefore consist of**

▪ **All fundamental daily living and supportive and and symptomatic care/ healthcare** activities as the general care to be rendered to all ill persons regardless of the communicable disease he/she suffers from.

▪ **All those specific therapeutic healthcare activities** set as based on and related to the diagnosis and course of the particular communicable disease.

The daily living and therapeutic care activities go hand in hand and are performed simultaneously or separately depending on the specific interventions and outcomes set.

When planning the culturally congruent and holistic healthcare interventions, the following activities have to be done, namely,

◈ stating the goals and objectives to be achieved through the care rendering
◈ establish the criteria by which the care rendering will be evaluated as well as the selection of the appropriate means to achieve the goals and objectives
◈ design the specific and individualized healthcare interventions to achieve the stated/desired outcomes relating to
  ✓ wellness care (enabling factors enhancing wellbeing),
  ✓ high-risk care (identifiable risk factors indicating preventive measures), and
  ✓ need-focused care (daily living activities and therapeutic healthcare to be performed or rendered).

Attention must specifically be given to all cultural factors that influences the scientific healthcare planned. To help the ill individual to become what he/she wants to become, must become and should become, the healthcare to be rendered must satisfy and be accepted by the ill person and his/her family. Therefore, all healthcare interventions must be in accordance with their cultural beliefs, convictions, norms and values, health behaviour, cultural health practices at primary, secondary and tertiary level and multi-dimensional lifestyle/pattern within the set boundaries for communicable diseases. To be able to achieve the preceding aim, the healthcare provider must do a comprehensive biomedical health assessment as well as a comprehensive culturally need assessment of the ill individual within his/her familial and community context. Simultaneously, the cultural interventions (based on the cultural diagnosis made) must be planned to be implemented. Thus, the goals and objectives of care rendering to be achieved **must include all cultural brokering and bridging interventions together with the scientific healthcare interventions that have to be rendered to the ill person and his/her family within their community context.**

After interpreting the data obtained regarding the ill person, his/her family and community and when compiling the healthcare plan, the healthcare practitioner has to consider

- the possibility that anti-microbial/antiviral therapy already has been commenced before the pathogen has been isolated and identified. All anti-microbial/antiviral treatment are to be commenced only after consideration was given to the side-effects, the cost, possible discomfort for the ill person, the route to be administered and duration of the treatment
- the information to be given to the ill person and his/her family as well as to the domestic worker (when necessary) regarding the particular communicable disease
- the measures to be taken to prevent the spread of the disease
- the tracing of contacts and carriers and the treatment to be given to them
- the availability of community resources for care rendering and rehabilitation
- notification, when the disease is a notifiable medical condition, and compliance with any other applicable legislation as well as the fact that the control programme will be monitored by either the Provincial or the National Department of Health
- quarantine and/or isolation regulations, and the enforcement of them
- the implementation and/or the enforcement of school exclusion regulations
- the introduction of a regime of prophylaxis for all involved (hosts [healthy, contact and carrier] and care givers)
- the measures to be implemented to maintain the health of the environment (physical-biological, psychological, socio-cultural, economical and others).

Not all ill persons suffering from communicable diseases require hospitalisation, therefore the healthcare provider must choose between home care or hospital care (see table 8.3). To make this decision the healthcare provider **must not** only rely on the data collected during the assessment phase but must **also consider** the disease/infection the ill person suffers from, risk factors in his/her environment and the support system available to the ill person. The specific data to be taken in account are

- ❖ the physical condition of the ill person - attention needs to be given to the properties of the specific infectious agent, the stage of development of the disease as well as the severity of the illness and the possibility of complications setting in

❖ the family of the ill person - the age of individual members, the susceptibility of the individual family members to the particular communicable disease and the ability of family members to care for the ill person

❖ the community wherein the ill person lives - the role that social, cultural, religious, occupational/school and other circumstances play in the lives of the individual and the family

❖ the environment - all factors in the environment (physical, biological, psychological, socio-cultural, economical and others) that had played a role (and is still playing a role) in the outbreak, contracting and spread of the particular communicable disease and in the maintaining of a healthy environment.

Table 8.3   DATA TO BE EVALUATED FOR EITHER HOME OR HOSPITAL CARE

RELEVANT DATA	DECISION
Is the degree of disease serious? Is the ill person's condition unstable? Is special care necessary, for instance, isolation?	When affirmative answers are given to more than two questions, the ill person has to be hospitalised
What type of communicable disease has been contracted	When certain serious diseases such as haemorrhagic diseases (Congo fever, Ebola fever etc.) and respiratory diseases (SARS, Avian flu, drug-resistant TB) are suspected, hospital care is compulsory regardless of any other considerations
WHEN HOME CARE IS CONSIDERED Are the living conditions adequate for taking care of the ill person? Is there a member of the family capable of taking care of the ill person? Is the food and water fit for consumption? Can the ill person and his/her family cope financially? Can the care-giver perform concurrent and terminal disinfection, when necessary? Will the rest of the family be able to support the ill person and the care-giver? Would the domestic helper or any other member of the family likely spread the disease?	If negative answers are given to more than three questions and the final question regarding the domestic helper/family members who are likely to spread the disease is in the affirmative, hospitalisation is indicated

Remember

1. The expected outcome goals and objectives and the care interventions must be accepted by the ill person and his/her family because if they do not accept it, they will not adhere to it (excluded are those circumstances where the ill person has to be isolated and/or legislative measures have to be enforced)

2. Documentation is a critical feature of all the phases of the healthcare brokering process to ensure an organized and systematic evidenced-base record of all data obtained (subjective, objective, historical and present), the healthcare that was rendered and the outcomes achieved. The healthcare plan has to be reviewed and updated continuously when changes in the ill person's health status occur, and/or when new or changed constraints in the environments (biological-physical, psychological, socio-cultural, economical, political etc.) occur, and/or after the causative pathogen has been identified

3. When a person becomes sick, he/she is scared and anxious – thus, the person wants to be surrounded what is culturally and familiar part of his/her everyday life. To obtain the best outcome for the ill person (whether child, adult or elderly), cultural brokering and healthcare brokering MUST BE DONE SIMULTANEOUSLY ON AN ONGOING BASIS by incorporating/merging of prescribed cultural customs and practices into/with scientifically-based healthcare interventions. Only when comprehensive, compassionate, holistic and culturally congruent healthcare is rendered, the needs of the ill person, his /her family and his/her community are fully met.

8.1.2.2 The fundamental healthcare interventions (general supportive and symptomatic) to be rendered to the ill person at home or in the hospital

As all the healthcare plans for all ill persons suffering from a communicable disease, must be comprehensive, compassionate, holistic and culturally congruent, a comprehensive healthcare plan consist of a number of components which must be adhered to. All fundamental healthcare (general supportive and symptomatic) to be rendered to all ill persons (see table 8.4) must always be accompanied by the specific therapeutic healthcare relevant to the particular communicable disease (as discussed under 8.1.2.3 and in theme IV under the various diseases). As cultural-care diversity and universality are so multi-faceted, only the biomedical aspects of care are described in full on the assumption that the healthcare provider will preserve, negotiate and restructure the healthcare to be rendered to maintain health, to protect health and to restore health by reaching a compromise with a newly formulated strategy, through the brokering and bridging of the barriers/conflicts/incongruence/ impositions that exist between diverse cultural health beliefs, types of lifestyles and scientific care interventions. Reference to culturally congruent practices and interventions to be taken in consideration are made where applicable.

Table 8.4   THE COMPONENTS OF A FUNDAMENTAL COMPREHENSIVE, HOLISTIC, CULTURALLY CONGRUENT HEALTHCARE PLAN

1. **Creating a therapeutic environment to render the necessary care in**
   - ❑ At home
   - ❑ In the hospital

2. **Standard precautions underlying the prevention of the spread of communicable diseases**
   - ❑ Protecting the health of the healthcare provider
   - ❑ Concurrent disinfection
   - ❑ Terminal disinfection
   - ❑ Giving health information to all interest groups
   - ❑ Management of carriers
   - ❑ Management of contacts
   - ❑ Eradication of vectors
   - ❑ Correction of environmental factors
   - ❑ Delousing and the disinfesting of fleas
   - ❑ Scrutinizing of cultural, social, recreational, occupational, religious and other practices for risk factors in promoting the spread of and/or preventing the control of communicable diseases
   - ❑ Notification according to law and enforcement of legislative measures

3. **Principles underlying the general fundamental healthcare to be rendered to all persons suffering from communicable diseases**
   - ❑ Rest and sleep
   - ❑ Nutrition and fluids
   - ❑ Oxygenation
   - ❑ Treatment of pyrexia
   - ❑ Relief of pain
   - ❑ Protection against injury
   - ❑ Psychological support
   - ❑ Prevention of complications

4. **General supportive and symptomatic care to be rendered to the ill person and his/her family**
   - ❑ **Physical care to be rendered to the ill person**
     - ▪ Promoting personal hygiene – body, skin, eyes, ears, mouth, nails
     - ▪ Monitoring of elimination
     - ▪ Providing a proper diet
     - ▪ Ensuring adequate rest
     - ▪ Ensuring adequate sleep

- Relieving of pain
- Checking of vital signs
- Observing for complications
- Administering of the prescribed chemotherapy and specific treatment regime
- Collecting of prescribed specimens for special and diagnostic tests

❑ **Socio-psychological care to be rendered to the ill person and his/her family**
❑ **Support to be given to the family**
❑ **Rehabilitation of the convalescent individual and reintegration into the family and into the community**
❑ **Support and care to be given when the ill person dies**

5. Meeting the unique age-related health needs of ill persons at home or in the hospital

❑ Infants
❑ Toddlers
❑ Children
❑ Adults
❑ Elderly persons

8.1.2.2.1   Creating a therapeutic environment to render care in

The aim of the care rendering to all ill individuals (infants, toddlers, children, adolescents, adults and elders) suffering from communicable diseases is directed at enhancing the defence mechanisms of the ill individual, the prevention of complications and the rehabilitation of the convalescent individual (or when the ill person dies, helping the bereaved family to adjust to individual, family and community life). All ill individuals must be cared for as a member of a family and a community, whether he/she is cared for at home or in a hospital. All care rendering interventions must be comprehensive (promotive, preventive, curative, rehabilitative), holistic, compassionate and culturally congruent in nature to maintain, protect and restore health. Grounded on the criteria for home-based or hospital-based care rendering (see 8.1.2.1), the ill person can be cared for at home or in a healthcare establishment (hospital).

❑ **Caring for the ill person at home**

When the ill person is cared for at home, the physical and emotional home environment becomes important as the caring is done by the family self. The role of the healthcare provider includes the therapeutic use of himself/herself within the healthcare provider-healthcare users-relationship as supporter, friend, giver of healthcare information and supervisor due to the fact the healthcare provider does not render the care herself/himself. During the caring process of the ill individual by the family, the normal housekeeping practices apply, for example, hand washing protocols, cleanliness and hygienic measures, fresh air, caring for pets, handling of food and food hygiene. When specific procedures/measures need to be done/taken, the care giver(s) must be taught how to do it. On the other hand, if any aspect in the home environment (such as insect and rodent infesting) negatively impedes on the health of the ill person, hospitalization is to be considered. The care giver and family must be supported during the period of caring, for example, by other family members, friends, professional providers, lay care givers, members of non-governmental organizations, traditional healthcare providers (also see 8.1.2.2.2 and 8.1.2.2.3). Regarding the care of the convalescent or disabled/chronically ill person at home, the interventions to be rendered is set out under 3.3.3. When palliative care is rendered to the ill/ dying individual at home, the same principles as above apply, accept that far more prompt interventions need to be taken as well as far more support has to be given to the care giver(s) and the family members because of changed responsibilities and roles, changes in financial and internal family resources and the stressors and strains of home caring. Situational depression in both the ill/dying person and care giver(s) is not uncommon as well as changes in the health status of the care giver(s). If necessary, modifications in the home environment for safety purposes need to be done, for example, high-rise toilet-seats, grab bars in the bath-room and much more. Lack of basic resources does not preclude home care, unless they are necessary for safety purposes.

❑ Caring for the ill person in the healthcare establishment - the hospital

When the ill person has to be admitted to the hospital, the physical, psychological and socio-cultural hospital environment plays an important part in the caring and recovery or dying process of the ill individual within his/her familial context. All care renderings in the hospital must include the healthcare interventions to care comprehensively, holistically and cultural-congruently for the ill individual and his/her family as well as all measures to create a therapeutic environment for the ill person to receive healthcare in and to prevent and control the spread of the particular communicable disease (see 8.1.2.2, 8.1.2.3 and 8.1.2.4). When complications had set in and the ill person is disabled or is chronically ill for the rest of his/her life, interventions on the tertiary level of prevention must be implemented as described under 3.3.3. When the ill person dies because of the pathogenesis of the communicable disease suffered from, the family has to be supported to adjust to individual, family and community life without the deceased family member.

In creating a therapeutic psychological and socio-cultural milieu/environment to render care to the ill individual within his/her familial/community context, the healthcare provider renders compassionate, humane, spiritual healthcare by using himself/ herself therapeutically through the use of his/her Self/Person/Being and corporality by being there for and with the ill person and his/her family - thus bringing meaning to the incomprehensibility of sickness or disability or death. Through linking phronesis (practical wisdom), praxis (integrating theory and practice), being (using the Self therapeutically), and doing (rendering comprehensive, holistic and culturally congruent care) the healthcare provider uses his/her humaneness to transcend interpersonal boundaries to meet and embrace the ill individual as a sick/ill human being that need care rendering and human dialogue. Through using the instrumental dimension of his/her corporality (intellect [by using the healthcare brokering process]; sensory organs of sight, smell, hear, touch, taste [taking in consideration of the spiritual-emotional and social aspects of the senses] and hands [when performing technical

339

procedures and rendering psycho-socio-spiritual care]) while helping the ill individual to become the person he/she must become, should become and can become in health/disease/disability/dying, the healthcare provider renders compassionate and holistic healthcare that satisfy both healthcare provider and healthcare user and his/ her family. The therapeutic use of their Self by the healthcare providers can only be actualized within the healthcare provider-healthcare user (ill individual and his/her family)-relationship as the healthcare provider-healthcare users (ill individual and his/ her family)-relationship grounds the therapeutic use of the Self. When the healthcare provider-healthcare users (ill individual and his/her family)-relationship has not been formed, the healthcare provider uses himself/herself un-therapeutically/neutrally that eventually may lead to the disintegration of the humaneness and self-actualization of the ill individual as person and as human being.

Within the milieu created by the healthcare provider-healthcare users (ill individual and his/her family)-relationship, the healthcare provider must use all relationships (family, friends, members of the multi-professional team [including traditional healthcare providers and lay care givers]) to support the ill individual and his/her family. The outcome of the treatment regime together with all relationships must also help the ill individual and his/her family to become self-caring and to become the persons they must become, should become and can become in health/disease/disability/dying. The management and control systems of the healthcare establishments, such as the vision and mission, organizational structures, human resource management, and quality control measures (including risks management), on the other hand, must underpin the therapeutic care of the ill person within his/her familial and community context. The more congruent and the more entwined the healthcare provider and the ill person and his/her family are with one another within the ill individual's familial and community context, the more meaningful and satisfying the care rendering will be for the ill individual and his/her family as well as for the healthcare provider.

During the care rendering period in hospital, infection control in the hospital is of the utmost importance as to prevent the spread of the particular communicable disease to susceptible co-patient and healthcare worker hosts, as well as to protect the ill individual suffering from a particular communicable disease from nosocomial infections. By isolating the ill individual the spread of the communicable disease can be controlled. By giving attention to housekeeping and sanitation measures regarding bed linen, disposal of waste (solid and liquid), proper cleaning and sterilization of contaminated articles, proper ventilation (natural and artificial) and/or air filtration and/ or ultraviolet germicidal radiation, as well as proper mopping and dusting to remove dust and other environmental reservoirs of infection, the spread of the communicable infections can be controlled. By strictly adhering to Standard Precautions/universal precautions, including barriers such as gowns, masks, gloves and body substance isolation, protection of healthcare workers from exposure to infectious agents and the ill healthcare user (patient) from cross-infection is accomplished.

Standard Precautions have to be used with all ill healthcare users regardless of whether the diagnosis is known as it pertains to (1) blood, (2) all other body fluids and secretions except sweat (whether containing visible blood or not), (3) non-intact skin and (4) mucous membranes. Transmission-based precautions, on the other hand, reduce the risk of airborne, droplet and contact transmission of specific pathogens and are used when caring for ill healthcare users with documented or suspected infections that is highly transmissible or which is of epidemiological importance for which Standard precautions may be insufficient. Airborne precautions are to be used to prevent transmission of pathogens in infected droplets (5μ or less in size [for example, *Mycobacterium tuberculosis humanis*]) or contained in dust particles. Special handling of air is of utmost importance, such as negative pressure, frequent air exchanges, direct-to-the-outside exhaust, HEPA air filters, or ultraviolet light radiation. Droplet precautions are used to prevent the contact of conjunctiva or mucous membrane of the nose and mouth with large-size (larger than 5μ) particle droplets containing pathogens generated by coughing, sneezing, talking or produced by procedures such as suctioning or bronchoscopy. Droplet precautionary measures include the following

- a fit-tested respirator and N-95 filtering face piece respirator/mask that are disposable to be worn by healthcare personnel when entering the unit/room
- gloves and gowns as well as eye protection (goggles or face shields) must be worn for all healthcare user contact within 1 (one) meter of the user as the infected droplets poses a risk for inhalation or settling on membranes. (When these droplets settle onto surfaces, it can no longer be inhaled except if disturbed into the air again)
- careful attention must be given to hand hygiene before and after all healthcare user contact or contact with items potentially contaminated with respiratory secretions
- disposable equipment such as stethoscopes, blood pressure cuffs, thermometers, etc. must be used
- healthcare personnel must also ensure that all ill healthcare users with respiratory infections or suffering from any other highly transmissible communicable disease wear masks when transferred from room to room or between departments. All respiratory secretions of infected individuals must be contained and burned. Personnel must wear the prescribed masks themselves when delivering care and/or examining a person with symptoms of a respiratory infection (particularly when fever is present), or with fever with/ without a rash is present, or when seeding of the lungs of the ill individual could has taken place as in Plaque, Haemorrhagic Fevers and Avian Flu.

Contact precautions are used to interrupt transmission of epidemiological important pathogens by direct contact (skin-to-skin) or indirect contact (skin-to-contaminated fomites). Contact precautionary measures include measures such as isolation in a single room with single-use, or dedicated-to-the-specific patient-equipment, together with the wearing of gown and gloves when entering the room of the healthcare user to render the necessary healthcare.

Note
1. Isolation measures to prevent airborne transmission cannot be implemented in the home situation, thus, all ill persons suffering from communicable diseases that are airborne transmitted (in the natural course of the disease or if the lungs of the ill person can become seeded due to the disease

pathogenesis) need to be admitted to a hospital where the necessary airborne precautions can be implemented. Enteric preventive measures, though, can be instituted at home, for example, the use of disposable cups, plates, knives and forks that can be burnt and toilet facilities that can be disinfected

2. Standard precautions must be used in combination with one or more of the Transmission-Based Precautions depending on the communicable disease diagnosed

3. Healthcare workers must promote their own health through living a healthy lifestyle and protect their health by strictly adhering to all Standard/universal precautionary measures and Transmission-based precautionary measures. The immunity status of all healthcare workers must be evaluated on a regular basis for the risk of contracting communicable diseases, such as Hepatitis B, Chickenpox, Diphtheria, Tetanus, Rubella, Measles, Poliomyelitis, and Tuberculosis in the occupational healthcare setting. Healthcare workers must make use of vaccines offered in the occupational setting to prime their immune system if they have not yet acquired natural-actively immunity against the abovementioned occupational diseases. When ill themselves or when female workers are pregnant/want to fall pregnant, they must be excused from rendering healthcare to ill persons suffering from communicable diseases. Healthcare workers must also be regularly evaluated for carriage status of communicable infections because they become healthy carriers. When occupational exposure to communicable infections/diseases occurred, healthcare workers must receive prophylaxis and follow up

8.1.2.2.2 Standard precautions underlying the prevention and control of the spread of the disease

The control and the prevention of the spread of all communicable diseases can be accomplished through measures aimed at the agent and/or the sources of infection. The use of ultra violet light to kill off certain infectious agents, for example, *Mycobacterium tuberculosis humanis*; the eradication of mosquitoes (source of infection) to prevent malaria infection; contact notification and chemoprophylaxis are examples of measures to be taken. In table 8.5 'Standard precautions underlying the control and prevention of the spread of communicable diseases' measures are set out that must be strictly adhered to as to prevent and control the spread of communicable diseases at home and in hospitals.

Table 8.5 STANDARD PRECAUTIONS TO BE INSTATED FOR THE CONTROL AND PREVENTION OF THE SPREAD OF COMMUNICABLE DISEASES

OBJECTIVES OF COMPREHENSIVE ACTIONS	CARING AT HOME	HEALTHCARE INTERVENTIONS IN A HOSPITAL
PROTECTION OF ALL LAY CARE GIVERS, TRADITIONAL HEALTHCARE PROVIDERS AND PROFESSIONAL HEALTHCARE PRACTITIONERS	✠ Inform family members how to care for the ill individual and how to protect family members, friends and neighbours ✠ Washing of the hands is the most effective measure to prevent the spread of infection at home. Hands should be washed before care rendering and after contact with body substances (blood, urine, faeces, sputum, vomitus or wound drainage) and before preparing food ✠ Instate clever devices and processes to make hand washing and personal hygiene routines easier and sustainable to prevent the spread and control of communicable diseases especially in informal and densely populated townships, for example, using of plastic bottles with a siphon tube stuck through the lid and a bar of soap suspended in a old pair of tights/leggings to enabled persons to wash hands after using the toilet and to wash hands regularly ✠ Care giver must wear gloves and smock/overall for protection. When disposable gloves are not available, use plastic bags to protect care giver's hands	❖ **Strictly adhere to all Standard Precautions to prevent the transmission of both identified and unidentified microbes** ❖ Wear gown, mask, gloves and eye protection within 1 (one) meter of the ill person ❖ Wash hands thoroughly before and after handling of the ill healthcare user ❖ Strictly adhere to respiratory hygiene and cough etiquette as well as to all enteric precautions ❖ Strictly adhere to all Standard/ universal Precautions for blood borne pathogens in healthcare units and in the laboratory

	✠ Inform all family members to cover nose and mouth when coughing or sneezing	
CONCURRENT DISINFECTION (WHERE APPROPRIATE, DISCUSSED FULLY IN THEME IV OF THE TEXT)	✠ When no diseases of the alimentary tract are involved, sewage waste can be disposed of in the usual/ every day/normal way ✠ Wash linen in hot soapy water. If laundry is soiled with blood, add a cup of bleach to detergent to disinfect the laundry ✠ Burn all waste when necessary, or discard in plastic bags ✠ Spills of blood and bodily substance(s) must be cleaned up using an effective household disinfectant ✠ Where diseases of the alimentary tract occur: • Wipe down toilet seat after use with an effective household disinfectant, and wash hands • When a bedpan is used, keep separate and place used toilet brush in an effective household disinfectant fluid • Dispose of secretions in flush toilets, pit toilets, septic tank or bucket toilets, or bury away from water supplies (take the normal flow off of the ground water table in consideration) • Clean bedpan with toilet brush and wash hands • Use disposable nappies for babies which must	❖ Use chemical solutions, autoclave or incinerator for burning to maintain concurrent disinfection ❖ Place secretions from the nose, throat and wounds into paper bags and incinerate ❖ Use disposable cups and plates as well as other disposable materials - burn after use ❖ When articles are used which may not be disposed of, disinfect in a chemical solution that has to be replaced regularly ❖ Place contaminated linen in containers supplied for this specific purpose and mark the containers as prescribed ❖ Ensure that each individual ill person has his/her own medical supply and equipment ❖ All mattresses and pillows must have special washable covers ❖ When water-borne sewerage is used, waste need not be disinfected – dispose in the usual manner ❖ Other types of sewerage systems – disinfect sewage waste chemically

	be burned or if cloth nappies are used, disinfect it in Dettol, Savlon, etc. Wash separately from other washing ▪ Keep eating utensils separate and wash separately (encourage the use of disposable eating utensils and burn after use)	
TERMINAL DISINFECTION	✠ Normal routine cleansing and ventilation of room	◈ As for home care ◈ If necessary, fumigation of room and equipment. Incineration of all used items
EDUCATING OF ALL CARE PROVIDERS (PROFESSIONAL, TRADITIONAL AND LAY) AND ALL OTHER SUPPORT FUNCTIONARIES	✠ Instruct members of the family to wash their hands after caring for the ill person and before the handling of food	◈ <u>Cleaners</u> - educate regarding the prevention of cross-infection and observing of isolation measures ◈ <u>Porters</u> - educate in correct handling of specimens and how to transfer the ill healthcare user (a mask to be worn by both ill healthcare user and porter, and porters to wear gown and gloves) ◈ <u>Laboratory staff</u> - notify them of disease[s] suspected, especially when the agent is a select agent such as in haemorrhagic diseases (Congo fever, Ebola fever), respiratory diseases (SARS, Influenza A-diseases), Plague, Meningococcal meningitis, etc. Prevent infectious pathogens from spreading in laboratory by working under stringent controlled laboratory conditions. Virus isolation studies and biological

		specimens for blood-borne pathogens on respiratory specimens must be conducted under the most stringent protection. ❖ <u>All healthcare practitioners in unit</u> - ensure that rules regarding hand washing and isolation measures are strictly complied with ❖ <u>Removal of linen/waste</u> - educate the workers to ensure that linen/waste is correctly handled in order not to become a source of infection **Strict adherence to all preventative measures to prevent personnel from contracting any disease**
MANAGEMENT OF CARRIERS	✠ The healthcare practitioner must contact the District Health Authorities or environmental health officers for further investigation ✠ Support carrier to comply with all legislative measures applicable (parents takes responsibility for child carriers) ✠ Healthcare provider (professional or traditional) must oversee the medical treatment to be taken by carriers as necessarily	❖ As for home care
MANAGEMENT OF CONTACTS	✠ The healthcare practitioner must assess the health status of all contacts and classify as either healthy, immune or susceptible ✠ Treat healthy, immune, and susceptible contacts as follows:	❖ As for home care ❖ As for home care

	▪ Bring school exclusion regulations to the attention of the head of the household ▪ When necessary, place contacts under quarantine ▪ Where necessary, inform employer/head of educational institution ▪ Do the necessary observations and tests ▪ When necessary, do vaccination or administer immuno-globulin or give prophylactic treatment ▪ When contact becomes sick, render care as for ill person	
ERADICATION OF BIOLOGICAL VECTORS AND IDENTIFICATION OF VEHICLES (WHERE NECESSARY)	✠ The healthcare practitioner must contact environmental health officials of District Health Authorities ✠ Scrutinize the general environment of the home to identify any objects that can serve as vehicles and/or biological vectors (e.g. pets)	❖ As for home care ❖ Scrutinize the general environment of the hospital to identify any objects that can serve as vehicles and/or biological vectors
RECTIFYING OF ALL PHYSICAL-BIOLOGICAL HAZARDS IN THE ENVIRONMENT (FOR EXAMPLE, SANITATION, CONTROL OF FLIES, WATER AND FOOD SUPPLIES)	✠ The healthcare practitioner must contact environmental health officials and/or District Health Authorities ✠ Routine barrier healthcare or nursing and medical care/isolation as well as high-grade barrier healthcare or nursing and medical care/isolation **can never** be implemented when family members render care to the sick individual at home as the family members are not	❖ As for home care ❖ Ensure engineering control of ventilation as to prevent air-borne droplets being transmitted throughout the hospital. ❖ Put routine barrier healthcare or nursing and medical care/isolation in place in general hospital units/wards to control the airborne transmission of infected droplets. ❖ Ensure environmental hygiene as well as all other measures to prevent cross-infection

	professionally educated to institute the above specialized isolation healthcare regimes	❖ Put in place waste control measures to prevent the spread of infections to the community ❖ For the control of gastro-intestinal communicable diseases, enteric precautions and disinfecting of the environment must be instated ❖ **High-grade barrier healthcare/nursing care/ isolation** is instituted for a specific group of communicable diseases that constitute a serious risk to all healthcare practitioners because they are transmitted via blood; fomites and airborne infected droplets (as seeding of the lungs can take place and profuse growth of the pathogen in the lungs can occur). High grade barrier/isolation care is **only** instituted in a specialized isolation unit for communicable diseases **(these measures can never be put in placed in general hospital wards/ units)** and the care has to be rendered by specialized trained healthcare personnel only. No visitors (family and friends) are allowed in this specialized isolation unit. All contacts (even entire communities) will be placed under quarantine
DISINFESTING OF FLEAS AND DELOUSING	✠ When necessary, perform de-flea-ing of fleas and delousing of ill person and his/her family	❖ As for home care

SCRUTINISING OF CULTURAL, SOCIAL, RECREATIONAL, OCCUPATIONAL, RELIGIOUS AND OTHER PRACTICES FOR FACTORS THAT POSITIVELY PROMOTE THE SPREAD OF COMMUNICABLE DISEASES	✠ Scrutinise rituals or customs or practices followed during life events (for example, pregnancy, birth, post-partum, childhood rearing practices, practices during dying and death, burial)	❖ As for home care
	✠ Scrutinise practices or rituals or customs followed during social gatherings	❖ As for home care
	✠ Scrutinise recreational and occupational activities that promote contact with animals and birds (farming, domestic, wild and exotic) as well as living organisms other than humans	❖ As for home care
	✠ Scrutinise sensitive occupations and their protocols	❖ As for home care
	✠ Scrutinise practices or rituals or customs followed during religious festivals or rituals or ceremonies	❖ As for home care
	✠ Scrutinise all practices and habits of all family members and/or friends and/or guests	❖ As for home care
NOTIFICATION ACCORDING TO LEGISLATION AND ENFORCEMENT OF ALL LEGISLATIVE MEASURES	✠ Ensure that the team member in charge of treatment attends to notification as demanded by law	❖ As for home care
	✠ Enforce, when necessary, all applicable legislative measures to prevent the spread of the disease over national and international borders and to protect the health of the nation (even if it means getting court orders against individuals, families and communities as well as calling in the national armed forces [civilian and military] to enforce the measures in communities)	❖ As for home care

8.1.2.2.3 Principles underlying the general fundamental supportive and symptomatic healthcare to be rendered to all ill persons suffering from a communicable disease

As the body reacts in a specific way (local and systemic) to the invasion by a specific pathogen(s), the body's defence mechanisms must be enhanced by all the supportive and symptomatic healthcare interventions that are to be rendered. The principles underlying the general healthcare and the rationale there for are discussed in table 8.6. All comprehensive, compassionate, holistic and culturally congruent healthcare brokering interventions must be rendered at primary, secondary and tertiary levels based on the prioritization of the diagnosis, the setting of aims, the individualization of the interventions set for health maintenance, health protection and health restoration and the evaluation set for healthcare rendering and cultural brokering. The most suitable person to execute the interventions (professional provider, member of family, ill person self, support person) must be identified and the necessary authority and responsibility must be delegated to the designated person. All limitations that may have a negative effect on the brokering process must also be identified and steps must be taken to change or rule them out. Lastly, the interventions must be communicated to all persons (professional, traditional, and lay care providers as well as to family members and friends) involved in the healthcare rendering process, with documentation of the execution of the interventions and the outcome of the healthcare rendered (healthcare and cultural brokering activities).

Please note that all fundamental healthcare to be rendered (routinely and general) must be based on scientifically practices as well as on prescribed socio-cultural health and other practices of the community, family and individuals. The cultural interventions must include culturally preservative and maintenance actions, cultural care accommodation or negotiation actions and cultural re-patterning or restructuring actions based on the brokering strategies of mediating, negotiating, intervening, sensitizing and innovation to maintain, prevent and restore health.

Table 8.6 THE PRINCIPLES UNDERLYING THE GENERAL FUNDAMENTAL HEALTHCARE TO BE RENDERED TO PERSONS SUFFERING FROM COMMUNICABLE DISEASES

PRINCIPLES UNDERLYING THE GENERAL HEALTHCARE RENDERING TO MAINTAIN AND PROTECT HEALTH	RATIONALE
REST AND SLEEP	Rest and sleep is a basic requirement for human beings. Sufficient rest and sleep is needed to maintain energy levels, restoration and maintenance of health and well-being. Changes in sleep and sleep-patterns do occur during sickness and as part of normal aging. This include a prolonged sleep latency (time to fall asleep), an increase in the number of awakenings during the sleep period - especially in aging, a decrease in slow-wave sleep and REM-sleep (rapid eye movement). These changes result in fragmented sleep and the experience of sleep deprivation. Other factors that may lead to sleep deprivation are physical problems such as pain, confusion, and many more, as well as certain drugs (for example, antihypertensive drugs) and environmental factors such as temperature, light, noise, type of bed and location. Because the quality of sleep can have far-reaching effects on the ill individual's general well-being, an assessment of the ill person's sleep-wake pattern must be done and specific interventions set to solve sleep problems to promote periods of rest and "naps". Infants and young children, on the other hand, tends to sleep more often and for longer periods when ill.
	As a considerable quantity of energy is required to fight infections and as this may be lacking when the ill person is over-active, bed rest is therefore recommended during the acute stage of the disease. During this time the ill person must be encouraged to exercise his/her extremities in order to promote circulation and maintain muscle tone. A sedative to encourage rest and sleep must only be administered under exceptional circumstances, that is, after all other strategies for combating insomnia and anxiety have failed and an assessment for signs and symptoms of complications [especially cerebral and neurological impairment] has been done.

NUTRITION AND FLUIDS	As a raised body temperature (fever) suppresses the appetite, the ill person reduces his/her nutrient intake. This decrease in nutrients results in the wiping out of the specific pathogen, as the infected cells die off because of starvation. Therefore, the monitoring and regulating of body fluid and electrolytes forms a crucial aspect of healthcare. Body fluid and electrolytes must be maintained within a limited range of tolerance as fluid or electrolyte deficit can lead to death. Fever causes fluid loss because of the evaporation of sweat from the body surface due to increased perspiration while phagocytosis requires energy. If energy is not provided, the body at first obtains it from its own glycogen stores and thereafter by catabolism of the body's proteins. These catabolic processes further undermine the defence mechanisms of the ill person. For this reason, persons with severe infections must be adequately provided with fluids, proteins and kilojoules. A full nutritional assessment (including macro-nutrients [proteins, fats, carbohydrates and fibre] and micro-nutrients [vitamins and minerals]) must thus be done to determine the nutritional status (especially the protein-status) of the ill individual as well as to determine whether an ill individual is malnourished or undernourished. As food and eating customs usually carry emotional and social significance, the assessment must also include a history of cultural foods to be eaten for maintaining health, for protecting health and for restoring health.
	The best method for administering kilojoules and fluids is per mouth. In the acute stage of the disease, the ill person usually has no appetite, and a fluid diet with high carbohydrate content should be offered. As soon as the ill person's appetite improves he/she should be offered a protein-rich diet to promote anabolism. To prevent the complications of an infection, such as shock and renal failure, an existing or potential fluid and electrolyte imbalance must be detected very quickly. Fluid replacement in therefore essential in an ill person with pyrexia.
	Communicable diseases almost always alter eating habits with important psychological and nutritional effects. It is often difficult to persuade children to take sufficient nourishment and fluids. For this reason parents must

	be informed and involved in the care of their children. It is recommended that small portions be given several times a day (6 to 8 times) and, where possible, for the adult to take the child on his/her lap to feed him/her. Of utmost importance is also to serve culturally accepted food for health restoration, health protection and health maintenance (for example, when hot food or cold food should be eaten, traditional food to be included, not serving foodstuff that are taboo) to the ill individual as sick persons very seldom eat "strange food" when sick. The family can also prepare food and bring it to hospital, if necessary. Sometimes it is better to serve 6 to 8 small meals than 2 to 3 big meals (for both adults and children).
OXYGENATION	An adequate quantity of oxygen is required to fight all types of pathogens. The environment wherein the ill individual is cared for must be clean and airy to ensure adequate oxygen supply. As infection is often associated with shock which curtails the oxygen supply to the tissues, oxygen must be administered to persons with hypoxia and/or hypoxemia. Certain pathogens, such as the Clostridium group, grow in anaerobic environments. Since these pathogens flourish in damaged and necrotic tissue, surgical debridement of wounds is performed to ensure adequate oxygenation of the tissues.
TREATMENT OF PYREXIA AND ASSOCIATED RIGORS	Infection goes hand in hand with pyrexia. Pyrexia benefits the body because an elevated body temperature not only enhances the ill person's immunological defence mechanisms but also kills off the infectious pathogen soon after the body raises its own temperature to fight the infection. The fever-induced lethargy also frees needed energy to enhance the immunological response. The ill person must therefore be cared for in a comfortable environment with the appropriate linen and clothing. Antipyretic drugs (when the body temperature is higher than 39,5°C), a high fluid intake and tepid sponging are some of the measures that can be used to lower the ill person's body temperature. Non-pharmacological approaches must be combined with pharmacological management of pyrexia. Sometimes the lowering of the body temperature with only antimicrobial and antipyretic drugs may result in the infection lingering longer and recuperation taking longer.

Please note

Antipyretic drugs must be administered very sensibly. When the body temperature is lowered to a point under the critical body temperature of 36,5⁰C, the immunological response (the innate and adaptive physiologic immunological responses) <u>cannot be activated</u> and maintained to induce phagocytosis and antibody-mediated and T-cell-mediated reactions to kill off the specific infectious agent. A low to moderated elevated body temperature (37,5⁰C to 38,5⁰C) can be well tolerated by most ill persons. If the ill person can tolerate a higher elevated temperature and <u>there are no indications of complications developing</u> (especially cerebral complications) the disease can be allowed to follow its natural course.

Drugs containing salicylate acid (for example, Aspirin, disprin, grandpa powders, etc.) <u>must never be given to children under the age of 16 years</u> as it can cause Reye's disease of the liver. It must also not be given to children who suffer from any virus infection.

Hyperthermia in pregnant women must always be treated because of the risk factors that maternal fever poses to the foetus (first trimester – neural tube defects and associated other birth defects with adverse outcomes; labour – neonatal seizures, encephalopathy, cerebral palsy, neonatal death, and adverse developmental outcome). All antipyretic medications must be given sensibly and with caution.

Signs of apathy and sleepiness in children or adults with pyrexia higher than 40⁰C are an indication of complications (particularly cerebral and neurological) setting in. Pyrexia higher than 40⁰C+ over a period of time and/or a very rapid rise in body temperature may cause feverish convulsions in children while hallucinations, delirium and restlessness can occur in ill persons of all other age groups.

Please Note

The body temperature **must never** be taken under the armpit - only under the tongue (mercury and digital thermometer) or in the ear canal (digital thermometer). A difference up to 5°C can occur between the body temperature readings taken under the tongue/in the ear and under the armpit, with the temperature reading taken under the tongue/in the ear proven as the most accurate body temperature. The difference in body temperature taken under the tongue and in the ear canal is less than 0,5°C to 1°C. The armpit has very little superficial blood vessels with the result that an incorrect body temperature reading is obtained. Superficial blood vessels are abundant under the tongue.

| RELIEF OF PAIN | Pain is multidimensional and entirely subjective. Pain can be evoked by a multiplicity of stimuli but the reaction to it cannot be measured objectively. Reactions to pain are therefore highly individual but the expression of and reaction to pain is influenced by the cultural and family background of the ill individual. Pain can only be described and evaluated by the person who experiencing the pain, namely, verbally by older children and adults. Pain experience in small children and adults not able to express themselves verbally, must be based on the non-verbal behaviour of the individual. It is therefore essential to understand the ill person's pattern of pain expression to evaluate his/her pain response. Pharmacological and non-pharmacological interventions must be used for the relief of pain.

Pyrexia is usually accompanied by headache which should receive treatment, since it leads to anxiety and restlessness, which in turn increases the body's oxygen consumption, resulting in a condition of shock. Analgesics can be given in small doses with intervals of 3 to 4 hours. A comfortable position, cold compresses and a dimly lit room contribute to the relief of headache. Other interventions to relief/reduce pain are therapeutic touch, using guided imagery, relaxation strategies, using cold and heat effectively, re-positioning, massaging, and therapeutic use of self by family members and/or healthcare providers.

Please note
*Before administering analgesics, every ill individual has to be assessed for signs and symptoms of neurological and cerebral impairment to exclude the possibility of encephalitis or meningitis. As many analgesics possess antipyretic properties, the same precautions are applicable as described under 'Treatment of pyrexia".
*Drugs containing Salicylate acid (for example, aspirin, disprin, grandpa powders etc.) <u>must never be given to children under the age of 16 years</u> as it can cause Reye's disease of the liver. It must also not be given to children who suffer from any virus infection. |
| PROTECTION AGAINST INJURY | Febrile individuals can become disorientated and confused, especially when they are of an advanced age. Assessment of the cognition and sensory perception of the ill individual must be done timely on a regular basis to determine when to institute special protective measures. |

	All ill persons (infants, children adolescents, adults, elders) must be protected against injuries and the family should be fully informed about it.
	As the risk of falling is very high in elderly individuals (resulting in injury and disablement as well as affecting the elder's functioning and quality of life) and increases when ill, assessment for the risk of falls must be done on a regular basis. The assessment tool must include aspects such as age; mental status; sensory (eye sight and hearing) and cognitive functioning; drug regimen; activity level and use of assistive devices, elimination; and history of falling within the last 6 months (and reasons thereto). Special attention must be given to the environment where the elderly are cared in, for example, well-lighted (although dimmed) environment during the night, while obstacles must be removed where the elderly move/walk such as slippery floors, wetness on floors, articles that has fallen on the floor etc.
PSYCHOLOGICAL-EMOTOINAL SUPPORT	The negative effects of isolation on an ill individual must not be underestimated. The aim of isolation and how it is accomplished must be explained to all ill persons and their families. In the care rendering of children, this aspect is of cardinal importance. Sedatives can be given, but only if there are no signs or symptoms of encephalitis/ meningitis or neurological impairment, and if there are no other strategies available to cope with anxiety and restlessness.
	Spirituality is of particular concern for all persons (even small children) who experience sickness/disease. Spirituality focuses on the meaning an individual attaches to life, particularly one's own life experiences as it represents a holistic integration of physical, social, psychological, cultural, sexual and theological experiences. For some ill individuals spirituality includes a connection with and commitment to a particular religious orientation and religious institution, while spirituality for other individuals means a "spiritual journey of life" that synthesizes the individual's inner contemplative experience and external human concerns (not believing in a specific religious dogma or belonging to a particular church). The experience of a

	communicable disease and a life crisis can precipitate a transformation or spiritual change, or cause a person to become more introspective and contemplative. Spiritual distress can result in a loss of physical, mental and social function. Hence, it is of utmost importance that healthcare providers are instrumental in supporting the spiritual well-being of the ill individual (regardless the spiritual beliefs and religious orientation of the healthcare provider self by being non-judgemental) by helping the ill individual to express himself/herself and to explore and find meaning in the experience of being ill. If the healthcare provider is not prepared to support the spirituality of the ill person, the provider must advocate for and refer the ill individual and his/her family to a provider/spiritual healer/pastor of choice.
PREVENTION OF COMPLICATIONS	Although most communicable diseases are acute illnesses that runs a short course with full recovery occurring usually (or terminating abruptly in death), complications do set in leading to disabilities. The disability is usually permanent as it is caused by non-reversible pathological alterations, and some disabilities may require a long or lifetime period of supervision, observation and care. As infection lowers the body's physiological resistance to other infections (secondary infections), special precautions must therefore be taken to prevent secondary infections (especially nosocomial infections when in hospital) and to obviate the complications of bed rest, such as deep venous thrombosis, and pulmonary embolism. Healthcare providers must thus assess the ill person on a daily basis for and recognize complications at an early stage and act accordingly. Any significant sign or symptom of any complication needs to be attended to immediately in order to prevent permanent disability. Should a temporary and/or permanent disability occur, rehabilitation must commence as soon as the ill person's condition permits. When necessary, refer the disabled individual to community resources on discharge.

8.1.2.2.4 The rendering of general routine fundamental healthcare – supportive and symptomatic

As the routine healthcare of an ill person suffering of any communicable disease does not differ from the care rendered to a person suffering from any other medical condition, all daily living activities and all therapeutic healthcare activities must be included in the care plan. A comprehensive healthcare plan consists of a number of components that must be adhered to, namely,

* the physical care of the ill person
* the psychological and social care of the ill person
* support to be given to the family
* rehabilitation of the convalescent person and reintegration into the family and the community
* support to be given when the ill person dies

Cultural and religious practices must be incorporated as far as possible into all healthcare interventions to be rendered. When the ill person is hospitalised, cultural tokens and customs can be allowed – even in high care isolation units (all items must be made of material that allows concurrent disinfection and terminally disinfection, or if disinfection is not allowed, incineration must then be allowed).

The routine fundamental healthcare interventions for all persons suffering from communicable diseases and their families are discussed under the following headings

✪ Physical care to be rendered to the ill person (Table 8.7)
✪ Psycho-social care to be rendered to the ill person (Table 8.8)
✪ Support to be given to the family (Table 8.9)
✪ Rehabilitation of the convalescent person and reintegration into the family and community (Table 8.10)
✪ Support and care to be given to the dying person and his/her family (Table 8.11).

Table 8.7   PHYSICAL CARE TO BE RENDERED TO THE ILL PERSON

OBJECTIVES OF COMPREHENSIVE ACTIONS	CARING AT HOME **Please note** **The caring is done primarily by members of the family with only support from the healthcare provider. Some interventions, however, must be performed by the healthcare provider self**	HEALTHCARE INTERVENTIONS IN A HOSPITAL
PROMOTING AND MAINTAINING OF PERSONAL HYGIENE	✠ Allow to take a bath/shower ✠ Sponge down when feverish and on request ✠ Hair may be washed as usually	◈ Allow to bath himself/herself and wash hair ◈ Give bed bath to and wash hair for ill person when unable to care for self ◈ Sponge down when ill person perspires excessively, and replace linen

CARING OF BODY SYSTEMS/ORGANS		
❖ *Skin*	✠ Wash skin with pure glycerine soap (or with glycerine soap infused with herbal tea extracts) as this will prevent dryness of the skin. Use a soft towel to dry skin	◈ As in home care
	✠ Rash - itchy: Any cream/ointment that relieves the itchiness, such as Anthisan cream, calamine lotion, cream containing vitamin E, as well as addition of bicarbonate of soda (baking soda) and/or salt to bath water	◈ As in home care
	✠ Dry skin - apply moisturising cream	◈ As in home care
	✠ Blisters - do not prick. Have ill person wear mittens	◈ As in home care
	✠ Scabs - prevent scratching by having ill person wearing mittens when necessary	◈ As in home care
	✠ Septic and other wounds Clean with luke-warm saline (1 teaspoon of salt in 1 litre of clean water) and apply an antimicrobial cream or antifungal cream or apply a mixture of Acraflavine (20-30 ml), honey (2-3 teaspoons) and Friars balsam (5-10 drops) or only honey (when very septic change dressing every 6 hours until sepsis has cleared up. When healing starts taking place leave dressing on for 12 hours, then 24 hours, then 36 hours, up to 72 hours. As soon as healing starts, reduces the cleaning with saline as it destroys the new tissue. Only clean	◈ As medically prescribed

	the healthy intact tissue). A pulp of pawpaw can also be applied to clear sepsis and then apply a healing balm or mixture or cream. The saline can be replaced by luke-warm black (no milk) herbal or rooibos or other types of tea. Healing wounds can also be painted with raw egg white and then exposed to direct sunlight for 5 to 10 minutes before applying the dressing	
❖ **Eyes**	✠ <u>Any discharge</u> (with the exception of pus and blood) – clean with swab soaked in cooled boiled water	◈ As in home care
	✠ <u>Purulent/bloody</u> discharge – consult a medical practitioner	◈ As in home care
	✠ <u>Photophobia</u> – darken room by drawing curtains or hanging a blanket in front of windows	◈ As in home care
❖ **Ears**	✠ <u>Any discharge of the ears</u> demands medical treatment	◈ As in home care
❖ **Mouth**	✠ <u>Brush teeth</u> as usual. When gums are painful, apply honey. When allergic to tooth paste or when tooth paste is not available, mix 1 teaspoon of salt and 1 teaspoon of bicarbonate of soda (baking soda) together and use as tooth paste. Make a paste with a bit of water and brush teeth	◈ When healthcare user is not able to care for own mouth, do it four-hourly for him/her ◈ If able to care for own mouth, as in home care
	✠ <u>Chapped lips</u> – apply lanolin or honey or glycerine or Vaseline balm	◈ As in home care

	✠ <u>Fever blisters and sores</u> in mouth – apply 1% gentian violet solution six-hourly with a damp swab or apply an antiviral cream or any other antibacterial oral suspension or honey. Serve food that is not very spicy or salty and avoid any acidic fruit and foods, or drinking of acidic fruit juices. When mouth is too painful/sore to eat a normal diet, a fluid diet can be served. A straw can be used to drink the fluid food as it protects the mouth mucosa (take care not to serve scalding hot food)	◈ As in home care
	✠ <u>Rinse mouth</u> with salt water, or with mouthwash, or mix in equal proportions honey, salt and fresh lemon juice (not preserved) in water to rinse mouth	◈ Rinse mouth with mouthwash
	✠ <u>Sore throat</u> can be treated with a mixture of turmeric (½ teaspoon), salt (2 teaspoons), honey and lemon juice (as much as deemed necessary while using only the juice of the fresh lemon fruit itself) – all dissolved in luke-warm water. Gargle with mixture every 2 hours. If condition does not clear up within 24 hours refer to medical practitioner	◈ Administer medically prescribed medication ◈ Assess sore throat every 6 hours and inform the physician
❖ **Nails**	✠ <u>Keep short and clean</u> ✠ When the person/child could <u>injure himself/herself</u> or prick the blisters by scratching, use mittens	◈ As in home care ◈ As in home care

MONITORING OF ELIMINATION (urinary and/or defecation function may be disturbed)	✠ Urinary function - refer all abnormalities, such as changes in appearance, composition, odour or frequency, for further medical treatment	❖ Test urine regularly or according to medical prescription ❖ Record intake and output as required
	✠ Defecation function Manage according to frequency, appearance and odour	❖ Defecation Function - Manage according to frequency, appearance and odour
	*Diarrhoea – evaluate diet. Give oral rehydration therapy (home-made - see chapter 11) or bought over counter). Give Probiotics, micro-nutrients (vitamins and minerals) and zinc as additional treatment. Refer for further treatment when necessary	❖ Diarrhoea - As for home care. Replace fluid loss by intravenous therapy. Administer medication as per medical prescription. Examine stools for the presence of blood or melaena. Attend to soiled linen according to protocols and standards of barrier healthcare
	*Constipation - increase intake of rough fibre and give stewed fruit such as prunes. Increase intake of fluids. Give 1-2 cups of green tea per day until normal bowl movement is established. Encourage mobility	❖ As medically prescribe ❖ As in home care
	✠ Manage diseases of the alimentary tract as indicated in Theme IV	❖ As in home care
	✠ Presence of infectious agents - concurrent disinfection. Use gloves	❖ As in home care
PROVIDING A CORRECT AND NUTRITIOUS DIET	✠ Abide by all cultural practices and preparations	❖ As in home care ❖ Family can provide food that is culturally acceptable and are allowed within the medical prescribed diet
	✠ Serve meals containing all six nutrient groups, namely, water, carbohydrates,	❖ A diet rich in proteins, minerals, vitamins, carbohydrates, fats and water are important

	proteins, fats, vitamins and minerals in the form of vegetables, fruits, and meat/fish, as well as the necessary micro- and macronutrients and enough <u>fibre</u> ✠ Offer <u>abundant fluids</u> with high carbohydrate content during the acute stage	❖ When necessary administer fluids intravenously. Record intake and output
	✠ <u>Increase proteins and carbohydrates in diet</u> as soon as ill person's appetite improves	❖ As in home care
	✠ <u>Prepare meals appetisingly and serve in an attractive manner</u> – hot or cold. Offer 6 to 8 smaller meals rather than 3 large meals per day	❖ As in home care
	✠ <u>Ensure that food is light and digestible and according to the ill person's taste and cultural preference.</u> Serve culturally accepted foods which are prepared according to culturally accepted practices	❖ As in home care
	✠ When the <u>temperature is elevated,</u> offer cold drinks and food or abide by culturally accepted practices	❖ As in home care
	✠ When <u>diarrhoea</u> occurs, decrease foods containing acid, for example, fruit juices	❖ As in home care
	✠ Prevent <u>constipation</u> by providing enough fibre and fluid in the diet	❖ As in home care
	✠ When <u>nauseous</u> give ginger (extract of ginger root, or in tablet form, or grounded ginger dissolved in water/tea) to drink to counteract nausea. Assess resolution of nausea after ginger was given. Assess effect of food intake	❖ When nauseous administer anti-nauseous medication as medically prescribed. Assess resolution of nausea after medication was given. Assess effect of food intake upon nausea and adjust food intake accordingly. Provide the necessary mouth care when

	upon nausea and adjust food intake accordingly. Assess skin tone and turgor for dehydration	necessary. Assess skin tone and turgor for dehydration
	✠ When <u>vomiting</u> occurs, administer anti-vomiting medication. Assess resolution of vomiting after medication was given. Assess effect of food intake upon vomiting and adjust food intake accordingly. Provide the necessary mouth care. Provide a clean emesis container after vomiting. Examine the vomitus for the presence of blood and immediately notify the physician. Attend to soiled linen when necessary. Assess skin tone and turgor for dehydration	◈ When vomiting occurs, administer anti-vomiting medication as medically prescribed. Assess resolution of vomiting after medication was given. Assess effect of food intake upon vomiting and adjust food intake accordingly. Provide the necessary mouth care. ◈ Provide a clean emesis container after vomiting and examine the vomitus for the presence of blood. Notify the physician immediately. Attend to soiled linen when necessary taking in consideration all barrier healthcare protocols and standards. Assess skin tone and turgor for dehydration 4-6 hourly

Dehydration of the ill person must be avoided at all costs. When the ill person is cared for at home, the members of the family have to be informed regarding the signs and symptoms of dehydration. When the ill individual is hospitalised, he/she must be observed hourly to four-hourly (1-4 hourly) for signs and symptoms of dehydration. Whenever necessarily, intravenous fluids must be administered as soon as possible, whether at home or in hospital.

Special attention needs to be given to the nutrition of the elderly as their taste is dulled. Many elders are also malnourished and their diet is often deficient in calcium, vitamins, iron and zinc. A multivitamin-mineral-probiotics supplement needs to be given additionally. It may also be necessary to give extra fluids to prevent dehydration as the elderly tends not only to be passively in bed, but also take diuretic drugs for chronic medical diseases.

Infants, toddlers and children also require special attention, as they become dehydrated very quickly. Extra fluids need to be given on an hourly to two (1-2) hourly basis, and in addition, the child needs also to be picked up and be cradled in the arms of the caregiver, or to be seated on the lap of the caregiver when being fed. As sick children tend to be very sleepy and sweaty when ill, the danger of becoming dehydrated is extremely great.

ENSURING ADEQUATE REST	✠ Allow ill person to rest according to his/her needs ✠ Complete bed rest is not always necessary	❖ When the ill healthcare user is on complete bed rest or partial bed rest, render care according to healthcare routine ❖ Promote rest by applying the necessary healthcare measures

ENSURING ADEQUATE SLEEP	✠ Promote sleep by applying appropriate healthcare measures
	✠ In case of insomnia
	  ▪ Evaluate for complications of disease (cough, diarrhoea, meningitis, encephalitis)
	  ▪ Remove cause of insomnia (itching, coughing, discomfort)
	  ▪ Care giver must reassure ill person and remain with him/her
	  ▪ If insomnia persists, refer for further treatment (particularly when the onset of complications is suspected)
		❖ As in home care
		
		❖ As in home care
		❖ Assess rest and sleep 12 hourly. Encourage verbalization of fear and/or insecurity – reassure the individual and inform him/her of progress made

EXERCISING TO PROMOTE HEALTH	✠ Encourage active or aerobic muscle exercises of extremities and torso to prevent muscle waste as result of inactivity, and to prevent vascular complications such as deep venous thrombosis ✠ Breathing exercises must be done on a regular daily basis as to prevent respiratory and cardio-vascular complications	❖ As in home care ❖ When the ill person is too ill or too old to do the exercises himself/ herself, the healthcare practitioner must do passive exercises for the ill healthcare user ❖ As in home care
RELIEVING PAIN	✠ Pharmacological approaches such as analgesics as well as adjuvant medications may be given for pain management ✠ Non-pharmacological approach (both alternative and complementary) such as	❖ Administer analgesics as medically prescribed ❖ When headache persist, obtain further medical treatment ❖ As in home care

	acupuncture, biofeedback, relaxation, hypnosis can also be used to alleviate pain	
	✠ A combination of pharmacological and non-pharmacological approaches can also be used to relieve pain	◈ As in home care
	✠ To alleviate headache, pharmacological and non-pharmacological approaches can be used as well as environmental strategies to ensure a restful environment. When headache persists, refer for further treatment	◈ As in home care
	✠ Immobilize painful, swollen joints and apply local heat. Give an analgesic when necessary	◈ As in home care

Pay attention to the use of salicylate acid because it is nephrotoxic and hepatotoxic. First monitor for signs of brain and neurological impairment before administering sedatives and/or medication inducing sleep. Drugs containing salicylate acid (for example, aspirin, disprin, grandpa powders etc.) must never be given to children under the age of 16 years as it can cause Reye's disease of the liver. It must also not be given to children suffering from any virus infection.

The pain sensory-perceptual function of the elderly becomes dulled with age. Elderly persons may therefore not complain of pain and practitioners must at times interpret the non-verbal behaviour of the elderly to ascertain whether the elderly individual has pain. The way the elderly sit, lie, and mumble, or their facial expression may be indicative of experiencing pain. Small children cannot always express pain and may cry continuously. Some small children may use other words than "pain" as being used in their family setting. Providers need to clear out the meaning of words used by small children with their parents/care giving parent/daily caregivers (nanny).

CHECKING VITAL SIGNS		
❖ *Temperature*	✠ Inform care-giver to take the ill person's temperature daily or observe for signs of fever or take temperature 4 hourly when necessarily. Instruct the care giver about the	◈ Take temperature every two to four (2-4) hours while the individual is seriously ill ◈ When the individual recovers, temperature may be taken twice (2) daily or daily

healthcare to be rendered when the temperature becomes elevated (39°C and higher) The use of a clinical mercury thermometer is not a necessity – a digital oral or ear thermometer or a temperature sticker is sufficient	❖ In case of an elevation in temperature, render care as in home care
✠ When an elevation in temperature develops, sponge down the ill person or let him/her take a tepid bath. Supply good ventilation. Contact a medical practitioner when higher than 39,5°C. Give antipyretics every four to six (4 to 6) hours according to age or weight, but not longer than 72–96 hours. Do not give more than the required dosage. Inform medical practitioner.	❖ As in home care
✠ Prevent the temperature to fall too low (under 36°C) as it impairs the immunological reaction – a moderate temperature (37,5°C.- 38,5°C) is necessary to stimulate and maintain the physiologic immunological reactions	❖ As in home care
✠ When any sudden drop in temperature occurs, obtain further medical treatment immediately (also see under mentioned information)	❖ As in home care

A constant elevation in temperature is usually an indication of complication(s) setting in. When the temperature does not drop within the normal time period according to the natural course of and signs and symptoms of the particular disease, further medical treatment should immediately be obtained. Elderly persons and neonates may sometimes be seriously ill without showing an elevation in body temperature.

Avoid excessive cooling down accompanied by shivering, discomfort and vasoconstriction. This has an adverse effect on the ill person as phagocytosis and the adaptive immunological responses are impaired in this way.

Should antipyretic remedies be administered, this has to be done every 4 to 6 hours to avoid the discomfort caused by alternative episodes of diaphoresis (excessive perspiring) and attacks of rigor. Drugs containing salicylic or acetylsalicylic acid/acetylsalicylate/salicylate/ASA (for example, aspirin, disprin, grandpa powders etc.) <u>must never be given to children under the age of 16 years</u> as it can cause Reye's disease of the liver. It must also not be given to children who suffer from any virus infection.

❖ *Pulse and respiration*	✠ Can be taken daily or four hourly, when necessary	◈ Must be taken every two to four hours while the ill person is seriously ill
	✠ The healthcare provider must check pulse and respiration daily	◈ When the ill person is recovering, pulse and respiration can be taken twice daily or daily
	✠ Observe the ill person for signs and symptoms of complications	◈ As in home care
	✠ Any sudden change in rhythm and volume of the pulse is considered a serious complication and must immediately be referred for further medical treatment	◈ As in home care
❖ *B l o o d pressure*	✠ Blood pressure is taken only when the nature of the illness demands it	◈ Blood pressure is taken according to the condition of the ill person and/or hospital routine
OBSERVING FOR COMPLICATIONS	✠ In order to observe for complications at the earliest possible time, the ill person should be continuously assessed by the healthcare provider. Question the care-giver/ill person continuously regarding additional complaints	◈ Observe for the smallest change in the physical, emotional and behavioural condition of the ill individual as it is an indication of complications setting in
	✠ All signs and symptoms shown by the ill person additional to the specific-general signs and symptoms of the clinical picture of the particular disease, need further medical attention	◈ As in home care

| ADMINISTERING THE NECESSARY MEDICINES | ✠ Drugs are to be administered according to prescription. The correct dosage must be given at the prescribed time. The course must be completed. Regularly observe for side-effects. Time conceptualisation of family and ill person must be taken in consideration, for example, clock time or sun time as well as the number of and time meals are eaten | ◈ As in home care |
| | ✠ When traditional or herbal medicine is taken, evaluate the interaction with the prescribed chemo-therapeutic drugs. If no harm comes, continue with traditional herbal medicine | ◈ As in home care |

Knowledge of the effect(s) of chemo-therapeutic drugs and traditional/herbal medicine is vital. In some cases the ability of the disease to be transmitted disappears within hours after commencing chemo-therapeutic treatment. It can also happen that the clinical signs and symptoms of the disease disappear, or that the clinical picture changes, while in some instances only the symptoms of the disease are relieved. Routine interventions have to be applied before, during and after administering of medicines, namely: continuous evaluation of the clinical picture of the ill person, correct administering of drugs prescribed, and observation for side-effects.

Failure of chemo-therapeutic treatment may have several causes
  ✓ **the ill person is not taking his/her medication or is taking it irregularly**
  ✓ **the ill person himself/herself has developed a resistance to the prescribed drug (over-prescribed previously)**
  ✓ **the drug(s) has not yet reached the site of the infection**
  ✓ **the dosage given/prescribed is not sufficient or treatment was discontinued too soon**
  ✓ **drugs are administered incorrectly (incorrect route for drug)**
  ✓ **the wrong drug is prescribed**
  ✓ **a different pathogen from the one isolated in the laboratory is the cause of the disease**
  ✓ **the specific infectious agent is resistant to the drug**
  ✓ **the infectious agent is present in an abscess**
  ✓ **super-infection(s) is/are present.**

Sometimes, elderly persons consume disproportionately more of all kinds of drugs because they experiencing more than one chronic illnesses. As numerous age-related physical changes occur in the elderly, healthcare providers must always be aware of the older person's response to medication. The absorption of the drugs is influenced by the presence or absence of nutrients, or by the decrease of hydrochloric acid in the stomach resulting in less absorption and efficiency of drugs that are depended on an acid medium for absorption. Absorption may also be altered because of the rate of transit through the gastrointestinal tract with age. The distribution of drugs within the body may also be affected because of the loss of lean body mass and the increased proportion of body fat. Fat-soluble drugs become stored in the body fat thereby decreasing the intensity of reaction while increasing the duration of reaction. The distribution of drugs in the bloodstream are affected by the amount of serum protein, especially albumin, as it serves as available binding sites for drugs (concentrations of bounded [inactive] drug distribution increases while unbound [active] drug distribution decreases when serum albumin levels are low). Although unbound drugs is metabolized by the liver, the drug metabolism is altered by lower levels of enzyme activity in the liver, resulting in prolonged or incomplete metabolism with an increased half-life, allowing the drug to exert its effect over a longer period of time. The decreased renal plasma flow to the kidneys, the decreased glomerular filtration rate, and the decreased number of tubules combine to result in inefficient excretion of active drugs, resulting in the accumulation of drugs to potentially toxic levels because of the decreased renal clearance. The decreased renal clearance and the changes in binding sites in the blood unite to prolong the elevated blood level and activity of many drugs. A further principle of drug interaction to be taken in account is the displacement of one drug by another from the protein-binding sites, for example, warfarin being displaced by aspirin. Both therapeutic and untoward response(s) of the elderly to drug medication must not only be regularly checked, but the drug level must be built up gradually, with the lowest dosage and the fewest number of drugs to be used first. The ongoing assessment of the elderly person's response to the drug regimen is based on the thorough drug/medication history and nutritional assessment to identify possible food interaction.

COLLECTING THE PRESCRIBED SPECIMENS FOR SPECIAL DIAGNOSTIC TESTS	✠ When special tests or investigations need to be done, explain the procedure to the ill person and his/her family, and interpret the results for them. Reassure them	❖ As in home care
	✠ Take specimens correctly	❖ As in home care
	✠ Handle specimens with care as to prevent contamination	❖ As in home care ❖ Notify laboratory staff beforehand

		(especially if certain extremely highly transmitted infections are suspected, for example, Avian influenza [bird flu] or Lassa fever etc.)

Table 8.8 PSYCHOLOGICAL-EMOTOINAL AND SOCIAL CARE TO BE RENDERED TO THE ILL PERSON

OBJECTIVES OF COMPREHENSIVE ACTIONS	CARING AT HOME	HEALTHCARE INTERVENTIONS IN A HOSPITAL
GIVING EMOTIONAL AND SPIRITUAL SUPPORT	✠ Support the family members to support the ill individual and the specific care giver by promoting the self-esteem of the ill individual and his/her family ✠ When necessary, the healthcare practitioner must support the ill individual as well as the specific care giver. ✠ When the care giver is not able to render the necessary care anymore, hospitalization must be considered for the ill individual	❖ Explain the protocols and standards of barrier healthcare to sick individual and his/her family and provide all appropriate information as necessary ❖ Help the sick person to verbalize his/her fears and anxieties as to support the ill person emotionally and alleviated his/her fears. ❖ Promote the self-esteem of the ill individual by promoting self-care ❖ If necessarily and if possible, personal and familial tokens as well as ethnic totems of custom are allowed. Ensure that the tokens and totems can be disinfected/ sterilized or incinerated as required ❖ Reassure the ill individual and his/ her family about all appropriate rehabilitation measures that will be instituted for social acceptance after discharge
ALLOWING VISITORS	✠ When necessary, restrict visitors, especially pregnant women (rubella) and infants (childhood diseases)	❖ When an ill individual is isolated, the person is deprived of personal freedom as his/her family and friends are not allowed to visit him/her. ❖ The healthcare practitioner must thus compensate for the lack of visitors by keeping him/her informed about his/her family and friends and if possible, ensure

		that he/she can contact them by telephone or radio/electronic means
ALLOWING PETS	✠ Pets can be allowed into the sick-room if it is to the ill person's advantage. Use discretion	◈ When recuperating from the infection in hospital, pets can be brought to hospital and re-uniting of pet and owner will be allowed on the hospital grounds (not in the care units/wards)
ENSURING EMPLOYMENT OR SCHOOLING	✠ In order to reassure the ill person, contact the employer to ensure that the ill person will not lose his/her job ✠ Introduce schooling to school-going children as soon as possible to prevent the child to fall behind in his/her schooling	◈ As in home care
PROVIDING OF RECREATIONAL AND OTHER LEISURE ACTIVITIES	✠ Promote play and other activities for children to prevent developmental lags ✠ Adapt activities to the general condition of the child/adult	◈ Arrange for familiar toys (which can be destroyed afterwards) to be brought in for the child to play with ◈ Promote play and other activities continuously to prevent developmental lags ◈ Cater for leisure activities for adults during the recovery period
IDENTIFYING THE SYNDROME OF HOSPITALISATION IN CHILDREN		◈ When it is at all possible, hospitalise mother and child together ◈ Observe child for reactions to hospitalisation and take the appropriate measures to ensure that the child can cope psychological during this stressful period ◈ Give honest answers to questions asked by the parents and keep them fully informed regarding their child's progress and care
RENDERING CULTURALLY CONGRUENT HEALTHCARE	✠ The cultural and religious customs of the family must be honoured if it does not threaten the safety and health of the ill family member and/	◈ As far as human possible honour the cultural and religious customs of the family and the ill individual without endanger the life of the ill individual or overthrow the

	or the family as unit. When the cultural and religious customs do endanger the ill person and/or the family as unit, the customs must be altered/changed to the satisfaction of both parties	measures put in place to prevent and control the spread of the communicable infection ❖ **Do not** remove any strings or amulets or chains or charms from the body of infants or young children when hospitalized except when it endangers the life of the child or the body site where the body strings or amulets or chains or charms are placed, must be used to administer treatment intravenously or intramuscularly. When the strings or amulets or chains or charms are to be removed, confer with parents/foster parents/guardians who must remove it

Table 8.9   SUPPORT TO BE GIVEN TO THE FAMILY

OBJECTIVES OF COMPREHENSIVE ACTIONS	CARING AT HOME	HEALTHCARE INTERVENTIONS IN A HOSPITAL
SUPPORTING THE FAMILY	✠ Effective home care acknowledges and incorporates the family's cultural and religious beliefs	❖ As in home care
	✠ Assess the expectations of the family regarding the illness of the family member, knowledge of the treatment plan, and their roles and responsibilities	❖ As in home care
	✠ Where necessary institute a therapeutic care plan for the family to work through their needs	❖ Support members of the family by regularly explaining the monitoring and care being rendered and reporting back on the ill person's progress and care
	✠ When possible, the extended family can be involved in the care rendering process	
	✠ Support spouse/both parents (father and mother)/only parent and all children as well as all other family members	❖ Assess the family's level of anxiety and ability to cope while encouraging family members to verbalize their fears
	✠ Take care that the main care	❖ Orientate the sick individual and

	giver does not exhaust herself/ himself. Observe the care giver for situational depression and take the necessary steps to help the care giver	family to protocols and standards of barrier healthcare
	✠ Observe the family for dysfunction due to disturbed family relationships. Institute the necessary therapeutic measures	◈ As in home care
	✠ Encourage the family and friends to ask questions	◈ As in home care
	✠ Allow members of the family to give voice to their fears and grief	◈ As in home care
	✠ Support the spiritual well-being of the family	◈ As in home care
	✠ Help the family to deal with their personal and emotional losses	◈ As in home care

Table 8.10 REHABILITATION OF THE CONVALESCENT PERSON AND REINTRODUCTION INTO THE FAMILY AND THE COMMUNITY

OBJECTIVES OF COMPREHENSIVE ACTIONS	CARING AT HOME	HEALTHCARE INTERVENTIONS IN A HOSPITAL
REHABILITATION OF THE INDIVIDUAL	✠ Allow more activities. Keep the convalescent person busy according to individual needs (particularly children)	◈ As for home care
	✠ Evaluate the person for psychological continuation of signs and symptoms of the disease	◈ As for home care
	✠ When disabilities have set in, assess the family's ability to care for the disabled family member and plan with the family to find solutions to perceived and actual healthcare needs within the context of their own unique lifestyle, for example, economic cost to care for	◈ As for home care

	the disabled family member and changed lifestyle	
	✠ Long-term care rendering of the permanent disabled individual may require structural remodelling of the home	◈ As for home care
	✠ Prevent social isolation of the family by instating a support network for the disabled person and his/her family	◈ As for home care
	✠ Explore and incorporate cultural network resources (friends, neighbours, church, and community groups) into the care rendering	◈ As for home care
	✠ Promote self care of the disabled individual and his/her family to restore and maintain health	◈ As for home care
	✠ Help the disabled individual and family to adjust to the treatment plan (for example, basic care needs; drug regime; nutrition; home environment; specific needs regarding transportation, exercises, socialization, occupation/schooling, cultural and family activities, and special equipment) and teach them the specific special skills they need for self-care	◈ As for home care

The healthcare provider must institute the necessary measures to prevent potential complications of the disease because it may result in temporary or permanent disabilities. In order to do so, the <u>healthcare practitioner must recognize complications at an early stage and act accordingly.</u> Any significant sign or symptom of any complication needs to be attended to immediately in order to prevent permanent disability. HEALTHCARE PRACTITIONERS NEED TO LISTEN TO THE COMPLAINS AND REQUESTS OF THE ILL PERSON TO IDENTIFY ANY SIGNS AND SYMPTOMS OF COMPLICATION(S). ALL ILL HEALTHCARE USERS MUST BE PHYSICALLY EXAMINED FOR SIGNS AND SYMPTOMS OF COMPLICATIONS ON A DAILY BASIS. Should a temporary

and/or permanent disability occur, rehabilitation must commence as soon as the ill person's condition permits. When necessary, refer the disabled person to community resources on discharge.

If a carrier state develops, the convalescent individual and his/her family should be assisted in working through the crisis. If the carrier has to change his/her job, help him/her to accept the situation and refer him/her to the appropriate community resources. Direct his/her attention to the necessary personal and legislative measures to which he/she has to subject himself/herself. If the carrier is a child, the parents/guardians/foster-parents will have to accept responsibility.

Table 8.11   SUPPORT AND CARE TO BE GIVEN TO THE DYING PERSON AND HIS/HER FAMILY

OBJECTIVES OF COMPREHENSIVE ACTIONS	CARING AT HOME	HEALTHCARE INTERVENTIONS IN A HOSPITAL
SUPPORTING THE DYING INDIVIDUAL AND HIS/HER FAMILY	✠ Support the spiritual well-being of the dying person and his/her family	◈ As in home care
	✠ Give special support to the dying person and his/her family before and during the process of dying until the family has completed the process of grieving by helping the dying person and his/her family to talk about their loss and impending death as well as to express their feelings about grieving with each other	◈ As in home care
	✠ Acknowledge and honour the dying person and family's beliefs and promote grieving without compounding their loss. Be cognisant of the acceptable expression of grief within the specific cultural context	◈ As in home care
	✠ Inform the family of the legislative aspects of handling the body (for example, cremation)	◈ As in home care
	✠ Prepare the family for an altered funeral or memorial service (for example, the body may already be buried/cremated)	◈ As in home care

	✠ Adhere to all cultural, familial and religious practices during the process of dying, burial and grieving	❖ As in home care ❖ When family is not allowed, work together with the family to adapt cultural and religious practice regarding death, dying and burial

8.1.2.2.5 Meeting the unique age-related health needs of ill persons at home or in a hospital

As the essence of all healthcare is the enhancement of the health of the ill person, his/her family and the community wherein they live, the unique health needs of the ill host, his/her family and the community wherein they live, must be met. To render holistic healthcare to the individual person, all healthcare interventions must be individualized as the healthcare differs for groups (families and communities whether healthy, ill, carrier, contact) and for individuals (whether healthy, ill, carrier, contact). Not only differ the age and roles of children and adults from one another, but each age group and gender group experience unique healthcare needs that have to be met. In the under mentioned table selected needs of children and adults are set out.

INFANTS (FROM BIRTH TO 2 YEARS OLD)
If necessarily, all infants should be hospitalised since they are usually very ill. Mother and child needs to be admitted as a unit (together) to hospital, except if the infant needs to be isolated. When doing a physical examination on the infant, the healthcare practitioner MUST start with non-invasive techniques, while leaving the invasive procedures, such as the examination of the throat and ears, until last. The examination must also be done at a slower rate as for adults, as the mother needs to reassure the infant continuously (it is sometimes better to let the mother hold the infant in her arms during the examination process). Keep in mind that the findings of what is considered normal or abnormal in a paediatric physical examination as the findings differentiate from those of an adult, for example, a positive Babinski reflex is normal in infants while a negative Babinski reflex is an abnormal finding in adults. Regarding the care rendering to the infant, the infant's feeding pattern must not be interrupted but either adapted as follows <blockquote>1 Do not discontinue breastfeeding. Rather put the infant to the breast more often, or let the mother express her milk and feed the expressed milk to the infant by dropper or cup-feeding. (This prevents the baby from being confused by the nipple when the mother starts breastfeeding again) 2 Do not introduce a mixed diet until the infant has recovered 3 Do not wean the infant of the breast or the bottle. Do it only after the infant has recovered 4 When the infant refuses either the breast or the bottle, he/she should be fed with a dropper or a cup 5 Offer feeds frequently, but only a small amount at a time, to prevent dehydration.</blockquote>

After the infant had recovered, the growth pattern of the infant must be assessed, namely, weight, height, head and chest circumference to determine whether the infant's own growth pattern shows a marked departure of the expected growth parameters.

Assessment of the infant's development in terms of developmental milestones (critical behaviours expected at specific ages) must also be done to detect developmental delays in the infant's neurological development (fine and gross motor development), personal-social development and language development. If necessary, further follow-up evaluations become a necessity as to help the infant to grow up within his/her own potential.

Support must be given to parent(s) as their ability to cope with the stresses and frustrations of parenthood, everyday life, and the illness of the infant/toddler/child/adolescent influence the emotional health of the infant/toddler/child/adolescent as the infant/toddler/child/adolescent is sensitive to the atmosphere around them and feels insecure and uncertain in a situation in which parents are under obvious stress. Parents need to become partners of the healthcare providers in the healthcare programme of the infant/toddler/child/adolescent and render the care to their child themselves (except if contra-indicated when the infant needs to be isolated). Parents also need to be informed about what to expect regarding the particular communicable disease and the treatment to be followed/instituted. When the infant/toddler/child/adolescent is disabled/chronically ill after resolution of the communicable disease had taken place, the parents must be helped to work through their loss, disbelief, anger, demystification and conditional acceptance as to normalize family life and quality interaction between infant/toddler/child/adolescent be sustained.

TODDLERS (2–6 YEARS)

Toddlers and older children react differently to their environment based on their individual temperament. The reactivity pattern (activity level, rhythmics, approach to new situations, adaptability, intensity of reaction, distractibility, attention span, threshold of response, and mood) of the toddler/child must be assessed as the characteristic features have implications for the child's interactions with other persons and healthcare to be rendered. For example, if the toddler/child is very active, and always into something, he/she needs close supervision. The placid child on the other hand may need more time to complete activities with the result more time needs to given to the toddler/child to respond and finish the activity. Toddlers, who have mastered independence in certain areas of development before becoming ill, may when ill, regress to more infantile behaviour – a normal behaviour pattern during illness. As soon as the toddler is recuperating, the toddler must be encouraged to regain the already-mastered independent tasks and behaviour patterns. The developmental milestones of the toddler need to be assessed on an ongoing basis to detect developmental delays and if necessary, developmental rehabilitation needs to be instituted as soon as possible.

Toddlers can be very demanding and do not want their mothers to leave the room. The toddler does not have to remain in bed all day long if he/she suffers from diseases such as varicella, rubella or pertussis. He/she may play in the house, provided there are no draughts and an even temperature is maintained. While convalescing, the toddler may play outside during the warmest hours of the day. Toddlers sometimes have to be fed until they start to feed themselves again. If necessary, have the child sit on the lap of an adult who can feed him/her. Offer small meals frequently. When the toddler wants to eat by himself/herself, offer meals which he/she can take in his/her hand. As toddlers/young children are stickers to routine because it gives them a feeling of security, the routine the toddler/young child is used to, can be followed when ill. When the routine was disrupted during the period the toddler/child has been ill, the normal routine within family life needs to be re-established as quickly as possible to promote the emotional health of the toddler/child. Disciplining patterns need to be re-instituted for the recuperating toddler/child as discipline could have been slacked down while ill. Parents and healthcare practitioners must work hand in hand to establish normal parenting activities for the convalescent toddler or child. If the toddler/child was hospitalized, healthcare practitioners need to fulfil the parenting activities for the parents when absent. Special attention must also be given to child safety practices in the home and the hospital and adequate supervision needs to prevail.

CHILDREN (7–18 YEARS)

The age of the child and adolescent influence the type of care to be rendered, for example, vaccination would receive more emphasis in the younger children while sexuality issues and substance abuse would be of greater concern with the adolescents. Because of vaccination of the infant and young child, "childhood communicable diseases" (for example, Measles, Mumps, and Chicken pox) are now becoming adolescent and young adult diseases that may result in serious ill adolescent/young adult individuals ending up with severe disabilities. Children/adolescents suffering from communicable diseases are usually excluded from school until such time they are not a source of infection anymore. As the education of the child/adolescent must be continued, healthcare providers must ensure that the child's schoolwork is not neglected. The help of his/her school friends and teachers must be enlisted. Because the child will be away from school for a prolonged period, any problems must be discussed with his/her teachers. Psychologically, it is to the child's advantage if his/her friends can visit him/her during his/her illness. Keep him/her busy during convalescence and allow him/her to go outside during the warmest part of the day. Parents need to be informed regarding the need to stay at home when the child/adolescent is ill.

Healthcare providers also need to ensure that that the child/adolescent receive the appropriate care to prevent complications. If the child/adolescent is disabled after recuperation, educational and vocational rehabilitative interventions need to be instituted. Healthcare providers also need to advocate for the disabled child/adolescent to prevent social isolation of the disabled child/adolescent.

ADULTS

The rendering of healthcare interventions to provide in the needs of the ill adult are influenced by many factors, such as gender, age (young adult, middle aged), marital status (married/unmarried, divorced [single parent]), sexual orientation (lesbian/gay), occupation, homelessness and many more. As such, women are prone to a number of genetically linked conditions that may complicate the natural course of communicable diseases. The outcome of pregnancy for both the ill mother and infant may also be extremely negative – certain infections in the mother may be worsen or reactivated because of the immune and hormonal changes during pregnancy. As the foetus has under-developed immune defences, the foetus may, when infected, be killed by the destructive activity of the infectious pathogen, leading to intra-uterine death of the foetus. The intra-uterine death of the foetus usually results in spontaneous abortion or stillbirth. If the foetus survives, the infant can be born with a congenital infection, and/or congenital malformations and/or congenital pathological body tissue(s) changes. The infant is generally small and fails to thrive. Because women usually assume caregiver roles within families, being ill becomes an emotional stressor which can negatively influence her health. Women sometimes also lack the support system that males have been able to build for themselves.

Because the health of men is not included as one of the health aims of the healthcare system, the health needs of men are not served well, leading to the phenomenon that men tend to encounter the healthcare system on an episodic basis. The pattern of physical health disorders and health-related needs of men differ from women, attributable to physiological differences between males and females, differences in health-related habits and health-seeking behaviour, differences in social roles, stress and coping mechanisms and differences in lifestyle. Cardiovascular disorders such as hypertension and ischemic heart disease are significantly higher among men than among women. Because of the stereotyped view of the masculine role, men experience social pressure to conform to the socialized view of men as being strong and invulnerable, resulting in difficulty to admit to health-related needs and frailties as well as to conform to health behaviours that do not conflict with good health.

Men cope differently with stress and tend not to voice their fears and worries. Some men also tend to delay seeking treatment for health-related disorders. Although most men live within a family situation, men may have difficulty in effectively interact with family members, with the result that their psychological needs are not always met. Different role expectations between husband and wife may result in marital conflict. Because younger males experience more embarrassment than older males about sexually related issues, younger males tend to delay treatment as long as possible.

Although men and women react differently to disability as the outcome of communicable diseases, disorders that affect the individual's sexuality, intellect and abilities have a profound impact on both men's and women's self-image and psychosocial functioning. After recovery from some communicable diseases such as meningitis, vocational rehabilitation may be necessary for disabled adults. When an adult falls ill from a communicable disease such as tuberculosis, healthcare practitioners must inform the ill person's employer of his/her condition and help the employer to keep the individual in the employment situation. Employers need to be encouraged to become part of the healthcare team rendering care to the ill/recuperating adult. When the individual is a carrier after he/she has recovered from the disease and has to change his/her job, he/she must be helped to deal with this crisis and to adjust to his/her new employment situation. The recovered person's attention must be drawn to legislation concerning carriers. Where necessary, community resources must be used to assist the recovered individual and his/her family to help them to live a fulfilling life in their community.

ELDERLY PERSONS

The health concerns for the elderly are multidimensional, requiring critical evaluation of what is normative and what is the result of the communicable disease. Elderly persons may be seriously ill without necessarily exhibiting the characteristic-specific clinical picture of the particular communicable disease. Subtle changes in appetite, or ambulation, or the onset of urinary incontinence, or an altered mental status (confusion), may be the initial and only clinical indicator of infection. A thorough baseline assessment of the elderly person's ability to carry out activities of daily living and performing instrumental activities of daily living thus needs to be done. In addition to the normal health dimensions indicators to be assessed; special attention must also be given to cognitive and sensory perception, risk of falling, depression and medication use. As such, functional disability correlates with physical illness, self-care ability, complications developing during hospitalization, and rehabilitative ability. All elderly persons who cannot be cared for at home since there is no one to take care of them there, or who cannot care for themselves, should preferably be hospitalised. Complications of a particular disease may also be disguised by other diseases that the elderly person may be suffering from. Elderly persons also tend to lie in bed without moving around and this may lead to serious complications.

Elderly persons who are hospitalized are also at increased risk for institutionalization as consequence of the loss of their ability to carry out activities of daily living and performing instrumental activities of daily living.

8.1.2.3   The specific therapeutic healthcare interventions to be set

The specific healthcare activities/interventions can only be set once the specific causative pathogen has been identified, because these interventions are specifically set for the particular communicable disease/infection as it is based on the specific identified causative pathogen. The specific healthcare interventions are fully described in chapters 9 to 14, as the specific therapeutic healthcare interventions to be set include all specific medical and other professional health care interventions relating to

✪ the cure of the disease
✪ the alleviation of the symptoms of the disease/infection
✪ the rendering of palliative care until the individual dies
✪ the activities to be set to be fulfilled to help the individual to cope with specific disabilities if complications have set in, and
✪ the setting of those specific control measures (locally, national and international) to control the spread of the particular communicable disease/infection and to prevent further outbreaks of the particular communicable disease.

All the specific healthcare interventions to be set are grounded in the specific diagnosis made, once the specific causative pathogen has been identified, or the complications already developed when the diagnosis is made. Underlying all the specific healthcare interventions to be set, are all the fundamental general supportive and symptomatic healthcare interventions already discussed under 8.1.2.1 and 8.1.2.2.

If the particular communicable disease/infection can be cured, specific chemotherapeutic drug therapy/anti-microbial drugs will be prescribed (see 8.2.2.2) or immunotherapeutic products may be administered (see 8.2.2.1). If symptoms are to be alleviated, specific immunotherapeutic products may be administered together with prophylactic anti-microbial drug therapy as well as other drug therapies, for example, anti-pyretic drugs, anti-inflammatory drugs and anti-epileptic drugs etc. whatever the specific need of the ill/disabled/dying individual may be. If no cure for the infection exists (for example, rabies, and Lassa fever) the fundamental supportive and symptomatic care must strictly be adhered to until the ill individual dies.

Inherent to the specific healthcare intervention are all those specified control measures to prevent the spread of the disease/infection, and all legislative measures applicable, as well as all those specified preventive measures to prevent further outbreaks of the disease/infection. The specified control and preventive measures also include all those international measures to be put in place to prevent communicable infections from spreading across the borders of the RSA, as well as all those specified measures to be implemented when a particular communicable disease is brought into the RSA as to prevent a outbreak of the particular communicable disease within the borders of the RSA, and to care for all ill/carrier/contact individuals.

8.1.3　The outcome phase – the evaluation of the healthcare rendered

The outcome phase is characterized by the systematic comparison of the ill individual's and his/her family's health status with the outcomes projected as well as the evaluation of the re-construction of the environment(s) done and the control measures instituted to prevent the spread of the communicable infection. The evaluation consist of two basic forms, namely, the **outcome evaluation** when an assessment is done of all the interventions executed (biomedical and cultural [care and cure activities], environmental and disease control), and **process evaluation** during which an examination is made of the quality of the actions taken and the processes used to achieve the outcome. As such, the following tasks must be executed when doing both forms of evaluation

❑ conducting the evaluation by setting the planned evaluative procedures for outcome and process evaluation into effect. The data collected are then organized for analysis

❑ interpreting the findings after comparison and analysis of the actual outcomes with the standards set. Judgement on the achievement of the set standards forms the basis for the following task of evaluation, namely, using the evaluative findings

❑ using the evaluative findings to make further decisions regarding the healthcare brokering process. When the outcome evaluative findings indicate that the interventions were effective and the objectives were met, the interventions can then either be continued or terminated as needed. When the outcome evaluative findings indicate non-achievement of the set objectives, another approach need to be tried, or the quality of execution of the set interventions need to be corrected as the execution of the interventions are incorrect. Lastly, changes to the other two components (assessment and care rendering) of the healthcare brokering process need also to be made, for example, expanding the assessment phase to gather more explicit or new data; or modify the interventions to meet new or changed constraints in the host and environmental situation.

8.2 IMMUNOTHERAPEUTIC PRODUCTS AND CHEMOTHERAPEUTIC PRODUCTS (ANTIMICROBIAL AGENTS) AVAILABLE FOR THE TREATMENT OF COMMUNICABLE DISEASES

Any alteration/change in the host and/or in the pathogen will eventually lead to the recovery (or death) of the individual and the control of the communicable disease. As the interactions between the host, the pathogen and immunotherapeutic products/ antimicrobial agents are interrelated (the links of the EPIDEMIOLOGICAL TRIAD OF COMMUNICABLE DISEASES MODEL), the administering of immuno-therapeutic products/chemo-therapeutic drugs lead to alterations in the interactions between the immuno-therapeutic products/antimicrobial agents and the pathogen as well as to alterations in the interactions between host and pathogen. By administering immunotherapeutic products (antiserum or non-specific gamma-globulin/ immunoglobulin), the resistance of the ill person is greatly enhanced. By administering antimicrobial agents to the host, selective toxicity is achieved by exploiting the differences in the structure and metabolism of the pathogen and the cells of the host because the specificity of an antimicrobial drugs resides in its ability to damage the pathogen (act at a target site present in the infecting pathogen) and not the host (the target site is absent in the cells of the host).

8.2.1 IMMUNOTHERAPEUTIC PRODUCTS

Various immunotherapeutic products agents are available for the treatment of communicable infections, such as non-specific cellular immunostimulants and antiserum. If antiserum/antitoxin against a particular communicable disease is available, it should generally be considered first of all as it is the best available product in the prescribed treatment regime.

8.2.1.1 Immunotherapy

Immunotherapy is an alternative to vaccination in those individuals who are already infected or are immunological compromised. Some situations exist where a different approach is necessary, for instance, the individual is already infected and a more rapid build-up of immune effector mechanisms than that occurs naturally is needed, or alternatively, the ill individual's immune system may be impaired and unable to respond either to infection or the vaccine, because of immunodeficiency or some specially resistant property of the pathogen.

8.2.1.1.1 Passive transfer of antibody via an antiserum or an antitoxin

Certain diseases such as tetanus and diphtheria are treated by the injection of preformed antibody whereby passive immunity is transferred to the ill individual. An antiserum already contains the specific antibody as it was obtained from either persons who have recovered from the specific communicable disease and whose bodies have formed antibody against the particular disease, or horses that were injected with the specific infectious agent and the body of the horse formed the necessary antibody. An antitoxin contains the necessary antitoxin to neutralize the specific toxin. Both these products/drugs offer only temporary passively-acquired artificial immunity since the body starts secreting the antiserum/antitoxin after 2–3 weeks. Antiserum/antitoxin (if available) is the best product/drug in the treatment regime since if offers the fastest way of helping the body to resist the infection. When a vaccine for the relevant disease exists, the person must always be actively vaccinated after his/her recovery (with the full dosages being administered) in order to stimulate the immunological response of the body.

<u>Please note</u>

Administering of an antiserum/antitoxin may elicit an anaphylactic shock reaction which can cause the death of the person. All the necessary precautionary measures have to be taken before the antiserum/antitoxin is administered. After administering the ill person should be intensively observed for serum sickness

8.2.1.1.2 Antibody in pooled normal blood serum - human immunoglobulin

Most normal persons have antibody to the causative pathogen in their blood serum. Human immunoglobulin is prepared from blood plasma of healthy donors after screening for hepatitis B and C and HIV. Human immunoglobulin, especially IgG, is an antibody-protein which plays an important role as prophylactic treatment in the prevention of infection, or as a treatment to enhance the physiological resistance of the body, especially after exposure, or as a treatment to decrease the severity of the disease. Human immunoglobulin or gamma-globulin can be given intra-muscularly or intravenously and dosages of as little as 5ml of IgG (100-400mg/kg) reduce the possibility for contracting of a particular communicable disease enormously.

8.2.1.1.3 Non-specific cellular immunostimulation

Some communicable diseases respond to treatment with non-specific cellular/molecular mediators that stimulate the immune system. Cytokines, a family of non-antibody specific molecules with diverse activity, such as interferon and interleukins, are effective in a number of viral infections as they contribute to the control of the infection and disease pathology in the body. Interferon is produced by body cells that were exposed to a virus infection as well as infections with rickettsiae, mycobacterium, and several protozoa. When interferon reaches other body cells, the physiologic resistance of cells against viruses are enhanced. As such, interferon has great therapeutic potential in the treatment and prevention of viral infections. It is, however, very expensive.

8.2.2 Chemotherapeutic drugs – antimicrobial agents/drugs

Antimicrobial agents/drugs, also referred to as antibiotics/antifungal/anti-protozoan/anti-helminthic, are derived from either natural products that are fermented, or from fermented natural products that are then chemical modified (semi-synthetically) to improve their antibacterial or pharmacological properties, or produced totally synthetically. **Antimicrobial agents** have either bacteriocidal (killing off of bacteria) or bacteriostatic (only inhibiting bacterial growth) action and target the following five target sites for their bacterial action, namely, the cell wall synthesis; protein synthesis; nucleic acid synthesis; metabolic pathways; and cell membrane function (individually or in combination). Each target site encompasses a multitude of synthetic reactions (enzymes and substrates), each of which are specifically inhibited by an antimicrobial agent. A range of chemically diverse molecules inhibit different reactions at the same target site. Because antimicrobial agents have diverse chemical structures, antibacterial agents are classified in classes (families) according the combination of their target site and their chemical structure.

The causative pathogen may develop resistance to antibacterial agents acquired by chromosomal mutation against a certain class of antimicrobial agents (cross-resistance) or via resistance genes on transmissible plasmids by coding for resistance determinants to unrelated families of antibacterial agents (multiple resistance). Resistance can also be acquired from transposons (jumping genes) and other mobile elements. The mechanisms of resistance encompass the following

✓ an alteration of the target site whereby the target site has a lowered affinity for the antibacterial agent but the site can still function adequately for normal metabolism to proceed, or alternatively,

✓ an additional target (for example, enzyme) may be synthesized, or

✓ the access to the target site may be altered (altered uptake or increased exit) by altering the entry (decreasing the permeability of the cell wall) or by pumping the drug out of the cell (efflux mechanism).

Enzymes such as beta-lactamases, amino-glycoside-modifying enzymes and chloramphenicol acetyl transferases, modify or destroy the antibacterial agent, thus producing drug inactivation.

Antifungal agents are limited and selective toxicity is very difficult to achieve in eukaryotic fungal cells than in prokaryotic bacteria cells. The treatment of fungal infections is hampered by problems of solubility, stability and absorption of the antifungal agent(s). Fungi develop resistance to antifungal agents with many similar mechanisms in operation as in bacteria.

When considering **antiparasitic agents**, the problems of very large number of different parasites capable of infecting man, the complexities of their lifecycles and the differences between them in their metabolic pathways, must always be taken in account. In general, antibacterial agents are ineffective against helminths although some antibacterial agents do possess anti-protozoan activity. Many antiparasitic agents carry the risk of significant toxicity while drug resistance is becoming an increasing problem.

Antiviral therapy consists of the administering of antiviral agents to the ill individual suffering of infections caused by viruses. Most antiviral drugs are virustatic rather than virucidal due to the difficulty of interfering with viral activity in the cell without adversely affecting the host because viruses are dependent on the host cell's protein synthesising machinery. For antiviral chemotherapy to be successful, the early diagnosis of viral infections with short incubation period, such as respiratory viruses, is critical. Antiviral resistance also occurs with varying prevalence in patient populations, especially anti-retroviral resistance across all the main classes of agents – nucleoside reverse transcriptase inhibitors; non-nucleoside reverse transcriptase inhibitors; and protease inhibitors.

Antimicrobial and antiviral agents are valuable drugs in the treatment of infections because of their specificity of the drug(s) being used. These drugs must be used appropriately (for prophylaxis or for treatment); must be correctly prescribed and must be correctly administered. It is therefore necessary for all healthcare providers to understand and be knowledgeable of the following aspects

✠ the site or likely site of infection

✠ the most suitable antimicrobial/antiviral agent to be prescribed for the specific infection (the wrong antimicrobial/antiviral agent will harm the ill individual and does not support the body's defence mechanisms)

✠ the pharmacology and the antimicrobial action of the agent

✠ the correct and appropriate route for administering (per mouth, per rectum, intravenously or intramuscularly, while taking into account the person's preferences, for example, tablet, cream, suppository, pessary or capsule)

✠ the desired drug-induced levels to be achieved in the tissues, taking in account the dosage intervals required to maintain the desired levels

✠ the route of excretion of the antimicrobial agent

✠ the risk of toxicity and side-effects/adverse effects of the antimicrobial/antiviral agent

✠ antimicrobial resistance

✠ allergic reaction shown by the host to any microbial/antiviral agent(s)

✠ other host factors that could modify the outcome

✠ the importance of completing the course of treatment.

8.3   KEY NOTES

❑ The assessments of persons suffering from communicable diseases include their families as well as the community and the environment in which they live, work or attend school.

❑ The healthcare of the ill person may be rendered at home or in a hospital, depending on the interaction between the health status of the host, environmental factors involved and the nature of the specific infectious agent involved.

❑ All healthcare interventions must be scientifically and culturally congruent in nature and be rendered at primary, secondary and tertiary level of healthcare rendering.

❑ All healthcare interventions planned for all hosts, (the individual [healthy, ill, contact, carrier], family and, if necessary, for the community) must include all the dimensions of health (bio-physical, psychological, socio-cultural, lifestyle, environment, and healthcare system).

❑ The healthcare plan must include both scientific fundamental and specific healthcare interventions as well as the culturally congruent interventions that satisfy both healthcare user(s) and healthcare provider(s).

❑ All healthcare planning and interventions (fundamental and specific) must take the age-related needs of the ill person and his/her family in consideration.

THEME IV

VICTORY FOR THE PATHOGEN - THE HOST HAS LOST THE BATTLE

The clinical manifestation of communicable diseases and the specific healthcare to be rendered

When the state of "balanced pathogenicity" between host and pathogens is disrupted, disease/infection arises. Depending upon whether the host defences are intact and competent or impaired, four types of infection can be distinguish based on the four different types of infecting pathogens, namely,

❑ diseases caused by pathogens (mostly viruses and certain bacteria) that possess specific mechanisms for attaching themselves to, or penetrating the body surfaces of normal healthy hosts

❑ diseases caused by pathogens that are introduced into normal healthy hosts by biting arthropods

❑ diseases caused by pathogens that are introduced into otherwise normal healthy hosts via skin wounds or animal bites

❑ diseases caused by pathogens that are able to infect a normal healthy host only when surface and/or systemic defences are impaired.

Furthermore, pathogens do not necessarily produce the same disease/infection in all infected individuals. The biological response gradient causes a spectrum that range from asymptomatic to mild, to serious, to fatal resulting in the death of the infected individual.

The signs and symptoms of infections are produced by the pathogens or by the host's immune responses. Symptoms that appear rapidly after acquisition of an infection are usually due to the direct action of the invading pathogen or its secretion/

toxins. Bacteria provoke most of their acute effects (symptoms) by releasing toxins or cause distress by inducing inflammation. Viruses in cells, on the other hand, cause metabolic "shut down" or lysis of the cells. The acute inflammatory response is the most important component of host protection as vascular permeability being vital for the rapid mobilization of cells and serum components such as complement and antibody. Inflammation is therefore intrinsically a healthy sign. Virulent bacteria such as staphylococci, however, can to some extent inhibit the acute inflammatory response. On the other hand, pathologic changes are often secondary to the activation of the immunological mechanisms that are normally thought of as protective – both the innate and the adaptive immune system can be involved. Tissue damage resulting from the adaptive immune responses cause "immuno-pathology" and is quite common in chronic and persistent infectious diseases.

All communicable diseases run a natural course with five distinctive stadiums, each of which is recognisable from the specific pathogenesis and reaction between the tissue of the body and the infectious agent as well as from the manner in which the signs and symptoms are clinically manifested (see chapter 7)

❑ The **first stadium** is that of pre-pathogenesis. At this stage the person has already been exposed to the infectious agent. Based on the body's innate and adaptive physiologic resistance, the person may become ill or may not. When the person becomes ill, the general and specific characteristic signs and symptoms will then clinically manifested

❑ The **second stadium** is that of pathogenesis which can be divided into four sub-stages, namely,

❖ **Early pathogenesis** - During this stage the person is already infected (as the disease has been contracted) although the clinical signs and symptoms (non-specific and typical/characteristic-specific) of the particular disease are not yet manifested. The person seems to be healthy. This stadium correlates with the incubation period and can last from a few hours to a number of days. The person can already transmit the particular disease to other persons

❖ **Prodromal stage (pre-clinical stage)** (early general discernible signs) - The signs and symptoms which appear during this stage are not typical of the disease. The person manifests the signs and symptoms of a general systemic illness (such as pyrexia) and already feels ill. Sometimes a prodromal rash may appear. This stage lasts until the characteristic signs and symptoms of the disease are manifested. During this period the infected person continues to transmit the particular disease to other persons

❖ **Characteristic-specific clinical picture (clinical stage)** - This starts with the manifestation of the characteristic-specific signs and symptoms of the particular disease. The clinical picture lasts as long as the clinical signs and symptoms are visible. The ill person continues to transmit the disease to other persons. (Note Some communicable diseases will only be transmitted as long as pyrexia is present. In other cases the disease is transmissible until the ill person has recovered)

❖ **Recovering stage (stage of resolution)** - During this stage the ill person recovers and the characteristic-specific clinical signs and symptoms disappear. When the ill person has recovered, he/she is immune (adaptive-mediated immunity with memory cells has been elicit) to the specific communicable disease. When no immunity with memory has been elicited, the person may contract the specific communicable disease once again. After recovering from certain specific communicable diseases a carrier state may develops.

All healthcare providers must have a thorough knowledge of the various communicable diseases, namely, the epidemiological data, pathogenesis and clinical manifestation of each particular communicable disease as well as the prevention and treatment thereof in order to render quality healthcare to the ill individual within his/her familial and community context and to all contacts and carriers. Epidemics can only be controlled and prevented if the epidemiological process is continuously implemented. All healthcare providers must thus at all times bear in mind that, despite all measures taken, outbreaks of communicable diseases do occur and will always occur. It is therefore necessary that the population be regularly monitored by all healthcare providers in order to lower the incidence of epidemics.

As there are more than 150 different communicable infections known to man, the clinical manifestations and diagnosis of the selected communicable diseases are classified and described according to the body system primarily involved at clinical level. The body-systems approach is used because infections caused by a wide variety of pathogens (bacteria, viruses, protozoa, rickettsiae, etc.) can be included on the basis of the clinical diseases/syndromes affecting the specific body system. Based on the body-systems approach and the microbiological classification of the causative pathogen, the epidemiological data, pathogenesis, clinical manifestation, diagnosis, complications, specific healthcare interventions (treatment) and preventive measures of selected communicable diseases are thus discussed in detail in Theme IV. Please note, that with any system of classification, grey areas and overlaps exist as many communicable infections cannot be readily pigeon-holed into any specific body system such as multi-system infections (diseases that are not obviously localized to one system of the body only).

Chapter 9

COMMUNICABLE INFECTIONS AFFECTING THE CENTRAL NERVOUS SYSTEM AND THE EYES

Diseases that affect the nervous system are usually of a very serious nature and when complications set in, they vary from slight to extremely serious, influencing to a great extent the quality of life of the infected person as well as his/her family. Some of these diseases are transmitted to humans by animals and are not transmissible between humans. The infected central nervous system also rarely assists in the transmission of the particular infection. Diseases of the eyes are highly contagious and all preventive measures against further spread have to be applied punctiliously. Enforcing preventive measures to prevent epidemics is of the utmost importance.

9.1 COMMUNICABLE DISEASES THAT AFFECT THE CENTRAL NERVOUS SYSTEM

The brain and spinal cord are protected from mechanical pressure or deformations by enclosure in rigid containers, namely, the skull and the vertebral column which also act as barriers to the spread of infections. The central nervous system is thus better protected against infection than other systems such as the respiratory or digestive systems, because it has no direct contact with the external environment. The blood vessels and nerves that traverse the walls of the skull and vertebral column are the main routes of invasion. Because of the complexity of the nervous system, invasion of the central nervous system occurs most commonly via blood-borne invasion. Invasion via peripheral nerves is less common while local invasion often also occurs from the olfactory tract, infected ears or sinuses, local injury or congenital defects.

Blood-borne invasion takes place across anatomical barriers as well as across the blood-brain barrier and the blood-cerebrospinal fluid-barrier to infect the cells of the nervous system. The blood-brain barrier consists of tightly joined endothelial cells surrounded by glial processes, while the blood-cerebrospinal fluid-barrier at the choroid plexus consists of endothelium with fenestrations and tightly joined choroid plexus epithelial cells. Pathogens transverse these barriers by
- growing across the barriers, infecting the cells that comprise the barrier
- being passively transported across the barriers in intra-cellular vacuoles
- being carried across the barriers by infected white blood cells.

When a specific pathogenic agent/microbe invades the central nervous system, the neural defence mechanisms are less able to defend the brain and nervous system than when the pathogen had penetrated other systems of the body. The result of any infection of the central nervous system is more serious and longer lasting.

The response of the central nervous system to invading pathogens is reflected by an increase in lymphocytes, mostly T-cells, and monocytes in the cerebrospinal fluid. A slight increase in protein also occurs. In viral infections the cerebrospinal fluid remains clear – "aseptic" meningitis. With pyogenic bacterial infections, an extremely rapid increase in polymorphonuclear leukocytes and proteins occur and the cerebrospinal fluid becomes visibly turbid – "septic" meningitis. With slower growing or less pyogenic bacterial pathogens, such as *Mycobacterium tuberculosis humanis*, less rapid changes occur.

The pathological consequences of infections of the central nervous system depend upon the pathogen causing the infection. Viruses that infect the neural cells sometimes show marked preference for specific neural cells. For example, polio- and rabies-viruses, invade neurons whereas other viruses invade the oligo-dendrocytes. Because there is very little extra-cellular space in the skull and spinal column, spreading occurs mostly direct from cell to cell along established nerve pathways. Viruses also induce peri-vascular infiltration of lymphocytes and monocytes resulting, sometimes, in direct damage to the infected neural cells. Invading bacteria and protozoa generally induce more dramatic inflammation events which limit local spreading, with the result that the infection is localized to form abscesses in the "vulnerable closed box" of the skull. Generally, in all cases of infection (bacterial and viral) of the central nervous system, a degree of inflammation and oedema that would be trivial in striated muscle, skin or liver, is life-threatening when it occurs in the "vulnerable closed box" containing the leptomeninges, brain and spinal cord. It also takes weeks after clinical recovery before cellular infiltrations are removed and histological appearances are restored to normal.

Antibody–mediated immunological and associated immune responses of the central nervous system components of the host develop as immune responses to viral meningitis and viral encephalitis. Infiltrating B-cells produce antibody to the invading viral-pathogen, with T-cells reacting with viral-microbial antigens to release cytokines that attract and activate other T-cells and macrophages, while inducing infiltration of the mononuclear cells. As soon as oligoclonal antibody production starts to take place, the infection becomes finally controlled. The production of oligoclonal antibody, together with the destruction of the infected neural cells and the viral spread cause immuno-pathology. The pathological condition evolves over the course of several days. In post-vaccinia encephalitis, the pathological condition evolves over the course of years as it is partly controlled by host defences – for example, sub-acute scleroses pan-encephalitis caused by Measles which has both a virological and immunological pathogenesis. With regard to bacterial infections of the central nervous system, local responses to bacterial antigens and toxins play an important part because bacteria cause more rapidly evolving pathological changes.

9.1.1 Infections of the meninges of the brain

Bacteria such as *Neisseria meningitidis, Haemophilus influenzae, and Streptococcus pneumoniae* cause bacterial meningitis, while viruses such as herpes-viruses, paramyxoviruses, enteroviruses, cause viral meningitis. Some of the bacteria, such as *Neisseria meningitidis,* is carried asymptomatically in the population and is attached by its pili to the epithelial cells in the nasopharynx of the carrier. Persons possessing specific complement-dependant bacterial antibody to capsular antigens are protected against invasion. On the other hand, persons with C5-C9 complement deficiencies show increased susceptibility to bacteraemia. Those most infected are young children who have lost the immunity acquired from their mothers, and adolescents who have not previously encountered the infecting serotype and therefore possess no type-specific immunity with memory. Person-to-person transmission takes place by airborne infected droplets, and is facilitated by other respiratory infections, often viral, that cause increased respiratory secretions. Conditions such as overcrowding and confinement such as prisons, military barracks and college dormitories contribute to the frequency of infection in populations.

Viral meningitis, on the other hand, is the most common type of meningitis and is a milder disease than bacterial meningitis. Person-to-person transmission takes place by airborne viral infected droplets. The enteroviruses are common causes of seasonal aseptic meningitis. Despite the fact that there are only a few antiviral drugs for treatment available, viral meningitis usually has a benign course and complete recovery is the rule. Viruses are isolated from the cerebrospinal fluid in less than 50% of cases and a virus isolated from the stool or throat of a child with mild meningitis may be of no etiologic significance.

9.1.1.1 MENINGITIS - BACTERIAL AND VIRAL

Meningitis is an acute infection of the meninges of the brain and/or the spinal cord caused by a variety of either bacteria or viruses. Meningitis is characterized by fever, neck stiffness and photophobia. Bacterial meningitis is life-threatening and needs urgent specific medical treatment

Epidemiological data	
Geographical distribution Occurring world-wide. In the RSA the incidence is sporadic or small epidemics occur	
Causative pathogen	

Bacterial
1. Meningococcal meningitis
   • *Neisseria meningitidis*
2. Bacterial meningitis
   • *Haemophilus influenzae Type* B
   • *Streptococcus pneumoniae*
   • *Mycobacterium tuberculosis humanis*
	Viral
	Viruses such as the paramyxoviruses, enteroviruses, arboviruses, herpes-virus

• Other bacterial pathogens such as fungi, protozoa, group *B haemolytic streptococci* and *Escherichia coli*.	

Incubation period
*Meningococcal meningitis: 2–10 days, usually 3–4 days
*Other types of bacterial meningitis: very short; 2–4 days
*Viral meningitis: depends on the specific pathogen causing the disease

Mode of transmission
*Horizontally - Airborne infected droplets for example, *Neisseria meningitidis*
*From a focus of infection elsewhere in the body via blood-borne invasion, for example, *Haemophilus influenzae Type B* and *Mycobacterium tuberculosis humanis*
*From skin or mucosal lesions elsewhere in the body via travelling up axons using the normal retrograde transport mechanisms that can move virus particles to reach the dorsal root ganglia, for example, herpes simplex virus

Period of infectiousness (communicability, transmission)
*Meningococcal meningitis - As long as Neisseria meningitidis is present in the nasal and throat secretions
*Other bacterial meningitis - 24–48 hours after commencement of effective chemotherapeutic treatment, the infection is no longer transmissible
*Viral meningitis - Depends on the specific infectious agent that caused the infection

Reservoir
Humans

Intermediaries
None

Carriers
Bacterial pathogens are found in the nasopharyngeal secretions, especially *Neisseria meningitides*

Immunity status
Uncertainty exists whether immunity with memory is elicited in bacterial or in viral meningitis

Susceptibility and resistance of host
Children and young adults are particularly susceptible to meningococcal meningitis and epidemics occur mainly in hostels, institutions and military camps. Immuno-compromised individuals are prone to fungal meningitis while premature neonates are prone to neonatal meningitis due to the immaturity of their immunological system (innate and adaptive). Elderly persons and young children (less than 2 years of age) are more prone to *Streptococcal pneumoniae* meningitis

Pathogenesis
Upon inhalation of the specific bacterial or viral pathogen, the specific pathogen invades the bloodstream to cause a bacteraemia/viraemia when localizing in the vascular endothelial cells. Via the vascular endothelial cells of the bloodstream,

the pathogen crosses the blood-cerebrospinal fluid-barrier to infect the meninges. Inflammatory demyelinising conditions occur in the dura mater, pia mater and arachnoid mater. The polymorphonuclear leukocytes and proteins as well as the lymphocytes (mostly T-cells) and monocytes in the cerebrospinal fluid increase. The cerebrospinal fluid may visibly stay clear (viral infection) or become visibly turbid (bacterial infection).

In all cases of bacterial meningitis, a purulent exudate is formed in the sub-arachnoid space which may either cover the entire brain and spinal cord or can be limited to certain areas. This exudate may be fluid or thick and can block the flow of the cerebrospinal fluid. The brain can also be infiltrated, causing it to swell, resulting in the flattening of the gyra and compressing of the ventricles. The infection of the brain may also cause an inflammation of the optic and other cranial nerves, leading to secondary inflammatory demyelinising conditions of the cranial nerves. When the flow of cerebrospinal fluid is blocked, internal or external hydrocephaly may develop.

❖ **Clinical manifestation**
The general clinical features of both bacterial and viral meningitis are the same but the manifestation of the infection by infants/young children and older children/ adults differ markedly
❋ **Babies and young children**
In infants, the signs and symptoms that develop are non-specific and therefore not as pronounced as is the case of adults. A stiff neck, which is a common occurrence in adults, develops seldom in babies except in advanced cases when opisthotonos occur
 • The signs and symptoms that develop in infants are
   ❋ Failure to thrive and develop
   ❋ Pyrexia
   ❋ Vomiting and diarrhoea
   ❋ Irritability followed by drowsiness (lethargy)
   ❋ Bulging fontanels when the infant is lying quietly and not crying
   ❋ Epileptic seizures
 • Headache and photophobia do develop in young children although they do not complain about these symptoms. Behaviour changes, such as shielding the eyes from light, refusing to open their eyes, irritability, crying, may indicate photophobia and headache
❋ **Adults and older children**
 • In older children and adults, the inflammation and swelling of the meninges causes pain when the neck or body is flexed. The pain is countered by a reflex muscle spasm of the extensor muscles of the neck and vertebral column. This extensor muscle spasm causes the classic sign of a stiff neck. (Stiffness of the neck is elicited when the hand of the examiner is placed under the ill person's head in an attempt to lift and bend the head to place the chin on the sternum. In mild cases, resistance to flexion is experienced only towards the completion of the neck flexion, while in severe cases the ill person can be lifted bodily off the bed without any head flexion taking place)

- Signs and symptoms that develop in older children and adults are
  - ❋ Rigor and pyrexia
  - ❋ Malaise and headache
  - ❋ Vomiting
  - ❋ Photophobia
  - ❋ General hyperaesthesia to all stimuli
  - ❋ Dysphagia
  - ❋ Meningeal irritation (including auditory stimulation)
  - ❋ Neck stiffness or nuchal rigidity (inability to flex neck forward due to rigidity of the neck muscles) and thoracic-columnar stiffness together with intensified symmetrical deep tendon reflexes and opisthotonos
  - ❋ Positive Brudzinski's signs
    - ♦ neck - in the supine position, hip and knee flexion occurs in response to the lifting/raising of the neck)
    - ♦ contralateral reflexes - when hip and knee of one leg are passively flexed on one side, the contralateral leg bends in identical reflex while reciprocal contralateral reflex occurs when the leg that has been flexed in response to the passive flexion of the contralateral hip and knee begin to extend passively
  - ❋ Bilateral positive Kernig's sign (resistance to straightening of knee [because of experiencing pain] when lying flat on the bed with leg and knee flexed)
  - ❋ Varying levels of consciousness such as delirium, drowsiness, stupor and coma, in accordance with the course of the infection and age of the individual
  - ❋ Muscle impairment with poor coordination, tremors, hypotonia and convulsions
  - ❋ Ocular impairment with venous congestion of the ocular fundi, pupillary oedema, pupils are unequal and react poorly to light, strabismus, diplopia with ptosis and paralysis of any of the eye muscles.

The specific clinical features of meningitis caused by different types of infectious agents are pathogen-specific. Only the most important pathogen-specific meningeal infections are discussed. When meningitis (especially bacterial meningitis) goes untreated or not treated in the early stages of the diseases, the fatality rate is extremely high.

❋ **Meningococcal meningitis**
- ✠ After an incubation period of one to three (1-3) days, the onset is sudden with a sore throat, headache, drowsiness, fever, irritability, neck stiffness, and photophobia
- ✠ A haemorrhagic skin rash with petechiae develops, reflecting the associated septicaemia
- ✠ In 35% of cases, the septicaemia is fulminating with complications due to disseminated intravascular coagulation, endotoxemia with shock and renal failure

✠ Acute Addisonian Crisis with bleeding into the brain and adrenal glands (Waterhouse-Friedrichsen syndrome) may develop in severe cases, resulting in the death of the infected person

✠ When recovery takes place, serious sequelae such as permanent hearing loss, intellectual disablement, may occur as well as amputation of limb(s) due to gangrene of the limb because of the occurrence of disseminated intravascular coagulation in the limb

✠ During outbreaks of meningococcal meningitis, the carrier rate may increase between 60-80% (the *Neisseria meningitidis* is carried in the nasopharynx where it is attached by its pili to the epithelial cells).

✱ Haemophilus B meningitis

✠ *Haemophilus influenzae type B*, a common secondary invader of the lower respiratory tract, causes meningitis in infants and young children when *type B Haemophilus influenzae* invades the blood and reach the meninges

✠ Although maternal antibody protects the infant up to three to four (3-4) months of age, a "window of susceptibility" develops as the maternal antibody protection wanes, until the infant produces his/her own antibody from two to three (2-3) years onwards as these antibody are T-cell independent

✠ After an incubation period of five to six (5-6) days, the onset is more insidious than that of meningococcal or pneumococcal meningitis

✠ Although the condition is less frequently fatal than meningococcal meningitis, haemophilus meningitis is commonly complicated by severe neurological sequelae such as hearing loss, delayed language development, intellectual impairment and epileptic seizures.

✱ Pneumococcal meningitis

✠ *Streptococcal pneumoniae* is a common cause of bacterial meningitis, particularly in children (under 2 years of age) and the elderly (especially in debilitated or immuno-compromised individuals)

✠ *Streptococcal pneumoniae* is a capsulate Gram-positive coccus carried in the throats of many healthy individual

✠ Susceptibility to infection is associated with low levels of antibody to capsular polysaccharide antigens as antibody opsonises the *Streptococcal pneumoniae* and promotes phagocytosis, thereby protecting the individual from invasion. (Note that as more than 85 different capsular types of *Streptococcal pneumoniae* exist, the protection is type-specific)

✠ Pneumococcal meningitis has an acute onset following pneumonia and/or septicaemia (especially in the elderly)

✠ The clinical features are generally worse than with meningococcal meningitis and haemophilus meningitis and the fatality rate is higher.

✱ Neonatal meningitis

✠ Neonates, especially those with low birth weight, are at an increased risk for meningitis because of their immature immunological status

✠ Neonatal meningitis is caused by a wide range of bacteria - especially *haemolytic streptococci group B* (carried sometimes by healthcare providers and other employees employed/private workers working in healthcare establishments or acquired by cross-infection in the nursery) and *Escherichia coli* (by routes of nosocomial infection when healthcare providers and other employees/ workers do not wash their hands properly). The neonate can also be infected by the mother when the infant, during the birth process, swallows maternal secretions such as amniotic fluid that is infected by *Haemolytic streptococci group B* which has colonized in the mother's vagina

✠ The infant manifest very seldom specific signs except for fever, poor feeding, vomiting, respiratory distress or diarrhoea

✠ Neonatal meningitis often leads to permanent neurological sequelae such as cerebral palsy, cranial nerve palsy, epilepsy, hydrocephaly, intellectual impairment. These sequelae results partly because of the difficulty to clinically diagnose meningitis in neonates and partly because of the inadequate drug-induced levels in the cerebrospinal fluid of the antimicrobial drugs.

❋ **Tuberculoid meningitis**
✠ Tuberculoid meningitis is caused by *Mycobacterium tuberculosis humanis* lodged in a focus of infection elsewhere in the body, although some infected persons have no clinical or historical evidence of such infection. In most cases, tuberculoid meningitis is associated with acute miliary tuberculosis

✠ In areas with a high prevalence of tuberculosis, tuberculoid meningitis tends to be seen more in young children - from birth to four (0-4) years old. In areas where tuberculosis is less frequent, most tuberculoid meningitis cases occur in adults

✠ Tuberculoid meningitis usually presents with a gradual onset (occasionally rapid) over a few weeks beginning with malaise, apathy and anorexia and proceeding within a few weeks to photophobia, neck stiffness and impairment of consciousness.

❋ **Fungal meningitis**
✠ Fungal meningitis is caused by *Cryptococcus neoformans* which invades the blood from the primary site of infection in the lungs and spreads from there to the brain to cause fungal meningitis

✠ Fungal meningitis is mostly seen in individuals with depressed cell-mediated immunity, for example, as in persons suffering from AIDS.

❋ **Viral meningitis**
✠ Viral meningitis is the most common type of meningitis and is a milder infection then bacterial meningitis

✠ Headache, fever and photophobia, but less neck stiffness, develop

✠ The cerebrospinal fluid is clear in the absence of bacteria and the cells are mainly lymphocytes, although polymorphonuclear leukocytes may be present in the earlier stages

✠ Viral meningitis usually has a benign course and complete recovery is the rule.

❖ **Complications**
- Paralysis
- Intellectual impairment
- Hydrocephaly
- Cerebral abscesses
- Blindness and/or deafness
- Ocular nerve paralysis
- Death
- Carrier status (meningococcal meningitis)

■ **Diagnosis**
- Isolation of the pathogen in and/or changes in the composition of the cerebrospinal fluid

■ **Prognosis**
- Bacterial - fairly good with antimicrobial treatment
- Viral - good.

■ **Specific healthcare interventions to be rendered**
- **Medical treatment**
  - ❖ Medical treatment must commence without delay without waiting for the results of the cerebrospinal fluid cultures
  - ❖ Chemotherapeutic-specific antimicrobial drugs are to be prescribed according to the treatment relevant to the specific infectious pathogen isolated
  - ❖ Analgesics are to be prescribed for headache
  - ❖ No specific antimicrobial drugs are available for the treatment of viral meningitis
- **General healthcare**
  - ❖ When the infected individual suffers from meningococcal meningitis, he/she must be cared for in isolation
  - ❖ When the infected individual suffers from other types of meningitis, bed rest in a quiet, darkened room
  - ❖ Fluid balance must be maintained – intravenous fluid therapy may be needed
  - ❖ Vital signs must be monitored and the temperature be taken every two to four (2-4) hourly to ensure early diagnosis of complications such as respiratory arrest, myocardial hypoxia, dysrhythmia and brain stem lesions
  - ❖ The level of consciousness of the ill individual must be observed hourly (1) until he/she shows signs of improvement, thereafter every four (4) hourly
  - ❖ A fluid balance chart must be kept
  - ❖ Rehabilitative care must be provided if the ill person is disabled after recovering

◆ **Preventive measures to be taken**
- ➢ Tracing of contacts and administering of prophylactic medication

> Tracing of carriers and administering of a short course of chemotherapeutic antimicrobial drugs (elimination of nasopharyngeal carriage of meningococci must be obtained)
> Preventing of overcrowding
> Meningococcal vaccine is available when necessary, such as for national servicemen and travellers or for high-risk groups (for example, children and healthcare workers) whenever epidemics occur. Routine vaccination is not advised
> An effective 7-valent conjugate pneumococcal vaccine is available for infants 2-23 months as well as for older children (24-59 months) who are at high risk. A 23-valent polysaccharide vaccine is available for children older than five (5) years

◆ **Measures to prevent epidemics**
   ⊹ According to regulation No. R2438 in the Government Gazette of 30 October 1987, any person who suffered from meningococcal meningitis may only return to educational institutions on presentation of a medical certificate
   ⊹ Contacts are allowed to return immediately, provided they take the necessary prophylactic drugs
   ⊹ Prophylactic treatment must be provided as required to all persons necessary
   ⊹ Carriers must be traced and treated
   ⊹ Hib vaccine can be administered to children who have not yet reached school-going age and attend pre-primary schools, Grade R, crèches, play groups or day care centres

◆ **Implications for disaster situations**
   ⊹ Meningococcal meningitis - epidemics can occur under conditions of sudden forced overcrowding

◆ **Compliance with international measures**
   ⊹ None

9.1.2 Infections of the substance of the brain and spinal cord

Infection of the substance of the brain and spinal cord occurs most commonly via blood-borne invasion. Invasion via peripheral nerves is less common, while local invasion from the olfactory tract, infected ears or sinuses, local injury or congenital defects occur sometimes. Infection of the brain and spinal cord, however, is a rare event because most pathogens fail to cross the blood-brain barrier to infect the substance of the brain and spinal cord.

When blood-borne invasion of the substance of the brain takes place, the microbes (for example, viral, bacteria, fungi, parasites) transverse the blood-brain barrier by
 • growing across it, infecting the cells that comprise the barrier
 • being passively transported across it in intra-cellular vacuoles
 • being carried across it by infected white blood cells

Once the infection has reached the meninges and the cerebrospinal fluid, the brain substance is invaded as soon as the infection crosses the pia mater, resulting in encephalitis. Characteristically, there are signs of cerebral dysfunction when the substance of the brain is affected, and a person with an encephalitic illness presents with abnormal behaviour, seizures and altered consciousness, nausea, vomiting and fever.

Sporadic acute focal encephalitis in older children and adults is caused by *Herpes simplex-virus-1* (HSV-1) when virus-reactivation in the trigeminal ganglia occur and the infection then passes back to the temporal lobe of the brain. Neonates acquire a primary and disseminated infection with diffuse encephalitis after vaginal delivery from a mother shedding *Herpes simplex-virus-2* (HSV-2) in her genital tract. When infected with the *Varicella-zoster-virus*, encephalitis occurs generally as a sequel to reactivation of the *varicella-zoster-virus*, while cytomegalovirus infection of the brain substance occurs either as a primary infection in-uteri, or when reactivation takes place as a complication of immuno-deficiency. Enteroviral and paramyxoviral infections can also invade the central nervous system in a complex stepwise series of bodily events after the specific virus had gained entry into the body. The *Human immunodeficiency retrovirus* (HIV-virus) also causes sub-acute encephalitis, often with dementia. Post-infectious virus encephalitis (for example, 1-2 weeks after normal Measles and Chickenpox, or Influenza-like illnesses) and post-vaccinia virus encephalitis (brain-derived inactivated rabies-vaccine, vaccination with non-infectious material leading to allergic encephalitis) also occurs occasionally and has possibly an auto-immune basis.

9.1.2.1   POLIOMYELITIS (POLIO)

Poliomyelitis is an acute viral infection that affects the meninges and the substance of the brain causing a characteristic inflammation reaction and manifest with muscle weakness or paralysis

---

Epidemiological data

Geographical distribution
Occurring world-wide. Epidemics occur particularly during summertime and autumn

Causative pathogen
The polio-virus, an enterovirus. There are three distinct serological (antigenic) types, namely, polio-virus Brunhilda, polio-virus Lansing, and polio-virus Leon. Very little cross-reaction exists between the three serotypes with the result that antibody to each type is necessary for protection. The polio-virus is resistant to unfavourable environment conditions and remains alive on contaminated hands and clothing, fomites, in sewage and on flies and cockroaches – a few weeks at room temperature and a few months when the climatic weather temperature varies between 0-8°C after which the virus dies

Incubation period
14 days but can be as long as 35 days

Mode of transmission
*Airborne infected droplets from nasopharyngeal secretions
*Ingestion of contaminated milk
*Faecal-oral transmission due to the fact that the polio-virus is excreted in the faeces (the polio-virus remains alive in stools for months). This is the most common mode of transmission

Period of infectiousness (communicability, transmission)
As long as the virus is excreted in the faeces or is present in the nasopharyngeal secretions

Reservoir
Humans

Intermediaries
Vectors - flies, cockroaches
Vehicles - contaminated hands and clothing, fomites, faeces

Carriers
Persons. The virus is present in nasopharyngeal secretions and faeces

Immune status
Life-long antibody-mediated immunity with memory against a specific serological type is elicited. A second attack rarely occurs. When it happens, it is due to an infection by a different serological type

Susceptibility and resistance of host
All persons of all age groups are susceptible if they have not been vaccinated. Causative factors during epidemics are pregnancy, malnutrition, low resistance, stress, exhaustion, and nasopharyngeal surgery such as a tonsillectomy. New-born babies have a natural passively-acquired immunity which will last for about six months owing to the antibody which crossed the placental barrier (if the mother had suffered from the disease or was vaccinated). Breast milk also contains polio-virus antibody

Pathogenesis

The polio-virus gains entry into the body through either the pharynx (inhaled) or via the intestines (ingested) where it replicates in the lymphatic tissue of the oropharynx or the gut-associated lymphoid tissue. From here it spreads via the lymphatic drainage system to the local regional lymph nodes and then into the bloodstream, spreading to the spleen and liver. In the viscera growth takes place causing a general viraemia which leads to a febrile illness. Due to the localizing of the polio-virus in vascular endothelial cells, the polio-virus crosses the blood-brain barrier and invades neurons of the cranial nerve (anterior horn cells) as well as the substance of the brain and spinal cord. The replication of the polio-virus in the substance of the brain and spinal cord causes petechial haemorrhaging in the brain stem and spinal cord with destruction of the infected neural cells. When the polio-virus spread through the central nervous system, encephalitis develops leading to flaccid paralysis of body muscles. The polio-virus also crosses the blood-cerebrospinal fluid-barrier and replicate in the cerebrospinal fluid with the result that meningitis develops. Impairment of the cranial nerves and the respiratory and cardiovascular centres in the medulla can also occur, with or without affecting the spinal cord. Impairment of the medulla is life-threatening but not necessarily fatal. Characteristic inflammatory reactions occur throughout the body and the liver, spleen and other organs are affected.

From the 5-6th day after infection had occurred, antibody appears and the virus replication becomes controlled. Life-long antibody-mediated immunity with memory against a specific serological type is elicited. A second attack rarely occurs. When it happens, it is due to an infection by a different serological type. The polio-virus is shed in the faeces from the 5th to up to 10th day (or longer) after it had gained entry into the body.

❖ **Clinical manifestation**
Poliomyelitis manifests across a wide spectrum and varies from a **sub-clinical infection** to a **non-paralytic** to a **paralytic disease**
The sub-clinical form of infection and the non-paralytic form of the infection occur in the majority of cases. This form is known as a minor attack and manifest as a slight infective condition with non-paralytic impairment. The clinical manifestations of the sub-clinical infection are characterized by a non-specific illness resembling influenza which lasts a few days
The paralytic form of the infection is characterized by the paralysis of the motor path of the nervous system (spinal or cranial). Depending on the areas of the central nervous system that have been invaded by the polio-virus, either a spinal impairment (when the cervical, thoracic or lumbar spinal cord is affected) or a bulbar impairment (when the cranial nerves and the cardiovascular and respiratory centres of the brain are affected) can be distinguished. The paralytic form of the disease is characterized by signs of meningeal irritation

The clinical manifestations of the sub-clinical form of infection, the non-paralytic form and the paralytic form of the disease are now discussed according to the degree and site of involvement.

General signs and symptoms of all forms of the disease (sub-clinical, non-paralytic and paralytic)
Sore throat, nausea, vomiting, headache and pyrexia lasting 1 to 4 days

✳ **Sub-clinical form of the disease** (Slight infective condition)
  • The onset is abrupt and lasts for a few hours or a number of days (2–6)
  • The abovementioned general signs occur, as well as abdominal pain and a slightly reddish sore throat
  • There is no involvement of the central nervous system
  • For about 2–3 weeks after the first signs and symptoms had appeared, the protein content of the cerebrospinal fluid remains high - an indication that slight inflammatory changes have taken place

✳ **Non-paralytic form of the disease** (minor attack, with slight invasion of the central nervous system without paralysis of the motor neurons)
  • The aforementioned general signs and symptoms develop as well as pain and stiffness of the neck, back and legs

- Headache increases in intensity
- The temperature elevation is more obvious and the condition of the ill person worsens
- Sometimes hyperaesthesia and paraesthesia develop
- The protein level of the cerebrospinal fluid increases
- Signs and symptoms of meningeal irritation develop

✱ **Paralytic form of the disease** (major attack – paralysis result because of spinal or bulbar invasion)
 ◈ **Spinal involvement**
   A biphasic phase occurs especially in children. The first and second phases may occur concurrently
   - The **first phase** is similar to the minor attack, followed by a period of one to seven (1–7) days during which the ill person feels better and appears to be well
   - During the **second phase** a recurrence of the same symptoms as in phase one, but in a far more severe form
     ❀ The ill person complains of hyperaesthesia, muscle pain or spasm of the impaired muscle groups
     ❀ The tendon reflexes may be normal or heightened
     ❀ Signs and symptoms of impairment of the central nervous system, such as anxiety, restlessness, drowsiness or coma develop
     ❀ Positive Brudzinski's signs as well as a positive Kernig's sign are present
     ❀ Paralysis sets in within a day or two (1-2) or up to seven to ten (7–10) days. Sometimes the paralysis is the first sign of the disease
     ❀ The paralysis is always preceded by stiffness of the neck and back. Some ill individuals may complain of a general weakness for two to three (2–3) days before paralysis sets in. No further paralysis occurs after the ill person's temperature has subsided. The paralysis is asymmetrical and flaccid. In 60% of cases the legs are affected and the arms in 25% of cases. Paralysis is predisposed by the following factors
       ⅄ Advanced age
       ⅄ Infection with serological type Brunhilda polio virus
       ⅄ Infection with the polio-virus causing an epidemic
       ⅄ Pregnancy
       ⅄ Excessive physical exhaustion just before or after the appearance of the first signs and symptoms
       ⅄ Local trauma – injections in a limb or surgery of the mouth, such as tooth extraction
       ⅄ Genetic susceptibility
   - An increase in the lymphocytes and monocytes as well as in the proteins in the cerebrospinal fluid occur which may last for up to eight weeks
   - Hypertension develops – lasting for approximately one (1) week
   - Decalcification of the bones, resulting from prolonged immobilisation, causes the formation of kidney stones

- The recovery phase is characterized by
  * The paralysis shows no improvement for a period of days or weeks
  * After a further month or two (1-2) months, atrophy of the paralysed muscles become apparent and the limb is smaller than the unaffected limb. Blood circulation is poor and the growth of the limb is retarded, with the result that it is shorter than the unaffected limb
  * Chest abnormalities may develop owing to paralysis of the shoulder and chest muscles
  * If spontaneous improvement becomes noticeable, such as the reappearance of the deep tendon reflexes and improved muscle strength, the peak is reached within 18 months, after which the residual paralysis is permanent

◈ **Bulbar involvement**
- Involvement of the tenth (10th) cranial nerve causes weakness or paralysis of the soft palate, pharynx and vocal cords
  * The first signs are a nasal intonation and hoarseness
  * The ill individual may refuse to eat or drink because he/she finds it difficult to swallow
  * Secretions accumulate in the throat and these are sometimes regurgitated through the nose
  * Laryngeal stridor is a life-threatening sign
  * Development of facial paralysis
- The involvement of the respiratory and cardiovascular centres in the medulla results in a gradual reduction of the vital functions of these two systems, leading to the death of the ill individual

❖ **Complications**
- Impairment of the respiratory muscles at a late stage of the disease
- Permanent flaccid paralysis
- Disabilities and deformities of the limbs
- Death may occur between one and two (1-2) weeks after the onset of the disease as a result of cardiovascular collapse

■ **Diagnosis**
- Clinical picture
- Culture of the polio-virus from throat and stool specimens

■ **Prognosis**
- Good

■ **Specific healthcare interventions to be rendered**
- **Medical treatment**
  ✪ No specific antimicrobial drug treatment may be prescribed
  ✪ Analgesics can be prescribed
  ✪ Orthopaedic surgery is done for correction of deformities
  ✪ Physiotherapy must commence as soon as the diagnosis had been made

- **Healthcare interventions**
  - ✪ The infected individual must be isolate for at least three (3) weeks and concurrent and terminal disinfection must be applied to prevent the spread of the infection
  - ✪ Complete bed rest must be ensured – the more activities allowed during the acute phase, the more extensive and severe the paralysis
  - ✪ Sedatives may be given to relieve anxiety (involvement of the cranial nerves or weakness of the respiratory muscles are contra-indications)
  - ✪ Body alignment must be maintained by
    - ✳ Providing a firm bed with a footboard to prevent drop foot or strap up the foot in the anatomic position
    - ✳ Allowing affected limbs to rest in a comfortable position. Prevent extension of paralysed muscles since this may result in permanent damage
    - ✳ Doing passive movement exercise two to four (2–4) times daily as soon as the ill individual has been admitted to hospital. (This prevents rigid immobilisation of the affected limb). Commence physiotherapy as soon as tenderness decreases
    - ✳ Applying moist heat to painful areas to relieve pain and spasms (hot baths may also be given)
    - ✳ Encouraging the ill person to use unimpaired muscle groups as much as possible without causing pain and exhaustion
  - ✪ Ensure the comfort of the ill individual by continually changing his/her position
  - ✪ Promote normal respiration by
    - ✳ Keeping the airway open
    - ✳ When respiration is weak, keep emergency tracheotomy tray at hand
    - ✳ Do regular postural drainage to get rid of accumulated secretions
    - ✳ Administering of oxygen when necessarily
  - ✪ Promote the ill individual's mental and emotional health as progress is slow
  - ✪ Provide facilities to limit disability by
    - ✳ Providing therapeutic nutrition
    - ✳ Providing rehabilitation facilities such as occupational therapy, physiotherapy, special orthopaedic appliances, psychological and social support, inclusive schools and special schools for learners with special educational needs, special vocational training and/or sheltered employment

- ◆ **Preventive measures to be taken**
  - ➢ Providing of health information about the necessity of early vaccination and modes of transmission of the polio-virus
  - ➢ Strengthening of the general resistance of the population through the enhancement of personal and environmental health such as the improvement of socio-economic conditions, good housing, garbage and sewage disposal, pure water and food supplies, and the pasteurization of milk
  - ➢ Avoid eating fruit or vegetables that have not been properly washed

> Prevent overheating and excessive cooling down of the body, particularly during spring and summer
> Vaccination of all contacts with TOPV or IPV/PV$_{(i)}$
> Tracing and treating of all carriers
> Epidemiological investigation of all cases of acute flaccid paralysis to prevent an outbreak of poliomyelitis

◆ **Measures to prevent epidemics**
   ＋ Regular mass vaccination campaigns to ensure a high herd immunity of communities through
      o Ensuring high infant vaccination coverage in the first year of life
      o Routine vaccination of all hosts (healthy, ill, contact, and carrier) when necessary
   ＋ Active surveillance for wild poliovirus through reporting and laboratory testing of all cases of acute flaccid paralysis among children younger than 15 years of age
   ＋ Targeted "mop-up" campaigns once the wild poliovirus transmission is limited to a specific focal area. By simultaneously vaccinating as many hosts as possible, the transmission of the wild poliovirus is blocked as the wild poliovirus is unable to infect another susceptible individual
   ＋ In terms of regulation No. R.2438 of 30 October 1987, individuals who had contracted poliomyelitis may only return to an educational institution on submission of a medical certificate while healthy contacts may return immediately
   ＋ Provide health information to motivate parents/guardians/foster-parents to have their children vaccinated
   ＋ Tooth extractions, tonsillectomies and any elective surgery, particularly of the nose and throat, must be avoided during epidemics
   ＋ Large assemblies of persons as well as visits to and from persons or families where the disease is prevalent, must be avoided

◆ **Implications during disaster situations**
   ＋ The crowding of non-immune groups of persons as well as inadequate sanitation can lead to epidemics

◆ **Compliance with international measures**
   ＋ Travellers need to comply with the regulations of the country of entry. If uncertain, polio vaccination advice and active vaccination can be obtained from travel clinics before leaving the RSA. Because of the setback in 2003 in the Global Polio Eradication Initiative of the WHO, certain countries are now classified as endemic and travellers to these countries need to be re-vaccinated (boosters) – children as well as adults

9.1.3 Infections of the central nervous system caused by animal-transmitted pathogens

Humans and animals share a common susceptibility to certain pathogens. A few infections of the human central nervous system are caused by animal-transmitted pathogens, ranging from viruses to protozoa to bacteria causing zoonotic infections in animals. When man is infected, the infection is zoonotic in nature as the non-human vertebrate host is the reservoir of infection. Human infection follows contact with the reservoir host, but man is not essential for the microbe's lifecycle or its replication in nature. Vector-borne zoonotic infections on the other hand are transmitted by blood-feeding arthropods. These vectors inject the pathogen into humans when they take a blood meal.

9.1.3.1 Vector-borne encephalitis

Humans live in daily contact, directly or indirectly, with many animal species, both vertebrate and invertebrate by sharing a common environment. The two classes of invertebrates or arthropods that make major contributions to disease transmission are the six-legged insects such as flies and the eight-legged ticks and mites. Arthropod-transmitted infections are the most common in tropical and sub-tropical geographical regions.

9.1.3.1.1 AFRICAN TRYPANOSOMIASIS (SLEEPING SICKNESS)

African Trypanosomiasis is a vector-borne infection of the central nervous system characterized by widespread enlargement of the lymph nodes, encephalitis, coma and death

---

Epidemiological data

Geographical distribution
The disease is prevalent in the tropical regions of Africa as well as in subtropical regions such as Zimbabwe and Botswana. Trypanosomiasis is also found in the tropical regions in South America (Chagas' disease caused by *Trypanosoma cruzi*)

Causative pathogen
Trypanosoma brucei rhodesiense and *Trypanosoma brucei gambiense* is a protozoan, a single-celled animal, of the genus Trypanosoma. *Trypanosoma brucei* remains extra-cellular, first in the tissues near the insect bite and then in the blood, where it divides rapidly and continuously

Incubation period
Trypanosoma rhodesiense - three (3) days to three (3) weeks
Trypanosoma gambiense - weeks or months

Mode of transmission
Horizontally - The bite of an infected tsetse fly (male or female) of the genus Glossina.
Vertically - Transplacental transmission takes place in humans

---

Period of infectiousness (communicability, transmission)
The disease is not transmitted from one person to another

Reservoir
Infected humans and animals (domestic and wild such as cattle, pigs, antelope/buck)
The tsetse fly is infected with the protozoan either during its normal development or when it sucks the blood of an infected animal. The protozoan reaches maturity within 21 days and is present in the saliva of the fly. A tsetse fly remains infected throughout its life-time (approximately 3 months). An infected fly does not become ill itself with the disease. Due to blood-sucking episodes by the tsetse fly, a person is infected with the protozoan. The infection lasts life-long, unless treatment had been given to destroy the protozoan in the individual's blood circulation

Intermediaries
Vectors - The tsetse fly, genus Glossina. The fly feeds during day light hours

Carriers
None

Immune status
No immunity with memory is elicited

Susceptibility and resistance of host
All persons of all age groups are susceptible

Pathogenesis

After a person has been bitten by a tsetse fly, the *Trypanosoma brucei gambiense* remains extracellular, first in the tissues near the insect bite and then in the blood. A swollen chancre develops at the site of the bite and lymphocytes accumulate at the site of the bite mark and interstitial oedema develops. Simultaneously, lymphocytes start to accumulate in the spleen and lymph nodes. The protozoan disseminates from the tissues to the blood where it multiplies rapidly and continuously leading to a bacteraemia and fever. Marked lymph-adenopathy is usually present between the second and the sixth month of the disease. Splenomegaly and hepatomegaly may also be present as well as myocardial involvement. During the second stage of the disease the central nervous system is invaded by the protozoan.

The natural course of the disease may last from one year in the case of infection with *Trypanosoma brucei rhodesiense*, to several years in the case of infection with *Trypanosoma brucei gambiense*. The *Trypanosoma brucei gambiense* survives freely in the blood because of its remarkable degree of antigenic variation based on switching between some one thousand different genes for the glycoprotein coat. A high concentration of IgM is found in the blood and later in the cerebrospinal fluid. IgM is mediated by plasma cells (the Mott cells) and is seen as a feature of the lymphocytic infiltrate ("perivascular cuffing") around blood vessels in the brain.

❖ **Clinical manifestation**
  ✱ The **acute stage** of the disease is characterized by
    • a swollen chancre (a hardened nodule, dark red in colour) that develops within a week or two (1-2 weeks), surrounded by oedema at the site of the bite
    • The following under mentioned signs and symptoms appear intermittently
      ✓ pyrexia and lymph-adenopathy (particularly the posterior cervical lymph nodes when bitten in the neck – Winterbottom's sign)
      ✓ oedema of the hands, feet and around the wrists and eyes and an erythematous rash that is of short duration
      ✓ pruritis of the entire body
    • The lymph nodes stay enlarged when the infection is well-established
    • Because the protozoan lives and multiplies in the blood, fever, splenomegaly and, quite often, signs of myocardial involvement, develops
  ✱ During the **second stage** of the disease (which may be early in the course of the disease or years after the acute stage) the central nervous system is affected (more acutely in the East African *Trypanosoma brucei rhodesiense* than the West African *Trypanosoma brucei gambiense*). Signs of meningo-encephalitis are manifest such as
    • changes in behaviour with delusions and psychological changes ('silent grief')
    • headache and tremors occurring at intervals
    • as time passes, the infected person appears weary, apathetic and lethargic
    • the infected individual develops a shuffling gait and speech becomes slow and mumbling
    • fibril tremors of the tongue and forearms are prominent
    • voracious appetite with weight loss
    • finally the stage of sleepiness is reached where it becomes difficult to rouse the infected individual
    • the infected individual becomes comatose with progressive marasmus due to insufficient intake of food
    • coupled with other infections, this condition leads to death

❖ **Complications**
  • Cerebral degeneration
  • Peripheral neuritis
  • Coma and death
  • Cured Trypanosomiasis can leave the individual with severe residual neurological and mental disability

■ **Diagnosis**
  ▪ A history of being bitten by a tsetse fly
  ▪ Blood and serological tests

■ **Prognosis**
  ▪ The disease is fatal if untreated
  ▪ With treatment the prognosis is good provided severe residual neurological and mental disability does not occur

■ **Specific healthcare interventions to be rendered**
- Specific antimicrobial and arsenic drug therapies are used for treatment during the acute stage, in the chronic stage, and for prophylaxis
- Side-effects of all drugs administered have to be observed and handled accordingly
- Observe for other underlying infective conditions
- Adequate hydration has to be ensured
- Follow-up visits after recovery must be encouraged
- When neurological and mental sequelae exist, rehabilitation must commence

◆ **Preventive measures to be taken**
- Control of tsetse flies by eradicating their natural habitat
- If fly control is unsuccessful, the region must be evacuated by humans
- Health information regarding
  - the nature and danger of the disease
  - personal measures to prevent being bitten by tsetse flies
  - destroying of the breeding places of tsetse flies
  - the use of insecticides

◆ **Measures to prevent epidemics**
- None

◆ **Implications for disaster situations**
- None

◆ **Compliance with international measures**
- None

9.1.3.2 Zoonotic viral encephalitis

A wide range of different viruses are transmitted from animals to man. Virus infections that are transmitted from animals that cause encephalitis are transmitted to humans in the saliva of the infected vertebrate animal. To be transmitted in the saliva, the virus always invades the central nervous system of the animal and then spreads from the central nervous system down the peripheral nerves to the salivary glands, from where it is shed into the saliva of the infected animal. Invasion of the limbic system of the brain of the animal causes a change in behaviour of the infected animal so that the animal becomes less retiring, more aggressive and more likely to bite, thereby transmitting the specific virus. This invasion of the limbic system is a fiendish strategy on the part of the viruses to promote their own shedding, transmission and survival. Humans infected from a zoonotic source, develop a severe febrile to fatal disease. Prophylactic vaccines for humans are not readily available (a vaccine for rabies in animals though is available), nor does any antimicrobial chemotherapeutic drugs exist.

9.1.3.2.1 RABIES (ALSO KNOWN AS HYDROPHOBIA)

Rabies is a zoonotic viral infection of the central nervous system of humans. The infection is characterized by muscle spasms, convulsions, hydrophobia and death

---

Epidemiological data

Geographical distribution
The disease occurs world-wide and is endemic to South Africa. The worst enzootic regions are the Free State and KwaZulu-Natal. The disease occurs in any climatic conditions and in any season

Causative pathogen
Rabies virus, a rhadovirus. The virus is excreted in the saliva of infected animals

Incubation period
Generally 4-13 weeks, but the duration are mostly non-specific and may last from one to three (1-3) months or even longer (up to 6 months). The incubation period is shorter in children. The extent, size and position of the wound also influence the duration of the incubation period. The further the bite is from the central nervous system, the longer the incubation period. When the infection originates from a wound to the head, neck or face, the incubation period is shorter

Mode of transmission
Being bitten by an infected animal and/or an abrasive skin wound, or abraded mucosa being licked by an infected animal
Airborne infected droplets from bats in caves visit by humans

Period of infectiousness (communicability, transmission)
The disease is very rarely transmitted from one person to another. The virus appears in the saliva of animals (wild or tame) 3–5 days before the characteristic signs of rabies are manifested by the infected animal. In bats the virus can be present for months without any sign of the disease. If an apparent healthy animal is still healthy after 10 days after biting a human, rabies is extremely unlikely

Reservoir
Wild vertebrate animals (including bats) and pets. The virus is present in the saliva of the infected animal and penetrates the human body by means of a skin wound or abraded mucosa

Intermediaries
Vectors - Dogs (wild or tame), cats (wild or tame), wolves, jackals, skunks, raccoons, meercats (mongoose or suricate), polecats, rats, bats and foxes. In the RSA the most important vectors are dogs, jackals, cats and meercats

Carriers
None

Immune status
No immunity with memory is elicited

Susceptibility and resistance of host
All persons are susceptible. Small children are bitten more often since they have no fear of playing with either tame or wild animals

---

Pathogenesis

The *rabies virus* gains entry into the body through an open wound or an abrasion in the skin or an abraded mucous membrane (mouth or eye). The *rabies virus* sequestered itself in muscle or subcutaneous tissues where it infects the muscle fibres and muscle spindles by binding to the nicotinic acetylcholine receptor. The *rabies virus* multiplies in the muscle tissue cells and then spread to the peripheral nerves (motor or sensory). After a latent period which may last for days, weeks, months or even years, the virus travels up the axons of the motor neurons or the sensory neurons of the peripheral nerves to reach the glial cells and neurones of the central nervous system where it further multiplies. Once in the brain, the rabies virus invades the neurons and spreads from cell to cell along established nerve pathways until large proportions of the neurons are infected. No cytopathic effect and almost no cellular infiltration occur. The distribution of the virus in the brain causes the clinical manifestation of the disease. The striking symptoms of the disease are largely due to the dysfunction of the infected cells, rather than to visible damage of the infected cells.

No detectable antibody-mediated or cell-mediated response develops, possibly because the antigen remains sequestered in the infected muscle cells. Hence, immunoglobulin is administered during the incubation period as to induce artificial passively-acquired immunity. Once infection of the brain has taken place, the infection is fatal. When recovery does occur, lifelong serious neurological sequelae remain.

❖ **Clinical manifestation**
The disease is characterized by a prodromal and an acute neurological phase
  ✹ **Prodromal phase (lasting 2 – 10 days)**
   • The clinical manifestation is non-specific with tiredness, mild pyrexia, headache, an aching body, sore throat, nausea and anorexia
   • Anxiety, nervousness, irritability and depression with or without any kind of change in behaviour
   • Hyperaesthesia and an increased sensitivity to bright lights and loud noised, excessive secretion of saliva, tears and perspiration, dilatation of the pupils, an increase in pulse rate and superficial respiration occur as a result of the involvement of the sympathetic nervous system
   • The most outstanding symptoms are abnormal sensations at the site of entry of the virus, including restricted or dispersed pain, sensations of burning or coldness, pruritis and paraesthesia

  ✹ **Acute neurological phase**
  During the acute neurological phase, two stages are apparent - a stage of excitability (which may last until the death of the infected person) and a stage where paralysis may occur
   • **Stage of excitability (1–3 days)**
     ◈ Anxiety and insomnia increase and the ill person does not want to be disturbed
     ◈ Pulse and respiration rates increase and body temperature rises to 40°C

◈ Although muscle tone is heightened, the muscles in the vicinity of the site of entry are weak. Muscle spasms and convulsion occur

◈ Involvement of the cranial nerves cause strabismus, diplopia, nystagmus, weakness of the facial muscles and hoarseness

◈ Hydrophobia (fear for water), the most classic diagnostic manifestation of the disease, is the most pronounced symptom during this stage. When the ill person tries to drink and swallow fluids, he/she is overwhelmed by a sensation of being painfully smothered. This symptom is caused by spasmodic contractions of the muscles involved in the processes of swallowing and respiration. The resulting choking leads to apnoea and cyanosis and death often occur during such an episode

◈ Manic behaviour, alternating with apathy, can be elicited by any kind of tactile, auditive, visual or other stimuli

- **Stage of paralysis**
  ◈ Hydrophobia disappears and the ill individual can swallow again, although with difficulty since paralysis of the muscles gradually sets in
  ◈ Progressive flaccid paralysis of the muscles of the affected limb occurs. This paralysis ascend in the direction of the muscles controlling respiration, chewing and swallowing
  ◈ The level of consciousness varies between confusion, disorientation, stupor and coma
  ◈ Death follows as a result of cardiac failure or paralysis of the respiratory muscles

❖ **Complications**
  - Increased cranial pressure
  - Convulsions
  - Dysrhythmia
  - Cardiac failure
  - Hypertension or hypotension
  - Hypothermia
  - Respiratory repression
  - Hypoxia
  - Death

■ **Diagnosis**
  - History of being bitten/licked by an infected animal or visiting of caves where bats live
  - Clinical manifestation
  - Confirmation of the diagnosis is done based on the presence of Negri bodies (characteristic intracytoplasmic inclusions) in the neurons of the infected animal when an autopsy of the brain, skin and corneal impression is performed
  - When it is impossible to examine the brain of the animal, Negri bodies will be found in the neurons of the individual's brain during an autopsy after the ill person had died

■ **Prognosis**
- There is no effective treatment after the first signs and symptoms of the disease have been manifested. The infected person usually dies

■ **Specific healthcare interventions to be rendered**
- Symptomatic and supportive
- Caring of the ill person must be done in an quiet, darkened room

◆ **Preventive measures to be taken**
- ➤ The incidence of rabies in animals have to be combated by means of
  - ◈ Legislation regarding the vaccination of animals against rabies and the imposition of punishment/fines
  - ◈ Registration, tax levies, and licensing of all domestic animals, particularly dogs
  - ◈ Limiting the number of animals that pet owners may keep in urban areas
  - ◈ Catching strange and stray animals in the streets and putting them down, particularly dogs
  - ◈ Prohibition on keeping wild animals as pets, particularly those known to be vectors
  - ◈ Putting down of all animals that were involved in biting humans three (3) times within a period of two (2) years
  - ◈ Notification to police stations, veterinarians, and animal protection societies of any animal involved in biting humans. These animals should be kept under observation until they have been declared healthy
  - ◈ Controlling the number of animals known to be vectors
  - ◈ Identification of sick/rabid animals. The following must be observed
    - ✠ change in behaviour, such as a wild animal suddenly appearing tame or a domestic animal becoming wild and restless
    - ✠ loss of appetite and increased salivating
    - ✠ problems with lapping up water or swallowing
    - ✠ strange behavioural signs appearing after 2–4 days later, such as convulsions, growling instead of barking. The animal will walk into objects, has a terrified expression in its eyes and will bite itself. The animal usually dies, but may be paralysed first and only die after a period of apathy and timidity

◆ **Prevention of rabies in humans**
- ➤ General prevention
  - ✪ Informing of the public to combat the disease in animals by voluntary vaccination of their pets (especially dogs) against rabies, identifying sick animals and emergency treatment of wounds caused by an infected animal. Children must be cautioned against playing with stray animals and taught to be extremely wary of any wild animal appearing to be tame
  - ✪ Compulsory notification of the disease in humans according to legislation
  - ✪ Prophylactic (pre-exposure) vaccinating of persons-at-risk can be done with Human Diploid Cell vaccine (HDCV). Three doses are administered.

A booster dose should be administered after one year and thereafter once every three years

✪ Wearing of gloves and protective clothing when working with sick animals

➢ <u>Treatment after infection had been acquired</u>

A person is considered to have been exposed when

✳ an rabid animal has licked a skin wound (cut or abrasion) or mucous membrane

✳ a child has been in contact with an rabid animal, even if there are no wounds on his/her body

✳ a person has been bitten by an rabid animal, even though it was through a layer of clothes

✪ **Treatment of the bite wound**

⋏ Treatment of the wound should commence as soon as possible after exposure, since the cleansing of the wound increases the possibility of eliminating the virus. The virus may be present in the wound area for a long time, even after the wound has healed

⋏ The wound should be allowed to bleed freely unless the bleeding is of a life-threatening intensity

⋏ The wound should also be washed several times with warm water and soap or any other disinfectant or alcoholic product (undiluted) or with hydrogen peroxide

⋏ Following this, the person who was bitten must be taken to a doctor with the **utmost urgency** for further wound treatment (particularly surgical enlargement and debridement of the wound area)

⋏ If the wound is left untreated for a fortnight after exposure, the infection is fatal

✪ **Systemic treatment**

⋏ Every person in a high-risk area who has been bitten by an animal must be considered as infected. These persons and, if necessary, their contacts (particularly children) must be vaccinated with human diploid cell vaccine (HDCV)

⋏ Persons **who consumed not-boiled milk** from an rabid cow, as well as all persons who have been **bitten by an animal that has only recently been vaccinated** (inoculation in animals is not always successful) **must be vaccinated** (1ml HDCV must be administered intramuscularly on the first day, then on days 3, 7, 14 and 30. A repeat dose on day 90 will be necessary only for those cases that have had the rabies antiserum administered. If adequate pre-exposure vaccination has been given, only 1ml vaccine is administered on day 1 and day 21)

⋏ Human rabies immunoglobulin must be administered within 72 hours after serious exposure. The first vaccination dose of HDCV is administered simultaneously with the human rabies immunoglobulin. Should the person only report for treatment more than a week after having been exposed, the human rabies immunoglobulin is not administered - only the course of five doses of HDCV for vaccination against rabies

⅄ Pregnancy is not a contra-indication for vaccination and the baby also has to receive prophylactic treatment after birth

Note

✳ Anti-rabies vaccination is not always successful and the person may become ill after systemic treatment

✳ It may sometimes be necessary to hospitalize a person during vaccination owing to the severe side-effects of the vaccine or the human rabies immunoglobulin

✳ When the animal involved could not be caught, prophylactic treatment must be started immediately. All prophylactic treatment is terminated when the person becomes ill

◆ **Measures to prevent epidemics**

⬇ Voluntary vaccination of all animals kept as pets against rabies according to the prescribed vaccination schedule

⬇ Campaigns to be held for vaccination of all animals (especially dogs) roaming free in informal and formal settlements by state and non-governmental organisations (NGO) if the owner cannot be identified

⬇ **When rabies in animals is diagnosed in a specific area, all designated animals as proclaimed in the *Government Gazette* in the demarcated area, must be compulsory vaccinated by the State Veterinary Services. A certificate of vaccination is issued to be kept by the owner and shown on inspection**

⬇ **The removal of any designated animal kept as a pet from a demarcated area without the necessary vaccination certification issued by the State Veterinary Services, is prohibited. The necessary arrangement must be made beforehand with the relevant authorities (that is, both in the "area of leaving" and "area of entry")**

⬇ **To prevent designated animals from being taken/transported illegally to a known endemic zoonotic area or clean (not-endemically infected) area, owners/drivers of all vehicles leaving such a proclaimed demarcated area have to submit to compulsory vehicle inspection by traffic officers or other designated officials**

⬇ **All dogs (and/or other animals) roaming free in the proclaimed demarcated area after notification was made of rabid animals involved in biting episodes, must be put down**

◆ **Implications during disaster situations**

⬇ Disaster planning must include provision for vaccination of animals against rabies

◆ **Compliance with international measures**

⬇ Compliance with legislation regarding the quarantine and vaccination of animals that are taken out of or brought into the country

9.1.3.3   Zoonotic bacterial encephalitis

Bacteria of animal-origin in nature that cause encephalitis in humans multiply mostly extra-cellular and generally secrete powerful exotoxins. The exotoxin that the bacteria releases, acts on the nervous system as the bacteria themselves do not invade the central nervous system. The toxin of *Clostridium tetani* has the characteristic A+B structure, the B subunit binding to ganglioside receptors on nerve cells while the internalized A subunit of the tetanus toxin is carried by axonal transport from the point of production to the central nervous system. In the central nervous system the A subunit of the tetanus toxin interferes with the synaptic transmission in inhibitory neurons by blocking the release of neurotransmitter. This allows the excitatory transmitter to continuously stimulate the motor neurones, causing spastic paralysis.

9.1.3.3.1   TETANUS (LOCK-JAW)

Tetanus is a serious neurological infection caused by a zoonotic bacterium and characterized by intermittent painful tonic spasms of voluntary muscles (particularly the masseter muscles) and convulsions

---

Epidemiological data

Geographical distribution
Tetanus occurs world-wide. It is a relatively unusual disease in industrialized regions, but more prevalent in farming and underdeveloped areas where contact with the excreta of animals takes place more readily and vaccination is inadequate

Causative pathogen
Clostridium tetani, a Gram-positive anaerobic bacillus

Incubation period
Usually 10 days but may last from 3–21 (even 50) days, depending on the severity of the infection and the type of wound

Mode of transmission
*The spores of *Clostridium tetani*, being wide spread in soil and originate from human or animal excreta, gain entry into the body through a wound or burnt wound(s) or an insignificant wound that does not even merit treatment when a person is injured
*In Tetanus neonatorum the spores gain entry through the umbilical cord of the new-born infant when manure is applied to the cord before it has healed. (It is a custom of some cultural groups to apply cow dung to the umbilical cord). When unhygienic practices are followed when the umbilical cord is cut, spores of *Clostridium tetani* can also gain entry when the instruments used to cut the cord, are contaminated with the bacterial spores
*Puerperal and post-abortus tetanus occur when the spores gain access through the genital tract during an unhygienic home delivery or an unhygienic non-spontaneous abortion
*Persons with burns are also at risk. The *Clostridium tetani* flourishes in necrotic tissue where it is assured of an anaerobic environment
*Since *Clostridium tetani* is also present in the gastro-intestinal tract, tetanus can also be associated with abdominal surgery

---

Period of infectiousness (communicability, transmission)
The infection is not transmitted from one person to another

Reservoir
Animals - *Clostridium tetani* forms part of the normal bowel flora in the intestines of animals
Humans - *Clostridium tetani* is found in the bowel flora of 25% of humans
Soil - Tetanus spores are widespread in soil and originate from animal and human faeces

Intermediaries
Vehicles - contaminated illegal drugs and narcotics that is injected intravenously

Carriers
None

Immune status
If the person has been vaccinated, immunity is elicited but wanes when no boosters' dosages had been received

Susceptibility and resistance of host
Persons of all ages are susceptible. Vaccination affords protection if regular booster dosages are administered every ten (10) years (or more often)

Pathogenesis

Since *Clostridium tetani* can only multiply in anaerobic conditions, the spores survive in live tissue for weeks, months or years until optimum conditions for growth are attained. When necrotic tissue or the presence of a foreign body permits local and anaerobic growth, the *Clostridium tetani* produces a virulent exotoxin, tetanospasmin. The tetanospasmin is transported (carried) in peripheral nerve axons and via the blood or the lymph to the central nervous system where it binds with the neurons of the anterior horn cells and sympathetic ganglia. In the anterior horn cells, the tetanospasmin blocks the release of inhibitory mediators in spinal synapses, causing over-activity of motor neurons. It can also pass up sympathetic nerve axons and lead to over-activity of the sympathetic nervous system. Tetanospasmin has no effect on the sensory nerves, cerebral cortex or cerebellum. Tetanospasmin cannot be neutralized once it has bound to the neurons. The head and neck muscles are first to be affected, followed by the muscles of the torso and limbs.

❖ **Clinical manifestation**
   The disease can manifest systemically or locally. Tetanus neonatorum in the new-born infant always manifests as a systemic disease
   ✱ **Systemic tetanus**
      • The infection commences with exaggerated reflexes, muscle rigidity and uncontrolled muscle spasms
      • Progressive stiffness of the all voluntary muscles develops with the masseter and neck muscles to be affected first. Within 24–48 hours the rigidity (stiffness) spreads to the muscles of the rest of the body

- The first and most common sign and symptom of tetanus is trismus (locked jaw) with consequent inability to open the mouth due to the contraction of the jaw muscles. Trismus is followed by dysphagia, restlessness and "risus sardonicus" (contraction of the facial muscles with lifted eyebrows and a grimace giving the face a sneering appearance)
- This is followed by spasms of the muscles of the entire body. The spasms are irregular at first, but become more regular later on, last longer and are extremely painful
- Spasms of the neck and back muscles cause severe opisthotonos
- In serious cases the spasms can cause fractures, especially of the vertebrae
- When the respiratory muscles are involved, laringospasm develops with the accumulation of secretions in the trachea-bronchial tree leading to asphyxia
- Involvement of the sphincters causes retention of urine and constipation
- Pyrexia seldom develops and when it does, the brainstem is affected
- Tachycardia and sweating result from effects on the sympathetic nervous system
- The infected individual is usually fully conscious and suffers severe pain during a spasm
- Coma or death occurs as a result of exhaustion, cardiac failure and/or asphyxia
- The spasms clear up within weeks. Trismus is the last to disappear

* **Local tetanus**
  - Tetanus is restricted to the local wound area and spasms of the muscles of the affected limb occur only
  - When local tetanus spreads and cause systemic tetanus with convulsions, the infection can be fatal
* **Tetanus neonatorum** (tetanus of the new-born)
  - Tetanus neonatorum is caused by animal dung that is applied to the umbilical cord of the new-born infant before healing has taken place and/ or by instruments, contaminated with spores of *Clostridium tetani*, used for cutting the umbilical cord
  - The baby has difficulty in sucking as the masseter muscles go into spasm with dysphagia and trismus
  - Tonic muscle spasms of all the body muscles occur intermittently with opisthotonos. The spasms are followed by exhaustion, an ashen colour and completely flaccid muscles
  - The crying of the baby varies from short sounds to a hoarse choking sound
  - The infant's colour varies from normal to cyanotic to pale

Note

Any person who has not received booster dosages every 10 years since his/her vaccination as an infant and child is at risk to develop Tetanus when injured and infected. Depending on the immune status of the individual, the person may suffer from a less severe to very severe form of the disease. Hospitalization is mandatory

❖ **Complications**
- Pneumonia
- Atelectasis of the lungs
- Mediastinal emphysema
- Pneumothorax
- Fracture of the vertebrae
- Injuries to the tongue
- Torn muscles and ligaments
- The infected individual may die when convulsions occur

■ **Diagnosis**
- A history of injury – wounds, burns, small skin lacerations
- Manifesting of clinical picture
- If possible, isolation of *Clostridium tetani* from the wound
- The new-born baby presents with a history of having the umbilicus treated with animal dung and the *Clostridium tetani* may be present in the umbilical cord. If manure was not used, the history of the procedure followed to cut the umbilicus and/or cleaning the healing umbilicus should be indicative of contaminated instruments.

■ **Prognosis**
- The mortality rate in the case of systemic infection is very high (50%) even if the ill person is treated
- In local tetanus infection the prognosis is good, unless the toxin has spread throughout the body
- For babies suffering from Tetanus neonatorum the mortality rate is extremely high (95-100%)

■ **Specific healthcare interventions to be rendered**
All individuals suffering from tetanus must be admitted to an intensive care unit
- **Medical treatment**
  - ✪ Debridement and excision of the wound and removal of all foreign bodies from the wound
  - ✪ Administering of human antitetanus immunoglobulin or tetanus antiserum
  - ✪ Administering of sedatives and muscle relaxants for deep sedation of the ill person to control the muscle spasms
  - ✪ Administering of antimicrobial drugs to inhibit bacterial replication and to prevent secondary infection
  - ✪ Commencing of physiotherapy
- **Specific healthcare interventions**
  - ✪ The ill person should be cared for in a quiet, darkened room where all auditive, visual, tactile and other stimuli are to be eliminated or reduced
  - ✪ When a tracheotomy is performed, routine tracheotomy care must be performed
  - ✪ Nasogastric feeds or intravenous hyper-alimentation is administered to eliminate aspiration

✪ An intravenous line is maintained to facilitate the administering of chemotherapeutic drugs

✪ Catheterization of the bladder must be done

✪ A cleansing enema must be given and a flatus tube must be passed to prevent abdominal distension

✪ All procedures must be discontinued when spasms occur

✪ The ill individual has to be regularly (2 hourly) turned in bed and all movements have to be done slowly and carefully

✪ Convalescence is slow and the individual needs a great deal of moral support

✪ When recovered, the infected individual/infant must be fully vaccinated

◆ **Preventive measures to be taken**

➢ Providing of health information, and encouraging the administering of vaccination

✳ at the primary level of prevention with regard to the necessity of active vaccination with tetanus toxoid of babies from the age of six weeks

✳ on maintaining active protection by administering of booster dosages every 10 years

✳ on prophylactic administering of tetanus toxoid to all persons who are at risk of infection, for example, farm workers, members of the armed forces, police, young people attending camps, and anyone else who runs a higher than average risk of trauma or injury

✳ on maintaining of active protection of all women throughout their childbearing age by administering five (5) adequately spaced dosages of tetanus toxoid

➢ Vaccination of pregnant women must be administered as follows

All pregnant women and breastfeeding mothers (primigravidae and multigravidae) who have never been vaccinated before

✳ Three (3) dosage of 0,5 ml tetanus toxoid are administered intramuscularly with intervals of 4 weeks between the 1st and 2sd dosage and the 3rd dosage 6 months later. The first dose is administered during the first antenatal clinic visit. The gestation period is not taken into account. Should the woman go into labour before the course is completed, it must be completed postnatal. Booster dosages must be given on the first visit for antenatal care with all subsequent pregnancies till 5 dosages have been received

✳ All pregnant women (primigravidae and multigravidae) who have been vaccinated previously must receive one dose of 0,5 ml tetanus toxoid intramuscularly during the first prenatal visit until 5 dosages have been received with all subsequent pregnancies

✳ The tetanus-immune status of all mothers (their own tetanus vaccination) must be checked when the mother brings her baby for his/her first postnatal visit to the clinic. If the mother has not been vaccinated, the necessary tetanus toxoid vaccine should be administered. At the same time the baby must also be vaccinated according to schedule

➢ Any person who has been exposed to contaminated soil when injured, must receive the following tetanus post-exposure prophylaxis

Type of wound	Person not immunized or partially immunized	Person completely immunized Time since last booster - 5 to 10 years	Person completely immunized Time since last booster - More than 10 years
Clean - minor	Begin or complete vaccination Tetanus toxoid 0.5 ml	None	Tetanus toxoid 0.5 ml
Major-clean or tetanus-prone	✓ In one arm - Human tetanus immuno-globulin 250 IU ✓ Other arm - Tetanus toxoid 0.5 ml	• Tetanus toxoid 0.5 ml	➢ In one arm - Human tetanus immuno-globulin 250 IU ➢ Other arm - Tetanus toxoid 0.5 ml
Tetanus-prone	✓ In one arm - Human tetanus immuno-globulin 500 IU ✓ Other arm - Tetanus toxoid 0.5 ml ✓ Antimicrobial therapy	• Tetanus toxoid 0.5 ml • Antimicrobial therapy	➢ In one arm - Human tetanus immuno-globulin 500 IU ➢ Other arm- Tetanus toxoid 0.5 ml ➢ Antimicrobial therapy
Delayed or incomplete debridement	✓ In one arm - Human tetanus immuno-globulin 500 IU ✓ Other arm - Tetanus toxoid 0.5 ml ✓ Antimicrobial therapy	• Tetanus toxoid 0.5 ml	➢ In one arm - Human tetanus immuno-globulin 500 IU ➢ Other arm - Tetanus toxoid 0.5 ml ➢ Antimicrobial therapy

➢ When a person has not been vaccinated previously or when the vaccination was not completed, artificial passively-acquired immune protection with human antitetanus immunoglobulin is indicated. Artificial actively-acquired immunity due to vaccination, however, should be started within 8 weeks

➢ All wounds should be thoroughly cleaned and disinfected with hydrogen peroxide as soon as possible. Debridement (cutting away dead and infected tissue in a wound) is imperative in order to prevent the multiplication of *Clostridium tetani*. Although penicillin and tetracycline is effective against the *Clostridium tetani*, good wound care remains a priority in preventive treatment

➢ The cultural custom of applying animal dung to the umbilicus of a new-born baby must be discouraged. All pregnant women must be taught how to care for their baby's umbilical cord until healed

◆ **Measures to prevent epidemics**
  ↓ No specific measures exist
  ↓ When a person was previously vaccinated and had received booster dosages but still contracts tetanus after injury, a thorough investigation of the case should be done to identify deficiencies in the preparation of the tetanus toxoid

◆ **Implications during disaster situations**
  ↓ Since traumatic injuries occur more often during disaster situations and war, there will be a greater need for human antitetanus immunoglobulin, tetanus antiserum and tetanus toxoid in these circumstances

◆ **Compliance with international measures**
  ↓ None

9.2 COMMUNICABLE INFECTIONS THAT AFFECT THE EYES

Because the outer surfaces of the eyes are exposed to the external world, the eyes are extremely accessible to infective microbes. Not only are the eyes a vulnerable epithelial surface, but because they are covered by eyelids, a warm, moist, enclosed environment is created in which infectious pathogens can quickly establish and set up a focus of infection. Although the eyelids and tears protect the external surfaces of the eyes, both mechanically and biologically, any interference with their functions increases the chance of a pathogen becoming established.

Eyelid infections are generally due to *Staphylococcus aureus.* When the margins of the eyelid are involved, blepharitis is caused. When the glands or follicles of the eyes are infected, styes or hordeolums are caused. The conjunctiva is particular susceptible and can be directly infected or can be invaded from other routes such as the blood or nervous system. The deeper tissues of the eyes can also be invaded from within, particularly by protozoan and worm parasitaemia.

9.2.1 Infections of the conjunctiva

A wide variety of viruses and bacteria cause conjunctivitis or pink eyes. Some infections are common in children and resolve quickly, while others are potentially more serious. Kerato-conjunctivitis caused by the *adeno-virus* or the *herpes simplex virus* or the *varicella-zoster virus* can result in severe eye and sight damage. An acute haemorrhagic conjunctivitis can follow infection with *enterovirus 70* and *coxsackie-virus A24*.

To establish infection of the conjunctiva, pathogens must avoid being rinsed and wiped away in tears. Pathogens attach themselves, via a specific mechanism, to conjunctival cells by which they prevent being rinsed and washed away. Contact lenses worn excessively leads to a reduction of the effectiveness of defence mechanisms the eyes, allowing pathogens to become established (especially when contaminated eye drops or cleaning solutions are used or contaminated lenses are inserted), resulting in corneal damage.

9.2.1.1 Chlamydial infection of the conjunctiva

Chlamydial infection of the eye is the most important eye infection in the world and more than six million persons worldwide are blind because of it. Chlamydia infection of the eyes is horizontally transmitted from person-to-person via direct contact with infected secretions, for example, by contaminated fingers and towels and by vectors such as flies. Poor access to water to wash the hands and face regularly favours chlamydia infection of the eyes. The eyes and lungs of a newborn infant may be infected after passage down an infected birth canal.

9.2.1.1.1 TRACHOMA

Trachoma is the result of chronic inclusion infection (re-occurring repeatedly) of the conjunctiva and cornea (kerato-conjuctivitis) that leads to blindness or visual impairment

---

Epidemiological data

Geographical distribution
Trachoma occurs world-wide but is endemic in some of the hot, dry regions such as the densely populated parts of Asia, Middle-East, Africa, and Latin America. In South Africa it occurs mainly in the Limpopo Province and the Eastern Cape

Causative pathogen
Chlamydia trachomatis. There are 8 different serotypes of the *Chlamydia trachomatis* responsible for inclusion conjunctivitis and another 4 different serotypes of *Chlamydia trachomatis* responsible for trachoma

Incubation period
5-14 days

Mode of transmission
Direct contact with secretions from the eyes, nose and throat of an infected person or from infected genitalia

Period of infectiousness (communicability, transmission)
For as long as the *Chlamydia trachomatis* is present in the lesions and secretions of the eye

Reservoir
Humans

Intermediaries
Vehicles - Fomites such as contaminated face cloths, towels, washbasins, bath water and eye make-up
Vectors - Flies spread the disease from one person to another in unhygienic conditions

Carriers
None

Immune status

Very few individuals have any immunity against *Chlamydia trachomatis*. No immunity with memory is elicited - thus the infection becomes chronic when not treated with antimicrobial drugs and re-infection occurs from time to time

Susceptibility and resistance of host

Children (particularly of preschool age) are extremely susceptible and are the main source of spreading the infection to others persons (especially chronic trachoma in adults and children). An infection acquired during childhood may sometimes clear up without any treatment. Lower socio-economic groups show a high incidence rate and race does not play a part

Pathogenesis

The *Chlamydia trachomatis* becomes attached to the epithelial cells of the cornea and conjunctiva by surface molecules that bind specially to receptors on the host cells. *Chlamydia trachomatis* produces a soluble antigen that causes necrosis of the cornea and conjunctiva resulting in the formation of connective tissue in the cornea and conjunctiva. The infection commences with diffuse hyperaemia on the palpebral conjunctiva that leads to the forming of vascular papulae and lymphoid follicles. Both the upper and lower eyelids become infected, but the lesions are mostly present on the superior tarsal plate. Mononuclear infiltration during the inflammation process leads to the formation of a pannus under the upper eyelid which can grow across the upper limbus of the cornea and may even reach the pupil area. The cornea becomes opaque. The corneal conjunctiva also becomes infected with the formation of follicles in the upper limbus. A superficial keratitis with corneal ulceration develops.

When the infection becomes chronic and re-infection occurs repeatedly, the **advanced stage** of the infection is reached (trachoma). Structural changes to the eyelids cause thickening and finally distortion – the retraction of the connective scar tissue causes distortion of the tarsal plate with either entropion, or ectropion or trichiasis of the eyelashes. As soon as the eyelids cannot close properly, the cornea dries out. Coupled with trichiasis, blindness follows.

❖ **Clinical manifestation**
  - The onset is usually gradual but it can also be acute
  - The infection manifests with
    ✪ complaints of eye irritation – itching and burning sensation
    ✪ photophobia and lacrimation
    ✪ swelling of the eyelids
    ✪ chemosis of the conjunctiva (conjunctiva are red, swollen, irregular and have a velvety appearance)
    ✪ a sero-mucous eye discharge – it can be so severe that the eyelids stick together
    ✪ pseudo-ptosis
    ✪ follicles visible on the palpebral conjunctiva as whitish-yellow spherical lesions
    ✪ visible capillary infiltration of the cornea from the limbus
    ✪ signs of keratitis and even corneal ulceration when the condition is left untreated

⊘ severe pain at the slightest touch of the eyes
- The infection can easily spread from the conjunctiva of one eye to the conjunctiva of the other eye

❖ **Complications**
- Corneal ulcers
- Blindness

■ **Diagnosis**
  ▪ Culture of the chlamydia trachomatis in conjunctival fluid or scraping

■ **Prognosis**
  ▪ Good when treated early
  ▪ Poor, when trachoma has developed

■ **Specific healthcare interventions to be rendered**
  ▪ **Medical treatment**
    ✠ Topical eye ointment and/or oral antimicrobial drugs are prescribed
    ✠ The follicles are ruptured to prevent the formation of lesions
    ✠ Cauterisation with silver nitrate or copper sulphate is sometimes performed
    ✠ Plastic eye surgery is done to repair complications such as entropion, ectropion and trichiasis
  ▪ Concurrent disinfection of all eye, nose and throat secretions, as well as genital secretions. Burning or disinfecting of all fomites
  ▪ **Eye care**
    ✠ Protect the eyes against bright lights
    ✠ Resting of the eyes
    ✠ Aseptic swabbing of the eyes with normal saline solution four hourly (4-hourly) before eye ointment is applied
    ✠ Atropine eye drops can be prescribed to prevent iritis
  ▪ **Rehabilitation and social aid**
    ✠ Providing of educational and vocational training to the blind person
    ✠ Securing of social aid in the form of a disability grant

◆ **Preventive measures to be taken**
  ➢ Mass screening in schools and at clinics – particularly in endemic regions by healthcare providers and by lay care groups trained to recognise trachoma in the early stages
  ➢ Health information to be given in respect of
    ✳ the improvement of the standard of hygiene
    ✳ the eradication of flies
    ✳ recognition of the early signs and symptoms of infection
    ✳ the importance of early diagnosis and treatment to prevent blindness
  ➢ Improvement of socio-economic living standards by means of education and the provision of jobs
  ➢ Improved housing to prevent overcrowding

◆ **Measures to prevent epidemics**
  ♦ Temporary closing of schools and public places to prevent an epidemic outbreak when a high incidence of the infection is reported in a specific area
  ♦ Launching of massive campaigns to detect, treat and destroy the source of infection

◆ **Implications for disaster situations**
  ♦ None

◆ **Compliance with international measures**
  ♦ None

9.2.1.2   Bacterial infections of the conjunctiva

Several bacteria, especially *Streptococcus pneumoniae*, *Haemophilus influenzae*, and *Staphylococcus aureus* cause conjunctivitis. A purulent discharge of the eye is characteristic of bacterial conjunctivitis. Styes (eyelid infection) and "sticky eyes" in neonates are caused by *Staphylococcus aureus* (the *Staphylococcus aureus* is transferred from the infant's own body or from a healthy infected adult, for example, from noses and fingers of adult carries).

9.2.1.2.1   OPHTHALMIA NEONATORUM (GONOCOCCAL CONJUNCTIVITIS)

Ophthalmia neonatorum (gonococcal conjunctivitis) is an acute infection of the conjunctiva of a new-born baby which the new-born acquires during vaginal delivery from an infected mother suffering from the sexually transmitted infection gonorrhoea

---

Epidemiological data

Geographical distribution
Occurring world-wide

Causative pathogen
Neisseria gonorrhoea

Incubation period
24 hours

Mode of transmission
The eyes of the baby are infected with *Neisseria gonorrhoea* during birth. The *Neisseria gonorrhoea* is present in the birth canal of the infected mother

Period of infectiousness (communicability, transmission)
For as long as the pathogen is present in the discharge from the eyes

Reservoir
Humans

Intermediaries
None

Carriers
None

Immune status
No immunity with memory is elicited. Infection with *Neisseria gonorrhoea* may also occur during a later stage in life

Susceptibility and resistance of host
Any baby, who is vaginally delivered from a mother suffering from gonorrhoea, is susceptible. Cross-infection can occur in the nursery between an infected neonate and non-infected neonates

Pathogenesis
Once *Neisseria gonorrhoea* has gained entry into the eyes during birth, an acute inflammation of the layers of epithelial and sub-epithelial cells of the conjunctiva develops. Oedema develops and the blood supply to the cornea is impeded. A severe purulent exudate is discharged. This may lead to several complications such as keratitis, corneal ulceration and corneal destruction, and blindness.

❖ **Clinical manifestation**
- An acute conjunctivitis with a purulent discharge develops within 24–72 hours after birth

❖ **Complications**
- Keratitis
- Systemic gonorrhoeal infection
- Arthritis
- Corneal ulceration and corneal destruction
- Blindness

■ **Diagnosis**
▪ Culture studies of the purulent discharge

■ **Prognosis**
▪ Good

■ **Specific healthcare interventions to be rendered**
▪ Administering of antimicrobial drugs and eye ointment (topical and/or systemic)
▪ Isolation of the baby with concurrent disinfection of all fomites
▪ Regular cleansing of the infected eye(s)
▪ Treatment of the mother and her contacts for gonorrhoea

◆ **Preventive measures to be taken**
➢ Providing of health infection regarding the prevention of sexually transmitted infections (STI's)
➢ Preventive treatment of the eyes of new-born infants by inserting 1% silver nitrate eye drops or the application of an topical antibiotic eye ointment
➢ Treatment of the parents (and their contacts) for gonorrhoea with antimicrobial drugs

◆ **Measures to prevent epidemics**
  + Isolation of the infant in the nursery
  + Adequate hand washing after handling of the infant
  + Strict adherence to Standard Precautionary measures and Transmission-based Precautionary measures, especially contact precautionary measures

◆ **Implications for disaster situations**
  + None

◆ **Compliance with international measures**
  + None

9.2.1.3 Conjunctival infections transmitted by blood or the nervous system

Several pathogens can invade the superficial tissues of the eyes after transport through the blood, for example, the *Measles virus* or, in the case of the *Herpes simplex-virus*, by movement along the trigeminal nerve. Reactivation of the *Herpes simplex virus* results in the development of keratitis with the formation of dendritic ulcers. The inadvertent use of topical steroids can aggravates conjunctival infections and the resulting severe ulceration leads to corneal destruction.

9.3   KEY NOTES

INFECTIONS OF THE CENTRAL NERVOUS SYSTEM

❑ Microbial invasion of the central nervous system [CNS] is very uncommon due to the presence of the blood-brain barrier and blood-cerebrospinal fluid-barrier which limit the spread of infection.

❑ Once infectious agents have traversed the blood-brain and blood-cerebro-spinal fluid-barriers, the pathogens generally cause neurological infection by involving the meninges and/or the brain substances (the anatomically defined compartments of the nervous system are interconnected or adjacent to one another, resulting in involvement of more than one in a given infection).

❑ Disease results from interference with the function of the infected nerve cells (for example, rabies), or from direct damage to the infected nerve cells (for example, poliomyelitis), or from the inflammatory sequel to the invasion of the central nervous system (for example, bacterial and viral encephalitis).

❑ Viral meningitis and bacterial meningitis are the most common infections affecting the central nervous system with infection of the brain substance a rarity.

❑ Infections/diseases of the central nervous system can also result when bacterial neurotoxins reach the central nervous system from extra-neural sites of growth (for example, tetanus) or from helminthic infections lodged in the brain substance.

❑ The sequelae of infections/diseases of the central nervous system are most of the time seriously and permanent in nature or even fatal.

INFECTIONS OF THE EYE

- ❑ The external surfaces of the eyes are extremely vulnerable to infections although they are protected by the eyelids and by bio-chemical factors such as lysozyme in tears.
- ❑ The consequences of eye infections are always potentially serious due to the fact that sight is dependent upon the presence of an intact transparent cornea and intact retina.
- ❑ Relatively few pathogens invade the retina and those that do, are potentially sight-threatening
- ❑ The pathogens that infect the conjunctiva have specific attachment mechanisms and the inflammatory responses elicited by the pathogens, though the conjunctiva is designed to limit invasion and repair damage, can sometimes irreversibly damage conjunctival and corneal surfaces.
- ❑ Some of the most serious infection-related diseases of the eye involve invasion by protozoan and helminthic parasites. The diagnoses often follows rather precedes the development of visual impairment.

Chapter 10

COMMUNICABLE DISEASES AFFECTING THE RESPIRATORY SYSTEM

The air that is inhaled contains millions of suspended particles, including pathogenic and harmless microbes. A variety of microbes lives harmlessly in the upper respiratory tract and oro-pharynx, colonizing the nose, mouth, throat and teeth and are well adaptive to live in these sites. The efficient cleansing mechanism of the respiratory tract prevents infection taking place. Although a distinction is made between the upper and lower respiratory tract infections, the respiratory tract from the nose to the alveoli form a continuum as far as infectious agents are concerned. There may, however, be a preferred "focus" of infection (for example, nasal-pharynx for corona-viruses) while other viruses such as the influenza-viruses infect all tissues of the respiratory tract. Communicable diseases affecting the respiratory system are generally transmitted by means of airborne infected droplets.

Two generalizations can be made about upper and lower respiratory tract infections, namely,
- ❑ most pathogens are restricted to the surface epithelium, but many other spread to other parts of the body, before returning to the respiratory tract and associated structures
- ❑ two groups of microbes can be distinguished - "professional" and "secondary" invaders (professional invaders are those that successfully infect the healthy respiratory tract as they are able to evade the local defences of the host. Secondary invaders only cause disease when the defences of the host are already impaired).

Two types of respiratory diseases can be distinguished, namely,
- ◆ infections that are restricted to/stay on the surface epithelium after gaining entry via the respiratory tract. The local mucosal defences are important and local spread takes place. The immune response is sometimes too late to be important in recovery and the incubation period is very short (a few days)
- ◆ infections that spread through the body after gaining entry into the body via the respiratory tract. Little to no lesion is formed at the site of entry and the causative pathogen returns to the surface for final multiplication and shedding after it had spread through the body. The immune response plays an important role in the recovery and the incubation period is long (weeks).

The signs and symptoms of a respiratory infection in adults are usually related to the respiratory tract, for example, a sore throat, earache, coughing, sputum production, pleurisy, and chest pain. In the case of young children, the signs and symptoms are not specifically related to the respiratory system. Children present with non-specific signs and symptoms that can be misleading, such as pyrexia, irritability, loss of appetite, vomiting and diarrhoea. Classic signs which are present in young children are stridor and croup.

10.1 COMMUNICABLE DISEASES AFFECTING THE UPPER RESPIRATORY TRACT

Although the upper and lower respiratory tract forms a continuum from the nose to alveoli, infections of the upper respiratory tract is mostly restricted to the surface epithelium of the nose, oro-pharynx, tonsils, larynx, oral cavity, cervical lymph nodes and salivary glands in the oral cavity.

10.1.1 Bacterial infections affecting the upper respiratory tract

A variety of bacteria such as *streptococcus (group A β-haemolytic); Corynebacterium; haemophilus influenzae (type B); borrelia Vincentia* and *Neisseria gonorrhoeae* are mostly responsible for the infections of the upper respiratory tract and associated structures. Each of these types of bacteria attaches itself to the mucosal surface via specific interactions between component molecules of the pili (fimbriae or adhesives) of the pathogen and the molecules in the cell membranes of the host. The presence of many pili help to prevent phagocytosis whereby the resistance of the host to the bacterial infection is reduced. Although immunogenic, the antigens of the bacteria can change, allowing the bacteria to avoid immune recognition. The bacteria sometimes invade the local sub-epithelial tissues.

10.1.1.1 DIPHTHERIA

Diphtheria is an acute disease characterized by typical systemic signs and symptoms and the formation of a false membrane that is caused by a fibrinous exudate on the mucous membranes of the upper respiratory passages. The disease can be life-threatening because of obstruction of the respiratory tract

---

Epidemiological data

Geographic distribution
Diphtheria occurs world-wide, primarily during the colder months

Causative pathogen
Corynebacterium diphtheriae

Incubation period
1–5 days but it may be as long as 10 days

Mode of transmission
Airborne infected droplets when the ill person sneezes, coughs, spits, talks or sings
Carriers

Period of infectiousness (communicability, transmission)
Until the *Corynebacterium diphtheriae* in excretions and lesions disappears after 3–4 days

Reservoir
Humans. The *Corynebacterium diphtheriae* is harboured in the nose and pharynx

Intermediaries
Vehicles - Fomites and contaminated milk

Carriers
Carriers harbour the *Corynebacterium diphtheriae* in the nose and pharynx

Immune status
Immunity with memory is elicited

Susceptibility and resistance of host
Babies acquire natural immunity passively from their mothers (if the mother was vaccinated or had suffered from the disease). This natural immunity lasts approximately six months. From the age of one year, every person is susceptible. Persons who had been vaccinated, should receive regular booster dosages.

Pathogenesis

Although the adhesion mechanisms are not understood, the *Corynebacterium diphtheriae* bind with the surface tissue cells of the respiratory tract after gaining entry. The bacteria multiply locally without invading deeper tissues or spreading through the body, but produce an exotoxin which binds to the specific receptors on the surface of the cells. The exotoxin destroys the epithelial cells and polymorphs causing a local inflammation reaction. An ulcer forms which is covered with a necrotic exudate forming a viscous/fibrinous membrane (false membrane) on the mucous membrane within 24–48 hours. The colour of the membrane varies from greenish-grey to black, depending on the quantity of blood it contains. The false membrane consists of a deposit of fibrin, white blood cells, red blood cells, tissue elements and the pathogen *Corynebacterium diphtheriae*. The membrane is formed across all anatomical barriers and if it is removed, it leaves numerous bleeding points. The mouth and breath have a distinctive malodorous smell. Extensive inflammation and oedema of the soft tissue below the membrane develop due to the local reaction to the exotoxin as well as the result of secondary infection. The intrusion of the membrane and the oedema in the limited space of the larynx leads to impeded breathing resulting in asphyxiation. The enlargement of the cervical lymph nodes, give rise to the "bull neck" appearance.

The exotoxin disseminates through the body via the lymph and blood. Although all the cells absorb the exotoxin, the exotoxin shows an affinity for the cardiac muscle (myocarditis), nerve tissue (myelin degeneration and peripheral neuritis) and the kidneys (tubular necrosis). A single *Corynebacterium diphtheriae* bacterium can produce 5000 exotoxin molecules per hour and the toxic fragment is so extremely stable within a cell that a single exotoxin molecule can destroy the cell.

❖ **Clinical manifestation**
The signs and symptoms vary in accordance with the organs of the upper airways involved and the quantity of exotoxin absorbed into the blood circulation. Two general types of diphtheria can be distinguished, namely, respiratory diphtheria (nasal, tonsillar, pharyngeal and laryngeal diphtheria) and non-respiratory diphtheria which includes haemorrhagic diphtheria, wound diphtheria and lesions of the conjunctiva, ears and genitals

✻ **Respiratory diphtheria**
All forms of respiratory diphtheria present with the following general signs and symptoms - a gradual onset with a slight elevation of body temperature, malaise, sore throat, lassitude and anorexia.

- **Nasal diphtheria (unilateral or bilateral)**
  - Typical signs and symptoms are a yellowish, watery, often bloody nasal secretion which is extremely malodorous
  - A persistent epistaxis may develop and a membrane can be visible
  - Nasal-pharyngeal diphtheria is the most severe form of the disease
  - Anterior nasal diphtheria is the mildest form of the disease when it occurs on its own because the exotoxin is less well absorbed from this site and the nasal discharge can be the main symptom. The ill person, however, is highly infectious

- **Tonsillar and pharyngeal diphtheria**
  - Within 24 hours after the onset of the general signs and symptoms, a visible membrane, greenish-grey to black in colour, is formed on the tonsils and mucous membranes of the pharynx
  - The throat of the person is extremely painful
  - Cervical adenitis and peri-adenitis follow. The enlargement and swelling of the lymph nodes causes the typical bull-necked appearance
  - The membrane gradually starts loosening by the 7th to the 10th day
  - When the membrane spreads to the rest of the pharynx, the uvula and the soft palate, the individual becomes seriously ill
  - Paralysis of the soft palate may occur

- **Laryngeal diphtheria**
  - Laryngeal diphtheria develops due to the spread of pharyngeal diphtheria
  - The ill person has a high-pitched cough and his/her voice is hoarse
  - When obstruction of the airways develops, the condition is fatal
  - Inspiratory stridor followed by supra-sternal, supra-clavicular and sub-costal retraction is characteristic of respiratory obstruction
  - When paralysis of the soft palate occurs, nasal speech results as well as problems with swallowing while food is regurgitated

- ♦ Paralysis of the soft palate can also, in exceptional cases, be accompanied by paralysis of the diaphragm and the respiratory muscles
- ♦ The membrane is coughed up within 6 – 10 days

✹ **Non-respiratory diphtheria**
- A false membrane is formed on any surface of the body at the point of entry by the pathogen, for example, genitals, ears
- General systemic signs and symptoms of malaise, an elevated body temperature and lethargy are present

NOTE

Persons who have been vaccinated as infants may develop an atypical clinical picture of the disease in later life while adolescents and adults become seriously ill and must be hospitalized

❖ **Complications**
- **Cardiac system**
  During the second week of the disease an acute myocarditis with dysrhythmia may develop. (This complication is reversible when the exotoxin is neutralized.) Cardiac failure or even myocardial infarction may occur approximately six weeks after the onset of the disease, leading to circulatory collapse and death

- **Neurological system**
  Motor paralysis develops when the neurological system is affected by the exotoxin. (Motor paralysis as well as its complications is reversible with the neutralization of the exotoxin.) The effect on the neurological system follows a specific pattern and depends on the quantity of exotoxin that was absorbed in the general circulation. Progressive paralysis may develop from the third to the tenth week and includes paralysis of the following structures
  - ♦ palate with changes in the voice and nasal pitch
  - ♦ eye muscles with diplopia and strabismus
  - ♦ muscles of the pharynx with dysphagia
  - ♦ muscles of the larynx and respiratory muscles with hoarseness, aphonia and respiratory suppression
  - ♦ muscles of the limbs with weakness and a tingling sensation

- **Nefrological system (Kidneys)**
  Albuminuria occurs when tubular nephritis develops

■ **Diagnosis**
- Clinical picture
- False membranes
- Culture studies - Throat and nose swabs or swabs of the membrane on the skin should be taken before antimicrobial drugs are administered

■ **Prognosis**
- Fair

- **Specific healthcare interventions to be rendered**
    - As soon as a diagnosis of diphtheria is suspected clinically, the ill person must be immediately isolated to reduce the risk of the specific microbial strain spreading to other susceptible individuals
    - **All healthcare workers must strictly adhere to all Standard Precautions and Transmission-based Precautions (Barrier nursing and medical care isolation – airborne, droplet and contact precautions) by wearing a mask when rendering healthcare. All ill healthcare users must wear a mask** when transported within different rooms/units or moved between different departments
    - The ill person must be isolated for not less than a minimum period of 14 days, or even longer, if necessary, until three subsequent nose and throat swabs taken 24-hourly, show negative culture reports
    - Simultaneous disinfection of all secretions from the ill person
    - When the ill person recovers, but still carries the pathogen for a period of more than 21 days, isolation measures must be maintained for a longer period in order to prevent the ongoing spread of the disease
    - Diphtheria antiserum is administered as soon as the ill person is hospitalized (even before the diagnosis is confirmed) in order to counteract the harmful effect of the exotoxin
    - Antimicrobial drugs must be administered in combination with diphtheria antiserum
    - Electrocardiogram (ECG) must be recorded on a daily basis
    - Prevent exhaustion by ensuring absolute bed rest for 4-6 weeks, but not less than 12 days. Avoid exhaustion at all times and by all means – the ill person is not allowed to do anything at all for himself/herself
    - Maintain hydration and nutritional status by ensuring that all food is soft and easily digestible with a high kilojoules value. When normal eating is impossible, administer nutrition intravenously
    - Detect complications early by
        * strictly recording all intake and output
        * monitoring temperature, pulse, respiration and blood pressure every half-hour to every four hours
        * observing colour of skin and fingernails and the degree to which the ill individual responds – every half-hour to every four hours
        * examining daily for signs of neurological impairment (see complications)
        * daily testing of urine for albumin
    - Report any abnormalities and instate the appropriate healthcare interventions
    - Maintain oxygen intake by supplying high humidity oxygen
    - Maintain an open airway and aspirate mucus whenever necessary (**_do not try to remove the membrane_**)
    - Keep an emergency tracheotomy tray at hand
    - When a tracheotomy has been done, tracheotomy care must be done extremely aseptically to prevent secondary infection

- Maintain personal hygiene by giving regular mouthwashes, preferably warm or very cold
- Keep teeth and lips clean and moist
- Carriers
  * Some individuals may remain carriers for six (6) months or even longer after recovering from the disease
  * Carriers present with a negative Schick test
  * All carriers are legally obligated to receive the prescribed medical treatment of taking antimicrobial drugs
  * If the carrier status persists, a tonsillectomy is advised

◆ **Preventive measures to be taken**
  ➤ Primary prevention
    - Health information regarding the importance of vaccination
    - Active vaccination of all children from the age of 6 weeks with diphtheria vaccine (DTP$_{[a]}$ or alternatively DTP$_{[a]}$-Hib or alternatively DTP$_{(a)}$-IPV or alternatively DTP$_{(a)}$-IPV-Hib from the age of six (6) weeks)

  ➤ Secondary prevention
    - Timely detection and notification of diphtheria
    - Tracing and treatment of contacts as well as legislative measures to be instated
      ✪ If the ill person is treated at home, all contacts must be placed under quarantine for the period of isolation
      ✪ Contacts may be released from quarantine when the initial isolation period has expired, even though the ill individual may still have to be isolated for a longer period of time
      ✪ Contacts, who wish to leave home to live elsewhere, may do so provided their nose and throat swabs are negative. When the father and/or the mother have to return to work, they are not allowed any contact with the ill person or with children outside the family circle. Persons, who handle food and/or work with small children, are forbidden all contact with the ill person. When they do come into contact with the ill person, they are excluded from handling food or caring for children for the prescribed period
      ✪ Contacts under the age of 10 years should receive a booster dose if they have been fully vaccinated at a younger age. If they had not been vaccinated, chemo-prophylactic treatment must be given and maintained for five days. The primary diphtheria vaccination course must be started simultaneously
      ✪ Contacts older than 10 years must be kept under observation for six days if they have been fully vaccinated at a younger age. When they had not been vaccinated, the Schick test must be done to establish the susceptibility of the contact for the infection and chemo-prophylactic treatment must be commenced. When the Schick test is positive, the primary diphtheria vaccination course is administered
    - High-risk groups, such as school children, must be monitored during an epidemic and contacts and carriers among them must be traced.

Susceptibility for infection can be established by doing the Schick test. This is done by injecting a small quantity of exotoxin intradermally. A red spot, 10mm in diameter, appearing within 24–48 hours, indicates a negative result. The spot will be red for 4–7 days. A second test can be done by means of an antitoxin titre test on a blood specimen

◆ **Measures to prevent epidemics**
  ♦ Vaccination with DTP(a) must be emphasized during the infancy period with booster dosages later in life
  ♦ When there is an epidemic outbreak, booster dosages must be repeated
  ♦ Persons who were not been vaccinated must be vaccinated
  ♦ Vaccination must be encouraged to prevent outbreaks in large gatherings of susceptible persons such as in young children cared for in crèches, pre-primary schools and hostels
  ♦ Strict adherence to the school exclusion regulations

◆ **Implications during disaster situations**
  ♦ Effective vaccination with either DTP(a) or other vaccine combinations containing DTP(a) for infants, with DT or Td for older children and purified diphtheria vaccine for adults

◆ **Compliance with international measures**
  ♦ None

10.1.2 Viral infections affecting the glands and lymphoid tissue of the oropharynx

Most of the viral pathogens are restricted to the surface epithelium, but some spread to other parts of the body before returning to the respiratory tract, oropharynx and the salivary glands from where it is shed to the exterior.

10.1.2.1 INFECTIOUS MONONUCLEOSIS

Infectious mononucleosis, also known as glandular fever (or "kissing sickness") is an acute or sub-acute disease of the lymphoid tissue and glands characterized by sore throat, painfully enlarged cervical lymph nodes, lassitude and a general feeling of malaise. The disease is self-limiting

---

Epidemiological data

Geographic distribution
The infection is prevalent the world over. Acute infectious mononucleosis occurs particularly in developing countries. The disease occurs sporadically as well as in epidemics

Causative microbe
The *Epstein-Barr virus* – the *Epstein-Barr virus* is structurally and morphologically identical to other herpes-viruses but ontogenetically distinct

---

Incubation period
5–10 days but sometimes 30 days or longer (4–7 weeks)

Mode of transmission
Through the oral-pharyngeal route – by means of direct contact with saliva during kissing

Period of infectiousness (communicability, transmission)
The exact period of infectiousness (communicability, transmission) is unknown but probably covers a period starting before the appearance of the symptoms until the pharyngeal secretions are no longer infectious. Pharyngeal secretions can be infectious for as long as a year after clinical recovery

Reservoir
Humans. The virus is harboured in the oropharynx and is species specific

Intermediaries
None

Carriers
Approximately one fifth of the population test positive for Epstein-Barr virus-antibody. The virus is harboured in the oropharynx

Immune status
Immunity with memory is elicited

Susceptibility and resistance of host
Every person is susceptible. The disease occurs mostly in young adults although young children and infants (0–6 years) are also affected

---

Pathogenesis

The *Epstein-Barr-virus* replicates in B-lymphocytes and certain epithelial cells and is shed in saliva from infected epithelial cells and possibly from lymphocytes in the salivary glands and from the oropharynx. Infection with the *Epstein-Barr-virus* results in a ubiquitous infection after the *Epstein-Barr-virus* (EBV) has attached itself to the C3d receptor on the B-lymphocytes and certain epithelial cells where the virus replicates. After infecting the epithelial cells of the mouth and oropharynx and possibly the lymphocytes in the salivary glands, the virus spread silently to B-lymphocytes in local lymphoid tissues and/or in other organs in the body (lymph nodes, spleen). Specifically activated T-lymphocytes respond immunologically to the infected B-lymphocytes and appear in the peripheral blood as "atypical lymphocytes". Lymph-adenopathy, nasopharyngeal lymphoid hyperplasia and splenomegaly follow.

The *Epstein-Barr-virus* not only infects the B-lymphocytes, but interferes with the immune defences through immuno-diversion of the T-cells of all specificities by polyclonal activation into immunologically unproductive activity, resulting in the production of a supply of B-cells in which the virus can grow. The *Epstein-Barr-virus* also interferes with the signalling between immune cells by coding for proteins that interfere with apoptosis (suicide or lysis is committed by the local cell when infected with a virus), permitting long-term infection of the cells. Viral latency in the infected cells takes place and when reactivation occurs, the virus appears in the saliva. In immunologically deficient individuals, reactivation may progress to cause clinical disease such as hairy tongue leukoplakia.

❖ **Clinical manifestation**
- In naturally infected infants and young children the immune response is weak and generally no clinical disease is manifested
- In older persons (14–20 years) the onset is gradual (4-7 weeks) with prodromal signs and symptoms of general malaise, headache, an elevated temperature, lassitude, loss of appetite (anorexia), sore throat with enlarged tonsils, pharyngitis, greyish-white exudate in the pharynx and/or petechiae on the hard palate
- Enlargement of the lymph nodes appears on the second or third day. The lymph nodes are firm, discrete and tender. The posterior cervical lymph nodes are the first to show signs of enlargement due to swelling, followed by the anterior cervical lymph nodes and lastly the axillary lymph nodes. Lymph-adenopathy of the entire body occurs only in very rare cases. A mild enlargement of the spleen occurs in about 50% of all cases. Blood tests show an increase in white blood cells, particularly in the lymphocytes and leucocytes
- Spontaneous recovery occurs within 2–3 weeks but the symptoms may persist for a few month

❖ **Complications**
- Complications occur very rarely, but those that may occur are
  - neurological impairment (aseptic meningitis and/or encephalitis)
  - rupture of the spleen
  - auto-immune haemolytic anaemia which subsides within 1-2 months
  - thrombocytopenic purpura with haemorrhages
  - airway obstruction due to oedematous pharyngeal and/or tonsillar inflammation
  - hepatitis
- As the virus can evade the immune defences, it is able to take up permanent residence in the immune system. Any immuno-deficiency in later life leads to reactivation of the infection. The virus re-appears in the saliva with no clinical signs and symptoms

■ **Diagnosis**
- Clinical manifestation
- Blood tests

■ **Prognosis**
- Good

■ **Specific healthcare interventions to be rendered**
- Symptomatic and supportive
- The infection is self-limiting and will clear up within a period of 2-5 weeks unless complications set in

- During convalescence, persons whose spleen and/or liver was enlarged, should avoid extreme activities and should not lift heavy objects
- When a person complains of continuous lassitude and depression, he/she should be encouraged to take adequate nutrition and resting periods

◆ **Measures to prevent epidemics**
  ↓ None

◆ **Implications for disaster situations**
  ↓ None

◆ **Compliance with international measures**
  ↓ None

10.1.2.2   MUMPS (EPIDEMIC PAROTITIS)

Mumps is an acute systemic viral disease and is characterized by localized oedema of the salivary glands which can be unilateral or bilateral

---

Epidemiological data

Geographic distribution
Mumps occurs endemically all over the world, with the highest incidence usually during springtime

Causative pathogen
Mumps-virus which is a member of the Paramyxoviruses – the only serotype of the single-stranded RNA Paramyxoviruses

Incubation period
On the average 17–19 days, although it varies from 12–28 days

Mode of transmission
Airborne infected droplets from the saliva of the infected host – close contact

Period of infectiousness (communicability, transmission)
The disease is transmissible from 6 days before the onset of parotitis until approximately 10 days afterward

Reservoir
Humans –   peak incidence is at 5-15 years or in crowded adult communities such as prisons, garrisons and ships

Intermediaries
None

Carriers
None

Immune status
Immunity with memory is elicited by either unilateral or bilateral mumps

---

> **Susceptibility and resistance of host**
> Due to the trans-placental transmission of natural passively-acquired immunity to infants from mothers who had become ill with mumps or were vaccinated against mumps, it is very rare for babies younger than one year old to contract mumps. Thereafter every person is susceptible. The immune status of persons who have been vaccinated against mumps diminishes with the passing of the time. Adolescents and adults become very ill when contracting mumps

Pathogenesis

The *paramyxovirus* gains entry into the body through the mouth and nose of the exposed person. The virus infiltrates the epithelial layer of the upper respiratory tract or eye where it replicates. From here the virus invades the blood circulation, spreading to lymphoid tissue cells (lymphocytes and monocytes) and reticulo-endothelial cells where the virus undergoes a lengthy period of growth. After approximately 7-10 days the virus re-enter the blood and localizes in the salivary gland(s) as well as in other glands and body sites including the testes/ovaries, pancreas, the thyroid and the central nervous system. Degenerative changes in the infected cells of the drainage ducts of the glands cause an accumulation of necrotic tissue. The resulting lymphocyte infiltration of the glandular tissue causes interstitial oedema. This, together with the leucocytes already present in the drainage ducts due to the infiltration, causes obstruction in the drainage ducts. After an incubation period of 18-21 days, the inflammation causes disease with unilateral or bilateral enlarged parotid glands. Although the parotid gland is usually the only glandular tissue affected by the paramyxovirus, the submandibular glands may also become enlarged. Recovery takes place within a week and life-long immunity with memory is elicited.

❖ Clinical manifestation

- The prodromal signs and symptoms of mumps are non-specific
  - ◆ Low-grade pyrexia, anorexia, malaise and headache develop. This period last 1-2 days
  - ◆ Complaints of pain near the ear lobe that is exacerbated by chewing together with tenderness and enlargement of the parotid gland(s) occur within 24 hours after the appearance of the first prodromal signs
- Although the parotid glands are not enlarged at this stage, this happens within the next day or two with a dramatic enlargement of either one or both of the parotid glands, displacing the ear lobe upwards and backwards. This sudden enlargement of the parotid glands is extremely painful. Enlargement of both parotid glands does not usually take place simultaneously, but within a few days of each other (bilateral mumps). It may also happen that only one parotid gland is affected (unilateral mumps)
- Persons with mumps sometimes experience trismus as a result of the enlargement of the parotid glands. The pain experienced by the person is exacerbated by chewing movements and in particular by the intake of acidic citrus fruit and juices
- During the first three (3) days of the disease the person's body temperature varies between 37⁰C to 40⁰C. As soon as the swelling of the parotid glands

reaches its peak, the pain; pyrexia and tenderness starts to resolve. After the swelling has peaked, the parotid glands resume their normal size within a week

- In about 10% of all persons suffering from mumps, the other salivary glands are also affected together with the parotid glands. When the other salivary glands are involved, it is the submandibular glands that are affected

NOTE

Persons who have been vaccinated as infants may develop an atypical clinical picture of the disease in later life while adolescents and adults become seriously ill and may need to be hospitalized

- ❖ **Complications**
  - Males
    Epididimo-orchitis is the most common glandular involvement besides the salivary glands. Between 20% and 30% of all adult males suffering from mumps, develop orchitis which can occur bilaterally or unilaterally. The latter is the most common occurrence. Epididimo-orchitis may often be the only sign of mumps in adult males. Epididimo-orchitis very rarely occur in boys who have not yet reached puberty. The onset of orchitis is sudden, with pyrexia which can reach 41^{0}C, rigors, headache, vomiting and pain in the testes. The testes are usually hot, swollen and tender. The testes can be swollen as much as four times their normal size before the swelling starts to subside. Tenderness of the testes remains until two weeks after the swelling has subsided
  - Females
    Oophoritis as a clinical manifestation of mumps may occur in adolescent girls and adult females. The ratio is much smaller than for orchitis. Oophoritis occurs in only about 10% of adult females suffering from mumps
  - Both males and females
    - ✓ Involvement of the central nervous system is a common manifestation of mumps and occurs on the average in 10% of all persons suffering from mumps. Meningitis may occur simultaneously with or without the absence of parotitis
    - ✓ Pancreatitis

- ■ **Diagnosis**
  - Clinical picture

- ■ **Prognosis**
  - Good

- ■ **Specific healthcare interventions to be rendered**
  - Supportive to relieve symptoms
  - Nutritious, soft foods, particularly during the period of swelling
  - Application of local heat and cold on swollen glands bring relief
  - Optimum oral hygiene

♦ **Preventive measures to be taken**
  ➢ Vaccination with the attenuated live virus should be recommended for all children older than one year
  ➢ Adolescent boys and girls and adult males who have not had mumps previously, should be encouraged to have themselves vaccinated

♦ **Measures to prevent epidemics**
  ⬥ None

♦ **Implications for disaster situations**
  ⬥ None

♦ **Compliance with international measures**
  ⬥ None

10.2 COMMUNICABLE DISEASES AFFECTING THE LOWER RESPIRATORY TRACT

Infections of the lower respiratory tract are usually more severe as infections of the upper respiratory tract and the choice of appropriate antimicrobial therapy is important and can be life saving. Lower respiratory tract infections are broadly divided into acute and chronic diseases. Among the acute infections, four major syndromes can be identified, namely, acute bronchitis; acute exacerbations of chronic bronchitis; acute bronchiolitis; and pneumonia. Influenza is a specific infection that, when severe, may proceed to bronchitis or pneumonia. Chronic infections of the lower respiratory tract include specific infections such as tuberculosis; conditions such as lung abscesses and infections in persons suffering from cystic fibrosis. Risk factors associated with exposure to pathogens that invade the lower respiratory tract are age (the young and the elderly), travelling, occupational setting, animals, underlying chronic medical conditions, underlying respiratory tract diseases, tobacco- and/or alcohol-dependency, homelessness, informal settlements with squatter housing and hospitalization.

10.2.1 Acute lower respiratory tract infections

Pathogens gain access to the lower respiratory tract by either inhalation of infected aerosolized material or by aspiration of the normal flora of the upper respiratory tract and/or by inhibiting of the normal cleansing mechanisms of the respiratory tract (for example, smoking). The size of the inhaled particles determines how far the pathogens travel down the respiratory tract – only those pathogens with a diameter less than 5μ reach the alveoli. Less frequently, the lungs become seeded with pathogens as a result of spread via the blood from other infected sites. Healthy individuals are susceptible to a wide range of infectious microbes possessing adhesions that allow the pathogens to attach themselves to the respiratory epithelium. Persons who are immuno-compromised may develop infections with microbes that do not cause infection in healthy individuals.

Because the lower respiratory tract has a limited number of ways in which it can respond to infection, the host response is limited to the following

- ✪ Lobar pneumonitis (pneumonia) whereby a distinct region of the lung is involved and the polymorph exudate that is formed in response to the inflammation response, clots in the alveoli and renders them solid (consolidation). The infection can spread to adjacent alveoli until constraint by anatomic barriers between lobes of the lung
- ✪ Broncho-pneumonitis whereby a more diffuse patchy consolidation of the lung takes place that can spread throughout the lung as a result of the original pathogenesis in the small alveoli
- ✪ Interstitial pneumonitis whereby invasion of the lung interstitial tissue takes place and is characteristic of viral infections of the lungs
- ✪ Forming of lung abscesses or necrotic pneumonia taking place - a condition in which there is cavitations and destruction of the lung parenchyma.

The outcomes common to all of the above conditions are respiratory distress resulting from the interference with the air exchange in the lungs and systemic effects as a result of infection in any part of the body.

10.2.1.1   Bacterial infections affecting the lower respiratory tract

Bacterial pathogens that cause acute lower respiratory tract infections possess the ability to overcome the cleansing mechanisms of the respiratory tract by attaching themselves firmly to the surfaces of cells forming the muco-ciliary sheet. Specific molecules (adhesions) on the pathogen bind to receptor molecules on the susceptible cell in the muco-ciliary sheet. Another way the pathogens gain entry into the body are by inhibiting the ciliary activity of the cells whereby the invading pathogenic microbes establish themselves in the respiratory tract or by producing various cilia-static substances of unknown nature.

10.2.1.1.1   WHOOPING COUGH (PERTUSSIS)

Pertussis is an acute and serious bacterial infection of the trachea-bronchial tree characterized by repetitive, severe spasmodic bouts of coughing which end in a protracted inspiratory wheeze (whoop). Copious clear, viscous secretions are coughed up

Epidemiological data
Geographic distribution   Pertussis occurs world-wide
Causative pathogen   *Bordetella pertussis*, a bacterium
Incubation period   Approximately 7–21days

Mode of transmission
Airborne infected droplets

Period of infectiousness (communicability, transmission)
Pertussis is highly communicable in the catarrhal stage before the paroxysmal coughing sets in. The period of communicability in untreated cases lasts from seven (7) days after exposure until three (3) weeks after the onset of the paroxysmal bouts of coughing. With antimicrobial drug therapy, this period can be shortened to seven days after commencement of treatment

Reservoir
Humans. The *Bordetella pertussis* is found in the secretions of the airways of the infected person

Intermediaries
Vehicle - Fomites

Carriers
None

Immune status
Life-long immunity with memory is elicited

Susceptibility and resistance of host
Everybody is susceptible. Natural passively-acquired immunity which is transmitted trans-placental when the mother had contracted whooping cough or was vaccinated against pertussis is inadequate and children under the age of one year are very susceptible. Vaccinated persons may sometimes experience an atypical attack which causes severe discomfort

Pathogenesis

Bordetella pertussis, when inhaled, attaches itself by fimbrial agglutinogens and filamentous hemagglutinin to the respiratory epithelial cells resulting in interference with the ciliary activity. The *Bordetella pertussis* now multiplies in the ciliated respiratory mucous membrane of the trachea, bronchi and bronchioles but do not invade deeper structures. The *Bordetella pertussis* produces a toxin with a variety of toxic factors, some affect the inflammatory process while other damage the ciliary epithelium together with an inhibition of defence functions, such as chemotaxis, phagocytosis and bactericidal killing – together resulting in necrosis of the mucous membrane. As a result of the necrosis, initially only watery clear mucus is secreted, which later becomes viscous. This viscous mucus can only be coughed up with the greatest difficulty - it irritates the mucous membranes and leads to paroxysmal bouts of coughing (a series of short coughs producing copious mucus, followed by a 'whoop' which is a characteristic sound produced by an inspiratory gasp of air) in an effort to get rid of the mucus. The local necrosis may be so widespread that the inflammatory process also occurs in the bronchi. When the viscous mucus cannot be coughed up, atelectasis and emphysema can develop. Anoxia, which occurs during the paroxysmal bouts of coughing, may lead to oedema and haemorrhages in the lung and brain tissue. These paroxysmal bouts of coughing may also lead to epistaxis, scleral haemorrhage, peri-orbital oedema, vomiting and aspiratory pneumonia.

❖ **Clinical manifestation**

The course of the disease can be divided into three stages, namely the catarrhal, paroxysmal and recovery stages, although overlapping of the clinical manifestations are fairly common

✳ The **catarrhal stage**
- The catarrhal stage lasts for one to two (1–2) weeks and is characterized by non-specific manifestations such as malaise, anorexia, clear nasal secretions, excessive lacrimation, conjunctivitis, bouts of sneezing and a low-grade pyrexia
- Although the disease is highly communicable at this stage, the clinical picture can be confused with less serious infections of the upper airways as well as with the prodromal manifestations of a number of other communicable diseases
- Late in the catarrhal stage the characteristic bouts of coughing develop. Initially it is a non-productive cough which increases in intensity and frequency, particularly at night

✳ The **paroxysmal stage**
- The paroxysmal stage is characterized by the paroxysmal bouts of coughing
- During the coughing bouts the person is extremely uncomfortable, while feeling relative well between bouts
- The bouts of coughing is characterized by the continuous repetition of violent fits of coughing during which the colour of the person's face changes from deep red to puce and the individual may even become cyanotic. Due to consecutive unsuccessful inspiratory efforts, the individual experiences respiratory distress to the extent that it appears that he/she is about to suffocate. The coughing fit ends when the individual succeeds with a tremendous effort to suck some air through the constricted glottis. This causes the loud "whoop"
- The individual often vomits after the whoop which helps to remove the viscous mucus
- The coughing bouts can occur as often as 50 times within a period of 24 hours. They are caused by internal as well as external stimuli
- This stage lasts for a period of three weeks

✳ The **recovery stage**
- During the recovery stage which lasts three to four (3–4) weeks, the bouts of coughing gradually recede
- Sometimes children experience coughing bouts for months afterwards, although not severely

NOTE

An atypical attack of whooping cough occurs in vaccinated persons. The person present with the typical paroxysmal bouts of coughing, lasting for four to six (4-6) weeks. Recovery is rapid. Atypical attacks are caused when the immune status of the person has been weakened with the passing of time and the person had been infected with a fairly virulent *B. pertussis* pathogen. Adolescents and adults become seriously ill and may need to be hospitalized

❖ Complications

- Secondary bacterial infections cause the development of otitis media and acute lobular pneumonia
- Broncho-atelectasis is presently a rare complication of whooping cough owing to the availability of anti-microbial therapy
- Complications of whooping cough that are not caused by secondary infections are related to the degree of severity of the disease. Epistaxis, petechiae or purpura of the skin and peri-orbital bleedings often occur due to anoxia and an increase in venous pressure. Brain haemorrhage is a rare complication
- Convulsions accompanied by severe pyrexia and long-lasting paroxysmal bouts of coughing can occur in children younger than two years
- Aspiration pneumonia may develop when the child inhales the mucus that is vomited at the end of a paroxysm
- An obstructed airway due to the accumulation of mucus, can cause atelectasis and emphysema
- The increase in the intra-abdominal pressure during a paroxysmal coughing bout may lead to abdominal and inguinal hernias as well as a rectal prolapsed
- Ulceration of the frenulum can also result from the persistent coughing

■ Diagnosis

- Clinical picture

■ Prognosis

- Good
- Infants under the age of two (2) years are seriously ill and may die from complications

■ Specific healthcare interventions to be rendered

Medical healthcare interventions

- Pertussis-gammaglobulin is administered to seriously sick babies or children under the age of two (2) years
- Antimicrobial drugs are administered to prevent secondary infection
- A cough suppressant is administered simultaneously with a mucolytic drug to relieve the cough

Specific healthcare interventions

- Supportive healthcare including
  - ◆ supporting of ill individual during paroxysmal coughing bouts
  - ◆ maintaining of the nutritional status and intake of fluids
  - ◆ maintaining of respiratory functions
  - ◆ careful observation for the development of complications
- Children under the age of one (1) years should preferably be hospitalized since they are seriously ill and malnutrition may soon follow
- Older children can be treated at home when no complications set in

◆ **Preventive measures to be taken**
> ➤ Vaccination with **DTP(a)** (Bordetella Pertussis acellular) or alternatively **DTP(a)-IPV** or alternatively **DTP(a)-IPV-Hib** from the age of six (6) weeks. (Passive protection of contacts with pertussis-immunoglobulin does not seem to be of much value)
> ➤ Prophylactic chemotherapy of close contacts

◆ **Measures to prevent epidemics**
> ➤ Vaccination with single dosage vaccine **DTP(a)** or any combination vaccine containing pertussis from the age of six weeks
> ➤ When being treated with antimicrobial drugs, infected children in crèches, play groups, pre-primary and secondary schools or in day care should stay at home for a minimum period of seven (7) days. A medical certificate should accompany the child on his/her return. When the child has received no antimicrobial treatment, he/she should be kept away from any educational or child care institution for a period of 31 days
> ➤ Contacts developing an infection of the upper airways within 21 days of exposure, should receive antimicrobial drug treatment
> ➤ Strict adherence to the school exclusion regulations have to be maintained

◆ **Implications during disaster situations**
> ⬩ Massive outbreaks can occur in refugee camps and similar temporary accommodation when a relatively large percentage of the children have not been vaccinated
> ⬩ Vaccinated children may also become ill

◆ **Compliance with international measures**
> ⬩ None

10.2.1.2 Viral infections of the lower respiratory tract

Viruses can invade the lungs from the bloodstream as well as directly from the respiratory tract. Many viruses cause pneumonia and accomplish infection in the presence of normal host defences. Healthy individuals are susceptible and most of the viruses have surface molecules that attach specifically to the respiratory epithelium. Although some viruses do not cause pneumonia, the viruses still damage the respiratory defences, laying the ground for secondary bacterial pneumonia. Sometimes the virus fails to spread significantly to air spaces, but remains in interstitial tissues to cause interstitial pneumonitis. The outcome of pneumonia is respiratory distress resulting from the interference with air exchange in the lungs as well as systemic effects due to infection in any part of the body. Transmission of influenza occurs by droplet inhalation and is restricted to the coldest months of the year. When complications set in such as pneumonia, the mortality rate rises, especially in the elderly. Influenza viruses damage the respiratory epithelium that predisposes the individual to secondary bacterial infection. Vaccines and antiviral agents are used to prevent influenza.

The influenza viruses can cause endemic, epidemic and pandemic outbreaks due to the inhalation of the infected airborne droplets. Influenza is caused by three types of influenza viruses, namely, influenza virus-A, influenza virus-B, and influenza virus-C. Influenza A-viruses cause epidemics and occasionally pandemics and has a natural animal reservoir, notably birds and pigs. Influenza B-viruses only cause epidemics and do not involve any animal host. Influenza C-viruses do not cause epidemics and give rise to only a minor respiratory illness. Characteristic to the influenza virus envelope/ membrane (the lipid bilayer of host cell origin into which virus proteins and glycoproteins are inserted) are the hemagglutinin (H) and neuraminidase (N) spikes or surface antigens (proteins) that are necessary for attachment to and adsorption into cells. For example, the hemagglutinin (H) and neuraminidase (N) spikes of the influenza A-virus envelope are host-specific antigens (notably avian species) and whereby the different strains of influenza A-virus are characterized. Influenza viruses undergo continuous genetic changes or mutations as they spread through the host species. This results in new strains to which humans have little or any/no prior immunity.

10.2.1.2.1 SEVERE ACUTE RESPIRATORY SYNDROME (SARS)

Severe Acute Respiratory Syndrome (SARS) is a respiratory infection caused by an associated corona-virus (SARS CoV), a new member of the corona-virus family. The new member of the corona-virus family came into existence when small mutations had taken place affecting the hemagglutinin (H) and neuraminidase (N) antigens of the corona–virus envelope and an antigenic drift had resulted. These changes enabled the corona-virus to multiply significantly in individuals with immunity to preceding strains and then re-infect the community as a new subtype

---

Epidemiological data

Geographic distribution
Severe Acute Respiratory Syndrome (SARS) occurs predominantly in Asia but has spread to the rest of the world via modern air travelling

Causative pathogen
An *associated corona-virus (SARS CoV)*, a new member of the corona-virus family

Incubation period
Approximately 2–10 days

Mode of transmission
Airborne infected droplets

Period of infectiousness (communicability, transmission)
As long as the virus is present in the respiratory tract

Reservoir
Humans. The SARS CoV–virus is found in the secretions of the airways of the infected person

Intermediaries
Vehicle - Fomites

Carriers None **Immune status** Immunity with memory is elicited **Susceptibility and resistance of host** Everybody is susceptible. Except for the tropics, influenza infection is mostly restricted to the coldest months of the year. During the coldest weather, individuals spent more time inside buildings with limited air space which favours transmission. At the same time, the natural resistance of many host may also be diminished due to colds and/or other respiratory infections

Pathogenesis

The initial symptoms of SARS are due to the direct viral damage and associated inflammatory response. The *SARS CoV* enters the respiratory tract in inhaled droplets and attaches itself to the cilialic acid receptors on epithelial cells via the hemagglutinin (H) glycoprotein of the virus envelope. As fewer virus particles are needed to infect the lower respiratory tract than the upper respiratory tract, the development of infection and complications follows quickly. Within 1-3 days after been infected, the cytokines mediated by the damaged cells and from the infiltrating leukocytes cause symptoms such as sore throat, diarrhoea, headache, rhinorrhoea, chills, malaise, fever (> 38°C), myalgia, a cough, shortness of breath or difficulty in breathing. Pneumonia sets in very quickly. The mortality rate is fairly high.

❖ **Clinical manifestation**
  - Feeling unwell - malaise
  - Sore throat
  - Diarrhoea
  - Chills
  - Headache
  - Rhinorrhoea
  - Hyperthermia - >38°C and higher
  - Myalgia (muscular aches and pains)
  - A cough which may produce sputum
  - Shortness of breath
  - Difficulty in breathing

❖ **Complications**
  - Secondary bacterial infection due to damage of the respiratory epithelium
  - Pneumonia
  - Death

■ **Diagnosis**
  - X-rays of the lungs
  - Abnormal crackling sound (rales) on auscultation
  - PCR detection of influenza viral RNA
  - Serology

■ **Prognosis**
  ▪ Fair

■ **Specific healthcare interventions to be rendered**
  ▪ The ill person must be cared for in a high-grade isolation unit and the principles of Standard Precautions, Transmission-based precautions and High-grade Barrier Isolation must be strictly adhered to
  ▪ Specific healthcare interventions are therefore mostly supportive and symptomatic
  ▪ The person's secretions, however, must be treated with great care and be burned

◆ **Preventive measures to be taken**
  ➤ Transmission via close contact from an infected person to un-infected persons is very high and occurs between family members, visitors and hospital staff caring for ill healthcare users suffering from SARS
  ➤ To prevent the transmission of all respiratory infections, including SARS, in healthcare establishments, the general measures set out in 3.2.3 - Modifying/reducing of risk factors in the environment, and the specific under mentioned measures should be implemented as a component of Standard Precautions as transmission of *SARS-CoV* disease in a single healthcare facility can have far reaching public health effects. Other measures of importance are
    ✠ Screening of all family members and friends who have been in contact with the ill person on a daily basis for fever and lower respiratory symptoms as they are at risk for SARS-CoV disease. When symptoms are present, control measures to prevent *SARS-CoV* transmission must be immediately instituted
    ✠ Adhering to Droplet Precautions by all healthcare personnel as to ensure that ill healthcare users suffering from respiratory infections wear masks when transferred from room to room and or between departments. Personnel themselves must wear masks when rendering care and/or examining a person with symptoms of a respiratory infection, particularly when myalgia, headache, sore throat, diarrhoea, rhinorrhoea (12-24 hours before the onset of fever) and fever is present. These precautions must be maintained until it is determined that the cause of the symptoms is not the infectious agent *SARS-CoV* that requires Droplet Precautions
    ✠ Screening for *SARS-CoV* of all persons with symptom onset of fever and lower respiratory infection within 10 days in the following conditions
      ▪ in radiographically conferred pneumonia of unknown origin
      ▪ has a travelling history to Asia (especially China [including Hong Kong], Taiwan, Korea, and Thailand)
      ▪ has been in close contact with an ill person with a history of resent travelling to one of those areas
      ▪ is employed in an occupation associated with risk for *SARS-CoV* exposure

- is part of a cluster of cases of atypical pneumonia without an alternative diagnosis
  - ✠ Rapid and prolonged isolating with Droplet Precautions of severe ill persons in an airborne isolation room or unit until recovered, or until it is determined that the cause of the pneumonia is not contagious
- ➢ Individuals suffering from a mild *SARS-CoV* infection can be safely isolated in locations other than acute-care healthcare establishments (hospitals) such as at home or in community facilities designated for isolation of ill healthcare users suffering from *SARS-CoV*. The same infection control measures for Respiratory hygiene and cough etiquette as well as Droplet precautions must be strictly adhered to

◆ **Measures to prevent epidemics**
- Because international air travelling enhances the spread of SARS to other countries and continents within hours, checking for respiratory infections with fever (>38°C and higher) in communities and at airports must be done when an alert has been sent out by the WHO
- Rapid identification of the SARS associated corona-virus can break the known chains of person-to-person transmission
- International networking and adherence to the global standard for investigation of disease outbreaks can prevent a pandemic outbreak of SARS
- Extremely strict adherence to all school exclusion regulations
- Extremely strict adherence to Standard precautions, transmission-based precautions and high grade barrier isolation
- Extremely strict adherence to all legislative measures
- Cultural practices have to be overruled when necessarily

◆ **Implications for disaster situations**
- None

◆ **Compliance with international measures**
- Notification to the World Health Organization that SARS has broken out in the RSA
- Strict compliance to all public health emergency plans put in place

10.2.1.2.2 INFLUENZA A-ILLNESSES: AVIAN INFLUENZA, SWINE INFLUENZA AND OTHER ANIMAL-ORIGINATED INFLUENZA A-ILLNESSES

All Influenza A-viruses are respiratory viruses that can cause endemic, epidemic and pandemic outbreaks. The Influenza A-virus is a typical orthomyxovirus (a single-stranded RNA genome) and the Influenza A-virus envelope possesses both hemagglutinin and neuraminidase spikes. The Influenza A-virus has an internal ribonucleoprotein (RNP) which is a group-specific antigen that differentiates it from the Influenza B-virus and the Influenza C-virus. The hemagglutinin and neuraminidase of the Influenza A-viruses are type-specific antigens and are used to distinguish between the different strains of the Influenza A-virus. The Influenza A-viruses easily undergo genetic changes – either an antigenic drift or an antigenic shift – as they spread through the host species. And because the Influenza A-viruses can infect both animals (birds and mammals) and humans, the Influenza A-viruses are able to re-assort and become mixed vessel transmissible viruses allowing the potential mixing of Influenza viruses A, B, and C and the emergence of new/novel strains of the Influenza A-virus.

Avian Influenza (Bird Flu)

Although the *Avian Influenza A-virus*, namely H1N1, H1N2, H3N2 H7N1 and H9N2, infect humans from time to time, epidemics of Avian Influenza caused by *Avian Influenza A-virus* occur on a regular basis in avian species such as poultry (chickens and turkeys), ostriches, and waterfowl (ducks and geese) as well as in pigs and whales. Avian species are the natural host and reservoir of most of the *Avian Influenza A-viruses*. Any genetic shift (sudden major changes) that occurs in the *Avian Influenza A-virus* envelope, affects both domestic and wild bird life and migratory birds can bring the new strain of *Avian Influenza A-virus* to densely populated areas of the world. As flocks of wild and migratory birds have no resistance to the new strain of *Avian Influenza A-virus*, transmission from bird to bird occurs rapidly and death on a large scale quickly follows.

The *Avian Influenza H5N1-A-virus* and H7N1 are new *Avian Influenza A-virus strains* as an genetic shift had occurred in the antigenicity of the H-surface antigen (hemagglutinin spikes consist of 16 types) and N-surface antigen (neuraminidase spikes consist of 9 types) of the *Avian Influenza A-virus* resulting in novel/new hemagglutinin genes that where derived from the *Avian influenza A-virus* genes. Associated with the change in the H and N surface antigens were apparently other genetic changes that had conferred increased pathogenicity and virulence as well as enhancement of the ability to spread rapidly from avian species to humans and from person to person. Humans lack protective immunity (anti-H5 antibody as well as anti-H7 antibody) against the new hemagglutinin surface antigens. Although *Avian Influenza A-viruses* possess the ability to infect humans without acquiring human influenza genes by re-assortment (recombination or mutation that occurs when the genes from human and bird viruses mix in an intermediate host, such as pigs or poultry, like the known circulating *Human Influenza A-viruses*, namely, H1N1, H3N2 and H1N2), the *H5N1-virus-A* has derived all its genes from *Avian influenza A-viruses* (product of three strains found in quail [H9N2], geese [H5N1] and teal [H6N1] that mutated when these birds came in contact with domestic poultry) without re-assortment with *Human Influenza A-viruses*. Because of the multi-basic cleavage site sequence of the *H5N1-virus-A*, the *Avian H5N1-virus-A* is highly pathogenic with host-receptor specificity that does not restrict its ability to infect, be absorbed into and replicate in humans. As the *Avian H5N1-virus-A* is now highly transmissible directly from-person-to-person via airborne droplets, re-assortment may already had taken place and the pathogenicity and/or virulence of the *Avian H5N1-virus-A* may has had further increased. When re-assortment of *Avian H5N1-virus-A* with one of the known human influenza virus-types occurs, an exchange of genes had already taken place resulting in another new strain that maintains the virulence of the *Avian H5N1-virus-A* but assumes the transmissibility efficiency of the human Influenza virus. As this re-assortment of the *Avian Influenza virus-A* has already occurred (the *Avian influenza virus-A* has re-assorted with the *Human Influenza virus-C* and the *H1N1-virus* affecting pigs [swines]), the probability of a pandemic of Bird flu in humans has thus greatly increased, especially with international air travelling enhancing the global spread within hours via person-to-person transmission.

Epidemiological data

Geographic distribution

Worldwide during a pandemic outbreak – the *Avian influenza H5N1-A-virus* has already been identified on all continents. International air and sea travelling enhances the global spread

Causative pathogen

Avian influenza H5N1-A-virus

Incubation period

Approximately 2–10 days

Mode of transmission

Horizontally - Airborne infected droplets
Transmission and spread occurs as follows

* From birds to humans
  * Aerosolized droplets landing on exposed surfaces of the human mouth, nose, eyes or inhaled into the lungs
  * Direct horizontal contact with infected birds or surfaces and objects contaminated by their faeces (large quantities of the virus are found in the faeces of infected avian species and contamination of soil occurs frequently)
  * Eating of raw poultry juices and products (meat and eggs) from infected poultry
* From human to human
  * Close contact with an ill person by minute airborne infected droplets when talking, sneezing, coughing, laughing, singing
  * International air travelling enhances the global spread of the *Avian Influenza H5N1 A-virus* via person-to-person transmission

Period of infectiousness (communicability, transmission)

As long as the virus is present in the respiratory tract

Reservoir

Avian species are the most natural host and reservoir of *Avian Influenza A-viruses*. Pigs and sea mammals (whales), however, can also be a reservoir as well as dogs (*Avian Influenza A-viruses* have already been isolated in the throats of dogs)

Intermediaries

Vehicle - Fomites

Carriers

None

Immune status

Immunity with memory may be elicited. Epidemics and pandemics occur due to the appearance of new strains of *Avian Influenza A-viruses* (including the *Swine Influenza A-viruses*) with the result that the given individual can be again infected with different strains

Susceptibility and resistance of host

Everybody (babies, children, adults, elderly – healthy, ill, disabled or dying) is susceptible to avian flu. Humans lack protective immunity (anti-H5 antibody as well as anti-H7 antibody) against new hemagglutinin surface antigens

---

Pathogenesis

The initial symptoms of Avian Flu are due to the direct viral damage and the associated inflammatory response. The *Avian Influenza H5N1-A-virus* enters the respiratory tract in inhaled droplets and attaches itself to the cilialic acid receptors on epithelial cells via the hemagglutinin (H) glycoprotein of the virus envelope. As fewer virus particles are needed to infect the lower respiratory tract than the upper respiratory tract, the development of infection and complications quickly follows. Within 1-3 days after been infected, the cytokines mediated by the damaged cells and the infiltrating leukocytes cause symptoms such as fever (> 38°C), myalgia (muscular aches and pains), coughing, shortness of breath or difficulty in breathing. Viral pneumonia very quickly sets in. Spreading of the *Avian Influenza H5N1-A-virus* to all body organs also takes place resulting in multiple organ failure. Multiple organ failure together with substantial tissue damage in the respiratory tract and lungs as well as a depletion of lymphocytes in blood, lung and lymphoid tissue together with a diminished production of pro-inflammatory cytokines, lead to the death of the infected person.

❖ **Clinical manifestation**
  - The *H5N1-Avian Influenza A-virus* causes a spectrum of clinical disease from mild respiratory infection to a severe to fatal disease
  - The replication of the *Avian Influenza H5N1-A-virus* with low pathogenicity is restricted to infection of the eyes and of the respiratory tract
    - ◈ Symptoms of respiratory infection such as sore throat, diarrhoea, headache, rhinorrhoea, chills, malaise, myalgia (muscular aches and pains), and coughing develops
    - ◈ The infection in the respiratory tract is cleared from the lungs by day 9 post-infected
  - The *Avian Influenza H5N1-A-virus* with a high pathogenicity, on the other hand, usually spreads systemically, infecting all major organs (including the brain) with death resulting 3-8 days after being infected
    - ◈ Avian flu starts with a fever (> 38°C), sore throat, coughing and respiratory distress and progresses very quickly to severe respiratory distress syndrome, secondary viral pneumonia and eventually multiple organ failure
    - ◈ Death occurs within 3 to 8 days

❖ **Complications**
  • Death

■ **Diagnosis**
  ▪ Culture studies done on nose swabs
  ▪ X-rays of the lungs
  ▪ Abnormal crackling sound (rales) on auscultation
  ▪ PCR detection of influenza viral RNA
  ▪ Serology
  ▪ The *Avian influenza H5N1-A-virus* can be isolated from throat washings taken 1-2 days after the onset of the disease and then cultured, although it takes several days

■ **Prognosis**
  Because humans lack immunity against *Avian Influenza H5N1-virus-A* death occurs within days after becoming ill

■ **Specific healthcare interventions to be rendered**
  The following standard precautions must be taken by all healthcare providers involved in the care of ill healthcare users with suspected or diagnosed Avian flu
  ▪ All persons who presents to a healthcare setting with fever and respiratory symptoms or a febrile respiratory disease and a history of travelling within the previous 10 days to a country with avian influenza activity, **must be isolated in an airborne high grade isolation unit**. (The unit/room should have monitored negative air pressure in relation to corridor with 6-12 air changes per hour. Exhaled air must be taken directly outside or if re-circulated, the air must be filtered through a high efficiency particulate air filter. A fit-tested respirator and N-95 filtering face piece respirator that are disposable must be used by healthcare providers when entering the unit/room)
  ▪ **When rendering care in the high-grade isolation unit, the principles of Standard precautions, Transmission-based precautions and High grade Barrier Isolation must be strictly adhered to**
  ▪ Specific healthcare interventions are mostly supportive and symptomatic
  ▪ Treatment consists of antiviral drugs and influenza vaccines. Treatment must be commenced within 48 hours and last for five days. Post exposure prophylaxis last for six (6) weeks
  ▪ Secretions of the ill individual must be treated with great care and be burned
  ▪ Careful attention must be given to hand hygiene before and after all contact with the ill individual or contact with items potentially contaminated with respiratory secretions
  ▪ Gloves, masks and gowns must be worn for all patient contact
  ▪ Disposable equipment such as stethoscopes, blood pressure cuffs, thermometers, etc must be used
  ▪ Eye protection (goggles or face shields) must be worn within 1 (one) meter of the ill individual

- All healthcare providers must adhere to Droplet Precautions by ensuring that all ill healthcare users suffering from respiratory infection wear masks when transferred from room to room or between departments
- **Healthcare providers must wear masks themselves** when delivering care and/or examining a person with symptoms of a respiratory infection, particularly when myalgia, headache, sore throat, diarrhoea, rhinorrhoea (12-24 hours before the onset of fever) and fever is present. These precautions must be maintained until it is determined that the cause of the symptoms is not the *Avian Influenza H5N1-virus-A* that requires Droplet Precautions
- All healthcare providers involved in the care of the ill person with Avian flu should be vaccinated with the most recent seasonal human influenza vaccine to prevent/reduce the likelihood of the healthcare providers being co-infected with both human and avian strains that can lead to re-assortment taking place resulting in the emergence of a new potential pandemic strain
- All precautionary measures must be continued for 14 days after the onset of symptoms or until either an alternative diagnosis has been made or diagnostic test results indicated that the individual is not infected with *Avian Influenza H5N1- A-virus*
- Any person not hospitalized and managed as an outpatient as well as any hospitalized patient suspected to suffer from Avian flu and discharged before 14 days have passed, must be isolated in the home setting according to "home isolation precautionary measures"
- Surveillance and monitoring of family members for fever, respiratory symptoms and conjunctivitis must be done on a daily basis
- All healthcare providers/personnel must be instructed to be vigilant for the development of fever, respiratory symptoms and/or conjunctivitis for one (1) week after the last exposure to Avian influenza-infected ill healthcare users. When any healthcare provider/employee becomes ill, medical care must immediately be seeked and prior to arrival, the healthcare facility has to be informed that he/she has been exposed to the Avian influenza virus. The healthcare facility must notify the occupational health and infection control department to instate the necessary precautionary measures
- All ill healthcare personnel must stay at home until 24 hours after resolution of the fever, unless an alternative diagnosis has been made or diagnostic test results has indicated that the individual is not infected with *Avian Influenza H5N1-A-virus*. While at home, ill personnel must practice good respiratory hygiene and cough etiquette to lower the risk of transmission of the *Avian Influenza H5N1-A-virus* to others

◆ **Preventive measures to be taken**
  ➢ To prevent the transmission of all respiratory infections in healthcare settings, including *Avian Influenza H5N1-A-virus*, the following measures should be implemented as one component of Standard Precautions and Transmission-based Precautionary Measures as transmission of *Influenza A-virus* infection in a single healthcare facility can have far reaching public health effects

* Implementation of infection control on a large scale as described in 3.2.3 - Modifying/reducing of risk factors in the environment, as well as
  ◈ Encouraging ill healthcare users to seek medical help as soon as possible
  ◈ Taking a full travelling history of the ill individual (including a travelling history of family members, friends and colleagues/co-workers or school mates/care-takers of non-school going children). If any doubt exist and a clear-cut diagnosis cannot be made, nose swabs for culture studies must be taken of all ill individuals
  ◈ considering all family members and friends who have been in contact with the ill person as at risk *for Avian Influenza A-virus* diseases and to be screened on a daily basis for fever and lower respiratory symptoms. When symptoms are present, institute immediately control measures to prevent *Avian Influenza H5N1-virus-A* transmission
  ◈ screening all persons with symptom onset of fever and lower respiratory infection for Avian flu within 10 days in the following conditions
    ▪ in radiographically conferred pneumonia of unknown origin
    ▪ has a travelling history to Asia (especially China [including Hong Kong], Taiwan, Korea, and Thailand)
    ▪ has been in close contact with an ill person with a history of resent travelling to one of these areas
    ▪ is employed in an occupation associated with risk for *Influenza A-virus* exposure
    ▪ is part of a cluster of cases of atypical pneumonia without an alternative diagnosis
➢ Rapid and prolonged isolation with droplet precautions of severe ill persons in an airborne isolation room or unit until recovered, or until it is determined that the cause of the pneumonia is not contagious
➢ Other measures to prevent the spread of avian flu are
  * Proper cooking of all parts of poultry (including eggs) and of pigs as the *H5N1-avian-virus-A* is heat sensitive and is not transmitted and spread via cooked food
  * Prevention of cross contamination by not mixing juices from raw poultry products with food items eaten raw
  * Food handlers must wear masks, wash their hands thoroughly, and disinfect all surface areas that come in contact with poultry or pigs
  * Culling of all domestic and farming poultry flocks (including ostriches) and/ or pigs when infected
  * The practice of misusing vaccines for the vaccination of poultry against *Avian influenza H5N1-virus-A* as well as other *Influenza virus-A* diseases must be prevented or stopped as well as the practice of diluting the vaccine when vaccinating of poultry is done
  * A medical or veterinary officer must be furnished with all information relating to the occurrence, spread, extermination or decrease on any premises in

the numbers of any animal/avian specie, or an increase in animal/bird carcasses and animal/bird product

* Complying with all legal measures introduced to prevent the spread of or extermination of or the reducing of Avian flu
* Placing of a demarcated geographical area under quarantine and restricting movement into, out of and within the demarcated area self of both humans and animals
* Any person who is present on premises or in an area placed under quarantine
    ◈ May not leave such premises or area before the expiry of the prescribed quarantine period without prior authorisation
    ◈ Shall subject himself/herself during such period to any medical observation, examination or supervision determined by an authorised medical practitioner
    ◈ Shall subject himself to all regulations relating to quarantine
* Instituting measures to be taken at inland borders, sea ports and airports with a view to preventing the introduction of Avian Flu via the import of infected poultry or meat into the RSA or the export from the RSA of any substance or thing such as to introduce Avian Flu into any area outside the RSA
* <u>Health information to be given to all persons/families/communities not to live closely together with poultry and pigs in their household – poultry and pigs should be kept in their own pens outside human dwellings and living spaces. Sick animals/poultry must be culled and the authorities must be informed when death of large numbers of animals/birds occur</u>

◆ **Measures to prevent epidemics**
    ⊥ Rapid identification of the *Avian H5N1-influenza-A-virus* to break the known chains of person-to-person transmission
    ⊥ International networking and adherence to the global standard for investigation of disease outbreaks to prevent a pandemic outbreak of Avian flu
    ⊥ The World Health Organization (WHO) encourages all countries to have public health emergency plans in place should an outbreak occurs, including active case finding of/looking for ill and infected individuals in the community, and adherence to the different levels of pandemic alertness issued by the WHO
    ⊥ Alerting of all cabin crew of trains, aeroplanes and ocean-going sea liners and cargo ships to the identification of passengers/crew with respiratory infections or who complain of not feeling well after takeoff from airports or leaving sea ports/ railway stations in countries where Avian Flu has been diagnosed in humans. Isolation measures (2-3 meters around the affected individual) must be instituted as well as strict adherence to Droplet Precautions and respiratory and cough etiquette
    ⊥ Extremely strict adherence to all school exclusion regulations
    ⊥ Extremely strict adherence to Standard precautions, transmission-based precautions and high grade barrier isolation
    ⊥ Extremely strict adherence to all legislative measures
    ⊥ Cultural practices have to be overruled when necessarily

◆ **Implications for disaster situations**
  ⊥ None

◆ **Compliance with international measures**
  ⊥ Notification to the World Health Organization that Avian Flu has broken out in the RSA
  ⊥ Strict compliance to all public health emergency plans put in place

A/H1N1 Influenza (Swine Flu)

Swine influenza is a highly contagious acute respiratory disease caused by one of several *Swine influenza A-viruses* that is species specific and is spread among pigs by aerosols, direct and indirect contact and asymptomatic carrier pigs. *Swine influenza viruses* are the most common of the H1N1 subtype with other subtypes that also circulate in pigs being H1N2, H3N1 and H3N2. Pigs can also become infected with *Avian influenza viruses* and *Human seasonal influenza viruses* as well as *other Swine influenza viruses*. When pigs are infected with more than one virus type at a time a genetic shift or re-assortment takes place. Pigs are the intermediate host for the new *A/H1NI Influenza A-virus 2009 strain* although the pigs as such do not die from the new A/H1N1 strain. Other susceptible animals for the *H1N1 Swine influenza A-viruses* are turkeys, ferrets, and cats.

The *Swine Influenza A-virus* causing A/H1N1-virus flu is the new *pandemic influenza A-virus 2009 strain* of the known *A/H1N1 Swine Influenza A-virus* consisting of mostly swine and partly avian and partly human antigens as an genetic re-assortment had taken place in the antigenicity of the H1-surface antigen and N1-surface antigen - resulting in novel/new hemagglutinin genes that where derived from all three influenza A-virus genes of human, avian and swine origin. As humans have no immunity to this novel *pandemic Influenza A-virus 2009 strain* of the *Swine A/H1N1 Influenza A-virus*, epidemics develops extremely rapidly, culminating rapidly into a pandemic. Humans mostly develop swine influenza when being infected by infected pigs, but when human-to-human transmission takes place epidemics and/or a pandemic rapidly occur. As the *Swine A/H1N1 influenza A-virus* has already mutated and will mutate again as it spreads across the world, the probability of causing a pandemic is greatly increasing. Because modern air and train transport supports the rapid human-to-human transmission of any novel/new strain(s) of the Swine *H1N1 Influenza A-virus*, many countries word wide is experiencing an increased influenza activity.

The signs and symptoms of the *pandemic A/H1N1-virus 2009 strain* Swine flu are similar to avian flu as described above or seasonal influenza. The clinical presentation ranges broadly from an asymptomatic infection to a severe pneumonia resulting in death. Mild or asymptomatic cases may escape recognition with the result that the true extent of the *pandemic A/H1N1-virus 2009 strain* Swine influenza amongst humans is unknown. The treatment of this *pandemic A/H1N1-virus 2009 strain* Swine flu is also similar to that of Bird flu. The death rate may also be very high. It is also safe to eat pork and pork products when pork meat and pork-derived products are properly handled, prepared and cooked. The *pandemic A/H1N1-virus*

2009 strain (Swine influenza A-virus) is killed by cooking temperatures of 170°C and the swine influenza virus has not been shown to be transmissible to humans when eating properly handled and prepared pork and other products derived from pigs. Pigs should also be routinely vaccinated against swine influenza and when swine influenza does occur in pigs, the pig population must be culled. Culling also applies to all others susceptible animals such as turkeys, cats and ferrets.

Because influenza can be more serious in pregnant women leading to influenza-associated deaths as well as adverse pregnancy outcomes with increased rates of spontaneous abortion and pre-term births and an increased risk for influenza complications for the mother as well as increased risk for adverse perinatal outcomes or delivery complications, all pregnant women suspected to be infected with the *pandemic A/H1N1-virus 2009 strain* must be tested for *Swine A/H1N1* influenza. Treatment of the mother should not be delayed pending the results and nor should treatment be withheld in the absence of testing as antiviral treatment is most effective when started within the first two days after the onset of symptoms. Although the risk for transmission of the *pandemic Swine A/H1N1-virus 2009 strain* through breast milk is unknown (probably rare), women who are not very ill with influenza should be encourage to initiate breastfeeding early and feed frequently (wearing a facemask) as infants who are not breastfeeding are more vulnerable to infection and hospitalization for severe respiratory illness. Unnecessary formula supplementation must be avoided as to ensure that the infant receives as much maternal antibodies as possible. Sick mothers who are able to express their milk for bottle/cup feedings by a healthy family member must be encouraged to do so. Antiviral medication treatment or prophylaxis is not a contra-indication for breastfeeding. Of importance and if possible, only healthy adults who are not showing any signs and symptoms of influenza-like illnesses should care for mothers and infants - including the preparation of infant feedings. All caregivers to mothers and infants should preferably wear a facemask - **a must when showing any signs and symptoms of influenza-like illnesses**. Furthermore, all infants should be kept away from persons who are ill and out of crowded areas. Parents and caregivers must at all time practice good hand hygiene and cough etiquette, limit the sharing of toys, and any item that has been in the infant's mouth must be thoroughly washed with soap and water.

NOTE
THE SAME MEASURES DESCRIBED ABOVE ARE APPLICABLE WHEN COMBATING EPIDEMICS OF *INFLUENZA A-VIRUS* IN LAND MAMMALS (ANIMALS) OR MARINE (SEA) MAMMALS OR WILD, TAME AND DOMESTIC BIRDS THAT HAS BEEN TRANSMITTED TO HUMANS OR INFLUENZA A-VIRUS DISEASES CAUSED BY NEW STRAINS OF *INFLUENZA A-VIRUSES* CONSISTING OF PARTLY ANIMAL, BIRD AND HUMAN ANTIGENS

10.2.2 Chronic infections of the lower respiratory tract

Chronic infections of the lower respiratory tract are mostly cause by pathogens that possess the ability to avoid phagocytosis by the alveoli macrophages and/or to avoid destruction after phagocytosis.

10.2.2.1   Mycobacterium infection of the lower respiratory tract

Many species of the mycobacterium are associated with disease, but the major pathogens of this genus are *M. tuberculosis humanis, M. tuberculosis bovis* and *M. Leprae*. Mycobacterium are Gram-positive bacilli (rods) that have a thick layer of peptidoglycan external to the cell membrane containing a variety of lipids (mycolic acids) which not only has a different chemical basis of cross-linking to the lipoprotein layer but also creates a waxy layer that gives considerable resistance to drying out and to other environmental factors. Mycobacterium are able to avoid phagocytosis by the host cells as it has a slimy surface created by an additional capsule of high molecular polysaccharides (this high molecular polysaccharides also determines the virulence of the mycobacterium). Mycobacterium can also avoid destruction after phagocytosis by surviving in the macrophages. Cell-mediated immunity is elicited as resistance to reactivation of a latent infection.

10.2.2.1.1   TUBERCULOSIS – DRUG-SUSCEPTIBLE AND DRUG-RESISTANT

Tuberculosis (TB), also known as the White Plague, is a chronic (sometimes acute or sub-acute) disease characterized by the formation of tubercles in any tissue or organ of the body. The lungs are most often the primary body organ that is affected. It affects both the apparently healthy individual (immuno-competent) as well as the immuno-compromised individual, being a serious disease. As such, tuberculosis is not only a medical problem but also a social and economic disaster of immense magnitude that occur the world over.

Please note
A distinction is made between **drug-susceptible tuberculosis** (TB) and **drug-resistant** TB. Drug-susceptible TB refers to the TB-disease caused by the drug-susceptible *Mycobacterium tuberculosis humanis* and is treated with first-line anti-tuberculosis drugs for a short period of time but not less than 6 months. The infected immuno-competent individual responds positively to treatment by first-line anti-tuberculosis drugs and resolution (recovery) of the infection is high and the prognosis is good. In immuno-compromised individuals (for example, individuals suffering from HIV+/AIDS) recovery is less favourable and treatment may last longer.

The iatrogenic (man-made) or drug-resistant form of TB is caused by different strains of the drug-resistant Mycobacterium *tuberculosis humanis*. (Resistant strains refer to those strains that differ from the sensitive strains in their capacity to grow in the presence of a higher concentration of a specific anti-tuberculosis drug). A distinction is made between new cases of drug-resistant-TB and re-treatment cases of drug-resistant-TB. In new cases of drug resistant-TB (primary resistance), the individual has been infected with one (or more) of the new strains of the drug-resistant *Mycobacterium tuberculosis humanis* and is not known as to previously suffered from TB. In re-treatment cases of drug-resistant *Mycobacterium tuberculosis humanis* (acquired resistance due to either relapse, failure or return after default), the sick individual is already on treatment but has developed drug-resistance to certain specific or to all anti-tuberculosis drugs (relapse), or failed to complete the treatment programme (failure) or has returned for further treatment after defaulting the treatment programme (return after default).

Drug-resistant TB are further classified in multiple drug-resistant-TB (MDR-TB), extensively drug-resistant-TB (XDR-TB) and completely/totally drug-resistant-TB (CDR/TDR-TB). In **multiple drug-resistant-TB or MDR-TB** the infected individual could suffer from either single-drug/mono-drug resistant-TB or combined-drug/ double-drug resistant-TB (a strain resistant to two specific first-line anti-tuberculosis drugs, isoniazid and rifampicin) or multiple-drug resistant-TB (triple → quadruple → more drugs - a strain resistant to more than two first-line anti-tuberculosis drugs). The different strains are transmissible to immuno-competent individuals with acquired adaptive cell-immunity to drug-susceptible TB; to immuno-compromised individuals (for example, ill healthcare users suffering from cancer and receiving chemotherapy); and to sufferers of active drug-susceptible TB. Treatment consists of a combination of first line and second-line anti-tuberculosis drugs or only second-line anti-tuberculosis drugs. Treatment last as long as 18-24 months and hospitalization may be necessarily. The treatment outcome for immuno-competent individuals is fair but much bleaker for immuno-compromised individuals within 2-5 years time. In **extensively drug-resistant-TB or XDR-TB** the infection is caused by the specific drug-resistant strain of *Mycobacterium tuberculosis humanis* that is resistant to all first-line anti-tuberculosis drugs as well as to more than 3 of the 6 classes of second-line anti-tuberculosis drugs. Treatment consists of only second-line anti-tuberculosis drugs for 24 months or longer. The treatment outcome for immuno-competent individuals is bleak and even bleaker for immuno-compromised individuals. The mortality rate is high (>70%) within 24 months and infected individuals have to be treated in special isolated healthcare units. In **completely/totally drug-resistant-TB or CDR/TDR-TB** the individual is resistant to all first-line and all second-line anti-tuberculosis drugs and at this moment in time there is no treatment available to treat CDR/TDR-TB. Mortality rate for persons suffering from CDR/TDR-TB is 100%. The drug-resistant *M. tuberculosis humanis* is extremely virulent and highly transmissible – transmissible to all persons who are immuno-competent and who have acquired adaptive cell-immunity to both drug-susceptible and drug-resistant *Mycobacterium tuberculosis humanis*; to all immuno-compromised persons and to all sufferers of active TB (drug-susceptible and drug-resistant). Because of the infectivity and seriousness of XDR-TB and CDR/TDR-TB, the welfare of the public/community takes precedence over the human rights of the individual.

The clinical picture and specific healthcare interventions of drug-susceptible and drug-resistant (MDR-TB, XDR-TB and CDR/TDR-TB) tuberculosis are more or less the same although the chemotherapy regime as well as the criteria for admission to hospital totally differs. The treatment outcome and prognosis of the disease become poorer when iatrogenic strains infect the individual or when the infected individual develops drug resistance himself/herself.

Epidemiological data

Geographic distribution
Tuberculosis is prevalent the world over

Causative pathogen
Human type - *Mycobacterium tuberculosis humanis* (drug-susceptible strain, drug-resistant strains)
Animal type - *Mycobacterium tuberculosis bovis*

Mode of transmission
Horizontally - Airborne transmission by inhalation of infected droplets
Mycobacterium tuberculosis humanis is coughed into the air in minute droplets from the tubercles with sinus formation in the lungs and is then inhaled by another individual
*Inhalation of *M. tuberculosis humanis* droplets in dust - The tuberculosis bacilli can live for up to six months in dust after having been coughed up, unless they are exposed to the direct rays of the sun. When the dust is disturbed (for example, when sweeping with a broom, when the wind is blowing or children are playing) the infected droplets in the dust is inhaled
Ingestion by drinking un-pasteurized milk from an infected cow; ingestion of infected droplets in dust or dust particles and by licking, sucking or swallowing fomites contaminated with *M. tuberculosis humanis* (mainly children)
Inoculation may occur during the performance of a post mortem examination. Babies may also be infected during birth by contaminated hospital equipment
Please note
Although tuberculosis is not vertically transmitted from mother to foetus as the *M. tuberculosis humanis* does not cross the placenta, a baby can be born with tuberculosis when the mother suffers from miliary tuberculosis and a placental focus or lesion has ruptured, infecting the foetal circulation

Incubation period
This varies from six weeks to years, depending on the time it takes for the primary lesion and/or metastatic infections to develop into the pronounced disease (susceptible drug TB). With drug-resistant strains the incubation period may be shorten

Period of infectiousness (communicability, transmission)
The communicability of the disease varies from one infected person to another. Horizontally communicability depends on the shedding of *Mycobacterium tuberculosis humanis* from the infected lesions in the body into the air. The shedding of the *M. tuberculosis humanis* depends on the position and type of the lesion (sinus formation from the lung lesion(s) to the airways must have taken place – open lung lesions) and the nature of the chemotherapy received. A person with open lung lesions who receives regular first-line chemotherapy for drug-susceptible TB can still secrete viable bacilli for approximately a month, but the disease is for all practical purposes no longer transmissible 24 hours after chemotherapy has commenced. In drug-resistant tuberculosis the drug-resistant *M. tuberculosis humanis* stays viable after second-line chemotherapy has been commenced and can be horizontally transmitted (due to open lung lesions) to all uninfected hosts (individuals who have never suffered from TB previously, to all infected individuals suffering from drug-susceptible TB and

to all other individuals suffering from drug-resistant TB not infected by the specific drug-resistant strain). A person suffering from any other form of tuberculosis (for example, kidney TB) cannot transmit *Mycobacterium tuberculosis humanis* horizontally as no sinus formation to the airways from the tubercle lesions in the kidneys could have taken place, except when the infected individual also suffers from TB of the lungs with sinus formation to the airways. Transmission now occurs as the sputum is smear-positive due to open lung lesions. When no sinus formation in the lungs has taken place (closed lung lesions with smear-negative sputum), no transmission can takes place except when sinus formation in the lungs develops (open lung lesions with smear- positive sputum)

Reservoir
Humans are the only reservoir of *Mycobacterium tuberculosis humanis* (both drug-susceptible and drug-resistant strains), while cattle and pigs are the reservoir for *Mycobacterium tuberculosis bovis*

Intermediaries
Vectors - None
Vehicles - Soil, air, fomites, dust

Carriers
Unknown

Immune status
Cell-mediated immunity, as a resistance to reactivation against a latent infection, is elicited after vaccination with BCG-vaccine or successful chemotherapy in drug-susceptible TB. But, depending on new strains/mutations and the virulence of the new strain(s) of the drug-resistant *M. tuberculosis humanis*, new infections can occur in persons who has been cured with successful first-line chemotherapy, or in persons who are still on treatment for drug-susceptible and drug-resistant TB (individuals who are not infected with the new specific drug-resistant *M. tuberculosis humanis*), or even in persons who have built up adequate cellular protection (cell-mediated immunity)

Susceptibility and resistance of host
All persons acquire a primary drug-susceptible tubercle lesion in his/her early childhood years. 85% of all persons regain their health completely without any medical therapeutic actions. After recovery these persons possess the necessary cell-mediated immunity to withstand further infections life-long of drug-susceptible TB. Resistance to drug-resistant TB has not yet been scientifically established

Regarding the other 15% of drug-susceptible infected persons, the disease (drug-susceptible TB) shows a latent period when it is not transmissible. Reactivation of the primary lesion occurs in unfavourable circumstances (intra-personal and/or in external milieu). Factors affecting the cell-mediated immunity of an infected person and thus leading to the endogenic reactivation of the dormant primary lesion, are the following
- Malnutrition and under nourishment
- Age – the very young child (whose immune system is not yet developed and whose immune reactions are inadequate); adolescents and adults (stress and other factors); and elderly people (whose immune response have diminished)
- Emotional as well as physical exhaustion and stress
- Diabetes mellitus
- Therapy that suppresses cell-mediated immunity such as corticosteroids and immunosuppressive therapy

- Malignancies such as leukaemia and Hodgkin's disease that suppress cell-mediated immunity
- Virus infections such as measles, influenza and the HIV-virus, which affect the cell-mediated immunity
- Diseases that lower pulmonary resistance such as silicosis
- Alcoholism
- Gastrectomy

Please note

✓ Individuals who have built up adequate cellular protection (cell-mediated immunity) but whose immune system is now (in later life) suppressed or compromised, for instance when infected by the HIV-virus or when taking immunosuppressive drugs, had adequate resistance previously to drug-susceptible *M. tuberculosis humanis*. In cases such as this, it is not a spontaneous endogenic reactivation taking place, but a "second" primary infection occurring at a specific time in the life of the person. Due to the compromised condition of the person's immune system now, his/her body cannot destroy the drug-susceptible nor the drug-resistant *M. tuberculosis humanis* and he/she becomes ill

✓ Although most persons have adequate resistance to drug-susceptible TB after vaccination with BCG vaccine, the disease (drug-susceptible and drug-resistant TB) occurs more and more in vaccinated persons. Reasons therefore are

  ◇ During the preparation of the BCG vaccine, the living pathogen is weakened to the extent that it cannot elicit a sufficient cell-mediated immune reaction any more. The person is therefore still susceptible to drug-susceptible and especially drug-resistant tuberculosis

  ◇ *Mycobacterium tuberculosis humanis* has undergone mutation and new extremely virulent strains have developed that are resistant to BCG vaccine and first-line and/or second-line anti-tuberculosis drugs. When a person is infected with the new strain, he/she becomes ill regardless of being vaccinated or previously treated successfully

  ◇ The combination of being administered the weakened BCG vaccine and being infected with the new *Mycobacterium tuberculosis humanis* drug-resistant strain(s)

  ◇ Injecting the BCG vaccine intradermally to the new-born infant as well as not taking in consideration that the vaccine is **extremely** sensitive to heat and light, including neon light

✓ Constant exposure to *M tuberculosis humanis* (drug-susceptible and drug-resistant strains) may be the reason why healthy persons, like healthcare providers who are continuously in contact with the pathogen, cannot always withstand invasion by either the drug-susceptible or the drug-resistant *M. tuberculosis humanis* and develop active tuberculosis. The continual and excessive exposure to the *M. tuberculosis humanis* depletes the cell-mediated immunity of the individual to the extent that **an infection** is caused

General pathogenesis of tuberculosis (infection in individuals encountering *M. tuberculosis* [drug-susceptible or drug-resistant *M. tuberculosis*] for the first time)
When the *M. tuberculosis humanis* gains entry into the body, it is phagocytised by the alveolar macrophages in which it survives and multiplies. Non-resident macrophages are also attracted to the site where they ingest the *M. tuberculosis humanis* and carry them to the local hilar lymph nodes. In the lymph nodes the immune response, predominantly a cell-mediated immunity response, is stimulated after the tuberculosis

antigen is processed. The lymphokines that are mediated by the sensitized T-cells activate the macrophages while simultaneously increasing their ability to destroy the mycobacterium. The infection is controlled by the cell-mediated immunity response and nearly all the pathology and the course of the disease is the consequence of the cell-mediated immunity response as *M. tuberculosis humanis* causes little or no direct or any toxin-mediated damage.

Due to the fact that tissue hypersensitivity and cell-mediated immunity only develop 4-6 weeks after invasion, *M. tuberculosis humanis* multiplies in the primary focus as well as in all the metastatic foci (other foci of infection in the body). To contain the *M. tuberculosis humanis,* the body forms "tubercles", small granulomas consisting of epithelioid cells and giant cells, to contain the *M. tuberculosis humanis* within. The pathologic process that occurs in the tissues and which leads to tissue hypersensitivity (cell-mediated immunity) is specific. The following specific processes take place, namely,

❏ **Formation of tubercles**

M. tuberculosis humanis causes a local area of inflammation and the lymphocytes and macrophages collect around this area in an effort to isolate the infection. Tubercles are formed around the *M. tuberculosis humanis*, in other words, a nodule develops consisting of a collection of epithelial cells, lymphocytes, fibroblasts and capillaries. The epithelial cells which are typical in the tubercle are highly specialised macrophages. These macrophages secrete fibroblast stimulating substances that lead to the deposit of collagen in the tubercle and finally results in the fibrosis of the tubercle. This hard tubercle is the body's successful tissue reaction in the process of isolating the *M. tuberculosis humanis*

❏ **Caseation, fibrosis and calcification of tubercles**

Due to the lysis enzyme action of the degenerative macrophages, tissue necrosis of the tubercle develops. This necrotic process is incomplete, however, causing the tubercle to change into a solid or semi-solid caseous (cheesy) mass (the so-called cold abscess) that is very unstable. Since the chemical environment and the oxygen tension in this caseous mass do not promote the growth of *M. tuberculosis humanis*, bacterial growth is inhibited. In a further effort of the body to isolate the infection, active connective tissue formation takes place around the caseous mass with the connective tissue replacing the necrotic tissue. The deposit of calcium in the caseous mass is the beginning of the healing process. As soon as fibrosis sets in (sterilization of lesions) healing of the tubercles have taken place. The individual's health depends to a great extent on the formation of these healed lesions

❏ **Healing process**

The process of healing of the tubercles commences spontaneously approximately 8 to 10 weeks after invasion when cell-mediated immunity has been elicited. Complete sterilization of all lesions (lung and metastatic foci) takes place and the individual recovers completely from the disease. The fibrotic and calcified lesions, *per se*, persist for a lifetime in the individual who is otherwise healthy and the healed tubercles show up on chest x-rays as radio-opaque nodules.

Please note:

When sterilization of the lesions are incomplete, *M. tuberculosis humanis* remains in the lesions, alive though latent. The latent TB infection is characterise by no symptoms, the individual does not feel sick and does not spread the infection to other persons but usually show a positive skin test reaction or a positive QuantiFERON-TB Gold test (QFT-G). Should the individual be exposed to situations of stress or disease that diminish the immune system (see natural endogenic cycle of tuberculosis in figure 10.1) and has not been treated for latent TB infection, the disease spontaneously reactivates. Reactivation occurs most commonly in the apex of the lungs. This site is highly oxygenated, thus allowing the mycobacterium to multiply more rapidly to produce caseous necrotic lesions which then spill over into other sites in the lungs. When the mycobacterium is not contained within these tubercles, they invade the bloodstream and cause a disseminated disease ('miliary' tuberculosis or extra pulmonary tuberculosis).

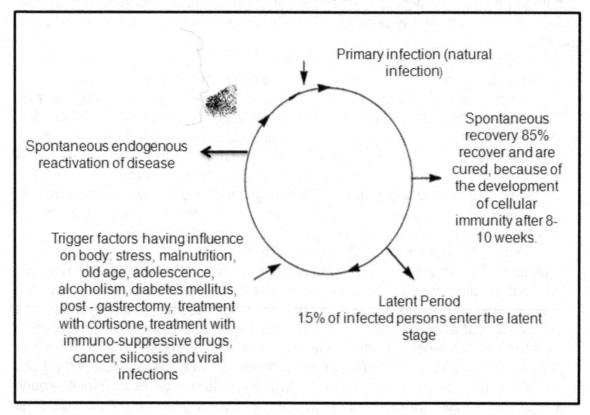

Figure 10.1 The natural endogenic cycle of drug-susceptible tuberculosis

Clinical manifestation of all forms of tuberculosis

Tuberculosis manifests systemically and locally as the *M. tuberculosis humanis* (drug-susceptible and drug-resistant *M. tuberculosis humanis*) possesses the ability to colonize almost any site in the body

* The systemic manifestations of the disease are associated with lassitude, general malaise, loss of appetite, nausea and rapid loss of weight, anaemia, severe night sweats, pyrexia and tachycardia
* The local manifestations of the tuberculosis lesions depend on the part of the body which is affected

- Lungs and bronchi – coughing, sputum, haemoptysis and dyspnoea
- Pleura – pleural pain, dyspnoea as a result of pleural effusion
- Larynx – hoarseness, dysphagia due to involvement of the pharynx
- Tongue – sometimes ulceration takes place
- Intestines – diarrhoea, mal-absorption of nutrients leading to malnutrition, intestinal obstruction
- Peritoneum – ascites, peritonitis
- Pericardium – pericardial effusion, pericarditis
- Kidneys and bladder – haematuria, increased urinary output
- Testes – epididimo-orchitis, painless swelling and sinus formation
- Uterus, fallopian tubes and ovaries – infertility, tube abscesses, amenorrhoea
- Brain – neurological signs of impairment
- Meninges – headaches as a result of meningitis
- Lymph nodes – enlargement of lymph nodes with formation of cold abscesses and sinus formation
- Suprarenal glands – signs and symptoms of Addison's disease
- Bones and joints – osteomyelitis, sinovitis
- Skin – lupus vulgaris, erythema nodosum
- Eyes – kerato-conjunctivitis

Please Note - The number of local manifestations of the tuberculosis lesions in other parts of the body other than in the lungs are on the increase

Please note

The abovementioned signs and symptoms may not necessarily be present in children. Some children present only with slight weight loss, general malaise and an inability to thrive/progress (although not always). A child with lung tuberculosis will not necessarily cough. Chest X-rays of the child will only show a "spot". Should a tuberculin test be done, however, the child will show a positive reaction (15 mm or more on the Mantoux test or grade III and IV in the Mono test). The prevalence of TB is similar in males and females until adolescence, when it becomes higher in males. In high-prevalence countries, however, women of reproductive age have higher rates of progression to disease stage than for men of the same age group. In women the disease also manifests at a later age resulting in a poor prognosis.

The specific pathogenesis of primary lung tuberculosis

Primary lung tuberculosis runs the following course

After invasion by *M. tuberculosis humanis* a primary focus of infection is formed in the central lung region where the largest airflow occurs. The *M. tuberculosis humanis* (drug-susceptible and drug-resistant *M. tuberculosis humanis*) multiplies and migrates via the lymph vessels to the hilar lymph nodes which react by becoming enlarged (the Ghon or primary complex consist of the lung lesion and the enlarged nodes). As soon as the *M. tuberculosis humanis* reaches the bloodstream a bacteraemia develops. The circulating *M. tuberculosis humanis* spreads to all those organs in the body with a high oxygen tension such as the apex of the lungs, kidneys, meninges, ends of long bones, vertebrae and glandular tissue, where metastatic foci develop. The individual shows no symptoms during this pathological process.

Tubercles are formed in the lungs, especially in the apex of the lungs. The caseous mass forms the typical cavities in the lungs. The caseous mass tend to liquefy and to form sinuses (open lung lesions) through which the *M. tuberculosis humanis*, via the bronchial tree, escapes to the outside environment. When no open lung lesions are formed, the caseous mass tend to remain spotted (sometimes coalescence occurs) without any sinus formation to the bronchial tree taking place (closed lesions) (see figure. 10.2). Where air comes into contact with these "open" caseous tubercles, an ideal environment is created for *M. tuberculosis humanis* to optimally multiply and complete healing cannot take place. In an effort to remove the pieces of caseous mass, the person develops a chronic cough. In open lung lesions *M. tuberculosis humanis* is present in the sputum (smear-positive sputum or sputum+). In closed lung lesions *M. tuberculosis humanis* is absent in the sputum (smear-negative sputum or sputum-) although the person present with the clinical picture of tuberculosis. X-rays show the typical tubercular cavities in both open and closed lung lesions.

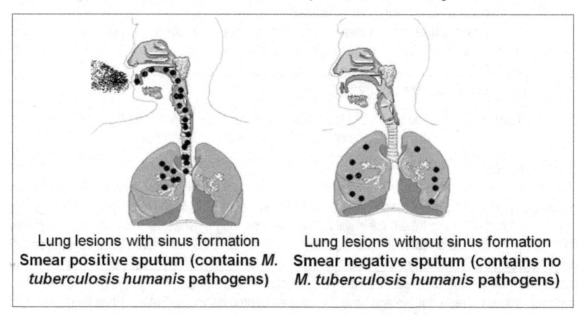

Lung lesions with sinus formation
Smear positive sputum (contains *M.*
tuberculosis humanis pathogens)

Lung lesions without sinus formation
Smear negative sputum (contains no
M. tuberculosis humanis pathogens)

Figure 10.2 Open lung lesions (sinus formations) and closed lung lesions in TB

❖ **Clinical picture of primary pulmonary tuberculosis**
- The disease develops gradually and takes its course over weeks or months
- At the initial stage only one or a few signs and symptoms may be present. (Most of the individuals present with more than one of the signs and symptoms.) This gradual development is the reason why most persons find it difficult to accept that they are suffering from the TB
- **The most common signs and symptoms of primary pulmonary tuberculosis are the following**
    ✪ The most important sign of pulmonary TB is an irritating chronic cough that becomes productive later on. The cough usually persists for a period of five weeks or longer before medical assistance is sought

✪ Loss of weight is another important early sign. In the progressive stage of the disease emaciation develops

✪ Anorexia that progressively increases is another early sign

✪ Lethargy and listlessness are typical symptoms

✪ Night sweats (cold, clammy sweating) occurring mainly during the night without pyrexia, is a typical sign. Night sweating is a result of the toxaemia which had developed

✪ Haemoptysis due to tissue destruction, is a late sign which can be copious or show blood spatters only

✪ Dyspnoea is another late sign which is caused by the pathology of the disease

✪ Chest pain is usually a sharp pleuritic pain, although it may also present as a dull ache

✪ Low-grade pyrexia which can be intermittent or recurring

✪ In a late stage the voice may grow hoarse

❖ **Complications**

The complications of *M. tuberculosis humanis* infection arise from the local dissemination of *M. tuberculosis*

• Miliary tuberculosis

• Metastatic foci formation in the kidneys leading to necrosis and destruction of the kidneys

• Tuberculosis-meningitis

• Pneumonia and broncho-pneumonia

• Chronic haematogenic, hepatic, skeletal, genital-urinary and gastro-intestinal tuberculosis and pericarditis

• Necrosis may erode blood vessels which can rupture and cause death through haemorrhage

■ **Diagnosis**

The diagnosis of tuberculosis is made on the grounds of the following (one only or in combination)

▪ **Clinical diagnosis**

✪ Every individual presenting with the systemic signs and symptoms of TB (whether a positive bacteriological sputum specimen could be obtained or not)

✪ Every individual found to be radiographic, bacteriological and cytological positive for TB

✪ All children younger than five years with an outspoken positive reaction to the tuberculin test

✪ All persons with a pleural effusion which reacts favourably to first-line anti-tuberculosis therapy after all efforts to make a diagnosis have failed

✪ All persons with a productive cough lasting for more than three weeks and at least two other signs and/or symptoms (such as weight loss, loss of appetite, dyspnoea, haemoptysis, chest pains, night sweats, lethargy) should be further tested for tuberculosis

✪ All persons who have undergone radiographic examinations and the X-rays is suggestive of tuberculosis

- **Bacteriological diagnosis**
  Adequate specimens of sputum or other substances should be collected for direct microscopy and culture. (The *M. tuberculosis humanis* may also be present in pleural and meningeal fluids, gastric secretions and urine.) Culture studies are more reliable than direct microscopy. Three sputum or other specimens – two for direct microscopy and one for direct microscopy and culture – are collected on three consecutive days, early in the morning as soon as the individual rises. (The person should have a clear understanding of the fact that the specimen must be of sputum and not of saliva.) All specimens **must** reach the laboratory within 4–7 days. Over weekends the sputum specimens may be kept in a refrigerator, but this practice is not recommended. A smear-positive sputum results confirms the diagnosis of open lesion (with sinus formation) pulmonary tuberculosis

<u>Please note</u>
1. In children, the diagnosis of pulmonary TB is especially difficult based only on smear microscopy and culture of sputum specimens because the disease is paucibacillary and sufficient sputum cannot always be collected for smear microscopy and culture
2. Smear-negative sputum results <u>do not mean the individual is not infected with</u> *M. tuberculosis humanis*. A smear-negative pulmonary TB-infection (closed pulmonary lesions with no sinus formation) must be diagnosed on other diagnostic tests such as signs and symptoms, or with X-rays, or on the exclusion of infections other than TB with broad-spectrum antibiotics. (Smear-negative pulmonary drug-susceptible TB is a slowly progressive disease with a low bacterial load and a fair prognosis)
3. Poor laboratory facilities in especially resource-poor setting and countries may also lead to a situation where the diagnosis of tuberculosis is jeopardize

- **Radiographic examination**
  Radiographic examinations (X-rays) of the lungs must always be accompanied by a bacteriological examination of the sputum to confirm the diagnosis. Please note that sub-standard radiography facilities such as poor film quality, low specificity and difficulty with interpretation in especially resource-poor settings and countries, may lead to a situation where the diagnosis of tuberculosis is jeopardized
- **Tuberculin skin tests**
  The tuberculin skin test has great diagnostic value as a screening test for tuberculosis and can be done on a large scale on children younger than 16 years. A strong positive skin reaction indicates the presence of viable *M. tuberculosis humanis* in the body. A variety of tuberculin tests are available, but the Mantoux test is considered the most reliable. (See preventative measures for interpretation of the test)
- **Histology**
  A biopsy can be done of those glands/nodes which are enlarged as a result of tuberculosis

- **Prognosis**
  - Good, when the individual is immuno-competent and the specific first-line anti-tuberculosis drugs are taken regularly for the prescribed period of time in drug-susceptible TB
  - Becomes poorer when the individual is immuno-compromised and infected with either the drug-susceptible or drug-resistant *M. tuberculosis humanis* strains or is immuno-competent and infected with drug-resistant TB strains

- **Specific healthcare interventions to be rendered in drug-susceptible and drug-resistant tuberculosis**

  To be successful, the healthcare therapy demands a multi-professional team effort involving healthcare providers, members of the family and members of the community as to meet the medical, economical and social needs of the ill persons and their contacts

  ➔ **The role of all healthcare professional and traditional practitioners and lay caregivers**

  Professional and traditional practitioners and lay caregivers working with individuals suffering from TB and their families, must use themselves therapeutically within the practitioner-healthcare user-relationship as to prevent reluctance of the infected healthcare users to attend clinics or to adhere to their treatment regime or to hide their condition from especially the caregivers and the rest of the world. Because the stigma healthcare users suffering from TB experience in the community extents into the clinics, the attitude shown by healthcare professionals, traditional providers and lay care givers when being unfriendly or hostile or uncaring together with long waiting times result in the denial of the infection by the sufferer, depression and anger in the sufferer and avoidance behaviour by the sufferer by bailing out of the programme all together. A patient-centred approach that includes facilitating access to treatment, deciding with the ill individual and his/her family the most convenient time and place for direct observation of treatment (DOT), and providing other social and medical services when necessary, is far more effective than tracing of defaulters. The use of incentives such as "thank you teas" for the ill individuals and their families, support groups, and award ceremonies on successful completion of treatment, can motivate individuals infected with TB to adhere to treatment and enhance the provider-user-relationship

  ➔ **All TB control programmes must be gender sensitive**

  Gender differentials exist in the reporting and diagnosing of TB while passive case finding also leads to failure to diagnose TB in women. The stigma associated with TB causes married women to be divorced by their husbands or when unmarried, never to be married or to be isolated/abandoned by their families. Husbands suffering from TB very often expect that their wives take care of them, but their infected wives very seldom receive care, resulting in married women hiding their symptoms instead of seeking help. Also, cultural and socio-economic factors play an important role in barriers to detection and successful treatment of TB in women. Women suffer more often from disproportionate poverty, have low social status, are less educated and must overcome more barriers to attain healthcare. Women very often find it more difficult to comply with treatment once symptoms subside, and when they do comply, they are often placed in an economically or socially precarious position. Although gender differentials in social and economic roles and activities result in differential exposure to *M. tuberculosis humanis,* TB in women always have serious repercussions for families and households because the health and welfare of children is closely link to that of their mothers. Because the health status of many women is unhealthier than men's, especially in terms of nutrition and immune status, women are at a higher risk to be infected with TB

➤ Accurate record keeping

Accurate record keeping (recording and reporting) is imperative for good planning as it measures both the successes and weaknesses of all current programmes for drug-susceptible and drug-resistant TB. Regular periodic audits must be done to monitor the necessary data records. Accurate record keeping of the health status of employees (professional, traditional and lay care) is also imperative so that employers can reduce their (the employees') risk of contracting TB by re-allocating them to other departments/units as necessarily

➤ Chemotherapy[1]

- ✪ Chemotherapy (specific anti-tuberculosis drugs) is the only effective way of combating active tuberculosis. The most important drugs presently in use are isoniazid, streptomycin, rifampin/rifampicin, pyrazinamide, streptomycin and ethambutol (first-line drugs for a short-course of 6 months in drug-susceptible tuberculosis). The first-line drug regime must consist of a combination of bactericidal (killing off of bacteria) and/or bacteriostatic (only inhibiting of bacterial growth) action-drugs (multiple drug therapy) and must be administered for 7 (seven) days a week for a period not shorter than 6 months to prevent drug resistance. Regular drug susceptibility tests for drug resistance should be done during the treatment period. (See drug-resistant TB for second-line chemotherapeutic regimes)

- ✪ Adherence by healthcare users (Patient adherence) to the drug regimen and the regular administering of medication under direct observation for a minimum period of six months (or longer) must be promoted and monitored (**DOTS** - short course of first-line anti-tuberculosis drugs for 6 months directly observed first-line anti-tuberculosis drug treatment, and **DOTS-Plus** treatment programme [longer course {up to 18-24 months} of combined first-line and second-line or only second-line anti-tuberculosis drugs under direct supervision in drug-resistant TB {MDR-TB}]). The best indicators of adherence include smear conversion from positive to negative; improvement in symptoms and clinical improvement. Neglect in taking the medication for the prescribed period or taking the medication irregularly or non-complying with the chemotherapeutic regime in totality leads to reactivation of the disease as well as the development of new drug-resistant strains of *M. tuberculosis humanis*

✪ Medication should be taken even when the individual feels better and no symptoms can be observed any longer. The individual should be regularly observed for side-effects of the medication

✪ For all practical purposes drug-susceptible TB is no longer considered to be communicable within 24 hours after chemotherapy has commenced. The *M. tuberculosis humanis* is weakened by the bacteriostatic drugs and cannot cause active drug-susceptible tuberculosis any longer

✪ The chemotherapeutic programme should also be adapted to the individual's needs. Factors such as distance from the clinic, working place and family circumstances must be taken into account. Other aspects that have to be taken into account are

✠ Chemotherapy should preferably be given under full supervision (**DOT** – directly observed treatment). Traditional healers, other community healthcare workers and community volunteers as well as family members and friends should be trained to become supervisors to monitor that the medication-regime is taken as prescribed until the course is completed. (Please note that using DOTS only for non-compliers is essentially flawed as clinicians cannot reliably identify adherent ill healthcare users – DOTS is a prerequisite for the optimum treatment of all persons suffering from drug-susceptible TB).

✠ Most ill individuals (adults and children) should be treated on an ambulatory basis where possible, whether the TB-infected individuals come to the healthcare clinic on a daily basis, or the TB-infected individuals visit the facilitators' homes in the area, or the facilitators visits the TB-infected individuals' homes in the area. All children with severe forms of TB (for example, TB-osteomyelitis, TB-meningitis, TB-spine, TB-peritonitis, miliary TB) **must be referred to hospital for management**

✠ Chemotherapy should be made as easy as possible for the individual and pre-treatment body weight must always be taken in consideration when prescribing the treatment regime

✠ **Daily chemotherapy is mandatory 7 days a week** during the prescribed treatment period in both the Intensive phase and the Continuation phase of the treatment regime for new cases (new smear or culture positive persons and new smear-negative persons or persons with extra-pulmonary TB) and the re-treatment of already treated cases (smear-positive defaulters, smear-positive failures, smear-positive re-treatment after interruption), regardless whether the ill individual suffers from drug-susceptible or drug-resistant TB and irrespective whether treated in hospital or at a clinic

✠ Interruption of work/schooling should be avoided by giving chemotherapy at the working place/school setting when possible

✠ Children younger than 8 years of age suffering from drug-susceptible TB (for example, uncomplicated intra-thoracic TB and pulmonary TB such as lymph gland and pleural effusion) must be treated according to protocol for a period not shorter than of 6 (six) months

✠ Children older than 8 years of age receive the same treatment regime as adults

✠ **Children with drug-resistant TB** usually have primary resistance transmitted from an index case suffering from drug-resistant TB. Drug susceptible testing must be used to guide the anti-tuberculosis drug regime although children with paucibacillary TB are often culture-negative. Nevertheless, every effort must be made to confirm drug-resistant TB bacteriological by the use of drug susceptible testing as to avoid exposing children unnecessarily to toxic drugs. Because only limited reported experience with the use of second-line anti-tuberculosis drugs for extended periods in children exist, the risks and benefits of each drug must therefore be carefully considered when designing a therapy regime. Adverse reactions to the prescribed anti-tuberculosis drugs must be closely monitored on an ongoing monthly basis. Frank discussion with parent(s)/family members is of critical importance from the outset of therapy. Furthermore, **body weight must be monitored monthly with adjustment of dosage as the child gains weight.** As treatment failure is difficult to assess in children, the weight of a child is of particular concern. The loss of weight or more commonly "failure to gain weight adequately" is often one of the first (or only) signs of treatment failure. Also, adolescents are at a high risk for poor treatment outcomes. Early diagnosis, strong social support, individual and family counselling and a close relationship with the medical provider may help to improve treatment outcomes in adolescents

✠ **TB sufferers (children and adults) who also suffer from any other medical condition**, for example, diabetes mellitus, AIDS, renal insufficiency, liver disorders, seizure disorders, psychiatric disorders, and substance dependence disorders (drugs and/or alcohol) **are at risk for poor treatment outcomes in both drug-susceptible and drug-resistant anti-tuberculosis drug regimes.** Some medical diseases can potentiate adverse reactions to anti-tuberculosis drugs while in others cases the anti-tuberculosis medical regime can interfere with the chemical action(s) of the medication prescribed for the specific medical condition. Drug-interaction must therefore be very closely monitored on an ongoing basis as well as the natural course of the underlying medical condition

✠ **Mandatory drug susceptibility testing for resistance** in any first-line and second-line anti-tuberculosis drugs must be done regularly according to protocol

✠ **Close monitoring and screening of ill healthcare users for common symptoms of adverse effects of first-line and second-line**

anti-tuberculosis drugs (rashes, gastro-intestinal symptoms, vomiting, diarrhoea, jaundice, ototoxicity, peripheral neuropathy, psychiatric ailments [psychosis, depression, anxiety, suicidal tendency], electrolyte wasting [palpitations and muscle cramping]) must be done by all healthcare practitioners and volunteer workers on a daily basis. Laboratory screening to detect more occult adverse effects (such as serum creatinine, serum potassium, thyroid stimulating hormone, liver serum enzymes); HIV- testing and pregnancy tests must be done on a regular basis according to protocol. **Proper management** (prompt evaluation, diagnosis and treatment) of adverse effects must be instituted as soon as possible (even in resource-poor setting) according to protocol. The continuation with the present regime when mild and not dangerous side effects appear, or the replacement of certain drug(s), or the adding of ancillary drugs to help, or the suspending of a drug to make the treatment less potent depends on the specific side effect(s) experience and the individual as person. **Health information must be given on an ongoing basis and a sustained trust relationship between the user and provider must be formed.**

➡ **Adequate sunlight, fresh air and nutritious foods are requirements for recovery.** Wasting can be limited when malnutrition (carbohydrates, protein, fat) and micro-nutrient deficiency (vitamins such as A, B-complex, C, D, E and K and mineral trace elements-deficiency such as zinc, manganese, selenium, copper, iron, magnesium, potassium and others) are corrected and then supplemented (taken extra in correct dosages) in an adequate and healthy diet. Small nutritious (healthy) and attractive meals served 6 to 8 times a day can correct or prevent malnutrition when taken together with the prescribed anti-tuberculosis drug regime. To maintain a healthy digestive system Probiotics can be taken together with the supplement of vitamins and mineral trace elements. The supplement of vitamins and mineral trace elements ensure optimal immune function in resisting disease

➡ **Establishing the degree of cell-mediated immunity** (for children under the age of 16 years only)
  ✪ The degree of cell-mediated immunity is established by the tuberculin skin test. With the skin test "Tuberculin Purified Protein Derivative" or PPD (a substance of the *M. tuberculosis humanis)* is injected under the skin. When sensitizing of the lymphocytes have taken place as a result of previous exposure to *M. tuberculosis humanis,* the macrophages and other cells accumulate at the injection site and swelling appears. This swelling reaction develops within 72 hours and indicates previous contact with viable *M. tuberculosis humanis* in the presence of cell-mediated immunity. The degree of positiveness (+) of the reaction (the test is read as a reaction of the skin) indicates the **intensity of the cell-mediated immunity**.
  ✪ When a child was not vaccinated with BCG vaccine and the tuberculin skin reaction is positive, the reaction is strongly suggestive of an acute

tuberculosis infection and chemotherapy should be considered. Infants and children up to the age of two years, whose tuberculin skin reaction is strongly positive, must receive chemotherapy. In children between the ages of 3 to 16 years, a strong positive skin reaction indicates viable *M. tuberculosis humanis* in the body, but does not necessarily indicate that the disease is active.

The interpretation of the tuberculin test and the suggested therapy are set out in table 10. 1.

Table 10.1 THE INTERPRETATION OF TUBERCULIN TESTS AND SUGGESTED THERAPY

MANTOUX-TEST (size of swelling when measured)	MONO TEST/ TINE TEST (outspoken swelling)	INTERPRETATION	SPECIFIC HEALTHCARE THERAPY
0 – 4,9 mm	0 (no swelling)	No reaction. No protection	Administer BCG
5 – 9,9 mm	I (slight swelling)	Doubtful. Poor protection	Administer BCG
10 – 14,9 mm	II (swelling readily visible)	Reactive. Good protection – no danger except in children under the age of two years	When there is a contact in the household whose sputum specimen is smear-positive, children under the age of 2 years must receive chemotherapy. Children between 2-5 years must receive chemotherapy for a period of 6 months. Children older than 5 years need not be treated
15 mm and more	III + IV (outspoken swelling and may be coalescent)	Strongly positive Viable *M. tuberculosis humanis* in body At risk to become ill or already ill	In children up to the age of 5 years, chemotherapy must be commenced. In children of 6 to 16 years old, chemotherapy must be considered based on clinical signs and symptoms

The causes of a negative/false-negative tuberculin skin reaction may be due to (in combination with or as single factor) no previous infection, another infective condition, recent vaccination against Measles, thyroid therapy, antihistamine therapy, malignancy and faulty testing techniques. The causes of positive/false-positive tuberculin skin reaction may be due to (in combination with or as single factor) infection with *M. tuberculosis humanis*, infection with other mycobacterium, BCG vaccination, a secondary infection at the injection site and faulty testing techniques

➔ **Health information to be given to all sick individuals**
It is important that ill individuals, their families and their communities be empowered to prevent primary and secondary infections through health promotion strategies

✪ All ill persons with active tuberculosis must be knowledgeable regarding the transmission of the disease (drug-susceptible and drug-resistant TB) and measures to be taken to prevent transmission of the infection

✪ The importance of taking of anti-tuberculosis drugs (first-line and/or second-line) regularly under supervision for the full prescribed period

✪ The extreme importance of covering the nose and mouth with the arm and sneezing or coughing into the elbow while disposing of all used paper tissues/other paper items through burning or incinerating

✪ The extreme importance of spitting any expectorated sputum in a disposable container or paper tissue that has to be burnt

✪ The extreme importance of avoiding of close contact with small children

✪ The extreme importance of not spitting on the ground but into paper tissues/other paper items that must be burnt

✪ The importance to avoid close contact with other persons by sleeping away (about 2-3 meter) from other family members and to air the room daily (if possible and if it is not too cold) or to use a fan in an open window to draw fresh air in and to blow contaminated stale air out

✪ All ill persons suffering from drug-resistant TB can be mandatory admitted to hospital for long periods of time until the disease is stabilized. The mandatory admission to hospital is legally enforceable by court order (up to 2 years or longer in accordance with the current treatment guidelines in place for drug-resistant TB)

➔ **Settings for treatment delivery**
Several treatment delivery settings exist for delivery of chemotherapeutic anti-tuberculosis drugs to infected individuals, namely, hospital, clinic, and community/home care facilities. Regardless of the mode of delivery, the management of the drug therapy depends on a steady supply of medicines to ill healthcare users free of charge through a reliable network of educated providers (professional, traditional and lay)

✱ **Community/Home care**

✪ Most ill individuals can be treated at home while taking responsibility for their own healthcare and for the taking of their medication (ambulatory treatment regime)

✪ Idleness and curtailment of activities must be avoided. The ill person must be encouraged to continue with his/her career or schooling

✪ Correct measures must be taken for doing away with sputum. Washing of the hands must become a habit

✪ Regular supervision (DOT/DOTS or DOT-Plus/DOTS-Plus) and follow-up visits to clinics or by the community healthcare provider (professional, traditional or lay) are very important as to ascertain adherence to treatment therapy

✪ All non-adherent ill healthcare users must be followed-up and providers (professional, traditional or lay) must work closely with the sufferer and his/her family to ensure the continuation of treatment

✪ When necessary, strict confidence must be maintained regarding the TB status and treatment of the ill person

✪ Other interventions to address socio-economic problems such as homelessness, hunger, and unemployment must be instituted to enhance adherence to the treatment regime

✪ To be suffering from TB is a devastating experience for both the infected individual and his/her family - therefore emotional and social support must be given by professional, traditional and lay care givers through support groups, counselling, and services delivered by non-governmental organizations

✱ **Hospitalization**
  ✪ Hospitalization is only considered in drug-susceptible TB when
    ◈ The ill person is a child
    ◈ The ill person is physically too ill to be treated as an out-patient
    ◈ A new case needs to be stabilized on medication
    ◈ There is a shortage of out-patient facilities
    ◈ The ill individual asks to be hospitalized (only in exceptional cases for a specific extraordinary reason)
    ◈ Early detection and identification of toxicity of drugs are undertaken
    ◈ The ill person suffers from tuberculosis-meningitis
    ◈ The ill individual also suffers from other disease (for example, diabetes mellitus, cardiac failure)
  ✪ In drug-resistant TB (especially XDR-TB and CDR/TDR-TB) hospitalization is mandatory. Mandatory detention could, however, result in an unexpected rise in incidence due to the restricted isolation capacities in hospitals
  ✪ In low resource facilities not built to prevent communicable infections that are transmitted by infected droplets, the following control measures need to be implemented (also see 3.2.3)
    ◈ The placement of ill healthcare users with TB must be planned within a nursing unit. Diagnosed cases of TB can share a room as long as there is adequate ventilation and superior cleaning of the room. When an individual suffering from TB is cared for in a room together with other ill healthcare users suffering from any other respiratory infection, the patient with TB must be cared for behind curtains

❖ Medical practitioners in both the public and private sectors must divulge the necessary information about the healthcare user's condition (diagnosed TB or suspected condition of TB) so that the necessary isolation arrangements for TB can be made

❖ Masks (N95) and protective clothing must be worn by all attending staff and ill infected healthcare users and the use of masks must be combined with reduced hospitalization time and a shift to outpatient therapy with DOTS

❖ It is mandatory that engineering control must be attained and maintained through improved ventilation management. The TB-infected patient(s) must be cared for next to the window(s) or closest to the air conditioner. The curtains around the patient's bed must remain drawn to minimise the spread of *M. tuberculosis humanis* throughout the room

❖ Rapid drug resistance testing of all TB ill healthcare users on treatment must be done on an ongoing basis

❖ On admission, screening of all ill healthcare users must be done to identify suspected or confirmed infection with *M. Tuberculosis humanis,* namely, lung x-rays together with an extensive cough assessment history [unexplained cough longer than 3 weeks] and health assessment history [history of possible exposure; previous history of TB with treatment failure; difficulty in breathing, loss of appetite and weight loss; night sweats with fever, general malaise without a specific cause, nausea while taking any drugs]. A history of haemoptysis, lung x-rays suggestive of pulmonary TB and a history of signs and symptoms suggestive of extra-pulmonary TB must be treated with caution and the ill healthcare user must be physically isolated until an alternative diagnosis has been made or diagnostic test results indicate that the individual is not infected with TB

(**Note** Informed healthcare users are sometimes wilfully dishonest about their current treatment regimes and thus do not disclose that they taking chemotherapy for TB or are under investigation for TB. When healthcare practitioners discover this omission by the infected healthcare user, interruption of treatment has taken place with an increased risk of drug-resistant TB developing. Healthcare users belonging to a medical fund very often deny/omit that they are being treated for TB or are under investigation for TB as they feel they must be treated at private healthcare establishments - establishments not built to treat, control and prevent tuberculosis infection)

❖ Health information must be given to all ill healthcare users regarding cough etiquette and sneezing hygiene to prevent the spread of TB by using paper tissues/other paper items only once when coughing; to safely dispose all used tissues/other paper items in a plastic bag destined for incineration; not to put used tissues/ other paper items or handkerchiefs back into a pocket or a handbag; to safely dispose of sputum by spitting in sputum containers and to report bloody sputum; not to cough and spit in public places; and wash/disinfect hands after coughing

◈ The correct disposal of all medical waste

◈ Bagging of used linen in a colour laundry bag to inform the staff not to shake or mishandle the bedding as to dislodge any dried sputum flakes and bacilli into the environment

◈ Hand disinfected gel must always be available at the bedside of the ill individual suffering from TB

◈ Mobile TB sufferers in the facility must be informed to use the bathroom facilities after the other ill individuals had used them. The bathroom and toilet windows must be left open to ensure adequate airflow, and any bodily spills have to be reported to the staff as to be immediately cleared away

■ **Specific healthcare interventions for contacts**

All the members of a family or all persons living in the same house as well as all persons working or sleeping within a radius of 5 metres of the ill person who is actively sick are seen as direct contacts

✠ All direct contacts of drug-susceptible TB sufferers should be treated as follows

☑ All contacts must be traced and examined. Chest X-rays and/or bacteriological examinations (in adults and children) or the tuberculin skin test (in children under the age of 16) must be done on those contacts reporting symptoms which might indicate tuberculosis. Although first-line chemoprophylaxis may be administered to adults, it is not generally recommended

☑ When the sputum of the ill person tested smear-positive, active case finding must be done of all children younger than 5 years of age. All children under the age of 5 years and weighing less than 5 kg, who are healthy contacts, must receive first-line prophylactic chemotherapy for 3 months. All children under 5 years of age who are healthy and weighing more than 5 kg must receive first-line chemotherapy for 6 (six) months. After 3 or 6 months of first-line chemotherapy a tuberculin skin test must be done. When the skin reaction is negative, BCG vaccine is administered. When the skin reaction is positive, prophylactic first-line chemotherapy is prolonged for a further three months

☑ Household contacts of ill individuals, whose sputum tested smear-negative, are at a low risk for contracting drug-susceptible TB. They do not need to receive first-line prophylactic medication. Chemotherapy will only become necessary when signs and symptoms of tuberculosis infection (sputum smear-positive because of sinus formation of lung tubercles) are shown

☑ Children over the age of 5 years and adults are only treated when they show signs and symptoms of TB infection

☑ Routine chemo-prophylaxis for children older than 5 years is not recommended

✠ All contacts of ill individuals who suffer from <u>drug-resistant TB</u> should receive the following therapy
  ✚ All contacts must be informed regarding the signs and symptoms of drug-resistant TB and the mandatory nature to report for chemotherapy when becoming ill
  ✚ Repeated physical examinations, culture and smears must be performed as well as monthly repeat chest X-rays be done on contacts of ill persons whose sputum is smear-positive until conclusive evidence of active TB is gained. Treatment must be started when diagnosed as symptomatic. A decision must be made to stop all investigations when asymptomatic and the results are inconclusive
  ✚ Contacts of ill individuals whose sputum are smear-negative must be treated according to the standard recommendations
  ✚ Children over the age of 5 years whose Mono-tuberculin-test tested negative and adults whose sputum tested negative, are treated according to the current recommended prophylactic treatment guidelines
  ✚ All children under 2 years old, who are contacts, must receive chemotherapy according to the current treatment guidelines regardless the status of their health may be. The chemotherapy has to include two (2) drugs that have been tested for sensitivity
  ✚ Children between the ages of 2 and 5 years who are contacts and whose Mono-tuberculin tests are positive, have to receive prophylactic multiple-drug chemotherapy
  ✚ HIV-positive contacts must undergo a multi-medication chemotherapy regime for a period of at least six months. According to laboratory tests, two of these drugs must have to been tested for susceptibility

■ **Specific healthcare interventions for non-pregnant women, pregnant women and breastfeeding mothers**
  ✱ <u>Non-pregnant women</u>
    All infected females of childbearing age should be tested for pregnancy upon initial evaluation. As such, pregnancy is not a contra-indication for treatment of active TB (drug-susceptible and drug-resistant TB) but the treatment of active drug-resistant TB poses great risk for the lives of both mother and foetus. A birth control measure is, however, strongly recommended for all non-pregnant women receiving anti-tuberculosis therapy for either drug-susceptible or drug-resistant TB because of the potential consequences for both mother and foetus resulting from frequent and severe drug reactions

  ✱ <u>Pregnant women and breastfeeding mothers suffering from</u> **drug-susceptible TB**
    ▪ Pregnant women receiving the usual first-line chemotherapy must continue with chemotherapy after the birth of the baby
    ▪ Should the mother be physically in a condition to breastfeed her baby, she should preferably wear a N-95 mask while doing so
    ▪ The baby is treated as follows

- ✪ Start immediately with first-line chemotherapy and continue for three month, then do a tuberculin skin test
- ✪ When the skin test reaction is negative, administer BCG vaccine
- ✪ When the skin test reaction is positive, continue chemotherapy for a further three months
- ✪ Repeat tuberculin skin test. If the skin reaction is negative, administer BCG vaccine
- ✪ When the skin reaction is positive, continue with first-line chemotherapy and test for medication resistance. After chemotherapy has been completed, administer BCG (as soon as the skin reaction to the tuberculin tests is negative) in order to stimulate adequate cell-mediated immunity (resistance)
  - If the mother's physical health status is poor, she should not breast-feed her baby. The baby must then be bottle fed
  - Mothers suffering from drug-susceptible TB and who are HIV+ should not breast feed their babies at all. The baby must receive bottle feeding directly after birth until such time that he/she receives a mixed normal diet. The baby must be tested and treated for TB as above as well as for HIV/AIDS

- ✸ Pregnant women and breastfeeding mothers suffering from **drug-resistant TB**
  - Pregnant women suffering from TB should be carefully evaluated, taking in consideration gestational age and the severity of the drug-resistant TB. As basis for the treatment regime, the risks and benefits of treatment must be carefully considered with the primary goal of smear conversion to protect the health of mother and child before and after birth
  - Since the majority of teratogenic effects occur in the first trimester of pregnancy, anti-tuberculosis (first-line and second-line) drug therapy may be delayed until the second trimester. Both mother-to-be and medical practitioner must agree to the postponement of treatment after analysis of the risks and benefits. Only oral anti-tuberculosis with demonstrated efficacy must be given. Injectable agents and ethionamide must be avoided at all cost
  - Mothers suffering from drug–resistant TB and their babies must be treated according the current treatment guidelines for drug-resistant TB (the mother must receive the full course of anti-tuberculosis treatment). Because the effects on infants have not been established regarding exposure to the full course of MDR-TB treatment for the mother (most anti-tuberculosis drugs are found in breast milk in concentrations equal to a small fraction of the therapeutic dose used for infants), it is recommended to provide infant formula options as an alternative to breastfeeding. The decision regarding breastfeeding must be made within the framework of the current treatment guidelines for drug-resistant TB. When the mother wants to breast-feed her baby and is physically in a condition to breastfeed her baby, she must wear an N-95 mask. Regular testing of the baby for multi-drug resistant-TB must be done according to protocol guidelines

Please note

The anti-tuberculosis drug-therapy regime the mother is taking must also be taken in account before the decision for breastfeeding the baby is taken, as some anti-tuberculosis drugs are contra-indicated for paediatric use or have never been tested for safe paediatric use. The presence of the anti-tuberculosis drugs used by the mother in her breast milk can sometimes be the deciding factor whether she may breast feed her baby or not (not her physical condition)

◆ **Preventive measures to be taken**

➢ **National TB preventive measures**

The preventive measures issued by the National Department of Health are focused on

- health information regarding tuberculosis
- therapy under supervision
- tracing of cases
- vaccination with BCG

These measures are intended to reduce the pool of infected individuals and protect all persons against infection

Community involvement and participation are prerequisites for the successful implementation of the preventive measures. SANTA is an organisation which renders invaluable services, amongst others by fund-raising and the distribution of food parcels to needy persons suffering from tuberculosis. On the request of the National Department of Health and with their full support, SANTA has instituted an intensive health informational programme regarding tuberculosis in order to heighten the population's awareness concerning tuberculosis. In this way, individuals and community members are encouraged to give assistance in the tracing of cases with symptoms that is suspicious of tuberculosis

➢ **General preventive measures to be taken**

⇨ Improvement of all socio-economic conditions in order to eliminate factors (such as overcrowding, unhygienic living and environmental conditions, stress, alcoholism, etc.) that can promote the spread of tuberculosis

⇨ Giving of health information to the public regarding the transmission of drug-susceptible and drug-resistant tuberculosis, all preventive and control measures, as well as the signs and symptoms of the disease

⇨ Regular weight control of employees is a rewarding and cheap procedure for tracing cases. Those employees with significant weight loss should be further examined. Employers should also be encouraged to supply meals to their employees and implement other measures in order to combat the predisposing factors of tuberculosis

⇨ Promoting of self-help programmes such as vegetable gardening and self-employment activities to heighten the community's responsibility for the prevention of tuberculosis

⇨ Availability of medical, laboratory and X-ray facilities for proper examination of ill persons (screening and diagnosing), the tracing of cases and contacts, and provision of chemotherapy

⇨ Inspection of dairies and ensuring the supply of safe, pasteurized milk

⇨ Health information to be given regarding the importance of good nutrition, balanced meals, breastfeeding, cultivating one's own or communal vegetable gardens, and school feeding schemes

⇨ Increasing the general standard of living by means of job creation, the implementation of community programmes for helping needy and homeless persons (such as feeding schemes), and the establishment of care groups to promote vaccination, as well as the cultivation of vegetable gardens and enhancing the standard of personal hygiene

⇨ Routine radiographic examination of all citizens of the RSA should be considered - the necessary facilities, funding and personnel must be made available

⇨ Health information to be given on family planning to prevent over-population and overuse of available resources

⇨ Measures must be implemented to upgrade the standard of housing. (Self-help programmes have to be promoted.) In informal settlements inhabitants should be assisted in building their houses in such a way that cross-ventilation is promoted

⇨ Regular health screening of all healthcare practitioners, traditional healthcare providers and voluntary healthcare workers must be done to prevent them spreading the disease from healthcare establishments to the community

> **Specific preventive measures to be taken**

◈ Primary cell-mediated immunity is elicited by vaccination with BCG vaccine to drug-susceptible TB. When a child has not been vaccinated after birth, BCG vaccine should be administered as soon as possible (preferably before the child is three years of age)

◈ Individuals suffering from drug-susceptible TB and who are in contact with children, for example teachers, must avoid working with children for a period of one month after drug-susceptible chemotherapy has commenced. When contracted MDR-TB the treatment protocols must be followed

◈ Health information to be given to the community regarding the importance of BCG vaccination and the early signs and symptoms of tuberculosis infection

◈ Early tracing and chemotherapeutic treatment of infected person by means of either the tuberculin skin tests (children) or having sputum specimens sent to laboratories for bacteriological and culture examination

◈ Observation and chemoprophylaxis treatment of contact persons

◆ **Measures to prevent epidemics**

⬍ An attitude of vigilance in recognising, tracing and treating new and reactivated cases, is of the utmost importance.

⬍ With regard to the above, attention must be given to the regular examination of large groups of persons working and living together, such as persons employed by the mining industry

- The correct method of administering BCG vaccine must always be very carefully followed, particularly in maternity units/wards, hospitals and clinics
- Strict adherence to the school exclusion regulations must be maintained in both drug-susceptible and drug-resistant TB by learners and by educators
- Infection control, based on administrative controls, environmental/engineering controls and personal respiratory protection, is of crucial importance to prevent drug-susceptible and drug-resistant nosocomial epidemics occurring in hospitals and caring facilities such as clinics, hospices, old age homes and palliative care facilities
- Culture and drug susceptibility testing of every individual suffering from TB (whether sputum smear-positive, sputum smear-negative or extra-pulmonary) on an ongoing basis
- Continuous and comprehensive approach to drug-resistance surveillance must become an essential component of all TB programmes as to plan appropriate interventions
- All professional healthcare practitioners {whether physicians, nurses, dieticians, physiotherapist, para-medical personnel, pharmacists, etc.} as well as traditional healthcare providers actively involved in patient care [regardless of practicing privately or in the public sector] must be educated regarding the local levels of TB drug-resistance and current TB-treatment guidelines. All healthcare providers must be able to do detection for tuberculosis (new cases) when treating the person for other ailments as a significant number of individuals with TB symptoms turn first to private physicians/other private healthcare providers, traditional healers or private pharmacists. All healthcare providers (whether practicing privately or in the public service) must also be able to identify not only any relapse in treatment (failure to improve) but also any medical errors in the prescribed chemotherapeutic regime as well as recognise non-adherence to the chemotherapeutic regime by the ill individual (failure and default). All healthcare providers (whether practicing privately or in the public service) must be knowledgeable how to address relapses, medical errors in the chemotherapeutic regime and patient non-compliance. All healthcare providers (whether practicing privately or in the public service) must record and report (documentation) adequately all treatment outcomes to support the national tuberculosis control programmes

Of utmost importance are
> **All healthcare providers (professional, traditional and lay) must strictly adhere to all Standard Precautions and follow proper procedure to protect themselves from being infected with either drug-susceptible or drug-resistant _M. tuberculosis humanis_**
> **Regular outreach educational programmes regarding diagnostic, surveillance and preventive activities in TB-programmes must be given to all healthcare providers to bring about the necessary clinician behavioural changes for active case-finding of TB-infection. Of cardinal importance is the ability and competence of**

professional healthcare practitioners to correctly diagnose all forms of tuberculosis; to collect specimens correctly for diagnostic tests; to correctly execute the necessary tests; to correctly interpret the results of all diagnostic tests done; to correctly prescribe the specific treatment regime and to correctly do the necessary documentation

◆ **Implications for disaster situations**
None

◆ **Compliance with international measures**
- Routine X-rays of individuals legally immigrating to the RSA from countries where the incidence of tuberculosis is very high
- The disease can be spread by illegal immigrants since their fear of being deported to their country of origin, prevents them from seeking healthcare treatment. In this way epidemics may be caused
- In the light of the prevalence and incidence of multiple-drug resistant-Tuberculosis cases globally, the country of entry has the right to demand radiography (X-rays) of the lungs (with or without sputum smear culture) for screening of all tourists, work seekers and immigrants before travelling to or at the port of arrival before issuing the necessary entry visa to the specific individual

Please note

1. Chemotherapy - All professional healthcare practitioners {whether physicians, nurses, dieticians, physiotherapist, para-medical personnel, pharmacists, etc.} as well as all traditional healthcare providers actively involved in the care of healthcare users [regardless of practicing privately or in the public sector] must be educated regarding the local levels of TB drug-resistance and current TB treatment guidelines. All healthcare providers must be able to do patient detection for tuberculosis (new cases) when treating the person for other ailments. All healthcare providers (whether practicing privately or in the public service) must also be able to identify not only any relapse in treatment (failure to improve) but also any medical errors in the prescribed chemotherapeutic regime as well as to recognise non-adherence to the chemotherapeutic regime by the patient (failure and default). All healthcare providers (whether practicing privately or in the public service) must be knowledgeable how to address relapses, medical errors in the chemotherapeutic regime and patient non-compliance.

DRUG-RESISTANT TUBERCULOSIS

The emergence of new strains of a pathogen that is resistant to antimicrobial drugs is a natural biological occurrence. The introduction of every antimicrobial drug/agent into clinical practice for the treatment of communicable and infectious diseases in humans (and animals) has been followed by the detection and isolation of resistant pathogens to antimicrobial drugs/agents in the laboratory, for example, microbes able to multiply in the presence of drug concentrations found in hosts receiving therapeutic doses. Such resistance is either a characteristic associated with an entire species or acquired through mutation. Resistant genes encode information on a variety of mechanisms that microbes use to withstand the inhibitory (bacteriocidal [killing off of bacteria] or bacteriostatic [only inhibits bacterial growth]) actions of specific antimicrobial drugs. These mechanisms confer resistance to other antimicrobial drugs of the same class and sometimes to several different antimicrobial drug classes. The *M. tuberculosis humanis* had over time acquired by either chromosomal mutation or from transposons (jumping genes) and other mobile elements or via resistance genes on transmissible plasmids, a specific resistance against only a certain class of anti-tuberculosis or multiple resistance by coding for resistance determinants to unrelated families of anti-tuberculosis agents.

The resistance of *M. tuberculosis humanis* to anti-tuberculosis drugs is man-made. The exposure to a single first line anti-tuberculosis drug, whether as a result of poor adherence to treatment, inappropriate prescription, irregular drug supply, or poor drug quality, suppress the growth of only those *M. tuberculosis humanis* bacilli susceptible to that specific anti-tuberculosis drug but permits the multiplication of pre-existing drug-resistant mutants. The ill individual develops **acquired resistance** when treated with first-line anti-tuberculosis drugs and the drug-susceptible *M. tuberculosis humanis* mutates to become drug-resistant or the multiplication of pre-existing drug-resistant mutants of *M. tuberculosis humanis* is permitted. Subsequent transmission of this drug-resistant mutant strains of *M. tuberculosis humanis* to other persons lead to a disease state that is drug-resistant from the outset (**primary resistance**). Therefore, the proxies of "resistance among new cases" and "resistance among previously treated case" have been adopted. Furthermore, drug-resistant TB are divided in <u>multiple drug-resistant-TB</u> (MDR-TB), <u>extensively drug-resistant-TB</u> (XDR-TB), and <u>completely/totally drug-resistant-TB</u> (CDR/TDR-TB). As such, the iatrogenic (man-made) form of TB (MDR-TB and XDR-TB – both new and re-treatment cases) is caused by different mutant strains of the susceptible-drug-resistant *Mycobacterium tuberculosis humanis* or of the multi-drug-resistant *Mycobacterium tuberculosis humanis*. CDR/TDR-TB is caused by further mutation of the already existing extensively drug-resistant *Mycobacterium tuberculosis humanis*.

(**Note** The mutations of *Mycobacterium tuberculosis humanis* are specific to drug resistance only and not a fundamental change in the behaviour of the microbe. Conferring further mutations of *Mycobacterium tuberculosis humanis* drug-resistant strains resulted in the new "super bug" *Mycobacterium tuberculosis humanis* that is not only totally/completely drug-resistant to all known anti-tuberculosis drugs but also differs in its genotype [on genetic level] to the multi-drug-resistant *Mycobacterium tuberculosis humanis*. The new "super bug" *Mycobacterium tuberculosis humanis* is more virulent and stronger than the other strains of *Mycobacterium tuberculosis humanis* and is likely to spread in the population).

Drug-susceptible TB as well as drug-resistant TB (both MDR-TB, XDR-TB and CDR/TDR-TB) are on the increase in all developed/industrialized, developing and under-developed countries and is caused by the interaction of numerous factors such as the deteriorating of the public health infrastructure; lack of a standardized therapeutic regimen; poor programme implementation; prolonged shortages of drugs and poor quality of drugs; inadequate resources; substandard case management in the private sector (maintaining of records, notifying of cases and evaluating of treatment outcomes); physician mismanagement (incorrect management of individual cases, difficulties in selecting the appropriate chemotherapeutic regimen with the right dosage and relying only on radiography without initial and follow-up sputum examinations); non-compliance of infected healthcare user to the prescribed treatment; and sufferers from TB being co-infected with drug-resistant tuberculosis and HIV-infection. Other factors contributing to drug-resistant TB are factors such as political instability; lack of political commitment to national TB control programmes; the increase of poverty and homelessness due to reductions in social services in industrialised countries as well as famine, wars, natural disasters and urbanisation in resource-poor countries; immigration from endemic areas; and demographic changes such as population growth. Drug-resistant TB is particular problematic because it threatens both the individual (chronic disability and death) and the community (drug-resistant TB is an infectious hazard in the community as persons with chronic drug-resistant TB represents an infectious reservoir for drug-resistant *mycobacterium tuberculosis humanis*). To avoid producing drug-resistant TB, clinicians need to understand the mechanisms leading to drug resistance; adhere to the recommended treatment regimens for drug-susceptible TB and the associated supervision strategies (DOTS and DOTS-Plus); and recognise the common treatment errors that results in the iatrogenic disease of drug-resistant TB.

✱ Multidrug-resistant tuberculosis (MDR-TB)

Multidrug-resistant tuberculosis (MDR-TB) is defined as a specific form of tuberculosis that is resistant to treatment with 2 most effective first-line anti-tuberculosis drugs. Acquired resistance of *M. tuberculosis humanis* is produced by a spontaneous unlinked chromosomal mutation with multidrug transporters mediating both intrinsic and acquired resistance to various drugs. Resistance to drugs must be confirmed through laboratory confirmation of in-vitro resistance to one or more first-line anti-tuberculosis drugs. Confirmed mono-resistance (single-drug/mono-drug resistant-TB) refers to the in vitro resistance to one specific first-line drug only; confirmed MDR-TB (combined-drug resistant-TB) refers to in-vitro resistance to the first-line drugs isoniazid and rifampin/rifampicin; while confirmed poly-resistance refers to in-vitro resistance to more than one first-line anti-tuberculosis drugs, other than both isoniazid and rifampicin. The virulence of the drug-resistant *M. tuberculosis humanis* heightens as it becomes unusually fit to survive.

Of utmost importance is the early recognition of ill individuals suffering from MDR-TB. The following persons should be tested for drug susceptibility/drug resistance
+ All infected individuals who do not respond to first-line chemotherapy, for example, still smear-positive after 2 months of treatment
+ All ill individuals whose condition deteriorate rapidly
+ All ill individuals whose resistance for certain first-line drugs have already been proved by laboratory tests

✚ All ill individuals who are considered high risks regarding multidrug-resistance such as
- ✴ persons with a history of having terminated previous chemotherapeutic regimes, or of not having completed the chemotherapeutic regime, or of taking medication on an irregular basis
- ✴ persons suffering from chronic diseases (for example, cancer, diabetes mellitus, renal failure, emphysema) or suffering from immune-suppressive disease (for example, AIDS and HIV-positive status due to the epidemiological association with MDR-TB and the propensity of these infected individuals to progress rapidly to active disease), or those who are using immune-suppressive drugs
- ✴ all persons who are dependent on or abuse the use of alcohol and/or drugs
- ✴ all contacts who were in an intimate relationship with someone who died of tuberculosis
- ✴ individuals with atypical clinical and radiological presentations or who suffers from non-well known infections such as *Mycobacterium avian complex* or *Pneumocystis carinii.*

All persons suffering from MDR-TB should preferably receive specialized healthcare interventions at relevant centres where DOTS-Plus programmes as well as hospitalization are provided. All persons suffering from MDR-TB are registered as category IV and Category V treatment outcomes. The treatment history of ill individuals suffering from MDR-TB must be thoroughly chronicled/documented by listing the site of drug-resistant tuberculosis disease (pulmonary or extra-pulmonary); all previous treatments; the person's adherence to all treatment regimens; bacteriological responses (including sputum conversion – 2 negative smears and cultures taken 30 days apart); clinical and radiological changes and drug susceptibility test results. The likely resistance pattern must be identified and a re-treatment regimen comprising of at least 4 anti-tuberculosis drugs with either certain, or almost certain, effectiveness must be prescribed. The standardized treatment regime must be given but can be individualized on the basis of previous history of anti-tuberculosis treatment and individual drug sensitivity test results. The re-treatment regimen must contain at least one to three first-line drugs tested for sensitivity as well as second-line drugs (drugs which the person has not received previously and the drug-resistant *M. tuberculosis humanis* pathogen is unlikely to be resistant to such as aminoglycosides, ethionamide, Quinolones, cycloserine and para-aminosalicylic acid) or only second-line anti-tuberculosis drugs. Anti-TB drug-susceptibility tests have to be done regularly - monthly to 3 monthly. The chemotherapeutic regime of this group of individuals lasts a very long time, sometimes as long as 18 to 24 months or longer. While on treatment, regular monitoring for side effects/adverse reactions must be done. As bacteriological response to treatment is the most reliable marker in treatment outcome, sputum specimens for bacteriological culture and microscopy must be collected - at first weekly and then monthly until three consecutive cultures are negative. Following on this, sputum specimens should be collected three-monthly. Persistently smear-positive sputum examination after 4 months treatment (or relapse) is an ominous sign that indicates the development of resistance to drugs in the current regimen. Resectional lung surgery and/or laser treatment of the caseous tubercles in the lung may benefit selected ill individuals suffering from MDR-TB in these circumstances. Nutritional support is of critical importance as MDR-TB is exacerbated by a poor nutritional status, low body mass index and severe anaemia. A good nutritional status may lessen adverse effects and morbidity as well as improve MDR-TB treatment outcomes.

The treatment outcome for persons suffering from MDR-TB is very poor. Six possible outcomes exist, namely,

◇ cured - the individual had completed an 18 month treatment and have had at least 5 consecutive smear-negative sputum cultures in the last month of treatment as well as consistent sputum culture of smear-negative status for the previous 11 months from samples collected at least 30 days apart in the final 12 months of treatment

◇ completed treatment but not cured – lack of bacteriological results exist with fewer than 5 cultures done in the final 12 months of treatment

◇ died – for any reason during the course of treatment for MDR-TB

◇ defaulted - treatment was interrupted for 2 or more consecutive months for any reason

◇ transferred out to another health district – treatment outcome is unknown

◇ failed treatment – two (2) or more of 5 cultures recorded in the final 12 months of therapy were smear-positive, or any of the final three cultures were positive, or a clinical decision was made to terminate treatment early because of poor response or adverse events. (When treatment is suspended, supportive care must be given to the ill individual suffering from MDR-TB and his/her family as to improve their quality of life).

The treatment failure rate (ill individual suffering from MDR-TB remains sputum smear-positive and culture-positive at the end of the treatment) in immuno-competent persons (CD4 and T-lymphocyte counts above 200/µl) is as high as 32-40% while the mortality (death) rate for immuno-suppressed individuals (for example, HIV-positive individuals) is as high as 90% with a median interval lapse of 2-4 weeks between been diagnosed with MDR-TB and dying (due to mal-absorption of anti-tuberculosis drugs resulting in sub-optimal therapeutic blood levels despite strict adherence to the treatment regimen). Only when TB is diagnosed early in HIV-positive persons and treatment is started promptly, the median survival time can be prolonged to 5-10 months. In resource-poor countries, cost-effective MDR-TB treatment is not always available and many MDR-TB sufferers are subjected to the natural course of TB as disease, namely, 55-65% of diseased immuno-competent persons die within 5 years after being diagnosed as MDR-TB positive, while immuno-compromised individuals die within 1-2 years (or less) after being diagnosed as MDR-TB positive.

Of paramount importance is the prevention of MDR-TB as the disease cost money and time. Nosocomial outbreaks of drug-susceptible TB and MDR-TB in healthcare establishments must be prevented through administrative, infection control and isolation measures. The prevention of the transmission of drug-susceptible *M.*

tuberculosis humanis and drug-resistant *M. tuberculosis humanis* must be done on three levels of control

◈ The use of administrative measures to reduce the risk of exposure (early recognition of potential MDR-TB cases, prompt laboratory diagnosis and immediate implementation of effective chemotherapy as well as isolation of ill individuals suffering from MDR-TB in special units away from other healthy or ill persons; comprehensive infection control plans [including the education of all staff, namely, line-, support-, and staff functionaries]; and health information to all sufferers on ambulatory care to prevent contact with the public and especially with susceptible children and individuals suffering from HIV-infection)

◈ The use of engineering controls to prevent the spread of *M. tuberculosis humanis* where ambulatory care is rendered (ventilated rooms, air filtration and ultraviolet air disinfection) as un-suspected, untreated persons with MDR-TB will enter hospitals despite all efforts to identify them

◈ Strict adherence by all healthcare personnel and other employees to hygienic hand disinfection practices and wearing of particulate respiratory protective equipment that fits the face tightly to prevent leakage between the face and the edge of the mask as to prevent inhalation of tiny [1-5μm] airborne infectious droplets such as high efficiency particulate filter respirators (special anti-tuberculosis face respirators) or disposable N95 particulate filter respirators. (Ill individuals suffering from MDR-TB must wear a surgical or a particulate respiratory mask when they have to leave the ward/unit/hospital for medically essential procedures).

Although the prevention of asymptomatic drug-susceptible TB-infection from progression to clinical disease by administering chemoprophylaxis is 93% effective in immuno-competent individuals, the preventive treatment of drug-resistant TB is far more problematic and controversial. The appropriate prophylactic treatment following exposure to MDR-TB is exacerbated by chemoprophylaxis. When the source patient/individual suffers from isoniazid-resistant *M. tuberculosis humanis*, all contacts who are at a high risk of active MDR-TB (for example, immuno-suppressed individuals) should receive rifampicin with or without a second drug for 6-9 months. Observation without preventive therapy is generally accepted for most individuals exposed to MDR-TB. Preventive treatment is only recommended for contacts likely to have been infected with MDR-TB who are at a high risk of progressing to active disease (for example, HIV+ individuals). The vaccination of immuno-competent healthcare personnel who are exposed to MDR-TB with BCG-vaccine proves to be marginally superior to screening and preventive treatment.

✳ Extensively drug-resistant tuberculosis (XDR-TB) (Also referred to as "Ebola on steroids")

Because of the selection of populations of drug-resistant *M. tuberculosis humanis* by incomplete or inappropriate drug therapy, a new strain (or strains) of the drug-resistant *M. tuberculosis humanis* had developed. Factors that have had caused the new strain(s) are host genetic factors; health provider factors such as physician error (inappropriate prescription), management factors such as irregular drug supply and/or poor drug quality and patient-related factors such as non-compliance during treatment. Extensively multi-drug resistant tuberculosis (XDR-TB) is an extreme form of MDR-TB and is caused by this new extremely virulent strain that is resistant to 2 (and more) effective classes of second-line anti-tuberculosis drugs (and/or even third-line anti-tuberculosis drugs). The new extensively drug-resistant strain causes a disease condition that is drug resistant from the outset (primary resistance/resistance among new cases) and the disease condition is transmitted to all persons (new cases and re-treatment cases) who have no physiologic immunological resistance to the new XDR-TB-pathogen. XDR-TB is widely distributed globally, poses a public health threat and opens up the possibility that epidemics (even a pandemic) of virtually untreatable TB may develop. The overwhelming burden of XDR-TB (both "resistance in new cases" and "resistance among previously treated cases") is, as with TB itself, extremely high in resource-poor countries whilst the prevalence of XDR-TB (especially "resistance in new cases") in resource-rich settings and countries is on the increase.

The treatment of XDR-TB is complex, prolonged, costly and not very successful. The treatment of sufferers of XDR-TB consists of mandatory hospitalization and the administering of susceptible second-line anti-tuberculosis drugs for 24 months or longer. Treatment protocols must be followed to the letter and ill healthcare users leaving the isolated area must wear masks to protect the public, co-ill healthcare users and other healthcare workers. Anti-TB drug-susceptibility tests have to be done regularly [monthly to 3 monthly basis] to detect the development of "completely/totally drug-resistant TB (CDR/TDR-TB)". The treatment outcomes of ill healthcare users with MDR-TB and XDR-TB in resource-limited setting can be positive provided that DOTS or DOTS Plus is in place as well as food, transport, housing, social, educational, and financial support are available. The major barriers to the treatment of multidrug-resistant TB are the high cost of quality-assured second-line anti-tuberculosis drugs as well as extensive laboratory and monitoring requirements, adverse events associated with second-line drugs, difficulties in ensuring adequate patient support during the long treatment course and the risk of resistance to second-line drugs. The fatality rate is very high in both immuno-competent and immuno-compromised individuals regardless of treatment. Because multidrug-resistant TB is a ubiquitous disease, MDR-TB and XDR-TB are increasing alarmingly, while the resistance on individual and populations levels are continuously amplifying. When "completely/totally resistant TB (CDR/TDR-TB)" sets in, the ill person dies because no anti-tuberculosis treatment is available at this moment in time. When CDR/TDR-TB is transmitted into populations, a global pandemic of catastrophic proportions may follow.

The compulsory/enforced isolation/detaining/quarantine of sufferers of XDR-TB is justifiable because the protection of the health of the public takes precedence over the rights of the individual. Current health legislation in the RSA empowers the authorities to detain ill healthcare users with diseases "until the disease no longer poses a public health threat" and the National Department of Health is legally required to protect the health of the population. As long periods of hospitalisation may be necessary to stabilise ill persons until they are not more infectious, all reasonable measures must be taken to provide the recommended healthcare and the ill person must adhere to it voluntary before any restriction will be instituted. When the ill person refuses treatment, justifiable isolation/detention becomes necessary until such time the patient is not infectious any more. Enforced hospitalisation/quarantine of ill healthcare users with XDR-TB and CDR/TDR-TB is therefore only justified as the last resort after all voluntary measures to isolate the individuals have failed. Confinement would have to be until death or, conceivably, indefinitely until the ill person has been cured/became not infectious any longer as XDR-TB is/can be an incurable and an untreatable disease. Furthermore, restriction must take place with sufficient legal procedural safeguards; applied within a human rights framework (according to the Bill of Rights as enshrined in the Constitution); is in the interest of a legitimate objective of general interest; is based on scientific evidence and limited in duration and subject to review. Hence, tough isolation measures, mandatory when necessary, are thus justified to contain XDR-TB and CDR/TDR-TB, a deadly contagious disease that can be/is incurable, to prevent a potentially explosive global health crisis. When individuals suffering from XDR-TB are not detained in a medical facility and treated, they may develop "Completely/Totally drug-resistant TB (CDR/TDR-TB)" and spread CDR/TDR-TB - a disease that is from the onset totally untreatable and incurable at this moment in time.

The prevention of the transmission of *M. tuberculosis humanis* in XDR-TB and CDR/TDR-TB must be done on three levels of control, namely,

❖ The use of administrative measures to reduce the risk of exposure (early recognition of potential XDR-TB cases, prompt laboratory diagnosis and immediate implementation of effective chemotherapy as well as isolation [in special units] of the ill individual from other healthy or ill persons; comprehensive infection control plans [including the training of staff]; and health information to prevent contact with the public and especially with susceptible children and individuals suffering from HIV-infection when on ambulatory care)

❖ The use of engineering controls to prevent the spread of *M. tuberculosis humanis* (ventilated rooms, air filtration and ultraviolet air disinfection) as un-suspected, untreated persons with XDR-TB will enter hospitals despite all efforts to identify them

❖ Strict adherence to hygienic hand disinfection practices and wearing of particulate respiratory protective equipment that fits the face tightly to prevent leakage between the face and the edge of the mask (to prevent inhalation of tiny [1-5µm] airborne infectious droplets) such as high efficiency particulate filter respirators (special anti-tuberculosis face respirators) or disposable N95 particulate filter respirators by all healthcare and other personnel. Sick infected healthcare users must wear a particulate respiratory mask when leaving the unit for medically essential procedures

❖ Other measures also to be instituted are
  ✓ controlled laundry washing practices
  ✓ good waste management
  ✓ strict adherence to safe housekeeping rules and measures.

The programmatic management of Drug-resistant Tuberculosis (MDR-TB, XDR-TB and CDR/TDR-TB) includes

- The strengthening of the basic care of TB (all forms) to prevent the emergence of drug-resistance
- Conducting of rapid surveys to detect cases of XDR-TB
- Ensuring the prompt diagnosis and treatment of drug resistant cases to cure existing cases and prevent further transmission
- Increasing the collaboration between HIV and TB control programmes to provide the necessary prevention and care to co-infected individuals
- An increased investment in laboratory infrastructures to enable better detection and management of resistant cases
- Increased research support for anti-tuberculosis drug development
- Promoting universal access to anti-retroviral drugs under joint TB-HIV activities.

❋ <u>Completely/Totally drug-resistant tuberculosis (CDR/TDR-TB)</u>

Completely/totally drug-resistant tuberculosis (CDR/TDR-TB) {also called super extensively drug-resistant tuberculosis [XXDR-TB]} is defined as the most severe form of drug-resistant tuberculosis that is resistant to treatment by all first-line, all second-line and all third-line anti-tuberculosis drugs. The development of this resistance is associated with poor management/treatment of TB (all forms) as a medical disease as well as the fact that CDR/TDR-TB has resulted from further mutations within the bacterial genome to confer resistance far beyond those seen in XDR-TB and MDR-TB. At this moment in time there is no treatment available to successfully treat CDR/TDR-TB and the mortality rate of individuals suffering from CDR/TDR-TB is 100%. This new strain of the extensively drug-resistant *M. tuberculosis humanis* is extremely virulent and highly transmissible – transmissible to all persons who are immuno-competent and who have acquired adaptive cell-immunity to both drug-susceptible and drug-resistant *Mycobacterium tuberculosis humanis*; to all immuno-compromised persons and to all sufferers of active TB (drug-susceptible and drug-resistant) regardless being poor or rich. Because of the infectivity and seriousness of CDR/TDR-TB, the welfare of the public/community takes precedence over the human rights of the individual. Thus, individuals suffering from CDR/TDR-TB are isolated in special healthcare facilities where strict barrier care is rendered until death. Only the minimal highly specialized trained healthcare providers must have contact with the ill person. Disposable equipment is mostly used and a hypochlorite solution must be used for cleaning while nothing should be removed from the room – all waste should be immediately incinerated as clinical waste.

<u>Please note</u>

All healthcare practitioners, all traditional healthcare providers and all voluntary healthcare workers as well as all other employees who are in close contact with drug-susceptible TB, MDR-TB, XDR-TB and CDR/TDR-TB are specifically protected by law under the Occupational Health and Safety Act of 1993. **Therefore**

- ✤ **All healthcare practitioners, all traditional healthcare providers and voluntary healthcare workers as well as all other employees must undergo regular** in-service education re the signs and symptoms and mode of transmission of TB as well as the prevention and control measures to strictly to adhere to

✠ **All healthcare practitioners, all voluntary healthcare workers, and all other employees must wear protective clothing such as the particulate anti-tuberculosis face respirators or the disposable N95 particulate filter respirator.** Every individual healthcare practitioner and employee must be fit-tested to wear exactly the right size and design in a range of respirators as to ensure a tight seal between the mask/respirator and the wearer's face. Disposable particulate respirators can be re-used but must be discarded when the respirator is soiled; loose; or worn for longer than eight (8) hours. If the respirator is in a condition to be re-used, it must be stored in a clean and dry location

✠ **All healthcare practitioners, all traditional healthcare providers and all voluntary healthcare workers as well as all other employees must know their HIV-status in order to avoid putting themselves at risk. Those healthcare providers and employees who work in high-risk TB settings must be provided with confidential HIV counselling outside the workplace**

✠ **All HIV-infected healthcare practitioners, all traditional healthcare providers and all voluntary healthcare workers as well as all other employees may not work in a high-risk TB environment and be transferred to a low-risk TB environment**

✠ **All healthcare practitioners, all traditional healthcare providers and all voluntary healthcare workers as well as all other employees caring for MDR-TB, XDR-TB and CDR/TDR-TB ill healthcare users must undergo compulsory (3-6 monthly) screening consisting of a verbal screening, a physical examination that includes weighing, x-rays of lungs (chest radiography), screening of symptoms, and sputum specimens for bacteriological culture and microscopy**

✠ **Any complaint of symptoms of tuberculosis must immediately be investigated and treatment must be commenced**

✠ **When healthcare practitioners, traditional healthcare providers and voluntary healthcare workers as well as other employees become ill (regardless being an acute or chronic medical disease) and the individual's immunity status becomes compromised, the individual employee must be transferred out of the high-risk TB setting and allocated elsewhere. Follow-up investigations must be done until the results exclude drug-susceptible TB or MDR-TB or XDR-TB or CDR/TDR-TB**

✠ **Female healthcare practitioners, and/or female traditional healthcare providers, and/or female voluntary healthcare workers, and/or other female employees who plan a pregnancy must be transferred out of the high-risk TB setting and environment 12 months or longer before falling pregnant. The same follow-up investigation must be done until the results exclude drug-susceptible TB or MDR-TB or XDR-TB or CDR/TDR-TB**

✠ **When a female practitioner or a female traditional healthcare provider or a female voluntary healthcare worker or a female employee falls pregnant while still working actively in the high-risk TB setting and environment,** she must be immediately transferred out of the high-risk TB setting and allocated elsewhere. The necessary investigations must be done until the results exclude drug-susceptible TB or MDR-TB or XDR-TB or CDR/TDR-TB

✠ When a healthcare practitioner and/or traditional healthcare provider and/or a voluntary healthcare worker and/or an employee become ill with susceptible TB or MDR-TB or XDR-TB or CDR/TDR-TB, the worker and his/her contacts must be treated according to the set protocol. The necessary support must be given to the ill individual employee and his/her family.

10.4   KEY NOTES

❑ Although the respiratory tract is continuous from nose to alveoli, the respiratory tract is divided into an "upper" and a "lower" part based on the type of infections occurring in the different parts.

❑ In upper respiratory tract infections such as Pertussis, the *B. pertussis* colonizes the ciliated respiratory epithelium and the pertussis toxin and other toxic factors are important for virulence. Antimicrobial drugs play a peripheral role while vaccination is effective.

❑ Infections of the lower respiratory tract are spread by the airborne route (airborne infected droplets – except helminths/flukes) and can be acute or chronic. These infections tend to be severe and can be fatal (e.g. tuberculosis). Lower respiratory tract infections are caused by a wide range of pathogens – usually bacteria or viruses but also by fungi and helminths.

❑ Influenza A-viruses cause endemic, epidemic and pandemic outbreaks as result of the capacity of the virus for antigenic drift and antigenic shift. Influenza-A infections are acute in onset, are clinically severe and may be even fatal. The viral damage to the respiratory mucosa predisposes the infected individual to secondary bacterial pneumonia. Antiviral drugs are available but are of limited efficacy.

❑ Various species of helminths pass through or localize in the lungs at some stages of their lifecycle. Damage is limited unless the parasite load is high and the damage is usually immuno-pathological in nature.

❑ Tuberculosis, a major killer disease in children and adults, is becoming more common and more clinically severe – especially the drug-resistant forms of TB. Anti-tuberculosis treatment in drug-resistant tuberculosis is becoming less and less effective and the mortality rate is rapidly rising. TB is also associated with AIDS due to immunodeficiency. Although TB has been declared a global emergency over a decade ago, tuberculosis (case finding, diagnosing, treatment and prevention) did not receive the attention it needed with the result it has spread rapidly, especially in developing and under-developed countries. The poor management of ill individuals on TB treatment has resulted in drug resistance to available drugs and the emergence of MDR-TB, XDR-TB and CDR/TDR-TB - virtually untreatable forms of TB. Women and adolescent girls are at an increased risk of tuberculosis (progression to disease) during their reproductive years because of biological (gender rates of infection), social-economic (health and nutrition status, gender differentials in reporting and diagnosing TB as well as in passive case finding) and cultural (female gender role fulfilling and activities) factors.

Chapter 11

COMMUNICABLE DISEASES AFFECTING THE GASTRO-INTESTINAL TRACT

Communicable diseases of the gastrointestinal tract are very common. Indigestion of pathogens causes many different infections. Some of these infections are confined to the gastro-intestinal tract or are initiated in the gut before spreading to other parts of the body. A wide range of microbial pathogens (bacteria, viruses and parasites) are capable of infecting the gastro-intestinal tract. Many pathogens are acquired via faecal-oral transmission. For an infection to occur, the specific pathogen must be ingested in sufficient numbers or must possess properties to elude the host defenses of the upper gastro-intestinal tract and reach the intestine. Here the pathogen remains localized and cause disease because it multiplies and/or produces toxin or has penetrated through the intestinal mucosa to reach the lymphatics or the bloodstream. The damaging effects of infection on the gastrointestinal tract are the result of

- ❖ physiological action of bacterial toxins
- ❖ local or distant to site of infection (for example, cholera)
- ❖ local inflammation in response to superficial invasion (for example, shigellosis, amoebiasis)
- ❖ deep invasion to blood and/or lymphatics as well as dissemination to other sites (for example, hepatitis A, typhoid fever and paratyphoid fever - the enteric fevers]
- ❖ perforation of mucosal epithelium after infection (for example, peritonitis, intra-abdominal abscesses).

The spread of intestinal infections is assured when public health and hygiene is poor, the pathogens appear in the faeces of sufficient number of persons and there are susceptible individuals in the vicinity. Diarrhoea gives the transmission an additional advantage, because of the recycling of faecal material back into the mouth by hands and fingers while contamination of milk, water, food, soil, surfaces (vehicles) and flies (vector) promote the faecal-oral spread of the pathogens on a large scale. Most individuals suffering from gastro-intestinal diseases are not hospitalized. This group of diseases can, however, be life-threatening to infants, young children and elderly persons, particularly when dehydration is preceded by malnutrition or undernourishment.

General clinical manifestation of gastro-intestinal infections

The **general signs and symptoms** accompanying gastro-intestinal infections are nausea, vomiting, diarrhoea, abdominal discomfort, pain and tenesmus. The

systemic signs and symptoms are malaise, headache, pyrexia and rigor. The signs of dehydration vary with the age of the individual and the quantity of fluid lost.

When a history is taken it must be clearly established what the ill person's concept of diarrhoea is. The physical examination reveals local or diffuse tenderness of the abdomen as well as increased bowel sounds. The examination must include a visual examination of faeces in order to observe for the presence of blood or pus in the stools. Diarrhoea with blood and pus in the stools is the result of enterotoxin production, whereas the presence of blood and/or pus cells in the faeces indicates an invasive infection with mucosal destruction.

Pathogenesis of gastro-intestinal infections

The small intestine plays an important role in the digestion and absorption of large quantities of food and fluid (10–11 litres per day). Approximately 2 litres of fluid are passed on to the colon of which a large part is reabsorbed in order to produce a formed stool. This process of secretion and absorption of fluid is of the utmost importance for maintaining the fluid and electrolyte balance of the body.

Infections of the **stomach** are mostly viral in origin or are caused by bacterial toxin. Vomiting and abdominal pain are common signs and symptoms but diarrhea seldom occurs. When the **small intestine** is infected, a large quantity of fluid is not reabsorbed but passed on to the colon which can only absorb two liters per day. The "surplus fluid" is secreted in loose stools. Abdominal pain is very seldom associated with the loose watery stools or the passing of blood or pus. However, dehydration develops very quickly, and may even be fatal. Infections of the **colon** results in its content not being reabsorbed and the surplus fluids (± two litres) are continually passed as loose stools. This condition is accompanied by severe abdominal pain, cramps and tenesmus. Small stools containing blood and mucus are passed often. Systemic reactions such as pyrexia, toxemia and peritonitis occur as a result of the extent of the damage to the mucous membrane of the colon. Dehydration does not develop.

11.1 DIARRHOEAL DISEASES CAUSED BY BACTERIAL AND VIRAL INFECTION

Diarrhoeal diseases are a group of infections that are contracted by the ingestion of specific pathogens which remain localized in the gastro-intestinal tract. The severity of the diarrhoea depends on the causative pathogen, the number of pathogens ingested, duration of exposure to the pathogens and the number of exposures. Infections of the gastro-intestinal tract range in their effects from a mild self-limiting attack of diarrhoea to severe, sometimes fatal diarrhoea. There may be associated vomiting, fever and malaise. As such, diarrhoea is the body's protective mechanism to get rid of infective pathogens and harmful substances. The diarrhoea is the result of an increase in fluid and electrolyte loss in the intestinal lumen, leading to the production of unformed or liquid faeces as reaction of the host's to forcibly expel the pathogen from the body. Diarrhoeal diseases are the major cause of morbidity and mortality in young children, the elderly and immuno-compromised individuals.

It is generally impossible to distinguish on clinical grounds between the different pathogens – however, information about the ill person's recent food intake and travelling history and microscopic examination of the faeces for pus and blood can provide helpful clues. When outbreaks of diarrhoea occur, appropriate epidemiological investigation is needed to put control measures in place. It is also extremely important to investigate food, milk, and water hygiene as food act as vehicle for the pathogen or provide conditions in which the pathogen can multiply to produce numbers large enough to cause disease.

11.1.1   GASTRO-ENTERITIS

Gastro-enteritis is the term used to describe the syndrome of infection of the stomach and the intestines. Gastro-enteritis is an acute disease characterized by diarrhoea, nausea, vomiting and abdominal discomfort

---

Epidemiological data

Geographical distribution
Occurring world-wide

Causative pathogen
Bacteria such as *Escherichia coli*, *Yersinia*, *Campylobacter*, *Clostridia* and *viruses* such as the *Rotaviruses and Norwalk-related viruses*

Incubation period
24–48 hours or longer (days)

Mode of transmission
Person to person - faecal-oral transmission by means of the hands
From animals to humans - faecal-oral transmission by means of the hands via faecal material through contact with the animals themselves or through contact with their excretions in the environment

Period of infectiousness (communicability, transmission)
This depends on the causative pathogen. The *Rotavirus* can still be excreted 2–3 days after the acute phase while other viruses are only excreted during the acute phase

Reservoir
Humans and domestic animals such as cattle, goats, pigs, dogs, cats, chickens as well as rodents such as rats

Intermediaries
Vectors - Flies
Vehicles - Contaminated food, water and milk (human consumption)
Food or water contaminated with infected faecal excretions of animals
Food contaminated by flies
Surfaces contaminated with faecal material

Carriers
None

Immune status
Although an immune response with memory is elicited, it does not last long. Re-infection may occur. Immunity to endemic virus-gastro-enteritis lasts between 24 to 48 months

Susceptibility and resistance of host
All persons are susceptible although infants and toddlers are particularly susceptible. The following host-related factors play a role in the susceptibility for gastro-enteritis - personal hygiene, gastric acidity and other physical barriers, normal enteric micro flora, intestinal motility, diminished innate resistance as well as a diminished adaptive specific intestinal resistance

---

Pathogenesis

The different bacteria responsible for causing bacterial gastro-enteritis use several distinct pathogenic mechanisms for attachment to epithelial cells of the small intestines because they differ in virulence factors that allow bacterial attachment. Disruption of the microvillus (an attaching-effacing mechanism of action), the release of powerful plasma-associated entero-toxins, endocytosis, tissue destruction, inflammation, necrosis and ulceration, results after attachment has taken place. The diarrhoea is the result of an increase in fluid and electrolyte loss into the gut lumen leading to the production of unformed or liquid faeces by which the pathogen is expelled by the body (and in doing so, aids its dissemination).

The non-bacterial gastro-enteritis and diarrhoea are usually caused by viruses, especially the *Rotaviruses*. The *Rotaviruses* multiply in the intestinal epithelial cells, damaging the transport mechanisms in the gut, and the loss of water, salt and glucose causes diarrhoea. The infected cells in the intestines are destroyed resulting in villous atrophy. The villi become flattened, resulting in the loss of both surface area for absorption and the digestive enzymes and the raised osmotic pressure in the gut lumen causes diarrhoea. Neither inflammation nor loss of blood occurs. For reasons unknown, respiratory symptoms such as cough and coryza are quite common. *Rotaviruses* are well-adapted intestinal infectious agents and as few as 10 ingested particles can cause an infection. The faeces are laden with enormous quantities of infectious particles. Other viruses may have different mechanisms of diarrhoea. Disruption of normal bacterial flora of the gut (usually due to antimicrobial treatment) allows pathogens normally absent or present in small numbers to multiply and cause antibiotic-associated diarrhoea.

❖ **Clinical manifestation**
  • Gastroenteritis is an acute disease and the signs and symptoms vary from slight to moderate
  • At times, as a result of dehydration, it can be severe enough to cause the death of the ill person
  • Nausea, vomiting and diarrhoea occur, as well as pyrexia of 37,9°C and higher
  • Dehydration with concomitant electrolyte imbalance is common

- Abdominal cramps and myalgia occur in cases of endemic virus gastro-enteritis

❖ **Complications**
  - Dehydration which can be fatal

■ **Diagnosis**
  - Clinical picture

■ **Prognosis**
  - Fair, provided the condition is treated
  - The mortality rates for babies and toddlers are very high

■ **Specific healthcare interventions to be rendered**
  - **Symptomatic and supportive**. Diarrhoea and vomiting can be self-treated for up to **3 (three) days** in adults and older children providing replacement with oral rehydration takes place and stools are not blood-stained and no fever develops
  - Fluids are supplemented intravenously (electrolyte solution) when dehydration has set in
  - **It is advisable not to give any binding agent** as it destroys the normal flora of the intestinal tract. Binding agents prevent the intestinal tract from flushing out the infectious agent. Antimicrobial drugs destroy the intestinal flora which can cause serious medical conditions such as the mal-absorption of nutrients
  - **Antimicrobial drugs must be used extremely selective** and the administering of anti-diarrhoeal drugs must be abstained. Under no circumstances must infants under the age of 2 be given anti-diarrhoeal drugs containing atropine. **Toddlers and young children under the age of 12 years should only be given anti-diarrhoeal drugs containing atropine under medical supervision.** Adults taking anti-diarrhoeal drugs containing atropine should do so with the greatest of care. (Anti-diarrhoeal drugs containing atropine inhibit peristalsis of the intestine, resulting in large quantities of fluid accumulating in the intestinal tract which can lead to the rupture of the intestines)
  - **Increase orally the Required Daily Allowance (RDA) of the mineral Zinc** as it helps to reduce the severity and duration of the acute diarrhoeal episode. Zinc also prevents subsequent episodes of diarrhoea in the follow 2-3 months. Give 20mg Zinc (zinc sulphate/gluconate/acetate, [tablets or syrup]) per day for 10–14 days (infants under the age of 6 months must be given 10 mg per day for 10–14 days). Remember Zinc must be taken with care and given in combination with Copper (I mg Copper with 15 mg Zinc)
  - **Oral rehydration therapy (ORT) must immediately be commenced** at the first sign of diarrhoea (watery stools) as the electrolytes prevents dehydration by enhancing the absorption of fluids into the blood and replaces the electrolytes that are lost because of the diarrhoeal stools. **Do not wait until later – ORT is to be given after each stool and between stools.** Reduced osmolarity solution oral rehydration salts (ORS) containing low concentrations of glucose (13.5 gm/litre), salt (2.6 gm/litre) and potassium chloride (1.5 gm/litre) should be given ad lib (as much as possible by mouth) as it treat and

prevent diarrhoeal dehydration, reduce stool output, and shortens the duration of diarrhoea. (It is advisable that a child be held on the lap of an adult while being fed with a teaspoon)

Prepare own Sugar–salt solution as follows when no readymade ORT is available

- 1 litre of boiled or treated water (see prevention)
- 2.5 ml (½ teaspoon – small teaspoon) salt
- 6x5 ml (6 teaspoons [small tea spoon]) sugar {not artificial sweetener}

Take 1 (one) full cup (200 ml) of the ORT after each loose stool starting immediately when diarrhoea/gastro-enteritis occurs and keep taking it as long as the diarrhoea persist. Children under the age of 2 years must be given 50-100ml (¼-½ cup) solution after each loose stool

Note

1. Readymade ORT (in combination with Probiotics or on its own) should be taken as prescribed on the packet. Cooled boiled or treated/clean cold water must be used for dissolving the content of the sachet
2. In case of emergency and no ORT is available or prepared, flat coca-cola (without any bubbles) can be taken until such time ORT becomes available
3. Check hourly for sign and symptoms of dehydration (skin turgor test can be done as well obvious sign of dehydration, namely, sunken eyes, lethargy and much more). Increase the volume of ORT immediately to treat dehydration and immediately admit to a healthcare centre

- **Probiotics** (the good microbes living in the intestines in a capsule) can be taken ad lib per mouth (orally) by all individuals (infants, children, adults and the elderly) during and after an episode of diarrhoea as it eliminates the microbial pathogen while enhancing the body's immune system as well as restoring the normal indigenous bacterial flora of the intestines. (For babies and young children the capsule can be opened and the content added to a milk feed or normal diet of the child or added to the ORT fluid that are given)
- **Under no circumstances should an infant's milk feeds (bottle feeds) or feeding per breast (breastfeeding) be stopped**, since this can lead to malnutrition which can prolong the recovery period and cause other medical conditions. Neither should **milk feeds be diluted**. Adults should be given a normal diet. (Foods which can lead to gaseousness should be avoided, as well as too much roughage)
- **A thin gruel made from culturally accepted ethnic foods** (for example, rice, oats, sweet potatoes, maize products, barley, etc) may be given as supplementary feeds
- **Solid foods can be given to the ill individual within 3–4 hours after having started with oral rehydration therapy**. Avoid roughage and foods which tend to form gases. As soon as the ill individual has recovered, a normal diet can be taken. Give small portions of food often – 6 to 8 meals per day. **NB: Increase the number of meals to 6 to 8 per day for infants, children and adults during and after the diarrheal episode for 10 to 14 days**

- **Alternate meals and oral rehydration therapy** (the oral rehydration compound forms the basis) together with a fluid diet as follows (when volumes of fluids and body mass can be measured)
  - ◈ 0 - 1 years old   120 ml/kg/day
  - ◈ 1 – 2 years old   100 ml/kg/day
  - ◈ 2 – 4 years old   85 ml/kg/day
  - ◈ 4 – 10 years old   70 ml/kg/day

  When the ill individual's condition is serious – administer 50–20 ml/kg above the maintenance therapy and normal feeds
- **When the ill person eat or drinks almost nothing, continues to pass watery stools, is very thirsty, vomits often/continuously, has a fever, shows blood in the stools, does not respond to treatment, or when the condition worsens, admit immediately to a healthcare institution**
- **Observe for other symptoms requiring medical treatment**, for example, bloody stools
- **Medical attention must be seek** under the following circumstances
  - ✳ Infants under the age of 12 months with diarrhoea that lasted more than 1 day and/or vomiting for more than 1 day as replacement of fluids are prevented
  - ✳ Infants with signs of moderate to severe dehydration, for example, limp, non-alert, sunken eyes, dry mouth and eyes as well as mucosa, and not passing urine
  - ✳ Infants younger than 3 years of age or elderly over 75 years who have diarrhoea for longer than 2 days duration
  - ✳ Older children and adults with diarrhoea that lasted longer than 3 days
  - ✳ Presence of blood of mucus in the stool or "oily" stools
  - ✳ Diarrhoea accompanied by severe vomiting and fever (in this case, the risk of dehydration is high)

◆ **Preventive measures to be taken**
  - ➢ When infants and toddlers attend crèches or day care centres, it is advisable that they are cared for at home until the diarrhoea has cleared up
  - ➢ To protect infants against severe *Human Rotavirus* gastro-enteritis, infants can be orally vaccinated with the *Human Rotavirus* vaccine from the age from of 6 weeks
  - ➢ A high standard of personal hygiene, in particular in respect of washing of hands, must be maintained
  - ➢ Safe drinking water must be supplied and used. When microbial/bacteriological contamination of water is suspected, or confirmed, or when any uncertainty consists regarding the safety/purity of the water, all supply of drinking water (including ice) should be boiled for 5-10 minutes and cooled before drinking or used. Water can also be treated with chlorine-based tablets/solution (bleach) such as Jik, Milton – 5ml chlorine to 10 litres water and leave it for 12 hours before consumption or 5 (five) drops of any household bleach containing chlorine to 1 litre of water and used after 30 minutes. This also applies to all

water used for preparing of formulas (baby food and nutritional formulas), juice and other drinks diluted with water (including ice)

➤ Safe and hygienic sanitary facilities must be provided
➤ Adequate food hygiene must be ensured at home and in the food industries
➤ Infesting of flies must be controlled
➤ Carriers need to receive adequate treatment
➤ When pets are kept or other farm animals grace in the vicinity, adhere to the following measures
  • promote the health of the animals, such as deworming every six months
  • isolate sick animals and give adequate treatment. Keep children away from sick animals
  • keep animals away from water and food sources
  • keep strange animals away from living quarters and surroundings
  • bury or otherwise destroy animal faeces on a daily basis. When compost heaps are used, ensure that they are out of reach of children
  • protect the play areas of children from all animal excretions. Disinfect sand in the sandpit every week or keep sand covered with a plastic covering
  • do not allow animals in the areas where food is prepared or where the family eat
  • do not feed animals from utensils used by humans
  • wash hands with soap and water after contact with animals and before eating or preparing food
➤ When travelling, abide by the following principles
  ◈ Keep water purification tablets at hand and boil filtrated water. When surface water needs to be drunk, boil or use chlorine-based purification of water first. Iodine and ascorbic acid should only be used in extreme circumstances
  ◈ Peel and boil all fruit and vegetables and eat only piping hot food. Avoid eating products from a street vendor unless it is served piping hot from a wok. Do not eat salads except when prepared personally
  ◈ Do not use ice cubes for drinks and beverages. Do not eat ice cream
  ◈ Do not eat shellfish, raw or rare meat and fish and do not drink un-pasteurised milk
  ◈ Eat in restaurants and hotels or prepare own food personally. Do not buy food from street vendors

◆ **Measures to prevent epidemics**
  ⬌ Proper personal hygiene – washing of hands after using the toilet
  ⬌ Provision of effective sanitary facilities
  ⬌ Tracing of sources
  ⬌ Recognition and treatment of disease
  ⬌ Do not use sewage waste water for permaculture (irrigation of vegetables and fruit) – use only grey water from wash basins and baths/showers
  ⬌ When solid sewage are buried – take the natural flow of the water table in account

◆ **Implications for disaster situations**
  ⬇ When any disaster occurs that damages the water supplies and sanitation facilities of a community, a better than average change exists that an outbreak of gastro-enteritis will occur

◆ **Compliance with international measures**
  ⬇ None

11.1.2   CHOLERA

Cholera is an acute bacterial disease characterized by diarrhoea, massive loss of fluid and electrolytes followed by dehydration and impairment of electrolytes

---

Epidemiological data

Geographical distribution
Occurring world-wide. Since 1980 the disease occurs epidemically in South Africa and it is endemic to Limpopo, Mpumalanga, and KwaZulu-Natal. Epidemics occur seasonally, reaching their peak during summertime

Causative pathogen
Vibrio cholerae. The El-Tor biotype causes cholera in South Africa. The properties of the microbe are
  ✳ It can live for four weeks in sewage and chlorinated clean, clear water
  ✳ It can live 1 – 2 days in fresh river water as a free-living inhabitant
  ✳ It can live up to 7 days on vegetables
  ✳ It can live for up to 4 weeks in dairy products
  ✳ It can live for up to 4 weeks on meat or fish
  ✳ It is resistant to salt, but sensitive to acid
  ✳ It is easily destroyed by heat, desiccation and disinfectants
  ✳ It cannot live more than 2 days on dry surfaces

Incubation period
From a few hours to five days

Mode of transmission
*Faecal-oral transmission (also when hands are contaminated with excessive perspiration from the peri-anal area of the carrier)
*By being exposed to contacts of sick persons (very rarely)

Period of infectiousness (communicability, transmission)
From approximately three weeks after ingestion of the Vibrio to recovery or for as long as the infectious agent is present in the stools. The *Vibrio cholera* disappears from the stools a few days after the clinical picture has cleared up (also see Carriers below)

Reservoir
Humans

Intermediaries
Vectors - Flies
Vehicles - Contaminated food, water and milk
        Contamination of food by flies

Carriers
A carrier state does occur, even when a sub-clinical infection condition has been contracted (1-20%). This state may last for a few months or for several years. (There are approximately 25 carriers [who are asymptomatic or have moderate diarrhoea] for each new case reported to healthcare services). Asymptomatic human carriers are the major reservoir of the infection

Immune status
Immunity with memory against a specific serological type is elicited

Susceptibility and resistance of host
All persons are susceptible. In endemic regions, most persons acquire a certain measure of immunity with memory by the time they reached adulthood

Pathogenesis

As the *Vibrio cholerae* is sensitive to stomach acid, large doses need to be ingested to cause the disease unless the host is achlohydric or is taking antacids. Because the *Vibrio* possesses additional virulence factors, the *Vibrio* can on ingestion, survives the host defences and attaches itself to the small intestinal mucosa by producing mucinase when binding with specific receptors on the epithelial cells in the ileum and jejunum. The *Vibrio* releases an entero-toxin which stimulates the intestinal tract to secrete an alkaline substance in which the *Vibrio* multiplies. The entero-toxin affects the entire intestinal tract. However, no acute inflammatory response occurs and neither the intestinal wall nor the enterocytes are damaged.

The typical "rice-water" cholera stool is attributed to the secretion of mucus from the epithelial cells. No blood or white blood cells are found in stools. The loss of fluid may, however, comprise 8–10% of the body weight within a very short period of time.

❖ **Clinical manifestation**
   - The onset of the disease is sudden with abdominal cramps and acute diarrhoea that increases in severity within hours
   - Within a few hours the severity of the diarrhoea causes the ill person to lose one litre per hour (24 litres of fluid in 24 hours)
   - The massive amount of watery, non-odour, and non-bloody diarrheal faeces consist mostly of large quantities of mucus (the so-called rice-water stools)
   - Blood may sometimes be present in the diarrheal faeces
   - Vomiting can also occur
   - Because of the fluid loss, dehydration starts within hours resulting in anuria, metabolic acidosis (loss of bicarbonate), hypokalaemia (loss of potassium) and hypovolemic shock resulting in cardiac failure
   - The temperature is normal and may even be subnormal

- A bacteraemia does not develop and no enterocytes or white blood cells are found in the stools
- Hypotension, acidosis and shock set in and the ill person may die when he/she is not treated

❖ **Complications**
  - Renal failure and death
  - Vascular collapse
  - Liver failure
  - Shock because of the severe dehydration
  - A carrier state may develop

■ **Diagnosis**
  - Clinical picture
  - A stool culture or rectal swabs are sent for a serum agglutination test as laboratory confirmation of *Vibrio* in the faeces

■ **Prognosis**
  - The mortality rates are high in untreated cases (40 – 60%)
  - With treatment the ill person recovers soon

■ **Specific healthcare interventions to be rendered**
  - Acidosis, hypokalaemia and dehydration must be treated. Early rehydration brings about a dramatic difference in the prognosis of Cholera and can be done in community clinics without the need for hospitalisation
  - Although antimicrobial drugs are not a necessity, antimicrobial drugs (tetracycline) can be given to reduce the time of excretion of the *Vibrio cholerae*
  - Recognition of and differentiation between Cholera and other types of diarrhoea based on the following
    ✳ number of stools per day increase rapidly in cholera
    ✳ the ill person presents with watery diarrhoea that has the typical rice-water appearance (greyish in colour and containing particles of material – typically only in Cholera)
    ✳ when the number of persons with diarrhoea and vomiting increase rapidly day by day, the possibility of an outbreak of Cholera should be taken into account
  - **Start immediately with oral rehydration therapy** (fluids and electrolytes). The following amounts of ORT should be administered within the first four hours after the onset of the disease
    ◈ 0 – 4 months   200 – 400 ml
    ◈ 4 – 11 months   400 – 600 ml
    ◈ 1 – 4 years   600 – 1 200 ml
    ◈ 5 – 14 years   1 200 – 3 300 ml
    ◈ 14 years and older 2 200 – 4 000 ml
  - ✱ **Do not wait until later – ORT is to be given after each stool and between stools.** Reduced osmolarity solution oral rehydration salts (ORS) containing low concentrations of glucose (13.5 gm/litre), salt (2.6 gm/litre) and potassium

chloride (1.5 gm/litre) should be given ad lib as it treats and prevent diarrheal dehydration, reduces stool output and shortens the duration of diarrhoea. (It is advisable to hold a child on the lap of an adult while feeding with a teaspoon) Prepare own ORT solution as follows if no readymade ORT is available

> 1 litre of boiled or treated water (see prevention)
> 2.5 ml (½ teaspoon of a small teaspoon) salt
> 6x5 ml (6 small teaspoons) sugar (not artificial sweetener)

Take 1 (one) full cup of the ORT after each loose stool starting immediately when diarrhoea starts and keep taking it as long as the diarrhoea persist. Children should be given 50-100 ml (¼ - ½ cup) solution after each loose stool **Note**: readymade ORT should be taken as prescribed on packets

- Within 3–4 hours of having started oral rehydration therapy, offer the ill individual solid foods. In the beginning, roughage in foods and all gaseous foods should be avoided. As soon as the ill person starts recovering, a normal diet can be served. **NB: Increase the number of meals to 6 to 8 per day for infants, children and adults during and after the diarrheal episode for 10 to 14 days**

- **Do not stop** breast-feeding or milk feeding per bottle for infants, nor dilute any milk feeds

- Although there is no need for strict isolation, enteric precautions should still be taken to prevent other ill persons or healthcare practitioners contracting the disease

- Because of the nature of the diarrhoea, all healthcare practitioners must wear plastic aprons when attending to ill persons as these can be scrubbed down with disinfectant after contamination

- Faeces and soiled linen must be soaked for 10 minutes in a solution of phenol

- In cases of severe dehydration, the fluid and electrolyte balance has to be restored by administering a solution of Ringer's lactate intravenously

◆ Preventive measures to be taken

> ➢ Prevention is based on water purification, sanitation and food hygiene
> ➢ Notification is important in order to prevent the spread of the disease
> ➢ In endemic regions all persons with persistent diarrhoea have to be treated as potential cholera cases
> ➢ Tracing and treatment of carriers until three (3) rectal swabs are negative
> ➢ Prophylactic vaccination is only 50% effective and the relative immunity lasts for 2–6 months only. Travellers to endemic regions sometimes make use of this vaccination but the possibility of becoming a carrier is great
> ➢ Preventing contamination of drinking water at communal washing and bathing facilities by promoting the use of disposable drinking cups (Styrofoam). Burn all used containers
> ➢ Use only water that has been purified for human consumption. Health information should be given when purified drinking water is not available. Water intended for drinking purposes should be boiled for 10 minutes or treated with sodium hypochlorite. (Home chlorination can be done by using Milton, Jik or any other household bleach containing chlorine. Five (5) drops of

any of these substances to one litre (1 litre) of water can be used for drinking purposes after 30 minutes (or 5 ml to 10 litre of water after 12 hours.) This also applies to all water used for the preparation of formulas (baby food and nutritional formulas), juice and other drinks diluted with water (including ice)

➤ When water is taken from rivers/lakes/springs for human consumption, the water must be collected from an area higher/above the area where washing are done and bathing takes place

➤ Adequate sanitation and sewage disposal must be ensured. When sewage waste has to be buried, the flow of the water table must be taken in account

➤ Ensuring satisfactory personal hygiene. The public should be encouraged to wash their hands after using the toilet and before handling of food and drinks

➤ Supervision of contacts for approximately five (5) days (no quarantine measures are necessary)

➤ Control/prevent infesting of flies

➤ Should an epidemic outbreak occurs, discourage the gathering of masses of individuals such as for festivities and burials

➤ Ensure that the deceased are removed and buried immediately according to legislative regulations

➤ In areas where contaminated rivers run into the sea, sea foods (oysters, mussels, etc) should not be eaten since it is infected

◆ **Measures to prevent epidemics**
  - Provide safe drinking water
  - Ensure proper sanitation and safe disposal of solid waste
  - Giving of prophylactic chemotherapy is not advised. In exceptional cases prophylactic chemotherapy can be administered to contacts when transmission had taken place horizontally
  - Establish emergency care centres (for example, schools, community centres, clinics) and ensure that sufficient treatment facilities and materials (for example, anti-microbial drugs, intravenous transfusions, etc) are available
  - Identify and treat ill individuals in the early stages of the disease and isolate them from other persons
  - Immediately instate enteric precautions and disinfect the environment of the ill individual such as bed linen, drinking and eating utensils, etc.
  - Vaccination is not advised since it offers only limited protection (three to six [3–6] months) and travellers may contract a sub-clinically form of the disease leading to a carrier state
  - Give health information regarding identification of the condition, proper handling of faecal and urinary secretions, ensuring the use of safe drinking water, safe handling and preparation of food and drinks, maintaining of satisfactory personal hygiene and administering of oral rehydration therapy
  - Placing limitations on travelling is unnecessary since it cannot prevent the spread of the disease. A large number of travellers are also carriers

◆ **Implications for disaster situations**
  - None

Compliance with international measures

- Some countries demand cholera vaccination before allowing entry into the specific country

11.1.3 SHIGELLOSIS (BACILLARY DYSENTERY)

Shigellosis (also known as bacillary dysentery) is a serious bacterial disease characterized by an invasive inflammation of the mucosa of the colon and rectum resulting in the presence of blood and mucus in the diarrhoeal stools

---

Epidemiological data

Geographical distribution
Occurring world-wide

Causative pathogen
Shigella dysenteriae – most serious
Shigella flexneri – severe infection
Shigella boydii – severe infection
Shigella sonnei – mild infection

Incubation period
1–4 days

Mode of transmission
Faecal-oral transmission by means of hands from one person to another

Period of infectiousness (communicability, transmission)
1–2 weeks

Reservoir
Humans. The shigella is harbored in the intestinal tract
Animal reservoirs - none

Intermediaries
Vectors - Flies can contaminate food
Vehicles - Contaminated food and water

Carrier state
A temporary/recovery carrier state may occur for a few weeks but permanent (chronic) carriage is unusually

Immune status
Immunity with memory against a specific serological type is elicited

Susceptibility and resistance of host
All persons are susceptible. As the shigellae appear to be able to initiate infection from a small infective dose (10–100 organisms), the disease is most prevalent among large gatherings of persons where food is not hygienically handled or stored properly; and where sanitary facilities are unsatisfactory; and in camps, crèches, overcrowded institutions and refugee camps

---

Pathogenesis

The shigella attaches itself to and invades the mucosal epithelium of the distal ileum and colon causing inflammation and ulceration. However, the pathogen very seldom penetrates the intestinal wall or migrates to the bloodstream. Within 12 hours after swallowing the shigella, toxaemia develops due to the multiplication of the bacteria in the colon. Abdominal pain, cramps and fever occur at this stage of the infection. The temperature subsides after 2–3 days while the abdominal pain and tenderness increase due to the bacterial invasion of the mucous membrane of the colon. Necrosis of the mucous membrane occurs which leads to blood, mucus and pus being present in the stools. The infection is self-limiting but dehydration can occur especially in the young and the elderly. Complications are associated with malnutrition.

The *Shigella dysenteriae* specie-pathogen produces a shiga-toxin, which causes damage to the intestinal epithelium as well as damages the glomerular endothelial cells – the latter leading to kidney failure (haemolytic-uremic syndrome).

❖ **Clinical manifestation**
- The symptoms range from mild to severe depending on the species of Shigella involved and on the underlying state of health of the infected individual. Shigellosis is primarily a paediatric disease and when associated with severe malnutrition it may precipitate complications, such as protein deficiency syndrome
- The onset is sudden with headache for a short period (1- 4 days), lassitude and fatigue, pyrexia, anorexia and abdominal discomfort followed by colicky abdominal pain and watery diarrhoea
- Vomiting can occur at first but does not last long
- The diarrhoea may last for a week or even longer and in severe cases may contain blood and mucus. The rectum is red and inflamed
- Less severe cases, which occur more commonly, are characterized by loose stools and malaise lasting a day or two
- Many cases are asymptomatic although the person excretes the specific pathogen

❖ **Complications**
- Severe dehydration that can cause death
- Convulsions
- Septicaemia and pneumonia
- Haemolytic-uremic syndrome

■ **Diagnosis**
- The Shigellsa is isolated by means of a bacteriological examination of the faeces

■ **Prognosis**
- Good, depending on age, resistance and early treatment of the condition
- The mortality rate amongst young children is high

■ **Specific healthcare interventions to be rendered**
- Chemotherapy – antimicrobial and anti-colic drugs

- Semi-isolation of ill person (enteric precautions)
- Oral rehydration therapy
- When the dehydration does not clear up, fluids are administered intravenously
- Concurrent disinfection of excreta
- Application of protective ointment to anus
- Tracing of contacts and carriers and treating them
- Correcting of environmental factors

◆ **Preventive measures to be taken**
  ➤ Adequate personal hygiene, in particular washing of the hands after using the toilet and before preparing food and eating of food
  ➤ Provision of adequate sanitary facilities and sewage disposal
  ➤ Provision of clean water and food supplies
  ➤ Controlling of infesting of flies

◆ **Measures to prevent epidemics**
  ♦ Health information concerning personal hygiene, environmental hygiene and food hygiene must be given on a continuous basis as epidemics can easily break out where large masses of individuals gather
  ♦ Persons who are in remission (temporary carriers) are not allowed to handle food intended for public consumption

◆ **Implications for disaster situations**
  ♦ None

◆ **Compliance with international measures**
  ♦ None

11.2　SYSTEMIC DISEASES INITIATED IN THE GASTRO-INTESTINAL TRACT

Although this group of infections are acquired by the ingestion of the pathogen, the pathogen disseminates (spread) to other organs and body systems causing a serious to fatal systemic disease. Complications occur frequently.

11.2.1　TYPHOID AND PARATYPHOID FEVER

Typhoid/paratyphoid fever is an acute enteric disease characterized by bacteraemia with reticulo-endothelial involvement and the formation of micro-abscesses as well as ulcerations in the distal ileum

Epidemiological data
Geographical distribution Occurring world-wide especially in hot climates with a high rainfall. Mild and atypical infections occur particularly in endemic regions. In the RSA, typhoid/paratyphoid fever occurs endemically in KwaZulu-Natal, Limpopo and Mpumalanga

---

Causative pathogen
Salmonella typhi or *Salmonella paratyphi*

Incubation period
1–3 weeks, on the average 10–14 days

Mode of transmission
Faecal-oral transmission

Period of infectiousness (communicability, transmission)
The disease is transmissible for as long as the pathogen is secreted in the urine and faeces of an individual - that is up to the end of the convalescent phase

Reservoir
Humans. The pathogen is harbored mainly in the gall-bladder or in the bladder

Intermediaries
Vectors -Flies
Vehicles - Contaminated water and food

Carriers
A permanent/chronic carrier state (fecal and urinary) develops after a sub-clinical or clinical attack. *Salmonella typhi/parathyphi* is harbored in the gall-bladder or bladder of the carrier. In some cases the person may be an intermittent carrier who only sporadically secretes the pathogen making it difficult to trace the carrier

Immune status
Immunity with memory is elicited

Susceptibility and resistance of host
Everybody is susceptible. Persons who have achlorhydria are particularly vulnerable as well as young children and young individuals between the ages 5–15 years

---

Pathogenesis

The *Salmonella typhi* or *Salmonella parathyphi* is able to survive the gastric acid and the antibacterial defences of the stomach and small intestines. After ingestion, *S. typhi* or *S. paratyphi* penetrates the gut mucosa through the Peyer's patches, probably in the jejunum or distal ileum. Once through the mucosal barrier, the *S. typhi* or *S. parathyphi* reaches the intestinal nodes and invades the lymphoid tissue of the ileo-cecal region causing reticulo-endothelial hyperplasia and hypertrophy. Here the *S. typhi* or *S. parathyphi* enters the macrophages and multiply within the macrophages (*Salmonella typhi/paratyphi* is an intracellular parasite that is not killed off by phagocytosis but invades the phagocytes and multiplies in the phagocytes). From the lymphoid tissue the macrophages transports the pathogen to the mesenteric lymph nodes and then, via the thoracic duct, to the bloodstream where the pathogen is finally discharged into the bloodstream. A transient bacteraemia now develops which clears up at the end of the first week. The signs and symptoms that are manifested during the first week of the natural course of the disease is the result of this specific progress of pathogenesis.

During the second week of pathogenesis, the *S typhi* or *S parathyphi* penetrates the reticulo-endothelial system seeding the spleen, bone marrow, liver (Kupffer cells) and Peyer's patches and multiplies within the reticulo-endothelial system. A second bacteraemia develops now when the *S. typhi* or *S. parathyphi* re-enters the bloodstream from the reticulo-endothelial cells while infecting other organs such as the kidney. Infection of the biliary tract occurs simultaneously and the salmonella multiply further as it is resistant to bile. When the infected bile is secreted into the intestinal tract, secondary infection of the digestive tract with millions of salmonellae takes place, causing a strong inflammatory response in Peyer's patches.

The most outstanding characteristic of the pathogenesis of typhoid/paratyphoid fever is the ulceration of the lymph follicles (Peyer's patches) in the small intestine. Inflammation with hyperplasia of the follicles occurs. Within a week or two, necrosis of the follicles follows due to the oedema and vascular obstruction which had developed. This leads to sphacelation. The typical "pea soup" stools (watery stools with necrotic follicles) are present. During this period of sphacelation, haemorrhage and/or perforation of the intestine may occur. The liver and spleen are enlarged and bronchitis is a common concomitant.

- ❖ **Clinical manifestation**
  - ✱ **First week (prodromal stage)**
    - The prodromal stage is characterized by a transient bacteraemia
    - The onset is gradual with flu-like symptoms such as a slight pyrexia, malaise, headache, anorexia, insomnia, epistaxis, aching limbs and constipation or diarrhoea
    - The pulse rate does not increase in proportion to the elevation in temperature
  - ✱ **Second week**
    - At the end of the first week the so-called "rose spots" appear on the chest, under the nipple line and on the abdomen. This is a pink maculo-papular rash lasting a few hours to 2 – 3 days and is not extensive (2 – 30 spots)
    - The temperature elevates/rises systematically and reaches a peak at 39⁰C to 41⁰C with a bradycardia
    - The abdomen is distended with splenomegaly and hepatomegaly
    - The ill person passes loose "pea soup" stools and the condition leads to dehydration
  - ✱ **Third week**
    - Toxaemia develops and the ill person becomes comatose
    - During the comatose stage, the ill individual exhibits the typical typhoid fever picture known as the "typhoid state" where the ill person slips down in the bed and stares aimlessly at the ceiling (coma vigil)
    - The ill person mumbles, is delirious and plucks at the bedclothes (carpology)
    - Incontinence of faeces and urine occurs and tachycardia is present
  - ✱ **Fourth to Sixth week**
    - The ill person's condition improves and the temperature subsides gradually. Recovery is slow and relapses may occur

❖ **Complications**
- Secondary to the local gastro-intestinal lesions - intestinal haemorrhage and intestinal perforation
- Associated with toxaemia - myocarditis as well as hepatic and bone marrow damage may occur
- Secondary to a prolonged serious illness - pulmonary complications may develop
- Myocardial infarction may occur without any obvious reason or explanation
- Resulting from multiplication of the *S. typhi* or *S. paratyphi* in other sites - meningitis, osteomyelitis or endocarditis may be caused
- A carrier state may develop – temporary/recovery carrier state develops for several weeks after recovery, or a permanent/chronic carrier state develops (in 1-3% of cases) when the *S. typhi* or *S. paratyphi* is shed for longer than a year, or an intermittent/transient carrier state develops when the *S typhi* or *S paratyphi* is shed intermittently. *S. typhi* and *S. paratyphi* is excreted in the faeces and urine

■ **Diagnosis**
- Clinical picture
- Positive blood culture during the first week
- Positive Widal agglutination test from the second week
- Positive urine and stool cultures from the second to the third week

■ **Prognosis**
- Good with treatment

■ **Specific healthcare interventions to be rendered**
- Chemotherapy. The classic picture of typhoid fever is seldom seen at present since the clinical picture of the disease changes dramatically when antimicrobial drugs, particularly chloramphenicol or other antimicrobial drugs, are administered. Within 48 hours after the commencement of treatment, the ill person's condition improves and his/her temperature is often normal by the fifth (5th) day. Complications such as those listed above, may still occur. However, when the ill person receives effective treatment timely, the possibility that a carrier state will develop rapidly diminishes
- Enteric precautions must be taken with concurrent disinfection (sometimes semi-isolation is necessary)
- Complete bed rest
- Accurate observation of vital signs
- Observation for signs of haemorrhage and other complications (especially myocardial)
- Careful rehydration of the ill person – prevent hypervolumia of the cardiovascular system and other systems of the body, do not serve gaseous forming food, nor give too much roughage

- Tracing of contacts and carriers. Urine specimens and rectal swabs have to be collected from carriers
- Treatment of carriers – three consecutive negative swabs cultures indicate successful treatment

◆ **Preventive measures to be taken**
  - ➤ Personal hygiene – washing of hands after use of toilet and before handling of food
  - ➤ Prevention of typhoid fever is based on the purification of water and the instatement of sanitation and food hygiene
  - ➤ Health inspections must be done in places where food preparation for public consumption takes place
  - ➤ Appraisal of the health status of all persons who handle food for carrier state. All positive food handlers must be excluded from employment in the food and catering industries until negative cultures are obtained. When being a permanent/intermittent carrier the individual must be helped to obtain employment in safe occupations
  - ➤ Preventing the contamination of food by flies
  - ➤ Notification of typhoid/paratyphoid fever
  - ➤ Although vaccination against typhoid/paratyphoid fever exists, prevention is based instead on the abovementioned measures as well as on active supervision of all ill and recovered persons and the treatment of carriers. (Immunity with memory is of short duration and may create a false sense of security)
  - ➤ Only grey water from baths/showers and wash basins may be used for perma-culture (irrigation of plants and vegetables)

◆ **Measures to prevent epidemics**
  - ⬦ As under preventive measures to be taken

◆ **Measures during disaster situations**
  - ⬦ When any disaster occurs that damages the water supplies and sanitation facilities of a community, a better than average change exists that an outbreak of typhoid/paratyphoid fever will occur
  - ⬦ Prevention of epidemics is once again based on efforts to supply safe drinking water to communities and establishing of safety measures regarding sewage disposal rather than launching a mass vaccination campaign

◆ **Compliance with international measures**
  - ⬦ None

11.2.2   VIRAL HEPATITIS

Viral hepatitis is a serious infection of the liver characterized by diffuse inflammatory changes and necrosis of the liver. There is a broad spectrum of clinical illness ranging from asymptomatic, symptomatic with malaise, anorexia, nausea, abdominal pain and jaundice to acute life-threatening liver failure

---

Epidemiological data

Geographic distribution

Hepatitis occur the world over. Hepatitis A has a seasonal incidence, peaking during the summer months. Epidemics which are spread through water and food, occur particularly in the developing countries

Causative pathogen

Hepatitis A-virus, Hepatitis B-virus , Hepatitis C-, D-, E-, F- and G-virus

Incubation period

Hepatitis A – 21–35 days (4 weeks), sometimes 15–50 days
Hepatitis B – 60–90 days, sometimes 42–180 days
Hepatitis C – 2 months
Hepatitis D – 2–12 weeks
Hepatitis E – 6–8 weeks

Mode of transmission

Hepatitis A-virus   Faecal-oral transmission through close contact between people
Ingestion of contaminated food and water.
Intimate anal intercourse

Hepatitis B-virus   The hepatitis B virus is a hepadna virus which contains three antigens, namely, HB surface antigen, HB core antigen, HBe antigen. The virus is present in the body fluids, blood, tears, saliva and the seminal and vaginal secretions of persons suffering from the disease and of carriers. The virus is therefore be transmitted by
  o   Blood transfusions
  o   Contaminated syringes and needles and equipment
  o   Droplets of saliva when kissing
  o   Sexual intercourse
  o   Skin lesions and the conjunctiva
  o   Vertically from mother to child when infected mothers transmit the virus during pregnancy and labour and while breastfeeding the baby

Hepatitis virus C, D, E, F and G

Faecal-oral transmission – *Virus E*

Blood transfusions and saliva – *Virus C + D*

Contaminated needles and syringes – *Virus C + D*

Ingestion of contaminated food and water – *Virus E*

Period of infectiousness (communicability, transmission)

<u>Hepatitis A</u> -   Type A virus is present in the excreta 1–2 weeks before symptoms appear until the
first week (sometimes second and third week) after the appearance of jaundice

---

<u>Hepatitis B</u> - Type B virus is present in the blood for several weeks before the first appearance of signs and symptoms and remains transmissible during the acute stage of the disease as well as when the chronic carrier state occurs

Reservoir
Humans – All serological types

Intermediaries
Vehicles – water and food (*virus A, E*)

Carriers
A carrier state occurs in hepatitis B, hepatitis C, hepatitis D (concurrent with hepatitis B)

Immune status
Immunity with memory to hepatitis A or hepatitis B is elicited

Susceptibility and resistance of host
All persons are susceptible to all types of hepatitis viruses
Virus A hepatitis mainly attacks children and young people
Persons at risk of virus B hepatitis - New-born babies, young children, healthcare workers, personnel and residents of institutions, sexually promiscuous persons, ill healthcare users receiving blood products, contacts and families, drug addicts, persons in endemic regions, persons who are exposed to hepatitis B by the nature of their careers such as policemen, members of the armed forces, firemen, healthcare providers

Pathogenesis

Hepatitis-viruses A, C, D, E, F and G. All these viruses have the same pathogenesis. After the virus has gained entry into the body, it replicates in the gastro-intestinal tract from where the virus infects the liver cells leading to oedema of the liver cells, necrosis of the liver cells and infiltration of the mononuclear cells of the parenchyma and portal vessels. The virus migrates from the liver into the biliary tract and infiltrates the gall bladder with a varying degree of infection. From the gall bladder the virus is excreted as part of the bile to reach the intestinal tract and the virus appears now in the faeces. Small amounts of the virus enter the blood stream at this stage. Because of the damage to the liver cells, the liver cannot transport bilirubin into the bile in the gall bladder, causing an increased level of bilirubin in the body fluids resulting in the yellow (jaundiced) tinge of the skin, sclera and mucous membranes. Regeneration of liver cells is rapid but fibrous repair can lead to cirrhosis (permanent damage due to an infection that persists). Viral hepatitis A is milder in young children than in older children and adults.

Hepatitis B-virus – after entering the body, the virus reaches the blood and then the liver where the result is inflammation and necrosis. Much of the pathology is immune mediated as infected liver cells are attacked by virus-specific T-cells. As liver damage increases, clinical signs of hepatitis appear. Viral hepatitis B is more severe than viral hepatitis A.

❖ **Clinical manifestation**
  ✳ <u>General signs and symptoms of all hepatitis viruses</u>
    • Pyrexia, malaise, anorexia, nausea and abdominal pain
    • Tenderness of the upper right-hand quadrant occurs
    • In the pre-icteric stage (jaundice) the liver may be palpable (hepatomegaly)
    • Stools are pale as a result of the absence of bile pigment while the urine is dark (yellowish-brown to greenish) in colour as a result of the conjugated hyper-bilirubinaemia
    • Jaundice appears after a few days (icteric stage)

  ✳ <u>Virus A hepatitis</u>
    • The onset is sudden
    • Virus is present in faeces 1–2 weeks before symptoms appear and during the first week (sometimes also second and third weeks)

  ✳ <u>Virus B hepatitis</u>
    • The onset is gradual and pyrexia may be absent
    • As the first virus-specific antibody is formed, there may be a brief prodromal illness with a rash and arthralgia. This is the result of the formation of immune complexes between HB surface antigen that is in excess and HB surface antibody in the circulation. The immune complexes are then deposited in the skin and joints
    • The disease varies from a very mild affliction which can only be confirmed by biochemical liver tests to very severe resulting in acute hepatic necrosis

  ✳ <u>Other hepatitis viruses</u>
    • The onset may be either sudden or gradual
    • If the latter is the case, a prodromal period occurs during which the person does not feel well and complains of non-specific symptoms

  ✳ <u>An asymptomatic form</u> of the infection can occur

❖ **Complications**
  • Relapses may occur
  • In the case of an infection that persists, chronicisity leads to liver cirrhosis with liver dysfunction
  • A carrier state can occur with virus B hepatitis as well as virus hepatitis C, D, E, F and G
  • Acute life-threatening liver failure can develop when more than half of the liver is damaged or destroyed
  • Hepato-cellular carcinoma can develop in hepatitis B

■ **Diagnosis**
  ▪ Liver function test
  ▪ Biochemical tests to identify the specific antigen as the respective forms of hepatitis can only be indicated serologically

■ **Prognosis**
  ▪ The individual usually recovers completely

■ **Specific healthcare interventions to be rendered**
  ▪ There are no specific drugs available for the treatment of hepatitis. The drug regime consists of multivitamins and essential phospholipids while an anti-inflammatory drug is sometimes prescribed
  ▪ Supportive and symptomatic
  ▪ Bed rest
  ▪ Proper preventive measures to prevent faecal contamination (hepatitis A, virus E to G types hepatitis)
  ▪ Virus B, C + D is resistant to boiling and general disinfection. Drastic methods should be used to destroy the virus on fomites such as burning, sterilizing by means of steam under pressure or the use of formalin
  ▪ Small nutritious meals (preferably cold) should be offered often to stimulate the person's appetite and improve his/her general resistance. A fat-free diet is not advised, since it inhibits the absorption of fat soluble vitamins (particularly vitamin K) which can lead to serious medical conditions such as blood clotting dysfunction
  ▪ For the relief of pruritis, creams containing antihistamine can be applied

◆ **Preventive measures to be taken**
  Virus A hepatitis as well as virus E to G serotype hepatitis
  The disease may occur in small epidemics where individuals live in close contact to each other. Prevention therefore has to focus on food and environmental hygiene such as
  ➤ Supplying safe drinking water
  ➤ Adequate sanitary facilities
  ➤ Ensuring good food hygiene
  ➤ Health information must be given to contacts regarding communal use of, for instance, eating utensils
  ➤ Passive vaccination of persons at risk with human y-globulin or active vaccination with hepatitis A-vaccine (Hep-A)
  ➤ Improving of personal hygiene, particularly washing of hands

  Virus B hepatitis as well as serotypes C and D hepatitis
  ➤ Persons who suffer from virus-B hepatitis are not permitted to donate blood
  ➤ Health information regarding personal hygiene such as using one's own tooth brush
  ➤ Health information to persons at risk regarding transmission by means of inoculation or contact through the mucous membranes and/or open wounds
  ➤ Effective sterilization of dental and other hospital instruments or the use of disposable equipment
  ➤ Careful handling of all intravenous and blood transfusion equipment, syringes, needles, etc

> Active vaccination of persons at risk and contacts with hepatitis B-vaccine (Hep-B)
> Active hepatitis-B virus vaccination of all persons from the age of six (6) weeks or older
> Carriers have to use condoms during sexual intercourse
> Hepatitis B-immunoglobulin must be administered within 48 hours after being exposed. The vaccine must be administered afterwards. Hepatitis B-immunoglobulin must also be administered to children of mothers who are carriers or are blood positive; to persons working in healthcare settings who have been accidentally pricked with a needle and to contacts. This should be followed up with active vaccination within six (6) weeks

◆ **Measures to prevent epidemics**
   None

◆ **Implications for disaster situations**
   None

◆ **Compliance with international measures**
   None

11.3   INTESTINAL PARASITAEMIA WITH PARASITES

Many species of protozoan and worm (helminths) parasites live in the gastro-intestinal tract but only a few are a frequent cause of serious pathology. The different life cycle stages include cysts, eggs and larvae. New parasitizing depend mostly upon horizontally contact (direct and indirect) with faecal material. The stages of protozoan parasites passed in faeces are either already parasitic or become parasitic within a short time. These parasites are usually acquired by swallowing parasitized eggs or larvae in faecal contaminated food and water. Worm parasites with two major exceptions (pinworm and dwarf tapeworm) produce eggs or larvae that require a period of development outside the host before they can parasitize the host. Transmission occurs as follows

- some species are acquired through food and water contaminated with parasitic eggs or larvae or picked up horizontally via contaminated fingers/hands
- some species have larvae that actually penetrate through the skin and then migrate eventually to the intestines
- some species are acquired by eating animal meat or animal products containing parasitized eggs.

The symptoms of intestinal parasitaemia range from very mild, to acute, to severe, to chronic diarrheal conditions associated with parasite-related inflammation, to life-threatening disease caused by the spread of parasites into organs of the body.

In many parts of the world intestinal parasites is accepted as a normal condition of life. The rate of parasitaemia most of the time reflects the standard of living, hygiene and sanitation.

11.3.1 Protozoan Parasitaemia

Protozoa are single-celled worms that parasitize the intestines as extra-cellular parasites. Extra-cellular protozoa feed by direct nutrient uptake or by ingestion of host cells. The pathology is caused by the host's response. Reproduction in humans is usually asexual, giving the potential for a rapid increase in numbers, particularly when the host defence mechanisms are impaired as in young children. Extra-cellular protozoa such as the amoebae, evade immune recognition of their plasma membrane by consuming complement at the cell surface. Extra-cellular protozoa are transmitted by ingestion of food or water contaminated with transmissible parasitic eggs and cysts.

11.3.1.1 Dysentery

Dysentery is a protozoan enterocolitis (inflammation involving the mucosa of both the small and large intestine) characterized by loose/diarrheal stools containing blood.

11.3.1.1.1 AMOEBIC DYSENTERY

Amoebic dysentery is an acute or chronic protozoan parasitaemia characterized by inflammation and ulceration (small localized superficial ulcers or formation of deep confluent ulcers in the entire colonic mucosa) of the mucus membranes of the colon and is accompanied by diarrhoea. Blood and/or mucous and/or pus is present in the stools

---

Epidemiological data

Geographical distribution
Occurring world-wide, particularly in tropical and subtropical regions

Causative pathogen
Entamoeba histolytica, a protozoan. The resistant encysted forms of the amoebae remain viable in a moist intermediary for as long as a month and act as the parasitized stage

Incubation period
3-4 weeks, sometimes 5 days to a few months

Mode of transmission
Oral-faecal transmission from the hands of one person to those of another
Oral-faecal transmission as a result of anal sexual activity

Period of infectiousness (communicability, transmission)
The disease is transmitted for as long as the amoebae are present in the intestinal tract. It may last for years

Reservoir
Humans. The protozoan cysts are present in the lumen of the intestinal tract

Intermediaries
Vectors - Flies and cockroaches can contaminate food (These insects live off human faeces. The cysts pass undamaged through the digestive tracts of the insects)

Vehicles - Contaminated water and food

Ingestion of food (especially raw vegetables) and drinking of unpurified water that were contaminated by the faeces of an infected individual

Carrier state

A carrier state does occur

Immune status

Parasitaemia does not elicit immunity with memory – re-infection can occur

Susceptibility and resistance of host

All persons are susceptible. Whether the person will become ill or not, is determined by factors pertaining to the individual self such as age, bacterial intestinal flora, nutrition, sources of iron and cholesterol levels. Only a small percentage of parasitized individuals develop acute symptoms

Pathogenesis

The *Entamoeba histolytica* lifecycle consists of three phases

❑ After being swallowed, the resistant parasitized encysted cysts pass, intact, through the stomach and excyst in the small intestines where they reproduce. The cysts penetrate and adhere to the epithelium of the intestinal tract and due to their lysinogenic effect on tissue they damage the epithelium by phagocytosis and cytolysis. When invading the mucosa, they feed on both the host's tissue and red blood cells, giving rise to amoebic colitis. The cysts cause lesions in the intestine varying from non-specific hypertrophy to ulceration of the mucous membranes.

❑ During the trophozoites stage, the cysts live in the large intestines on the mucosal surface. When the cysts mature, they release trophozoites into the small intestine when conditions are favourable. (Trophozoites are easily destroyed by the high pH and enzymes in the stomach, but the cysts remain unaffected.) The trophozoites penetrate the tissue of the colon and are capable of destroying leucocytes. Consequently, inflammatory cells are only found at the outer edges of the ulcers. The trophozoites also migrate to the liver where they cause abscesses and liver fibrosis. Necrotic areas may occur in the liver as a result of the obstruction of the portal blood vessels. As result of the obstruction of the portal blood vessels of the liver, abnormalities in the functions of the liver develop. When the infection spreads to the liver, the disease is serious.

❑ With time cysts are gradually formed by the mature trophozoites that are present in the lumen of the colon. The cysts are passed within the faeces of an individual.

❑ Reproduction of the amoebae during the trophozoites stages is by binary fission. There is periodic formation of resistant encysted forms which pass out of the body. These resistant cysts are able to survive in the external environment and act as the parasitizing stage. Infection occurs when food or drink is contaminated either by parasitized food handlers or as a result of inadequate sanitation.

❖ **Clinical manifestation**

Two forms of the disease exist, namely intestinal and hepatic amoebiasis

✴ **Intestinal amoebiasis**

Intestinal amoebiasis varies from asymptomatic to obvious and can be either acute or chronic in nature

⬥ **Acute amoebic dysentery**
- Abdominal pain
- Pyrexia
- Diarrhoea with blood, pus and mucus present in the stools

⬥ **Chronic or sub-acute amoebic dysentery**
- Irritation of the colon with abdominal discomfort and pain
- Intermittent diarrhoea or no diarrhoea. When diarrhoea develops, the stools are loose and contains mucus and/or blood
- Anorexia
- Malaise

✴ **Hepatic amoebiasis (extra-intestinal amoebic dysentery)**

Hepatic amoebiasis is a disease of the liver which develops within days or even years after intestinal amoebiasis occurred. It is characterized by
- pain in the upper right-hand quadrant or in the chest or in the epigastrium
- pyrexia
- tenderness of the liver and the liver is palpable
- weight loss occurs and paleness is present
- diarrhoea with mucus and blood in the stools occur
- the functions of the liver are abnormal

❖ **Complications**

✴ **Intestinal amoebiasis**
- Obstruction of the bowel due to lesions in the colon
- Haemorrhoids
- Perforation of the colon with consequent peritonitis

✴ **Hepatic amoebiasis**
- Formation of abscesses in the liver
- Spreading of the liver abscesses to the pleural cavity and the lungs
- Hepatitis
- Peritonitis
- Empyema
- Pericardial involvement
- Brain abscesses

■ **Diagnosis**
- A microscopic examination of a warm stool specimen reveals the amoebae. Please note that when the stool cools down, the amoebae form vesicles which cannot easily be recognised
- A sigmoidoscopy reveals the ulcerations

■ **Prognosis**
- Good, if no complications set in and treatment commences early
- The mortality rate amongst children is high

■ **Specific healthcare interventions to be rendered**
- Antiparasitic drugs
- Supportive and symptomatic healthcare
- Tracing of carriers and treating them
- Tracing of sources
- Concurrent disinfection of stools
- Measures to control infesting of flies and cockroaches

◆ **Preventive measures to be taken**
➢ Adequate personal hygiene, in particular, washing of hands after using the toilet and before preparing food and eating
➢ Provision of adequate sanitary facilities and sewage disposal
➢ Provision of clean water and food supplies
➢ Precautions to ensure that vegetables and fruit are not grown in contaminated soil and irrigated with contaminated water. Raw vegetables and fruit must be washed before eating. Contaminated vegetables and fruit should preferably be soaked in salt water for at least 20 minutes. Only grey water must be used for perma-culture (bath/shower and water of wash basins to be used for plant and vegetable irrigation)
➢ Controlling the infesting of flies and cockroaches
➢ Tracing and treatment of carriers

◆ **Measures to prevent epidemics**
- Parasitized persons must be kept under observation since the disease is not always cured by antimicrobial and other drug treatment and may re-occur
- Health information concerning personal hygiene, environmental hygiene and food hygiene must be given on a continuous basis
- Persons who are in remission and carriers are not allowed to handle food intended for public consumption

◆ **Implications for disaster situations**
- None

◆ **Compliance with international measures**
- None

11.3.2   Helminthic parasitaemia

Helminths are parasitic worms that cause intestinal parasitaemia. The mode of transmission predisposes children in particular to parasitaemia. In the RSA the most common helminthic diseases are caused by nematodes (roundworms, threadworms and hookworms) and Cestoids (tapeworms). Worm parasitaemia produces chronic mild intestinal discomfort rather than severe diarrhoea or other conditions. Parasitaemia leads to hypersensitivity responses and may reduce responses to vaccination. Each parasite has a number of characteristic pathologic conditions linked to it. The transmission of helminths occurs in four distinct ways, namely, by swallowing parasitic eggs or larvae via faecal-oral route; by swallowing parasitic larvae in the tissues of another host such as animal meat; by active penetration of the skin by larvae during the larval stage; and by the bite of an infected blood-sucking insect vector. The outer surfaces of helminths provide the primary host-parasite interface and the helminths have develop protective mechanisms to prevent the host damaging their outer surface. Because of the magnitude of parasitic worms that can parasitize humans, helminthic parasitaemia will not be discussed.

11.4   KEY NOTES

❑ Gastro-intestinal pathogens are transmitted via the faecal-oral route. Pathogens may invade the intestines causing systemic diseases (for example, typhoid/ paratyphoid fever) or multiply and produce locally acting toxins and damage only the gastro-intestinal tract (for example, cholera). The number of organisms ingested and their virulence attributes are critical factors in determining whether an infection becomes established or not.

❑ Diarrhoeal diseases (for example, viral and bacterial gastro-enteritis) cause high morbidity and mortality especially in young children and the elderly. Diarrhoea, the most common symptom of gastro-intestinal infections, ranges from mild and self-limiting to severe with consequent dehydration and death.

❑ The major bacterial causes of diarrheal infections are *E. coli*, salmonellae, shigellae, *V. cholerae*. Salmonellae have a large animal reservoir and spread via the food chain

❑ *Vibrio cholera* and Shigellae have no animal reservoir but spread via contaminated food, contaminated drinking water and unhygienic faecal waste disposal.

❑ Indigestion of food or water contaminated with *S. typhi/paratyphi* results in systemic enteric fever (typhoid/paratyphoid fever).

❑ Hepatitis is caused by viruses (for example, *hepatitis A to G*) via the faecal-oral route and indigestion of contaminated food and water. Excluded are hepatitis B, C and D that are transmitted by blood with hepatitis B also by the sexual route. Infection with *hepatitis B* and *C-viruses* often leads to chronic hepatitis or liver cancer.

❑ Diagnosis of microbiological gastro-intestinal infections are usually impossible without laboratory investigations although the assessment history, especially the travelling and food history, provides useful pointers.

❑ Many protozoa and helminths live in the intestine but relatively few cause severe diarrhoea. Parasitic infections can also involve the liver (liver flukes) leading to serious hepato-pathology.

❑ Infection of the biliary tree is usually secondary to obstruction. The normal intestinal flora cause mixed infections that may extend to form liver abscesses and septicaemia. Peritonitis and intra-abdominal sepsis follow contamination of the normal sterile cavity with intestinal microbes. The presentation is acute and the infection can be fatal.

❑ Disruption of the normal bacterial flora of the intestinal tract (usually due to antimicrobial drug treatment) allows microbes normally absent or present in small numbers to multiply and cause antibiotic-associated diarrhoea.

❑ A carrier state may develop as complication of certain gastro-intestinal diseases.

Chapter 12

COMMUNICABLE INFECTIONS AFFECTING THE SKIN

In addition to being a structural barrier, the skin is not only colonized by an array of microbes that forms its normal flora but also serve as an important source of colonization of certain bacteria and viruses. The relatively arid areas of the skin are colonized with fewer microbes (predominantly Gram-positive bacteria and yeast) while in the moister areas, the microbes are more numerous (more varied including Gram-negative bacteria). The microbial load of the normal skin is kept in check by various factors such as the limited amount of moisture that is present; the acid pH of the skin; the surface skin temperature that is not optimum for many pathogens; the salty sweat that kills many microbes; chemicals like sebum, fatty acids and urea that prevent attachment to the skin, and the competition between the different species of the normal flora that inhibits the growth of pathogens. Any alteration in these factors upset the ecological balance of the commensal flora predisposing the skin to infection.

Microbial infections of the skin result from any of three lines of attack, namely,
❏ breaches in the intact skin, allowing infection from the outside
❏ skin manifestations of systemic infections that arise as a result of blood-borne spread from the infected focus to the skin or by direct extension, for example, draining sinuses from body lesions
❏ toxin-mediated skin damage due to the production of a microbial toxin at another site in the body (for example, scarlet fever, toxic shock syndrome).
The skin spreads infections by shedding or direct contact. Dermatophytes (fungi such as those that cause ringworm) are shed from the skin and also from the hair and the nails, depending on the type of fungus. The normal individual also sheds desquamated skin scales into the environment depending on physical activities such as exercise, dressing and undressing. Staphylococci may be present in these skin shedding. Transmission by direct contact with skin lesions or with contaminated fingers or hands is much more common than following release into the environment.

Communicable diseases that affect the skin or manifest with a skin rash are very common and outbreaks of epidemics occur easily. When the skin infection and lesions are caused by bacteria that had gained entry into the skin through breaches in the intact surface of the skin, transmission takes place via direct contact with the infected or pustular skin lesions. When the disease is caused by viruses and certain airborne bacteria, entry into the body is usually gained by means of the mucous membranes of the respiratory tract and transmission between persons takes place by means of airborne infected droplets. Where the disease/infection is caused by the bite/sting of an animal or insect, transmission between persons is rare except in cases where a septicaemia/viraemia/bacteraemia is present and profuse growth of the pathogen in the lungs of the ill person has taken place – transmission now occurs via airborne infected droplets (for example, during coughing, speaking, singing and kissing).

12.1   BACTERIAL INFECTIONS OF THE SKIN

Bacterial infections of the skin can either involve the epidermis on its own, or only the epidermis and dermis of the skin, or all the deeper layers of the skin as well as the underlying soft tissue. Some infections may even involve several components of the soft tissues. The skin lesions that can develop are

- abscess formation such as boils and carbuncles as a result of infection and inflammation of the hair follicles in the skin (folliculitis). These skin lesions are normally not transmitted between persons although sinus formation may take place due to eroding of the overlying skin
- infections that spread such as impetigo, erysipelas, and cellulitis. Some lesions such as impetigo is highly contagious and small epidemics may result
- necrotic infections such as fasciitis of the soft tissues below the dermis. When the blood supply is interrupted, gangrene develops due to ischemia of the tissues. When the infection was caused by anaerobic pathogens, gas gangrene develops as result of the fermentative metabolism of the microbes and the gas is palpable in the tissues.

The most common pathogens that cause skin lesions are *streptococcus pyogenes; staphylococcus aureus; dermatophytes fungi; clostridia* as well as *anaerobes and micro-aerophiles*. These pathogens gain direct entry into the skin and/or soft tissues through breaches in the intact skin that range from microscopic to major trauma which may be accidental (for example, lacerations or burns) or intentional (for example, surgery).

12.1.1   IMPETIGO

Impetigo is an acute streptococcal (sometimes mixed) infection that affects only the epidermis and presents as a bulbous (blisters) or a crusted and/or pustular eruption of the skin

---

Epidemiological data

Geographic distribution
Impetigo occurs worldwide. Seasonal climatic conditions (summer/autumn/spring); heat and humidity favour the growth of the pathogen(s). It is also more common in areas where overcrowding occurs and under poor hygienic living conditions

Causative pathogen
Streptococcus pyogenes (group A streptococci) alone
Staphylococcus aureus and *Streptococcus pyogenes* as a mixed infection caused by both pathogens

---

Incubation period
1–5 days, usually 24-48 hours

Mode of transmission
Exogenous source - contact with a person suffering from impetigo or with a septic lesion
Auto - infection (self-inoculation) from a carrier site (for example, the nose)

Period of infectiousness (communicability, transmission)
Until all scabs have fallen off and all skin lesions have healed

Reservoir
Humans. Various factors plays a role in the development of streptococcal skin infections such as race, age, minor trauma, insect bites and vectors, personal hygiene and other skin diseases

Intermediaries
Vehicles - Fomites such as handkerchiefs, babies' nappies, towels, toys, clothing, bed linen

Carriers
Staphylococci are usually transmitted by carriers who harbour the pathogen in the nose while the streptococci are usually transmitted by carriers who harbour the pathogen in the pharynx. The infected person himself/herself may harbour the pathogens in his/her nose or throat with colonization occurring after the skin had become infected

Immune status
No immunity with memory is elicited

Susceptibility and resistance of host
The infection mainly affects young children and elderly persons whose resistance is generally low. Small outbreaks of epidemics can sporadically occur in hospital wards, hostels, camps and schools where children group together

Pathogenesis

The skin is directly penetrated by either *Strep. pyogenes* and/or *Staph. aureus* after direct contact with other persons with infected skin lesions. The pathogens may sometimes first colonize and multiply on the normal intact skin before invasion through minor breaks in the epithelium of the skin takes place. The type of skin lesion that develops is determined by the type of pathogen causing the infection. At first all skin lesions develop within 24-48 hours as an intense inflammatory response and presents as pinkish-red round maculae which enlarge rapidly. As a rule the lesions are not itchy.

❏ When the infection is caused by staphylococci (including *Staph. aureus*), blisters (vesicles) develop in the maculae. The vesicles suppurate rapidly and form pustules which rupture. A thin, flat crust is formed over the lesion. The lymph glands are not enlarged as a rule. Toxin production by *Staph. aureus* causes a serious skin infection.

❏ Streptococcal infection seldom causes blisters. The *Strep. pyogenes* triggers especially a marked inflammatory response as the immune system (innate and

537

adaptive) attempts to localize the infection. The pathogen produces a number of toxic products and enzymes which help the pathogen to spread in the skin tissue. Suppuration develops rapidly and a thick, elevated yellow crust is formed. The regional lymph glands are involved resulting in lymphadenitis and lymphangitis. Streptococcal infections sometimes affect the deeper layers of the skin and cause the development of cellulitis which may leave lesions on healing. Untreated cases of streptococcal infection may develop glomerulonephritis as complication.

❑ A mixed infection is fairly common caused by staphylococci and streptococci. Pustular lesions develop that often merge to form large crusts. Pus escapes from under the crusts when pressure is applied. The crusts are fairly loose and when removed, it leaves a bare, raw area. On healing, a temporary area of erythema is visible.

❑ Bulbous impetigo of the newborn (pemphigus neonatorum) is an extreme staphylococcal infection of the epidermis caused by *Staph. aureus* and/or by a strain of *Staph. aureus* that produces a specific toxin known as "exfoliating or scalded skin syndrome toxin or specific epidermolytic staphylococcal toxin" which destroys the intercellular connections in the skin. The infection is characterized by large superficial blisters covering the entire body or large areas of the body of the newborn. The vesicles may form pustules with pus escaping. When the blisters burst, loss of fluid from the damaged surface may also occur. A thin, flat crust is formed over the lesion. The newborn may develop pyrexia, sometimes diarrhoea, and a septicaemia or toxaemia which may be fatal. The appearance may be confused with localised scalded skin syndrome (Ritter's disease).

❖ **Clinical manifestation**
- Initially, maculae are formed, followed by vesicles, pustules and finally crusts
- Lymph nodes can be enlarged
- Skin lesions develop mainly on the face and exposed parts of the body but other parts can also be affected
- The skin lesions can be few or in abundance, large or small
- Systemic involvement does not occur except in infants
- The condition is sometimes secondary to or concomitant with eczema, ringworm, head lice, insect bites, scabies or even chicken-pox
- On healing, permanent lesions may be left in the skin
- Infants and young children may develop malaise and become irritable

❖ **Complications**
- Glomerulonephritis (streptococcus)
- Empyema
- Meningitis (*staphylococcus aureus*)

■ **Diagnosis**
- Clinical picture
- Identification of the specific pathogen in skin lesions

■ **Prognosis**
- Good

■ **Specific healthcare interventions to be rendered**
  - Chemotherapy – antimicrobial drugs
  - Soften the crusts with a normal saline solution and treat with an antibiotic ointment or cream
  - Cover lesions until the crust falls off
  - As soon as the crusts have fallen off, the skin lesions may be painted with an antiseptic solution and left open

◆ **Preventive measures to be taken**
  - Nasal carriers of *staph aureus* can be treated with nasal creams containing an antimicrobial drug
  - Regular nose and hand cultures to be taken of **all healthcare practitioners and other employees (including medical practitioners)** working in maternity wards (ante-natal, delivery and postnatal), paediatric wards, neonatal and paediatric intensive care units. When the practitioner is a carrier, antimicrobial therapy must be commenced. When the carriage state does not clear, the practitioner must be allocated to other occupational settings
  - Rigorous adherence to hand washing procedures

◆ **Measures to prevent epidemics**
  - Children with impetigo should not attend educational institutions until they are completely free of the infection. When they do attend school, the lesions should be covered
  - Adults with impetigo may only visit public places if the lesions are covered
  - Strict adherence to the school exclusion regulations must be maintained

◆ **Implications for disaster situations**
  - Impetigo spreads rapidly amongst large groups of persons

◆ **Compliance with international measures**
  - None

12.2   MYCOBACTERIUM INFECTIONS OF THE SKIN

Mycobacteria are Gram-positive bacilli (rods) that have a thick layer of peptidoglycan external to the cell membrane. The outer envelope contains a variety of lipids (mycolic acids) that not only have a different chemical basis of cross-linking to the lipoprotein layer but also create a waxy layer that gives considerable resistance to drying out as well as to other environmental factors. Mycobacterium are able to avoid phagocytosis by the host cells as it has a slimy surface created by an additional capsule of high molecular polysaccharides (this high molecular polysaccharides also determines the virulence of the mycobacterium). Mycobacterium can also avoid killing off after phagocytosis by surviving intra-cellular in the macrophages. Cell-mediated immunity is elicited as resistance to reactivation of a latent infection.

12.2.1　LEPROSY (LEPRAE, HANSEN'S DISEASE)

Leprosy is a chronic skin disease characterized by gross deformities of the skin and the superficial peripheral nerves. Involvement of other organs of the body may also develops

---

Epidemiological data

Geographic distribution

Leprosy is prevalent world-wide and the largest percentage of cases occurs in Asia, Australia, South America and Africa. The disease is endemic in in South Africa

Causative pathogen

Mycobacterium leprae

Incubation period

Leprosy is not highly contagious as prolonged exposure to the infected source is necessary. The average incubation period is estimated to be 2–10 years which makes it very difficult to control the disease

Mode of transmission

Prolonged exposure to an infected source is necessary. Transmission occurs as follows
*Inhalation of airborne infected droplets. Large numbers of *M. leprae* are present on the mucosa of
  the nose, throat and mouth of an untreated person with lepromatous leprosy
*Direct contact through broken skin when prolonged close physical contact occurs
*By using contaminated instruments during ceremonial tattooing

Period of infectiousness (communicability, transmission)

With effective antimicrobial chemotherapy approximately 99% of the *M. leprae* in the body are killed off within seven (7) days after chemotherapy has been commenced. Transmission by airborne droplets is eliminated in this way. It takes, however, sometimes years before all *M. leprae* in the skin are killed off

Reservoir

Humans. The vast majority of infected persons do not present with outspoken clinical features, thus forming a reservoir for the *M. leprae*. It is estimated that the reservoir consists of more than 25% of the inhabitants of an endemic region

Intermediaries

Vehicles - Fomites such as contaminated handkerchiefs, bandages. (It could not yet be proved that the disease can be transmitted by contaminated food and eating utensils)

Carriers

None

Susceptibility and resistance of host

Elderly persons and children younger than 15 years are particularly susceptible. Approximately 80% of all leprosy sufferers are adults. There is no difference in susceptibility according to gender until puberty – thereafter the incidence is higher in men than in women. All races are susceptible

---

to leprosy although the disease occurs more often in persons with dark skin colour. The reason for this is unknown. Leprosy is not hereditary although a genetic susceptibility is being investigated. Leprosy occurs mostly in regions where poor diet, poor personal and environmental hygiene, poverty and overpopulation are common circumstances

Pathogenesis

Very little is known about the mechanism of pathogenicity of *M. leprae* as the bacillus cannot be grown in artificial culture media. *M. leprae* grows extremely slow and grows better at temperatures below 37°C. *M. leprae* shares many pathobiological features with *M. tuberculosis humanis* but the clinical manifestations of the disease are quite differently. *M. leprae* grows intra-cellular, typically within the histiocytes and endothelial cells of the skin and the Schwann cells of the peripheral nerves, hence, its concentration in the skin and superficial nerves. The *M. leprae* cannot penetrate the central nervous system directly proximal to the dorsal ganglions - therefore, the central nervous system is never affected. However, *M. leprae* does infiltrate the corneal branch of the fifth cranial nerve and the facial branches of the seventh cranial nerve.

The reaction of the body to the invasion of *M. leprae* is cellular as a cell-mediated immune reaction is elicited. Depending on the presence or absence of the immuno-biological cell-mediated reaction in the body of the infected person, the spectrum of disease activity is very broad – the disease may clear up, or it may remain stable though infectious, or it may progress into lepromatous leprosy or tuberculoid leprosy. Intermediate forms of the dimorphic type may also occur and may progress to either extreme lepromatous leprosy or extreme tuberculoid leprosy.

M. leprae flourishes in the cooler parts of the body and the first lesions normally appear on the face, back or limbs. Minimal sensory changes can be observed and are considered the earliest clinically observable form of leprosy. As soon as the peripheral sensory nerves are affected, a gradual to total anaesthesia develops. Impairment of the motor nerves follows as large peripheral branches of nerves are affected.

The **non-infectious, tuberculoid (numb)** form of leprosy affects only the nerves, in particular the sensory and autonomous peripheral nerves as the *M. leprae* multiply in the nerve sheaths. When large mixed types of nerves are affected, paralysis may occur. Nerve lesions are usually single and asymmetrical. The nerve thickens due to cellular infiltration and may be irregular or spindle-shaped. Anaesthesia (loss of sensation) occurs in the affected nerves followed by muscular weakness, atrophy of the muscle tissue and destructive degeneration of nerve tissues. Due to the affliction of the nerves, deformities and tropic ulcerations develop. The latter is the result of the insensitivity of the affected tissue to pressure and injuries. Sometimes the skin may also be involved. A few single or scattered lesions may appear. The size of the lesions varies and displays a clear, sharp, elevated outline. These skin lesions are usually rough, dry, hairless, numb and hypo-pigmented. No systemic involvement of the body occurs. The tuberculoid form usually affects persons with a good cell-mediated immunity (a vigorous cell-mediated immune response is elicited leading to phagocytic destruction of the mycobacterium and exaggerated allergic responses). With chemotherapeutic treatment the person reacts positively and recovers rapidly.

The **infectious nodular or lepromatous** type manifests mainly with skin lesions. In lepromatous leprosy the skin as well as the nasal mucosa and septum is usually effected. The *M. leprae* also rapidly multiplies in the blood and manifest as a systemic disease with multiple organ involvement (due to the multiplying of *M. leprae* in the body), although the infected person presents with no pyrexia, no leukocytosis, no anaemia or no any other signs of a systemic infection. Small peripheral nerves are not destroyed and loss of sensation is not present in the early stage, nor does the infiltrate spread. The skin lesions are multiple tiny symmetrical maculae which spread across the entire body. They grow quickly, can merge, are shiny, erythematous and have indistinct boundaries. The lesions usually appear first on the cooler parts of the body but spread later across the entire body. When they remain untreated, they grow into thick skin nodules, the so-called lepromas which appear particularly on the forehead, earlobes, eyebrows, nose, and jaw areas. The person's eye-lashes and the hair of the eyebrows fall out and unnatural wrinkles form to present the typical "lion-faced" appearance. Many extra-cellular *M. leprae* are visible in the lesions. Gross deformities together with thickening and enlargement of the nostrils, ears, and cheeks develop. There is progressive destruction of the nasal septum while the septum is loaded with *M. leprae*. The lepromatous form usually effects those persons with a lack of cell-mediated immunity.

Note
Anaesthesia, trophic ulcers, palsies, deformities and loss of function may be concomitant with all forms of leprosy. The course of the disease is slow and death is usually due to other causes

❖ **Clinical manifestation**
- Because *M. leprae* grows extremely slow, the onset of leprosy is gradual and the first and most common complaints for which the infected individual seeks medical help, are
  - Skin lesions that change colour and are painless. The infected person complains that the lesions are cosmetically unattractive
  - Loss of sensation that leads to physical injuries such as burns, abrasions and cuts with ulceration and delayed healing
  - Muscle weakness. This is often the first complaint of a infected individual and if the person does not receive chemotherapy and medical treatment, paralysis of the muscles may develop
  - Itching. Dispersed itching of the skin appears for a short while before the skin lesions appear. It is seldom associated with leprosy
  - Swelling of hands and feet may occur although, once again, it is seldom associated with leprosy
  - Pain is a rare symptom but may initially be present in the affected peripheral nerves

- ◆ Bone changes, particularly in the fingers and toes, are already serious complications of leprosy, but unfortunately these are seldom the first complaints
- ◆ Palpable peripheral nerves that may be observed by the person himself/ herself or may be identified during a physical examination
- Depending on the presence or absence of cell-mediated immune response, tuberculoid leprosy or lepromatous leprosy or intermediated forms of leprosy develops
  - ✹ Tuberculoid leprosy presents with
    - ✠ Blotchy red lesions with anaesthetic areas on the face, trunk and extremities
    - ✠ Palpable thickening of the peripheral nerves
    - ✠ Repeated trauma and secondary bacterial infection of the local anaesthetic areas as the affected individual is rendered prone by the anaesthesia
    - ✠ Tuberculoid leprosy can progress across the spectrum towards lepromatous leprosy in some individuals
  - ✹ Lepromatous leprosy present with
    - ✠ Extensive skin involvement with large numbers of *M. leprae* in affected areas
    - ✠ Loss of eyebrows and thickening and enlargement of the nostrils, ears and cheeks resulting in the typical leonine (lion-like) facial appearance as the disease progresses
    - ✠ Progressive destruction of the nasal septum. The nasal mucosa is loaded with *M. leprae*
    - ✠ Gross deformities - a characteristic of late lepromatous leprosy. The deformities result primarily from the infectious destruction of the naso-maxillary facial structures and, secondarily, from pathological changes in the peripheral nerves that are predisposed to repeated trauma and subsequent super-infection with other pathogens
  - ✹ Individuals suffering from intermediated forms such as borderline lepromatous leprosy or borderline tuberculoid leprosy may progress to either extreme

❖ Complications
- Deformities of limbs and skin
- Blindness

■ Diagnostic tests
- Alertness to the possibility of leprosy when confronted with dermatological, neurological or/and multisystem complains
- Specific diagnostic tests to be done include
  - ✠ Skin smears of lesions
  - ✠ Biopsies of skin lesions and/or thickened nerve branches
  - ✠ Nose and throat swabs
  - ✠ Nasal scrapings

- **Prognosis**
  - Tuberculoid leprosy – fair to good and in some individuals the disease is self-limiting
  - Lepromatous leprosy - poor

- **Specific healthcare interventions to be rendered**
  - **Specific medical healthcare interventions**

    The management principles of the prescribed chemotherapeutic regime for the individual suffering from leprosy comprise the following
    - Hospitalization is rarely necessary
    - Should infected individuals be hospitalized, they are isolated for a period of 8–11 weeks until they have been declared non-infectious according to the chemotherapeutic regime. Following this, instruction is given regarding the nature and duration of the chemotherapeutic regime. The infected individuals are then treated as out-patient healthcare users under supervision of a community healthcare provider (professional or traditional or lay care giver)
    - Administering of multiple drug therapy (multidrug therapy). The disease is not transmissible 2–3 days after antimicrobial chemotherapy has been commenced
    - To prevent non-compliance with the chemotherapeutic regime (since the regime can last as long as two years or longer) the marking points regarding poor/non-compliance should be built into the programme and should receive continuous attention
    - An acute immunological reaction may occur during the period that chemotherapy is administered, namely, Erythema Nodosum Leprosum (ENL). ENL is usually an immunological complication which is characterized by pyrexia, malaise, dispersed red, hot, elevated or nodular rash, acute neuritis, swollen joints, albuminuria, and itching of the body. New skin lesions or nodules multiply rapidly, pain occurs in the eyes, nerves and legs as well as neurological impairment such as paralysis and swollen joints and limbs. When ENL occurs, hospitalization is necessary and the sufferer is considered a medical emergency. The immediate specific healthcare interventions comprises
      - ∗ Painkillers, especially drugs containing aspirin
      - ∗ Anti-inflammatory drugs
      - ∗ Corticosteroids for the treatment of neuritis
      - ∗ The existing chemotherapeutic programme should under no circumstances be terminated
      - ∗ The prescribed drug regime must include Dapson (a sulphonamide) as it is the most important bacteriostatic drug against leprosy and must be administered for a period of five (5) years. (When a sulpha drug allergy is present, prescribe a different combination of drugs.) To prevent the individual from poor/non-compliance with therapy (and to avoid building up a resistance to the anti-mycobacterial drugs prescribed) the

chemotherapy regime for leprosy should form part of the community healthcare service delivery

- **General healthcare interventions**

  Since most sufferers from leprosy are only diagnosed after complications have set in, all healthcare interventions are symptomatic and supportive

  ✠ **Rehabilitation**

  Rehabilitation is a multi-professional team effort and must be implemented as soon as the diagnosis has been made

  ✴ **Physical rehabilitation and care**

  ◈ <u>Treatment of any form of ulceration</u>, particularly plantar ulcers. This is usually the result of injuries sustained due to loss of sensation in the limbs. The infected individual must be taught to identify and avoid the causes such as burns and pressure

  ◈ <u>Specific treatment of dry, chapped skin</u> by daily washing in lukewarm salt water and massaging cream or oil into the skin

  ◈ <u>Daily foot care</u> is very important

  - ⅄ Examine all pressure points – red or hot areas are signs of the forming of ulcers
  - ⅄ Examine shoes daily for nails, sand, dust and stones. Remove these
  - ⅄ Exercise the ankle wrist joints to prevent dropped feet
  - ⅄ When foot problems occur, avoid excessive walking
  - ⅄ Dry thoroughly between the toes – examine skin areas between the toes daily for infections, broken skin or moist spots
  - ⅄ Always wear shoes
  - ⅄ Avoid taking large steps
  - ⅄ Avoid walking long distances

  ◈ <u>Pay attention to the type of shoes worn</u>. Shoes have to fit comfortably to prevent friction. Open sandals are ideal. The tips and soles of shoes have to be reinforced to protect the toes. Soft, genuine leather should be used and nails or wire must not be used for stitching. When the feet are already deformed, special shoes should be made to measure. Inner soles made from sponge rubber, or sheepskin or microcellular material are recommended. Velcro should be used for buckles and straps instead of metal or other stitching materials

  ◈ Give special attention <u>to all pressure points of the body</u>

  ◈ <u>Caring of the hands</u>

  - ⅄ All injuries must be considered as serious
  - ⅄ Protect the hands when working/playing
  - ⅄ Bandage injured fingers and immobilize them when necessary
  - ⅄ Be on the lookout for hot and sharp objects
  - ⅄ Hand exercises must be done daily

  ◈ <u>Caring of the eyes</u>

  - ⅄ Do eyelid exercises daily

- Inspect eyes daily for redness, infection, excess lacrimation or any other abnormality. Obtain medical help as soon as possible
- Protect eyes by wearing sunglasses
- Wash eyes daily in clean water
- Use eye-drops (for example, Eye gene, Natural tears) daily, in the morning and at night
- Wear a hat outdoors and in the sun
- Do not rub the eyes
- When the eyes are infected, consult a doctor

❖ <u>Physiotherapy must be done daily</u> to prevent contractures, to keep the wrists mobile, strengthen affected muscles and prevent muscular atrophy and stretching

❖ <u>Reconstructive and plastic surgery are done to</u>
- Correct lagophthalmos, entropion or ectropion
- Correct difficulties in closing of the mouth caused by paralysis of the facial nerves
- Correct/improve claw hands and feet and/or loss of joints by lengthening and transplanting tendons
- Effect cosmetic correction of facial lesions such as thickened eyebrow, pinna and ear lobes, removal of wrinkles and reconstruction of the nose and jaw

❖ <u>Giving of health information to the family and community</u>
- Have the infected individual, his family and the community join the non-governmental organizations such as the Leprosy Mission
- Give health information regarding leprosy
- Help the family not to reject the infected individual
- Teach the family how to maintain the "self care programme" in order to help the infected family member

* **Psychosocial rehabilitation**
  ❖ This includes the prevention of social isolation of the infected individual by appropriate employment, schooling (when necessary) and reinstatement in the community
  ❖ One of the most important tasks of all healthcare providers is to supply the public with the necessary knowledge regarding leprosy in order to prevent ignorance, stigmatising and prejudice which is often more difficult to handle than the disease itself

◆ **Preventive measures to be taken**
  ➢ There is no vaccine available against leprosy or specific preventive measures to implement
  ➢ <u>General primary preventive measures include</u>
    ✤ Improving the general physical resistance of all persons
    ✤ Maintaining of good personal hygiene

⚕ Combating overcrowding and poor housing (this restricts close physical contact between persons)

⚕ Vaccination of all children with BCG vaccine. The incidence of tuberculoid leprosy in certain developing countries has drastically been lowered since vaccination with BCG was introduced

➢ <u>Secondary prevention is presently the highest priority in the care of persons suffering from leprosy and comprises the following</u>

⚕ Early diagnosis and administering of chemotherapy immediately

⚕ Tracing of contacts and administering of chemotherapy, when desirable or necessary

⚕ Regular control of the administering of chemotherapy and follow-up visits to monitor the infected individual's general health and progress

◆ **Measures to prevent epidemics**
  ⬥ Adherence to the school exclusion regulations

◆ **Implications during disaster situations**
  ⬥ None

◆ **Compliance with international measures**
  ⬥ None

12.3   PARASITIC INFECTIONS OF THE SKIN

The skin is a major route of entry for parasites which may
  ❑ penetrate directly (for example, schistosomes, nematodes)
  ❑ be injected by blood-feeding vectors.

Many of these parasites leave the skin almost immediately, but some remain there and others may become trapped. A few parasites actually exit the body through the skin. Pathologic responses to parasites associated with the skin range from mild to disabling severe. Invertebrate vectors such as insects, ticks and mites (the bloodsuckers) are the most important vectors spreading infection. Certain ticks, lice and mites live on blood or tissue fluids from humans, feeding non-selectively or host-specific on humans. The feeding processes and the inevitable release of saliva give rise to skin irritation which becomes more intense as the body responds immunologically to the proteins present in the saliva. When populations of lice and scabies mites that spend the greater part or the whole of their lives on the human body accumulate, severe skin conditions are caused. These conditions arise from
  ◈ the activity of the parasites themselves
  ◈ their production of excreta
  ◈ the oozing of blood and tissue fluids from the feeding sites
  ◈ the host's immunological responses.

12.3.1   SCABIES

Scabies is a parasitic infested skin condition presenting with a characteristic skin rash caused by the scabies mite that burrows into the skin and cause irritation. Secondary infections may follow scratching

---

Epidemiological data

Geographic distribution
Scabies occurs world-wide

Causative pathogen
The mite, *Sarcoptes or Acarus scabiei*. The female mite lays her eggs in burrows under the skin where it hatches 3-4 days later. The larvae leave the burrow and hide in the hair follicles of the skin. After 4-6 days when the adult stage is reached, the mites mate and the cycle is repeated. In infants and children the burrows are clearly visible as meandering, pinkish elevations of the skin which are only a few millimetres in length. Sometimes the dark faeces of the mites are visible at the opening of the burrow. In adults it is difficult to see the burrow – it may not be visible to the naked eye

Incubation period
Usually 1– 4 days

Mode of transmission
Contact with an infested person

Period of infectiousness (communicability, transmission)
For as long as living mites appear on the skin

Reservoir
Humans

Intermediaries
Vehicles - Clothing, bed linen and personal items shared with an infested person

Carriers
None

Immunity status
No immunity with memory is elicited

Susceptibility and resistance of host
All persons are susceptible, regardless of their personal state of hygiene. The condition is, however, more prevalent where overcrowding occurs and when personal hygiene is poor. The condition spreads rapidly in schools, hostels and camps

---

Pathogenesis
The scabies mite generally burrows in the skin body folds such as the inter-digital web space of the fingers, the wrists, elbow and knee folds, axilla, groins and around the waistline. The area of infection can, however, spread to cover large areas of the body from the original site. In infants, the entire body is affected, including the face

and palms of the hands. The genitals of little boys may also be affected. A vesicle or pustule forms in the skin at the site of the burrow. An immunological reaction develops and an extremely itchy erythematous-papular rash develops around the burrows. The extent of the rash bears no relation to the number of parasites present on the skin as it is an immunological reaction. Secondary infections may follow scratching. In immuno-compromised individuals or in persons who are unable to care adequately for themselves, very heavy infections may develop. Under these conditions there is extensive thickening and crusting of the skin.

❖ **Clinical manifestation**
- An erythematous-papular rash which is extremely itchy (particularly at night) develops on any part of the body
- The affected person is not systemically ill but a secondary infection presents concomitant with pyrexia, headache and malaise
- If the skin lesions are broken when scratched and become infected, pustules appear which later rupture and form scabs. (The septic skin lesions may hamper the diagnosis)

❖ **Complications**
- Secondary infections

■ **Diagnosis**
- Clinical picture
- The female mite is visible under a magnifying glass, particularly around the hair follicles where they feed and shelter
- The mite can be microscopically identified from a skin scraping, particularly when this is taken from the entrance to the burrow in the skin

■ **Prognosis**
- Good

■ **Specific healthcare interventions to be rendered**
- All members of the family and all contacts must receive treatment
- All bed linen, towels, face cloths and clothing that may possible have been infested, have to be washed and ironed
- Toilet articles and toys have to be disinfested
- The local treatment to destroy the mite is as follows
  - ✠ Taking of a hot bath while washing the skin thoroughly with a specific soap such as Tetmosol soap
  - ✠ Thoroughly drying of the skin with a rough towel
  - ✠ Applying a 25% benzyl-benzoate preparation such as ascabiol or any other 1% gamma benzene hexachloride preparation to the entire body
  - ✠ Dressing in clean clothes and changing of all used bed linen
  - ✠ Repeating the procedure after 24 hours and again after one week in order to destroy any mites which may still have hatched
  - ✠ The use of Tetmosol soap is recommended to prevent re-infestation
  - ✠ Septic skin lesions must be treated with an antimicrobial cream/ ointment

♦ **Preventive measures to be taken**
  ➢ Combating overcrowding and unhygienic personal habits
  ➢ Avoiding physical contact with persons who have itchy rashes
  ➢ Identifying and treating all sources of infesting
  ➢ Protecting of healthcare providers when treating infested cases by wearing gloves and washing of hands with Tetmosol soap or a similar product
  ➢ Scratching of the skin by the infested person must be prevented. Children should wear mittens
  ➢ Avoiding the use of infested bed linen, towels and face cloths
  ➢ Parents and teachers should be informed regarding early identification of the condition

♦ **Measures to prevent epidemics**
  ⬥ Children with untreated scabies are not allowed to attend educational institutions
  ⬥ Public gatherings must be avoided during epidemics of scabies
  ⬥ Contacts must be examined and treated
  ⬥ Strict adherence to the school exclusion regulations must be maintained

♦ **Implications during disaster situations**
  ⬥ Scabies spreads rapidly amongst large groups of persons

♦ **Compliance with international measures**
  ⬥ None

12.4 MUCOCUTANEOUS LESIONS CAUSED BY VIRUSES

Viruses by themselves are metabolically inert – they replicate only after having infected a host's cell(s) and parasitized the host's ability to transcribe and/or translate genetic information. Not only infect viruses every form of life but they also cause some of the most common and many of the most serious diseases in humans. The most common forms of virus transmission are
◈ via inhaled droplets (for example, measles)
◈ in food and water (for example, hepatitis A)
◈ from bites of vector arthropods (for example, Yellow fever).
The process of attachment to the host's cells depends first upon the operation of general intermolecular forces and then there after upon more specific interactions between the molecules of the nucleocapsid (in naked viruses) or the virus membrane (in enveloped viruses) and the molecules of the host cell membrane. In many cases there is a specific interaction with a particular host molecule which acts as a receptor for the specific virus. After fusion of the viral and host membrane or the uptake into the phagosome, the virus particle is carried into the cytoplasm across the plasma membrane. As soon as the envelope and/or the capsid are shed and the viral nucleic acid is released, the virus is no more infective. This "eclipse phase" persists until new complete virus particles re-form after replication. Viruses are difficult targets for antimicrobial chemotherapy but can be controlled by effective vaccines.

Muco-cutaneous lesions that are caused by viruses can be divided into

❑ Those in which the virus remains restricted to the body surface at the site of the initial infection (for example, papilloma-virus [warts])

❑ Those in which the virus causes mucocutaneous lesions after spreading systemically through the body (for example, herpes simplex virus infection [cold sores], coxsackie-virus, erythro-virus, measles-virus, rubella-virus and other arthropod transmitted viruses)

Infections that spread systemically can in turn be divided into

✠ those in which the vesicular skin lesions are sites of virus replication and are infectious (for example, smallpox, shingles)

✠ those in which the maculo-papular skin lesions are non-infectious and immunologically mediated. The virus is shed from other sites (for example, from the respiratory tract as in measles, rubella, and other arthropod transmitted viral diseases).

In many systemic viral infectious diseases, the skin rash has a characteristic distribution - with the exception of zoster (the reason being unknown). The skin rash is caused by the viraemia which develops in the body. The typical skin rash can also appear on the mucous membranes of the mouth as well as in other organs of the body. The complications of systemic viral infections with a skin rash are often serious and may even be fatal. Transmission between persons does not normally occur through contact with the skin lesions. Hospitalization is not always necessary.

12.4.1 Systemic viral infections causing a maculo-papular skin rash

12.4.1.1 MEASLES (MORBILLI)

Measles is an acute viral disease characterized by coryza, Koplik's spots and a general maculo-papular rash that lasts approximately one week. The disease is self-limiting but highly transmissible

---

Epidemiological data

Geographic distribution
Measles is prevalent world-wide

Causative pathogen
The *measles-virus*, a member of the genus Morbilli virus of the family Paramyxoviridae

Incubation period
10 days on average although it may vary from 8–13 days. The maculo-papular rash usually appears 14 days after being infected with the virus

Mode of transmission
Horizontally - Airborne infected droplets

Period of infectiousness (communicability, transmission)
From the late catarrhal stage until the temperature subsides – approximately 2 days after the onset of the maculo-papular rash

Reservoir
Humans. The virus is present in the pharyngeal secretions as well as in the blood and urine of the infected person

Intermediaries
Vehicles: Fomites although inactivation occurs as the *measles-virus* dries out on surfaces

Carriers
None

Immunity status
Immunity with memory is elicited
Pregnant women, who have had Measles or were vaccinated against the disease, transmit natural passively-acquired immunity (which last a few months) via the placenta to the unborn foetus

Susceptibility and resistance of host
Every person is susceptible. Artificial active vaccination only lasts a number of years. Vaccinated children may experience an atypical attack of Measles later in life. All infants belong to the high-risk group and during an epidemic all infants may contract the disease – even neonates

---

Pathogenesis

After being inhaled, the *measles-virus* attaches itself to the mucous membrane of the upper and lower respiratory tract at unknown sites where the *measles-virus* starts to replicate. The measles-virus now disseminates in large numbers into the blood causing a primary viraemia resulting in the leukocytes becoming infected by the virus. From the blood the measles-virus spreads, by means of the infected leucocytes, to the sub-epithelial and local lymphatic tissues without causing detectable lesions or symptoms. During the next few days, the *measles-virus* slowly spreads and multiplies in all lymphoid tissues in the body including the spleen. About one week after being infected, the infected reticulo-endothelial cells die off while releasing large numbers of *measles-viruses*. The leukocytes are now re-infected and a secondary viraemia is caused. The *measles-virus* disseminates now to a variety of epithelial sites such as the lungs (temporary respiratory illness), the ear (otitis media), oral mucosa (Koplik's spots), skin (maculo-papular rash), and intestinal tract (although no lesion or diarrhoea develops, the infection of the gastro-intestinal epithelial site may lead to exacerbating malnutrition, halting of growth and impairment of recovery). During this phase, the catarrhal phase, the entire mucosa of the respiratory tract, the gastro-intestinal tract and eyes are infected while the infection of the upper respiratory tract goes concomitant with coughing. Secondary bacterial infections may develop because of the oedematous mucous membranes and reduced movement of the cilia, (especially in the respiratory tract) with subsequent otitis media, pneumonia, gastroenteritis and corneal ulceration. The ill individual is highly infectious because of the large numbers of *measles-viruses* being shed in the respiratory secretions.

The cell-mediated immune response is elicited at this stage to combat the growth of the *measles-virus* in the lungs and elsewhere – without the cell-mediated response the *measles-virus* continues to grow and gives rise to giant cell pneumonia.

Two days before the appearance of the skin rash and a few days after the onset of the infection of the upper respiratory tract, Koplik's spots appear on the oral mucosa. Koplik's spots are minute white spots (resembling grains of salt) on the inflamed buccal mucosa and are present until approximately two days after the skin rash had appeared. The typical measles skin rash is a maculo-papular rash which clears up within 5–10 days. The rash does not itch and is caused by the cell-mediated immune response when the *measles-virus* invades the cells of the epidermis and the oral mucous membranes (Koplik's spots). An antibody-mediated immunological reaction with memory is elicited which last life-long. The skin rash does not appear in ill individuals suffering from a deficiency in cell-immunity and the infected person becomes seriously ill. The exception is persons suffering from agammaglobulinemia who experience the normal course of measles and develop normal cell-mediated immunity with memory. The person suffering from agammaglobulinemia can be protected by vaccination.

❖ **Clinical manifestation**

The disease is characterised by two pronounce phases, namely, the catarrhal phase and the phase of exanthema (skin rash)

✱ **Catarrhal phase commences 9-10 days after infection had occurred**
- The catarrhal phase lasts four (4) days on average and is the first sign of measles
- During this phase the person is seriously ill and experiences general lassitude, pyrexia, anorexia, conjunctivitis and respiratory symptoms (coryza), a persistent non-productive cough, runny nose with concomitant bouts of sneezing and laryngitis
- These signs are caused by the *measles-virus* and not by a secondary infection
- The catarrhal phase of Measles is often confused with an acute upper respiratory tract infection due to its clinical manifestations
- However, the appearance of Koplik's spots on the mucous membranes of the mouth excludes such a diagnosis
- Koplik's spots appear from the second day of the catarrhal phase and last until approximately two days after the measles rash had appeared. Koplik's spots appear mostly on the buccal mucous membranes of the cheeks. In severe cases the entire oral buccal mucosa can be covered with these spots

✱ **Period of skin rash (stage of exanthema)**
- The typical measles skin rash appears on the face, particularly behind the ears and neck and from there spreads to the rest of the body
- The rash initially consists of maculae, rapidly developing into a confluent maculo-papular rash. The rash is confluent on the face and neck but has a spotty appearance on the rest of the body

- The rash is brownish-pink in colour and after about five days it starts to clear up by means of a brown desquamation in those areas where it first appeared

✳ **General signs and symptoms**
  - The individual is very ill from the onset of the catarrhal phase until the third (3rd) day after the appearance of the rash
  - At this stage the ill person presents with hyperpyrexia (± 40°C), confluent Koplik's spots on the inflamed buccal mucous membranes, puffy eyelids, severe coryza with nasal secretions and coughing
  - Within 24–48 hours after the appearance of the skin rash, the body temperature drops rapidly while the conjunctivitis, nasal secretions and coughing rapidly resolve and the individual feels much better
  - If no complications occur, the disease lasts 7–10 days from the catarrhal phase until the rash has cleared up

NOTE

All persons who have been vaccinated against measles may experience an atypical attack of measles years later. The term "atypical" refers to the unusual signs and symptoms experienced by these individuals. During the catarrhal phase which lasts for 1-2 days, the person experiences low-grade pyrexia. The skin rash consists of irregular maculo-papular maculae which almost never forms a confluent rash. Children are not very ill (although some children do become seriously ill) and the characteristic cough may be absent. But the older the individual gets (adolescents and adults), the far more seriously ill the individual becomes when he/she contracts measles. The individual sometimes need to be hospitalized and complications that last life-long develop more often

❖ **Complications**

The complications of measles are divided into two groups, namely, those affecting the respiratory tract and those affecting the central nervous system. Owing to the serious nature of the complications, the disease is presently regarded as a serious health risk for infants and children. The disease occurs mostly in children between the ages of 10 months and three (3) years, especially those living in poor socio-economic circumstances

- **Respiratory tract**
  - ◈ Secondary bacterial super-infection(s) of the respiratory tract play an important role in the development of respiratory complications
  - ◈ Laryngitis with severe oedema of the larynx, vocal cords and epiglottis may occur. In this case, the ill person experiences laryngeal stridor and in severe cases restlessness, anxiety and severe dyspnoea may be present
  - ◈ Another respiratory complication is bronchitis. All individuals suffering from measles experience a persistent cough which is one of the last symptoms to disappear when the disease resolves. When the ill person develops bronchitis as well, severe tachypnoea is present
  - ◈ A further respiratory complication is pneumonia which is most often broncho-pneumonia. The cough intensifies and worsens and the ill person becomes dyspnoeic and even cyanotic

◈ Otitis media which is characterized by a red, bulging tympanic membrane is a related respiratory complication which may occur. The ill individual may not necessarily complain of earache

- **Central nervous system**
  ◈ As is the case in any disease characterized by pyrexia, convulsions may occur, particularly in children younger than four years
  ◈ Encephalitis is a less common but very serious complication of measles due to perivascular infiltration and demyelisation of the brain substance. When this occurs, the onset of measles-encephalitis is 4 - 6 days after the appearance of the skin rash. At this stage the ill individual without encephalitis is beginning to recover dramatically, while the ill individual with encephalitis becomes very ill. The pyrexia, which usually drops within 48 hours after the appearance of the rash, remains the same or becomes higher elevated - either gradually or suddenly
  ◈ Other neurological impairments are also present
  ◈ Very rarely, sub-acute sclerosing pan-encephalitis develops after apparent recovery from an acute infection. The *measles–virus* gains entry into the brain substance via perivascular infiltration during the acute phase of measles. The *measles-virus* growth is slow, often incomplete and partially controlled by host defences. After an incubation period of 1-10 years, the clinical disease of sub-acute sclerosing pan-encephalitis appears

- **Less serious complications**
  ◈ After an attack of measles some infants and young children may develop Protein-Energy-Malnutrition (Kwashiorkor) or marasmus
  ◈ Herpes stomatitis, cardiac and renal failure and blindness may occur
  ◈ In the first few months after recovery there is also a high incidence of respiratory tract infections
  ◈ Because of the high ratio of herd immunity under young children due to vaccination, Measles is now becoming a disease contracted by adolescents and young adults. Adolescents and adults contracting measles are severely ill and complications occur more often
  ◈ The overall clinical impact of measles is much more serious in malnourished individuals with poor access to medical care. The epithelial surfaces of the individual are more extensively infected and more serious sequelae result. Not only are the local mucosal defences of the malnourished individual impaired but the impairment of the individual's immune defences is further increased by the added impact of immuno-suppression by the *measles-virus*. Also, most malnourished individuals live in poor communities where they are exposed to a higher concentration of the *measles-virus* as well as high levels of bacterial contamination of the environment

■ **Diagnosis**
  ▪ Clinical signs

■ **Prognosis**
  ▪ Good, when properly treated

- The mortality rate is high in children below the age of two (2) years who suffer from malnutrition and live in circumstances of overcrowding

- **Specific healthcare interventions to be rendered**
  - Antimicrobial drugs are prescribed to prevent secondary infections. Antimicrobial drugs must only be prescribed when the person's general state of health is very poor
  - Supportive and symptomatic (home care and in bed)
  - Darken the room with blankets or blinds or curtains that do not let light in because the ill individual experiences severe light sensitivity
  - Observe for complications. When serious complications occur, the person must be hospitalized
  - Vitamin A should be administered to children with a poor health status

- **Preventive measures to be taken**
  - All infants must be vaccinated with measles at the age of 9 months and a booster dose must be given at 18 months. When an epidemic of measles breaks out, infants in the high-risk group must be vaccinated with the attenuated living measles virus vaccine from the age of 6 months. A booster dose must be administered when 18 months old. Should the young child older than 11 months be vaccinated with MMR vaccine the booster dose of measles at 18 months is not necessary
  - Healthy contacts must be vaccinated with the attenuated live measles virus within 48 hours after been exposed to the measles-virus
  - Susceptible contacts must be given immunoglobulin as passive protection within 48 hours after exposure. When the individual does not become ill, vaccination with the attenuated living measles virus vaccine must be continued
  - Enhancement of the immunological resistance of undernourished persons (especially children) by improving their nutritional status

- **Measures to prevent epidemics**
  - Isolation of individuals suffering from measles for 10 days
  - Vaccination of all healthy infants and older children with the attenuated living measles virus vaccine or MMR vaccine and giving of immunoglobulin to susceptible contacts within 48 hours after exposure to measles
  - Maintaining of strict adherence to the school exclusion regulations

- **Implications during disaster situations**
  - A high mortality rate occurs when there is an outbreak of Measles in a community which is particularly susceptible to Measles

- **Compliance with international measures**
  - None

12.4.1.2   GERMAN MEASLES (RUBELLA)

Rubella is generally a very mild (often sub-clinically) acute viral infection that causes a multisystem infection and is characterized by a macular skin rash and enlarged posterior auricular, occipital and cervical lymph nodes. Rubella has, though, a major impact when the unborn foetus is infected

---

Epidemiological data

Geographic distribution
Rubella is prevalent world-wide and the incidence is highest in springtime

Causative pathogen
Rubella-virus

Incubation period
16–18 days although it may vary from 14-21 days

Mode of transmission
Horizontally - Airborne infected droplets from nasopharyngeal secretions
Vertically - Trans-placental

Period of infectiousness (communicability, transmission)
5 days before appearance of rash until approximately three days after the skin rash erupted
In congenital Rubella the virus is transmitted by the baby for months after birth. The latter situation constitutes a serious risk for infecting pregnant women

Reservoir
Humans. The *Rubella virus* is found mainly in the respiratory secretions of infected persons. In congenital Rubella, the virus is present in all body secretions of the infant for several months although the infant often has a high concentration of antibody. The reason for this is unknown

Intermediaries
Vehicles - Fomites

Carriers
None

Immune status
Immunity with memory is elicited

Susceptibility and resistance of host
Everybody is susceptible, particularly children. Pregnant women who are immune to Rubella, transmit natural passively-acquired immunity, via the placenta, to the unborn baby which will protect the infant for several months

---

Pathogenesis
After silently gaining entry into the body via unknown sites in the respiratory tract, the *rubella-virus* infiltrates the local lymph nodes causing the characteristic lymph-adenopathy. The *rubella-virus* replicate for a period of time in the local lymphoid

tissue followed by dissemination, via the lymph drainage system, to the spleen and lymph nodes in the body. Further multiplication in these tissues takes place and one week later a viraemia develops with localization of the *rubella-virus* in the respiratory tract, joints, kidneys and skin. When a female is pregnant the *rubella-virus* may also localize in the placenta, especially during the first trimester of pregnancy. As soon as the skin rash appears, the *rubella-virus* disappears from the bloodstream. The systemic signs caused by the viraemia clear up at the same time. An antibody-mediated immune reaction with memory is elicited, lasting life-long.

❖ **Clinical manifestation**

With the exception of congenital Rubella, children suffer a far milder degree of Rubella than adults. The first sign of rubella in children is usually the skin rash, whereas adults and adolescents first experience a prodromal phase before the skin rash appears

✹ **Prodromal phase**
- The prodromal phase lasts approximately 1–5 days
- It is characterized by a low-grade pyrexia, headache, malaise, anorexia, mild conjunctivitis, coryza, sore throat, cough and lymph-adenopathy
- Red spots, the size of pin pricks, may appear on the oral mucosa of the soft palate of persons suffering from rubella. These spots are known as Forchheimer's spots
- As soon as the viraemia is resolved, all signs and symptoms of the prodromal phase disappear

✹ **Period of skin rash (stage of exanthema)**
- The skin rash that characterizes rubella initially consists of irregular pinkish to red maculae which develop into papulae
- The maculo-papular rash becomes confluent and the skin acquires a pinkish-red glow
- On the first day the rash appears on the face and torso, from where it spreads on the second day to the arms and legs. The skin rash clears up within three days

NOTE

Persons who have been vaccinated as infants may develop an atypical clinical picture of the disease in later life while adolescents and adults become seriously ill and may need to be hospitalized

❖ **Complications**
- Complications are not common
- Complications that occur are arthritis, haemorrhages due to thrombocytopenia and congenital rubella
- The teratogenic consequences of the *rubella-virus* during the first trimester of pregnancy (the rubella-virus crosses the placental barrier) lead to the congenital rubella syndrome in the foetus. This syndrome is characterized by congenital defects such as perception deafness, cataracts and cardiac abnormalities. The specific nature of the congenital defects concurs with the

specific development stage of the foetus when the mother became infected. For example, when the foetus is infected during the neurological developmental stage, the foetus develops neurological congenital abnormalities as well as intellectual disabilities

Serological confirmation that a pregnant woman had been infected with the *rubella-virus* during the first trimester of pregnancy is an indication for an abortion

■ **Diagnosis**
  - Clinical picture
  - A rising antibody titre against the *rubella-virus* in the blood
  - Culture for the presence of the *rubella-virus* in pharyngeal secretions and urine

■ **Prognosis**
  - Good

■ **Specific healthcare interventions to be rendered**
  - Symptomatic and supportive – no specific antimicrobial chemotherapeutic interventions
  - Isolation is not necessary
  - Women in the first trimester of pregnancy must avoid all contact with individuals with a systemic skin rash

◆ **Preventive measures to be taken**
  ➢ Vaccination of infants with MMR vaccine after the age of 11 months
  ➢ Vaccination with the attenuated live *rubella-virus*, particularly of non-pregnant pre-adolescent girls and women who have a low antibody titre immune status and who are contemplating pregnancy

  Please note
  A pregnancy test should be done before vaccination in order to eliminate the possibility of pregnancy. The pregnancy test is indicated for all women who are married or sexually active The only safe period during reproductive life for vaccination of any female is the post-partum period. Taking of a complete history of menstruation is fallible

◆ **Measures to prevent epidemics**
  ⬥ An outbreak of rubella in schools, army camps or other institutions justifies the implementation of a programme of vaccination of high-risk persons
  ⬥ Strict adherence to the school exclusion regulations must be maintained

◆ **Implications during disaster situations**
  ⬥ Poor hygienic conditions may lead to outbreaks of the disease
  ⬥ Active vaccination programmes must be launched.

◆ **Compliance with international measures**
  ⬥ None

12.4.2 Systemic viral infections causing a vesicular skin rash

12.4.2.1 CHICKENPOX (VARICELLA)

Chickenpox is an acute viral disease characterized by crops of vesicles that develop from maculae to papulae to vesicles and then scab over. The disease is highly communicable only by airborne infected droplets. The *varicella-zoster virus* is not present in the scabs and transmission does not occur via direct contact with vesicular fluid or the scabs

---

Epidemiological data

Geographic distribution
Chickenpox occurs world-wide. The disease is more common during winter and spring than during the other seasons of the year

Causative pathogen
Varicella-zoster-virus, a member of the alphaherpesvirus group

Incubation period
14 days, average of 7-23 days
Immuno-compromised individuals encounter a shortened incubation period

Mode of transmission
Horizontally - Airborne infected droplets from respiratory secretions and saliva
Vertically - Trans-placental

Period of infectiousness (communicability, transmission)
From 2 days before the skin rash appears until 7 days after onset when the vesicles have crusted

Reservoir
Humans

Intermediaries
Vehicles - fomites

Carriers
None

Immunity status
Immunity with memory is elicited

Susceptibility and resistance of host
All persons are susceptible. Adults tend to be more seriously affected than children

---

Pathogenesis
After the *varicella-zoster-virus* had been inhaled, infection of the respiratory tract, especially the pharyngeal, palatine and lingual tonsils, occurs. Neither symptoms

nor any detectable lesions at the site of entry into the body are manifested. The *varicella-zoster-virus* passes across the surface epithelium of the respiratory tract to infect both migratory T-cells of the immune system (T-cell tropism) within the tonsillar lymphoid tissues as well as lymphocytes, especially the mononuclear cells in lymphoid nodes. A primary viremia is caused and the *varicella-zoster-virus* is carried to reticulo-endothelial organs such as the liver - facilitated by the virus-mediated modulation of the major histocompatibility complex MHC-I and MHC-II expression. The *varicella-zoster-virus* slowly replicates in the lympho-reticular tissues for about a week resulting in a secondary viraemia. When infected T-cells enter the blood circulation, the *varicella-zoster-virus* is seeded out to the epithelial sites in the body such as the respiratory tract, the skin, the mouth, the conjunctiva, the alimentary tract, and the urinal-genital tract. The skin, the trunk, the face, and the scalp are, for unknown reasons, especially involved. From the before-mentioned epithelial sites, the T-cells infected with the *varicella-zoster-virus* exit through the capillary endothelium by the usual mechanisms for trafficking of migratory T-cells to infect sub-epithelial and finally the epithelial cells of the skin. Multi-nucleated giant cells with intranucleated inclusions are present in the lesions. In the oropharynx and respiratory tract the *varicella-zoster-virus* reaches the surface and is shed to the exterior to infect other individuals about 2 weeks after the initial infection.

When reaching the skin, the *varicella-zoster-virus* mediates the skin rash due to the failure of the *varicella-zoster-virus* to trigger up-regulation of inflammatory adhesion molecules on capillary endothelial cells in the skin. The skin rash passes through several phases, namely, macular, papular, and vesicular followed by scab formation. The vesicles are usually restricted to the epidermis, although the dermis may sometimes also be involved. The vesicles appear first on the trunk, then on the face and scalp, but less commonly on the arms and legs. They often come in 'crops' over the course of several days and all stages of lesions occur simultaneously – maculae, papulae, vesicles, break down, and scabbing over. They leave a small scar on the epidermis when they spontaneously fall off. The marks of the scars disappear within six (6) weeks and the skin retains its normal appearance. When the scabs are scratched off, permanent scars remain even though no infection had occurred. If the vesicles are broken, bacterial infection may take place. The bacterial infection spreads to the dermis of the skin and permanent scars are left. Apart from the skin, chicken-pox lesions may also occur in the lungs, liver, spleen, adrenal glands and pancreas. Lesions may also occur on the mucous membrane of the mouth cavity that is very painful. Four days after the onset of the disease a sufficient number of antibody (varicella-zoster-virus-specific antiviral T-cells) are present in the blood and the viraemia clears up. The disease clears up within a week but the scabs remain on the skin until they fall off naturally. **The scabs do not transmit the *varicella-zoster-virus.***

❖ **Clinical manifestation**
   Chicken-pox is usually more severe and more likely to cause complications in adults and immuno-compromised individuals

* **Prodromal phase**
  - The prodromal phase does not usually occur in children. The first signs of chickenpox in children are low-grade pyrexia (38^0C – 39^0C) (sometimes none) with a simultaneous skin rash (vesicles)
  - The prodromal phase which usually occurs in adults lasts a few days and is characterized by pyrexia, rigor and aching joints as well as a prodromal resembling an influenza-like illness
* **Phase of skin rash (stage of exanthema)**
  - The temperature rises to 38^0C.
  - The vesicular skin rash is characteristically centripetal in distribution and seen in areas of the body that is not exposed to pressure. The rash usually appears first on the trunk and then on the scalp and from there it spreads to the rest of the body. Sometimes two or three vesicles may appear on the trunk of the infected individual a few days before the actual rash appears
  - Within 10–24 hours the vesicular skin rash passes through the various phases, namely, maculae that change into papulae, followed by vesicles. The vesicle is filled with straw-coloured serous fluid. The vesicle breaks down and dries out within days, leaving a scab/crust formation
  - The lesions appear in a series of crops so that the various stages of the skin rash in their genesis appear concurrently on the body at any one time though each stage lasts 2–4 days
  - The grouping of the lesions is as follows - the lesions on the trunk form the first vesicles as the first maculae had appeared on the trunk. The lesions on the arms and legs form vesicles at a later stage
  - Pruritis of the lesions is present during all of the stages and is worst during the formation of scabs
* **Recovery phase**
  - This phase follows 4–5 days after the onset of the disease. The scabs fall off naturally

NOTE
Persons who have been vaccinated as infants may develop an atypical clinical picture of the disease in later life while adolescents and adults become seriously ill and may need to be hospitalized

❖ **Complications**
  - Secondary bacterial infection of broken vesicles is fairly common and a permanent scar is left
  - Permanent scarring of the skin occurs when the scabs are scratched off
  - Haemorrhagic Chickenpox - present 2-3 days after the onset of the rash with haemorrhage into the skin, epistaxis, and melaena or haematuria that can be present. Nothing is known about the pathogenesis of this serious complication
  - Complications that are less common are lymphocytic meningitis or encephalomyelitis and interstitial pneumonia or bacterial/viral pneumonia. In immuno-compromised individuals these complications can run a fulminating course resulting in death. Surviving individuals suffering from pneumonia

may recover either completely or be left with permanent fibrosis of the lungs. Other complications include cerebella ataxia, Guillain-Barre-Syndrome, Reyes syndrome, arthritis, myocarditis, renal and uretic damages

- Pregnant women who contract Chickenpox during pregnancy are at risk for the more serious complications such as pneumonia and encephalitis which can be fatal

- Maternal Varicella infection can be vertically transmitted to the foetus, although the *varicella-zoster-virus* rarely crosses the placenta. When the primary infection happens during the first or second trimester of pregnancy (first 20 weeks), the possibility exists that congenital defects develop such as skin scarring, hypoplastic limbs, and other stigmata involving the eyes and brain - "congenital varicella syndrome" when reactivation of the *varicella-zoster-virus* had apparently taken place in the uterus. An abortion is recommended

- In the late second to third trimester of pregnancy, the *varicella-zoster-virus* can cross the placenta, causing a congenital infection of the foetus. Foetal infection acquired in this way may result in the infant developing Chickenpox in the neonatal period. When maternal antibody has developed, the infection is generally without consequences and mild (only when the Chickenpox rash occurred more than 7 days before delivery as sufficient immunity would have been transferred to the foetus)

- Maternal Chickenpox during the second and third trimester may lead to the appearance of zoster later in life in a healthy infant at birth - with no evidence that the individual ever suffered from Chickenpox in his/her life-time

- When the mother is infected less than 7 days before delivery, the infant is exposed to the *varicella-zoster-virus* without maternal antibody crossing the placenta; the infant can suffer severe disseminated neonatal Chickenpox. Artificial passively-acquired protection with varicella-zoster immunoglobulin may prevent or attenuate the infection in the infant

- Babies born to sero-negative mothers who are infected in the perinatal period are also likely to suffer a severe disseminated neonatal infection as they do not have any protection of *varicella-zoster-virus*-specific maternal IgG

- Zoster (shingles) may result years later from reactivation of latent *varicella-zoster-virus* infection because the *varicella-zoster-virus* had gained entry into the sensory nerve endings from the mucocutaneous lesions during the primary infection and had established a latent infection in the sensory neurons in the cerebral or posterior dorsal root ganglia. Reactivation causes zoster (shingles) in the dermatome at the site of the reactivation such as the thoracic dermatome, because this site is the most common affected site for the original Varicella lesions

- Childhood zoster can occur in children whose mothers contracted Chickenpox during the second and third trimester of pregnancy or when the child self contracted chickenpox very early in life

- Thrombocytopenia can occur but it is usually symptomless

- In immuno-compromised individuals, particular children with leukaemia, Varicella can be a life-threatening disease

■ **Diagnosis**
- Clinical picture

■ **Prognosis**
- Good in immuno-competent individuals
- Serious to fatal in immuno-compromised individuals and neonates

■ **Specific healthcare interventions to be rendered**
- Symptomatic and supportive, particularly regarding the pruritis. Salt or bicarbonate of soda (baking soda) can be added to the bath water to soften the water. Use a soft soap like glycerine soap to wash the body surface. Dry the body lightly with a soft towel (take care not to break the vesicles). Eliminate external factors such as rough sheets and nightclothes that may exacerbate the pruritis. A cream containing vitamin E may be liberally applied to the body
- Prevent secondary bacterial infections by attending to personal hygiene and by keeping the fingernails of small children short. It may be best to let them wear mittens
- When the Chickenpox rash appears in the mouth, the ill person should have soft foods only
- The scabs/crusts do not transmit the disease. There is no need to burn the scabs. The scabs should be allowed to fall off naturally – when they are scratched off, permanent scars are left. Apply cream to the scabs to keep them soft
- Because Varicella can cause complications in adolescents and adults, anti-viral treatment should be offered, especially as new lesion formation, viral shedding and symptoms will be reduced
- Severe infections must be treated with intravenous acyclovir, especially in high-risk groups

◆ **Preventive measures to be taken**
➢ Vaccination of infants with varicella-zoster after the age of 12 months
➢ Artificial passively-acquired protection to high-risk persons by means of administering varicella-zoster immunoglobulin within 96 hours after exposure

◆ **Measures to prevent epidemics**
- There are no measures to be taken to prevent Chickenpox epidemics
- The disease has the potential to cause unmanageable situations in hospitals due to its communicability. It is therefore recommended that children suffering from Chickenpox and those who have been in contact with Chickenpox are not admitted to hospitals
- When a child should show signs of Chickenpox after having been admitted to hospital, the child should be immediately isolated (respiratory isolation) and discharge as soon as possible. When hospitalization of a child suffering from Chickenpox is necessary, the most strict isolation measures must be applied for the duration of the period of communicability. All other sick children who contract Chickenpox in hospital also need to be isolated or be discharged if their condition allows it
- Strict adherence to the school exclusion regulations must be maintained

◆ **Implications during disaster situations**
  ⬩ Epidemical outbreaks of varicella can be expected if children with Chickenpox are housed in close proximity

◆ **Compliance with international measures**
  ⬩ None

12.5 OTHER INFECTIONS PRODUCING SKIN LESIONS

Other systemic bacterial, fungal and rickettsiae infections also produce a variety of skin rashes or skin lesions such as *Salmonella typhi; Neisseria meningitides; Treponema pallidum, rickettsiae prowazeki, Streptococcus pyogenes; Staphylococcus aureus* and *Cryptococcus neoformans*. The skin rash is caused by the bacteraemia that develops in the body. The invasion of vascular endothelial cells in the skin provides the basis for the skin rash but is not the source of direct shedding to the exterior.

12.5.1 SCARLET FEVER (STREPTOCOCCAL SORE THROAT WITH A SKIN RASH)

Scarlet fever is a complication of an acute streptococcal infection of the pharynx and tonsils that is characterized by a sore throat and a papular skin rash

---

Epidemiological data

Geographic distribution
Streptococcal sore throat (with or without a rash) is common in high to mild temperature zones such as the subtropical regions. Apart from epidemics spread by food which may occur in any season, the highest incidence of scarlet fever occurs during late winter and spring. Sporadic cases may occur all year round

Causative pathogen
A lysogenic strain of *Streptococcus pyogenes (group A β-haemolytic streptococcus)*. The *Strep. pyogenes (group A β-haemolytic streptococcus)* possesses certain surface proteins (M and T) which is antigenic and differs from the M-type and T-type that are associated with skin infections. The M-proteins are important virulence factors because they inhibit opsonization and confer on the bacterium resistance to phagocytosis

Incubation period
2-4 days, sometimes 1–7 days

Mode of transmission
Airborne infected droplets from the infected person or carrier

Period of infectiousness (communicability, transmission)
*Untreated infected persons with scarlet fever transmit the *Strep. pyogenes (group A β-haemolytic streptococcus)* for a period of 10–21 days.
*Untreated cases of persons suffering from pharyngitis and tonsillitis with purulent throat secretions transmit the *Strep. pyogenes (group A β-haemolytic streptococcus)* for weeks or even months

---

*The communicability of *Strep. pyogenes (group A β-haemolytic streptococcus)* is curtailed with sufficient penicillin therapy to 24–48 hours

Reservoir
Humans

Intermediaries
None

Carriers
Healthy individuals are carriers of *Streptococcus pyogenes (group A β-haemolytic streptococcus)* and harbours the streptococcus in their nose and throat

Immunity status
Immunity with memory is elicited against an infection with a rash but not against other streptococcal infections

Susceptibility and resistance of host
Every person is susceptible. Children between the ages between 3 and 15 are extremely susceptible

Pathogenesis

After inhalation, the *Streptococcus pyogenes (group A β-haemolytic streptococcus)* gains entry into the body by attaching itself to the mucosal surface and invades the local tissues of the pharynx. From here it spreads to the lymph nodes, the blood, and the rest of the body. The lysogenic strain of *streptococcus pyogenes (group A β-haemolytic streptococcus)* produces a pyrogenic exotoxin, namely, streptolycin-O which is a super-antigen with a potent influence on the immune system coded for by a lysogenic phage. The toxin spreads through the body leading to a mild haemolysis of red blood cells and localizes in the skin to induce the characteristic diffuse punctuate erythematous skin rash (scarlet fever). The antibody-mediated immunity with memory that is formed, is specific to *the group A β-haemolytic streptococcus* and the person will not contract *Streptococcus pyogenes (group A β-haemolytic streptococcus)* with a skin rash again. However, the individual may suffer from other types of streptococcal pyogenes throat infections.

❖ **Clinical manifestation**
  The disease occurs in three phases
  ✱ **First phase**
    • A extremely sore throat, sudden pyrexia (39°C to 40°C), malaise and vomiting
    • The tongue is coated white, the throat is very red and there is usually an exudate on the tonsils that can be easily removed
    • The tonsillar lymph glands are enlarged and painful
    • Sometimes abdominal pain develops
  ✱ **Second phase**
    • Within 11–24 hours after the onset of the pharyngitis and tonsillitis, the reddish papular rash appears. It first appears on the face, neck and chest

and then spreads to the rest of the body. It is rare for the rash to spread to the palms and soles. It is particularly visible in the body folds (Pastia's sign). Seen from up close, the rash is spotty red but from a distance it appears to be a confluent red. The rash becomes pale when pressure is applied

- The lesions themselves are not serious, but signal an infection by a potentially harmful streptococcus causing serious complications
- Pyrexia stays elevated (39°C and higher) for days
- The tongue is heavily coated and the papillae are elevated (white strawberry tongue). After 2–3 days the tongue peels and becomes red and raw (red strawberry tongue)
- The face is flushed with a pale circle around the mouth (circum-oral pallor)

* **Third phase (recovery stage)**
  - Pyrexia gradually subsides
  - The rash fades and becomes pale over the course of a week and the skin starts to peel. Desquamation may take as long as 3–4 weeks. The hands and feet are the last to peel when involved

❖ **Complications**
  * **Early complications**
    - Tonsillar abscesses
    - Pyogenes throat infections
    - Otitis media and mastoiditis
    - Retro-pharyngeal abscesses
    - Sinusitis and cervical adenitis
    - Bronchitis and pneumonia
  * **Late complications**
    - Acute myocarditis
    - Endocarditis
    - Acute glomerulonephritis
    - Rheumatic fever
    - Rheumatic heart disease
    - Orbital abscesses

■ **Diagnosis**
  - Clinical picture
  - Positive *β-haemolytic streptococcal* throat swabs

■ **Prognosis**
  - Good, when medically treated immediately
  - Poor, if not medically treated properly

■ **Specific healthcare interventions to be rendered for the ill infected person**
  - Chemotherapy – antimicrobial treatment. **The antimicrobial drug regime is prescribed for 10–14 days and it is vital that the chemotherapeutic treatment be strictly adhered to for the prescribed period in order to prevent complications, especially renal complications**

- Antipyretic drugs
- Bed rest most of the time
- Strict mouth hygiene with regular mouthwashes every 4-6 hours
- Supervision of intake of fluids and output of urine to detect renal complications in the early stages. Test daily for albuminuria
- While the throat is still very painful, the diet should consist of milk and other soft foods which do not contain acids. Later, semi-solid foods may be given such as jelly or other foods which can be easily swallowed
- The ill person is not allowed to go to work or attend school for the duration of the disease
- Persons who have a sore throat or fever, should not handle food

■ Specific healthcare interventions for contacts and carriers
- There is no vaccine available for contacts, but contacts can be treated prophylaxis with antimicrobial chemotherapy
- Antimicrobial treatment is administered to all persons with a history of rheumatic fever in the family
- All carriers have to receive antimicrobial chemotherapy

◆ Preventive measures to be taken
- Health information to the public regarding the early diagnosis and medical treatment of streptococcal throat infections
- Inspection and control of dairies regarding the handling of milk, milk products and containers
- Boiling or pasteurising of milk
- Inspection and control of food handlers. Ensure that persons with sore throats and fever do not handle food
- Prophylactic chemotherapy with antimicrobial drugs for all carriers during outbreaks in institutions
- Isolation of ill individual when hospitalized
- Health information to all individuals regarding the use and disposal of paper tissues
- Preventing of overcrowding

◆ Measures to prevent epidemics
- In the event of groups of cases, notification must be done as well as immediate investigation for the possibility of contaminated milk or food
- In special circumstances, antimicrobial drugs may be prophylactic administered to groups – particularly to members of a household and immediate contacts or to persons who were exposed to contaminated milk and food
- Strict adherence to the school exclusion regulations must be maintained

◆ Implications during disaster situations
- Scarlet fever spreads rapidly amongst large groups of persons

◆ Compliance with international measures
- None

12.6   KEY NOTES

❑ The intact skin is an invaluable barrier to protect the body against microbial invasion.

❑ A wide range of microbes such as bacteria, fungi and viruses, gain access into the skin via breaches caused by trauma in the skin barrier while other microbes are introduced into the skin by arthropod vectors. Some parasites, on the other hand, initiate their own penetration into the skin (for example, bilharzia flukes).

❑ Once gained entry into the skin, the pathogens cause either local infections or disseminate through the body to distant sites causing systemic infections.

❑ Superficial infections of the skin are the most common infections in humans (for example, boils, impetigo, and ringworm).

❑ Invasion of pathogens deeper into dermal and sub-dermal tissues produce severe infections that can be rapidly fatal (for example, gangrene) or slow but progressive deformation and destruction (for example, leprosy).

❑ Many other pathogens invade the body via other routes and portals of entry, disseminate in the body and then localize in the skin or cause toxic or immuno-pathologic manifestations in the skin (for example, measles, chickenpox, scarlet fever).

Chapter 13

COMMUNICABLE DISEASES AFFECTING THE GENITAL-URINARY TRACT

Although the genital-urinary tract is a continuum, the communicable diseases that affect the urinary tract and the genital tract are not related to one another. Communicable diseases (sexual transmitted infections) that affect the genital tract and genital organs are transmitted through direct intimate contact between two persons which usually occurs during sexual intercourse (coitus). Communicable diseases of the urinary tract, on the other hand, are not related to sexual transmitted infections (venereal diseases). The urinary tract is one of the most common sites of bacterial infections. The majority of urinary infections is short-lived and is not transmissible between two individuals while severe infections may result in a loss of renal function as well as serious long term sequelae. Infection of the urinary tract also occurs through infection by parasites or worms such as Schistosoma. The possibility that diseases of the urinary tract may be accompanied by sexual transmitted infections is not excluded.

13.1 DISEASES OF THE GENITAL ORGANS AND REPRODUCTIVE SYSTEM (VENEREAL DISEASES OR SEXUALLY TRANSMITTED DISEASES [STD'S] OR SEXUALLY TRANSMITTED INFECTIONS [STI'S])

Sexually transmitted diseases (STD's) or infections (STI's) include all the specific sexually transmitted infections as well as the specific infections which affect the mucous membrane and skin of the genitals such as herpes genitalis, lymphogranuloma venereum, granuloma inguinale and genital warts. An individual can suffer from more than one sexual transmitted infection simultaneously such as syphilis and gonorrhoea, or syphilis, gonorrhoea and genital warts. Because almost all mucosal surfaces of the body can be involved in sexual activity, sexually transmitted infections not only involve the genitals (penis/vulva and vagina) but also other body sites such as the anal-rectal mucosa of the anus, the oral-pharyngeal mucosa of the mouth, and the hands of an individual.

The spread of sexually transmitted infections is inextricably linked with sexual behaviour. Pathogens shed from the genital-urinary tract are transmitted as a result of mucosal contact between two individuals

- through a discharge - the pathogens are carried in the epithelial surfaces
- from mucosal ulcers (sores) - the epithelium contains infected cells
- through semen – the presence of pathogens in semen plays a role in both homosexual and heterosexual transmission
- during birth, via the infected genital tract of the mother, to the new-born infant - pathogens are wiped onto the conjunctiva of the neonate or inhaled by the neonate leading to a variety of conditions, for example, bacterial meningitis, pneumonia, and conjunctivitis.

STI's are transmitted with far less speed and efficiency than other infections like viral infections that are transmitted via infected droplets. Close sexual contact by separate sexual acts is necessary to spread STI's from one person to another. Sexual promiscuity is therefore essential in the transmission of STI's from person-to-person. On the other hand, by maintaining monogamous sexual practices or a stable polygamous sexual practice without intrusion from outsiders, STI's can be prevented. Stable partners can do no more than infect each other regardless of frequent sexual activity. As almost all mucosal surfaces of the body can be involved in sexual activity, the pathogens can infect any site of the body. When genital-oral-anal contact occurs, intestinal infections can be spread directly between individuals despite good sanitation and sewage disposal.

Despite anti-microbial treatment, the incidence of sexually transmitted infections has increased during the past number of years. The most important factors leading to this phenomenon are

- ❖ increased density and mobility of human populations
- ❖ increase in social pathology (for example, prostitution, poverty, unemployment) and changes in social value systems
- ❖ socio-cultural customs of a community that are hard to change
- ❖ difficulty of engineering change in human sexual behaviour has led to increased levels of promiscuity and a permissive attitude towards premarital sexual intercourse as well as the number of sexual partners
- ❖ increasing use of and availability of contraceptives and techniques promoting permissive sexual behaviour
- ❖ the sexual health of commercial sex workers is not screened in South Africa
- ❖ asymptomatic sexually transmitted infections that are generally not treated, facilitate further cycles of infection and spread
- ❖ the appearance of drug resistant specific infectious agents that causes STI's
- ❖ the social stigma attached to STI's hampers not only infected individuals to obtain treatment but also the tracing of the contacts of the infected person
- ❖ most of the STI's do not stimulate an immune reaction with memory in the host and re-infections on re-infections occur
- ❖ non-existence of effective vaccines for prophylaxis of almost all STI's

◈ because all mucosal surfaces of the body can be involved in sexual activity, the specific pathogenic microbes have had increased opportunity to infect new body sites.

The World Health Organization recommends the following strategy for the prevention of STI's

❋ **Maintaining of responsible sexual conduct/behaviour through strict adherence to the ABC of sexual behaviour:**

- ◆ **A = Abstinence from all sexual activity until married or betrothal** in a stable relationship
- ◆ **B = Betrothal and be faithful to your partner** (do not sleep around or become involved in any form of promiscuous sexual activities)
- ◆ **C = condomize when promiscuous**

❋ Maintaining of stable monogamous or polygamous sexual practices as well as disallowing outsiders to enter any polygamous sexual relationship

❋ Encouraging the use of condoms, both male and female condoms. Condoms should be readily available and affordable

❋ Treatment of STI's should forms part of primary healthcare service delivery

❋ Providing adequate and correct treatment for STI's (syndrome/syndromic approach of disease management)

❋ Encouraging everybody to seek treatment as soon as possible after having been infected

❋ Tracing and treatment of all contacts of infected individuals

❋ Screening of clinical asymptomatic persons

❋ Health information is the most important way of bringing about a change in sexual behaviour and a decrease in the incidence of these infections. Health information should include the following

- ◆ Notification of contacts of being exposed and encouragement to submit to treatment (and completing the treatment course)
- ◆ Asymptomatic manifestation (no overt disease symptoms) of sexually transmitted infections. Many persons are unaware that they are suffering from a venereal infection. When the sexual habits of a person are such that he/she falls into the high-risk group, the individual should be subjected to screening tests on a regular basis
- ◆ The aetiology, clinical manifestation, complications and transmission (spread) of venereal infections
- ◆ Prevention by means of health information (for example, the dangers of promiscuity) and by emphasizing and encouraging the importance of maintaining monogamous or stable polygamous sexual practices. **Strict adherence to the ABC of responsible sexual behaviour**
- ◆ The value of using condoms when monogamous or stable polygamous sexual practices are not maintained
- ◆ The importance of early diagnosis and treatment (screening, such as taking blood specimen and swabs of discharges from the urethra, cervix and

rectum) which can be done on request in ante-natal clinics, family planning clinics, gynaecological and primary healthcare clinics

- Emphasizing the fact that immunity with memory is never elicited and re-infection can take place ad infinitum.

Note

1. Although STI's are not notifiable diseases, legislation makes it obligatory for persons suffering from a sexually transmitted infection(s) to undergo treatment until the disease is no longer transmissible. A person who has contracted a sexual transmitted infection(s) may not intentionally infect other persons or expose them to the specific sexual transmitted infection(s) and has to subject himself/herself to treatment until he/she can no longer transmit the infection(s). When the individual is treated by a private physician but does not report regularly for treatment, the private physician has to notify the District Health Authorities or the Provincial Department of Health who has to bring the requirements of the law to the attention of the person concerned. He/she is then ordered to report for treatment. If the person should withhold his/her cooperation, a warrant is issued by a magistrate on the recommendation of the medical health officer. This warrant compels the person to undergo treatment or to be isolated for treatment until the individual is no longer infectious

2. The treatment regime for all sexual transmitted infections is based on the syndrome/syndromic approach of disease management. The disease management or diagnostic approach is very difficult to follow in resource-restricted/resource–poor settings/countries because of its dependence on laboratory support that are often not available in remote and rural areas. Because the client cannot always wait/return for laboratory test reports days/weeks later, the STI goes untreated with the danger remaining of infecting sex partners. The syndromic approach, on the other hand, involves the recognition of signs and symptoms of a STI or syndrome of STI's and then prescribing treatment for the major causes of the syndrome. The syndromic approach enables treatment of most symptomatic sexual transmitted infections effectively during the client's first visit, even when access to sophisticated laboratory tests is not available. The syndromic case management is inexpensive, easy to use by all healthcare practitioners, does not require laboratory support, allows treatment immediately during the first visit (no delays or need for a return visit), and is highly successful. Disadvantages of the syndromic approach are that it does not address any asymptomatic sexual transmitted infections and that over-treatment of the client may occur when supplying the client with more drugs than actually necessary

3. The Bill of Human Rights and the Patients' Rights Charter are applicable in all care rendering to all infected individuals and the infected individual has the right to accept or refuse the treatment provided by the healthcare service delivery system

13.1.1 Sexual transmitted infections characterized by a discharge

As sexual transmitted infectious agents do not elicit an antibody-mediated with memory response, most pathogens elicit only an inflammatory response characterized by a discharge from the genital tract. The discharge is usually thick and purulent. Inflammation and swelling of the genital glands develop simultaneously.

13.1.1.1 GONORRHOEA

Gonorrhoea is a specific inflammation of the mucosa of the genital tract characterized by a yellowish-white urethral/vaginal discharge. The infection can be acute or become chronic

---

Epidemiological data

Geographic distribution
Is prevalent world-wide. Gonorrhoea is one of the most common communicable diseases on earth as women have a 50% and men a 20% change of contracting the disease after one single act of sexual intercourse

Causative pathogen
Neisseria gonorrhoeae – a human specific pathogen (not found in animals) that is sensitive to drying out and thus does not survive well outside the human host

Incubation period
2–4 weeks

Mode of transmission
Horizontally - Intimate sexual contact between two persons
Vertically - Mother to child during birthing leading to Ophthalmia Neonatorum

Period of infectiousness
For as long as the gonococcus can be cultivated

Reservoir
Humans. Asymptomatic persons serve as a source of infection - a serious risk for the spread of the infection

Intermediaries
None

Carriers
None

Immune status
No immunity with memory is elicited

Susceptibility and resistance of host
All individuals who are sexually active and promiscuous are susceptible

---

Pathogenesis

The *N. gonorrhoeae* usually enters the body via the mucosa of the vagina (women) or the urethral mucosa of the penis (men) although, because of other sexual practices, deposition of the gonococci also occurs in the mouth, throat and/or rectal mucosa. Because *N. gonorrhoeae* possesses special adhesive mechanisms that prevent it from being washed away by urine or vaginal discharges, it attaches itself to non-ciliated epithelial cells of the columnar epithelium of the urethra, prostrate, seminal vesicles, epididimis and associated glands in men, or in the columnar epithelium of the urethra, Bartholin's glands, cervix and Fallopian tubes in women. *N. gonorrhoeae* gonococci are also found in the rectal mucosa of both genders. The non-ciliated epithelial cells internalize the *N. gonorrhoeae* and allow them to multiply within intra-cellular vacuoles protected from phagocytes and antibody. *N. gonorrhoeae* also induces its own uptake and transport across urethral epithelial surface in the phagocytic vacuole. Because the gonococcus is capsulated, it is able to resist phagocytosis. During the next 3-4 days, these vacuoles move down through the cell and fuse with the basement membrane and discharge their bacterial contents into the sub-epithelial connective tissue. As *N. gonorrhoeae* does not produce a recognised exotoxin, a strong inflammatory response is induced by the *N. gonorrhoeae* (though the gonococci themselves are able to evade the consequences) and a yellowish–white inflammatory exudate is formed. The *N. gonorrhoeae* then invades the bloodstream and lymph spreading to other glands. Various virulence factors facilitate the spread of *N. gonorrhoeae* through the body. The clinical symptoms and signs of infection develop within 2-7 days after infection had taken place. Although *N. gonorrhoeae* elicits especially IgA-antibody, the gonococcus produces IgA-protease to combat the host's defences and thus allowing re-infection to occur with an antigenic variant.

❖ **Clinical manifestation**
- Gonorrhoea is asymptomatic in 60% of infected women and in 10% of infected men
- **Men** experience a sudden burning sensation during urination, three to five (3-5) days after infection, followed by a muco-purulent discharge from the urethra (thick, yellowish-white)
  - ◈ The glans penis is inflamed
  - ◈ After 10–13 days severe dysuria, persistent frequency of micturition, and haematuria occur
  - ◈ Prostatitis develops and prostate gland becomes oedematous
  - ◈ Retention of urine, pain, and pyrexia develop
  - ◈ Epididimitis is characterized by severe pain, tenderness, and swelling
- **Women** experience dysuria, frequency of urination, low backache, and a thick, yellowish-white vaginal discharge
  - ◈ Bartholin's glands are red and swollen and abscesses may form
  - ◈ The spread of the infection from the cervix to the Fallopian tubes is characterized by low abdominal pain
  - ◈ Acute salpingitis, pain, pyrexia, and formation of abscesses
  - ◈ The inguinal lymph glands are swollen and tender on palpation and the labia are red and swollen
- When the rectum is infected a rectal discharge is present in both male and female individuals
  - ◈ The person complains of a burning pain in the rectum or a persistent peri-anal irritation
  - ◈ Both men and women may suffer from asymptomatic proctitis

- When gonococcal pharyngitis occurs, infected persons (male and female) complain of a sore throat and on examination a mild exudate may be present
  ◈ Asymptomatic gonococcal pharyngitis can also develops

❖ **Complications**
  - Without treatment **men** may suffer from urethral stricture, chronic prostatitis, abscess formation, chronic epididimitis and sterility
  - Untreated **women** may develop salpingitis, abscesses, ectopic pregnancy and sterility
  - Systemic complications may develop in both genders such as septic gonococcal arthritis with swelling of the joints and skin lesions (erythematous papules that become pustular and haemorrhagic with necrotic centres)

■ **Diagnosis**
  - Clinical picture
  - Identification of the gonococci in smears from the urethra, cervix, rectum and throat

■ **Prognosis**
  - Good

■ **Specific healthcare interventions to be rendered**
  - Syndromic treatment with chemotherapy (antimicrobial drugs). Some genera/ strains of gonococci (a super bug) have became resistant to the standard antimicrobial drug regimen and therefore treatment with other classes of antimicrobial drugs according to protocol needs to be given
  - Contacts receive the same treatment
  - Follow-up cultures must be done after completion of the chemotherapy - for men seven days after completion (urethral discharge and/or rectal) and for women 7-13 days after completion (cervical and rectal discharge)
  - All persons with gonorrhoea must be treated for syphilis. Syphilis and gonorrhoea may occur simultaneously in the same person. Although penicillin cures both diseases the dosage for gonorrhoea is not sufficient to cure syphilis as well, and should be adapted accordingly (see syndromic treatment protocol)
  - Condoms should be used during intercourse

◆ **Preventive measures to be taken**
  ➢ Although gonorrhoea is not a notifiable disease, legislative regulations makes it statuary for any person suffering from a STI to undergo treatment until the infection is no longer transmissible
  ➢ All mothers and their babies who did not receive ante-natal medical care should be subjected to a screening test (TPHA) and all pregnant women should be subjected to the same test during their first visit to a ante-natal clinic
  ➢ All contacts of the infected individual must be traced and treated
  ➢ The use of condoms during intercourse is recommended (particularly when monogamous or stable polygamous sexual practices are not maintained)
  ➢ Health information re the ABC of responsible sexual behaviour

◆ **Measures to prevent epidemics**
 ⬇ None

◆ **Implications for disaster situations**
 ⬇ None

◆ **Compliance with international measures**
 ⬇ None

13.1.2 Sexually transmitted infections characterized by ulceration

Most of the pathogens that cause ulceration in the genital tract and on the genital organs are bacteria that multiply within the host to produce a very large number of progeny, thereby causing an overwhelming infection. Some of the bacteria can live outside cells, thus providing opportunities for growth, reproduction and dissemination. Many extra-cellular bacteria also possess the ability to spread rapidly through extra-cellular fluids or move rapidly over mucosal and skin surfaces resulting in a widespread infection within a relatively short time. A negligible inflammation is induced by most of the pathogens.

13.1.2.1 SYPHILIS

Syphilis is a chronic infection characterized by ulcerations with different stages occurring in the natural course of the disease. All the organs and systems in the body become infected as the disease progresses through these different stages while specific pathological changes take place within the different body sites. The degree of seriousness varies from complete asymptomatic latency to a rapidly progressive condition

---

Epidemiological data

Geographic distribution
Occurring the world over

Causative pathogen
Treponema pallidum – a spirochaete which is easily destroyed by chemical and physical agents. Heat, water, soap and drying out destroy the spirochaete immediately. *T. pallidum* can still not be cultivated in the laboratory in an artificial medium

Incubation period
9–90 days, on average 21 days

Mode of transmission
Horizontally - Close personal contact during sexual intercourse
Close personal contact with infective cutaneous, genital and mucous membrane lesions (extra-genital lesions caused by kissing, sucking, biting)
Blood and blood products during the late stage of the disease
Vertically - Transplacental infection – mother to child transmission in-utero

---

> **Period of infectiousness**
> Highly transmissible during the primary and secondary stages of early syphilis. During the late stage of syphilis the spirochaete is present in the blood only and is transmitted only by blood and blood products (not by sexual intercourse)
>
> **Reservoir**
> Humans
>
> **Intermediaries**
> Vectors - None
> Vehicles - Fomites such as contaminated needles
>
> **Carriers**
> None
>
> **Immune status**
> No immunity with memory is elicited
>
> **Susceptibility and resistance of host**
> All individuals who are sexually active and promiscuous are susceptible

Pathogenesis

T. pallidum gains entry into the body through minute abrasions in the mucous membranes and/or via a hair follicle in the skin, forming chancre(s) at the site of infection – the response of the host to the treponemes. The chancre is a small, painless lesion which develops at the site of infection and the live treponemes can be seen on dark-ground microscopy of the exudate (fluid) from the lesions. The chancre heals within 2 month without treatment. Unlike other bacterial pathogens, *T. pallidum* can survive in the body for many years despite a vigorous but ineffective cell-mediated immune response. The treponemes evade recognition because it is able to resist phagocytosis (due to absorbed fibronectin) and elimination (by maintaining a cell surface rich in lipid – a layer that is antigenically non-reactive). The antigens are only uncovered in dead and dying treponemes with the result that the host is then only able to respond immunologically. An ineffective cell-mediated immune response is elicited but re-infection with an antigenic variant is allowed.

The natural course of the disease can be divided into three stages. During the **primary stage** (lasting 1-3 months) local multiplication of the spirochaete results in the infiltration of plasma cells, polymorph and macrophage causing enlargement of the regional lymph nodes (the inguinal nodes). Healing of the regional lymph nodes occur spontaneously. During the first 2 to 10 weeks after infection had occurred, the spirochaete multiplies very slowly in the body and disseminates from the regional lymph nodes to the peri-vascular lymph vessels where a tissue reaction is elicited leading to endarteritis. The inflammation of the blood vessels causes necrosis and fibrosis in the surrounding tissue. In the beginning, the necrosis is superficial, causing erosion and leading to the formation of a primary granuloma (chancre). The chancre is initially a papule that then becomes a painless ulcer and, if not chemotherapeutic treated, heals within 6-8 weeks without any complications. During this period the infected individual is highly infectious.

During the **secondary stage** of the disease (lasting 2-6 weeks), a general infection of all the organs and systems of the body occurs as multiplication and formation of rubbery gummata lesions in the lymph nodes, liver, muscles, joints, skin, mucous membrane, and especially in the brain take place. A low-grade toxaemia, a skin rash, enlarged glands, aphthous mouth ulcers, and condyloma latum (secondary lesions that look like warts) develop. Not all persons infected with the *T. pallidum* develop the tertiary stage of the disease – a substantial proportion remains free of disease after suffering the primary or secondary stages of infection. Spontaneous resolution of the secondary stage takes place.

A period of latency lasting 3-30 years occurs between the second and third stage of syphilis while the Treponema lies dormant, in query, the liver and the spleen. When multiplication of the treponemes re-occurs, further dissemination and invasion with cell-mediated hypersensitivity occur. Gummas/gummatas (painless localized lesions comprising of granular tissues and with a rubbery consistency) are formed in any part or in any organ of the body during the **tertiary stage**. Apart from these lesions, degenerative changes of the nervous system (tabes dorsalis and general paralysis of the insane) and cardiovascular tissue (aortic lesions and heart failure) also develop (the damage is mostly due to the host response).

❖ **Clinical manifestation**
  Syphilis forms a continuum, but for the purpose of discussion it will be divided into early and late syphilis
  ✹ **Early syphilis**
    Early syphilis consists of the primary and secondary stages
    ● **Primary syphilis**
      - A chancre develops at the site of entry within 2-10 weeks. Single or multiple chancres usually develop on the external genitals
      - The chancre first appears as a papula which later becomes necrotic
      - The necrotic chancre exudes a small quantity of watery, yellowish discharge and a thin, greyish-yellow, slightly bloody scab is formed
      - The lesion is painless but becomes painful when a secondary infection takes place
      - The chancre heals with time (6-8 weeks) and forms a connective tissue scar which is palpable as a papula
      - Because of different types of sexual activity, chancres occur also extra-genitally – on the lips, tongue, fingers, skin, eyelids, nipples and anal canal. A chancre on the fingers can be very painful
    ● **Secondary syphilis.**
      4-12 weeks (sometimes six (6) months) after the primary infection had occurred, the progress of the disease is manifested by
      - Signs and symptoms similar to a flu-like illness with headache and fever
      - Myalgia

- Anaemia
- Alopecia
- General lymph-adenopathy of the inguinal, sub-occipital and axillary lymph nodes with unobtrusive, rubbery, painless swellings of the lymph glands
- Development over the entire body of a secondary mucosal-cutaneous syphilitic skin rash with a coppery glow as well as on the palms of the hands and the soles of the feet. The rash may be macular, papular, follicular or papulo-squamous
- Appearance of rounded mucosa lesions (greyish-white surrounded by a red areola) on the mucosa of the mouth. These lesions are known as aphthous ulcers
- Appearance of hypertrophic granulomatous lesions in all moist areas of the body, particularly in the anal-genital area and are known as condyloma latum
- Disappearance of all the typical dermal and mucosal symptoms and signs with time when the secondary stage of syphilis is left untreated. The disease now progresses to the latent stage of late (tertiary) syphilis

✸ Late syphilis (granulomatous tertiary syphilis)

The tertiary stage of syphilis is rarely seen or diagnosed these days owing to the treatment given to infected individuals early in the course of the disease. In untreated cases or those not properly treated, late tertiary syphilis develops 2-10 years (or even 30 years later) after being infected. At this stage the disease is not transmissible via sexual intercourse but can be transmitted though infected blood. Serological tests are mostly positive and may even be negative

- Skin, mucosa and bone gummata are formed. Gummata (see pathogenesis) occur in the skin, soft tissue, mucosa, bones, viscera, and tissue of the cardiovascular and nervous systems and cause tissue damage
- Cardiovascular syphilis. This usually occurs five or even 10-30 years after being infected. The aorta is often affected, its walls are weakened and a saccular aortic aneurysm is formed
- Neurosyphilis. This mostly occurs 2-35 years after being infected. Within 2-5 years after late syphilis had set in, signs and symptoms of acute syphilitic meningitis appear. A few years later signs and symptoms of meningo-vascular neurosyphilis appear with
  ◇ Irregular pupils and a poor reaction to light (Argyll Robertson pupils)
  ◇ Dementia paralitica
  ◇ Tabes dorsalis (locomotor ataxia)
  ◇ Personality changes

❖ Complications

Congenital syphilis

Pregnancy often masks the early signs of syphilis although the serological evidence of a treponemal infection in the mother is positive. When the mother is not treated, vertically transmission takes place and the treponemes can be detected in the foetal blood. The *T. pallidum* is able to cross the placental barrier to the foetus after 16-18 weeks of pregnancy causing congenital syphilis in the new-borne infant. Congenital syphilis is manifest as either a serious disease resulting in intra-uterine death, or congenital abnormalities that are obvious at birth, or a silent infection that only becomes apparent when two years of age (facial and tooth deformities)

The early form of congenital syphilis shown at birth resembles early secondary syphilis with skin and mucosal lesions and a skin rash. When nasopharyngeal lesions are present at birth, the nasal secretions are often bloodstained and are highly infectious. The rash is blistery in nature (the so-called syphilitic pemphigus). When an infant does not receive treatment at this early stage of the disease, late congenital syphilis develops, during which stage the cardiovascular and nervous system as well as the eyes and the bones are affected. Without treatment the infant shows within 2-8 weeks after birth the characteristic physical signs of congenital syphilis. The clinical picture of congenital syphilis manifests with an inability to progress, hepato-splenomegaly and lymph-adenopathy, rhinitis (snuffles), damaged upper permanent teeth with a serrated appearance (Hutchinson's teeth), malformed nails, a saddle nose (flat bridge) as a result of nasal lesions, sabre-formed tibiae, thickening of the skull bones, bald patches in the hair, blindness and intellectual retardation/impairment

- **Diagnosis**
    - The diagnosis is based on the syndromic clinical picture and microscopy
    - Serological tests, both the non-specific tests (such as VDRL [venereal disease research laboratory] and RPR [rapid plasma regain]) and the specific tests (the Treponemal antibody tests such as the TPHA [T. pallidum haemagglutination assay]) must be done for screening
    - Nobody should be diagnosed as syphilis infected on the grounds of only one test. Tests should be repeated ten days later and the diagnosis should be confirmed with an FTA-ABS (fluorescent treponemal antibody absorption)
    - The cerebrospinal fluid is examined to diagnose neurosyphilis
    - The serous exudate of primary and secondary lesions can be examined under dark ground microscopy immediately after collection or ultraviolet microscopy after staining during the transmissible stage of syphilis. Live treponemes can be seen

- **Specific healthcare interventions to be rendered**
    - Syndromic treatment with chemotherapy according to protocol
        - ✠ The treatment regime for persons who are allergic to specific antimicrobial drugs must be adjusted according to protocol
        - ✠ The treatment schedule must be adapted for pregnant women according to protocol due to the toxic effects of the antimicrobial drugs on the mother and/or the foetus. When the mother has been effectively treated and re-infection does not occur, it is unlikely that the infant will contract congenital syphilis

- ✠ The treatment regime **must** be completed – incomplete treatment can result in the development of late syphilis
- Contacts must be traced and receive the same treatment according to protocol
- Condoms should be used during intercourse
- Screening for other sexual transmitted infections
- Discouragement of oral sexual activity
- Follow-up must be done as follows for all individuals receiving treatment
  - ✠ After treatment for early syphilis, the infected individual is followed up after three (3), six (6) and twelve (12) months. Clinical and serological evaluations are to be done
  - ✠ Infected individuals with late syphilis are followed up for a number of years
  - ✠ Babies of sero-positive mothers are examined at birth and thereafter every month for a period of three (3) months

◆ **Preventive measures to be taken**
  - ➢ Although syphilis is not a notifiable disease, legislative regulations makes it statuary for any person suffering from a STI to undergo treatment until the infection is no longer transmissible
  - ➢ All mothers and their babies who do not receive medical care, should be subjected to a screening test (TPHA) and all pregnant women should be subjected to the same test during their first visit to a ante-natal clinic
  - ➢ All contacts of the infected individual must be traced and treated. This is particularly important where pregnant women are concerned in order to prevent re-infection, **since the foetus is repeatedly exposed to becoming infected**
  - ➢ The use of condoms during intercourse is recommended (particularly when monogamous or stable polygamous sexual practices are not maintained)
  - ➢ Health information regarding the ABC of responsible sexual behaviour

◆ **Measures to prevent epidemics**
  - ⊥ None

◆ **Implications for disaster situations**
  - ⊥ None

◆ **Compliance with international measures**
  - ⊥ None

13.1.3   Sexually transmitted infections caused by viruses

Virus particles enter the body through direct transfer, via sexual intercourse, from an infected host to an uninfected host. The outer membrane of the virus makes first contact with the membrane of the host (the skin and/or the mucosa of the genital tract). After fusion of host and viral membranes had taken place as well as the uptake of the virus into a phagosome had occurred, the virus is carried across the plasma membrane into the cytoplasm of the host's cells. Replication of the virus then starts to take place. New virus particles are released by cell lysis or by budding through the membrane of the host's cells. Some viruses such as the retroviruses and herpes-viruses become latent and needs a trigger to resume replication while others replicate at a slow rate to persist as a source of infection in symptomless carriers.

13.1.3.1   ACQUIRED IMMUNITY DEFICIENCY SYNDROME (AIDS)

Acquired Immunity Deficiency Syndrome (AIDS) is characterized by profound immunological deficiency, multiple super infections and unusual forms of certain malignant neoplasmas. AIDS is a chronic disease due to the progressive compromising/deterioration of the immune system

Note
1. Although HIV/AIDS occurs world-wide, it does not pose a threat to the health of the public and is therefore classified only as a STI – a sexual transmitted infection/disease that is not notifiable.
2. Persons suffering from other STI's are more susceptible to HIV-infection because the ulcerations and inflammation facilitate the transmission of the HIV-virus
3. The concentration of the HIV-virus is also very high in genital discharges and secretions making the HIV-infected individual extremely infectious

---

Epidemiological data

Geographic distribution
World-wide.

Causative pathogen
Human immunodeficiency virus (HIV). The *HIV-virus* possesses lymphotropic and neurotropic characteristics that cause gradual suppression of the immune system. The *HIV-virus* is a member of the lenti-virus, a genus of the retroviruses which cause slow, progressive, irreversible, fatal diseases. The virus is a delicate, labile virus which cannot survive for a long period outside the human body. The HIV-virus has mutated in two main groups of viruses which also have mutated to give a number of subtypes. The most common HIV-virus in South Africa is the HIV-1 and its subtypes

Incubation period
Unknown

Mode of transmission
The virus **is not transmitted** via the upper gastro-intestinal tract or the respiratory tract, nor can it be transmitted by food or water, insects, toilet seats, swimming pools, touching and hugging or personal contact
Horizontally - Sexual intercourse (heterosexually, homosexually and bisexually)
              Blood and blood products
              Organs and tissues of donors such as bone marrow, semen, kidneys, skin, cornea, etc
Vertically - Transplacental in-utero and intrapartum during delivery (20%) and through breastfeeding
            (11-16%)

Period of infectiousness
For as long as the virus is present in the blood and secretions

---

> **Reservoir**
> Humans – homosexual, bisexual and heterosexual individuals
>
> **Intermediaries**
> None
>
> **Carriers**
> Individuals may be infected with the virus without showing any signs of the disease. They are, however, capable of transmitting the virus to another person. Infected individuals are carriers for approximately 5–10 years during which period they infect other persons
>
> **Intermediaries**
> None
>
> **Immune status**
> No immunity with memory is elicited
>
> **Susceptibility and resistance of host**
> All individuals who are sexually active and promiscuous are susceptible. High-risk persons include heterosexual, homosexual, bisexual men and women who do not practice monogamous or stable polygamous sexual practices, commercial sex workers (men and women), and drug addicts who administer dependency drugs intravenously to themselves

Pathogenesis

The *HIV-virus* gains entry into the body in seminal/vaginal discharges/secretions from the infected partner via sexual intercourse (intimate mucosal contact). The pathogen, *the HIV-virus*, infects mainly CD4-receptor-bearing cells such as T_H-cells, monocytes, dendritic cells and microglia. The *HIV-virus* enters the host's cells by binding the viral gp120 envelope glycoprotein to the CD4 antigen-receptor and chemokine co-receptors on the host cell surface (the CD4 molecule acts as the high affinity binding site). Following this, replication of the virus starts to take place and new virus particles are released by budding through the host cell membrane. Productive replication and cell destruction does not occur until the T_H-cells of the adaptive immune system have been activated. In an attempt to respond to the HIV-antigens, T_H-cell activation of the adaptive immune system is greatly enhanced. Because monocytes, macrophages, Langerhans' cells and follicular dendritic cells also express the CD4-molecule, they may be first cells to be infected by the *HIV-virus*. As these cells are not generally destroyed, they act as reservoir for the infection.

During the first few months, virus-specific CD8-positive T-cells are formed that reduces the viraemia (the HIV load). This is followed by the appearance of neutralizing antibody. Because millions of infectious virus particles and infected lymphocytes are produced daily, the immune system begins to gradually suffer damage. The number of circulating CD4-positive T-cells falls steadily while the HIV load rises. By selectively infecting T4-lymphocytes in the lymph nodes, the *HIV-virus* damages those specific cells which would normally control the destruction and elimination of viruses. The cell-mediated immune responses to viral antigens also weaken (as judged by lymphocyte-proliferation) whereas the responses to other antigens stay/are normal. Eventually the individual loses the battle to replace the lost T-cells and the T-cell number falls more rapidly. Immunological abnormalities develop such as the absence of natural killer cells, reduction of cytotoxic cell activity, polyclonal activation of B-cells and functional changes in T-lymphocytes. Due to this suppression of the immune system, the body is extremely susceptible to opportunistic infections. Certain malignant tumours of the blood, skin and bones develop. Progressive neuro-degenerative infections or progressive immune deficiency diseases or both may develop. The clinical disease signs and symptoms of AIDS is an indirect result of infection with the *HIV-virus.*

❖ **Clinical manifestation of HIV-infection and AIDS in Adults**
  The clinical picture can be divided in different phase
  ❋ The primary HIV infection phase
    • About six weeks after being infected, sero-conversion takes place and the individual's HIV-status changes form HIV-negative to HIV-positive
    • The individual develops an disease state similar to glandular fever lasting 1-2 weeks
    • A "flu-like" disease or mononucleosis-type disease develops with a sore throat, headache, mild fever, fatigue, muscle and joint pains, lymph-adenopathy, gastro-intestinal symptoms and oral ulcers
    • Occasionally a rash may appear
    • The HIV viral load is very high and the individual is highly infectious
  ❋ *Clinical Stage 1 - The asymptomatic latent phase (window period or silent phase)*
    • The viral levels reach a set point (steady immune response of a CD4 count of 500-800) 16-24 weeks after infection
    • The infection nevertheless remains active in the body and continues destroying CD4-positive T-cells (with the CD4 count falling to less than 800)
    • A lower set point at this stage is an indication of a lowered viral load and a better prognosis for the individual
    • Although the individual is HIV-positive, no manifestation of any clinical signs and symptoms of the disease occur and the person leads, on the surface, a healthy life
    • Some individuals stay healthy for years while others may deteriorate rapidly within months
    • When the virus invades the central nervous system a self-limiting aseptic meningo-encephalitis may develops
  ❋ *Clinical Stage 2 and 3 -The phase of chronic virus infection*
    ✓ The minor symptomatic stage commences when the individual with HIV-antibody presents with one or more of the following symptoms
      • cervical, axillary, and inguinal lymph-adenopathy
      • recurrent attacks of pyrexia
      • herpes zoster
      • skin rashes, dermatitis, chronic itchy skin

- fungal infections – nails and skin
- recurrent oral infections
- recurrent or chronic upper respiratory tract infections such as otitis media, otorhoea, sinusitis, or tonsillitis
- weight loss (up to 10% of body weight) and not responding to standard therapy
- malaise, fatigue and lethargy

✓ The major symptomatic phase

During this phase the CD4-cell count becomes very low while the viral load becomes very high. Major symptoms and opportunistic infections appear because of an overgrowth of some of the natural flora with fungal infections and reactivation of old infections (for example, Tuberculosis [TB]) occurs. As the immune deficiency progresses more and more frequent and severe opportunistic infections develop

- Intermittent or constant unexplained fever lasting for more than a month
- Weight loss – significant (more than 10% of body weight) and unexplained and not responding to standard therapy
- Persistent and recurrent infections – Candida (oral and vaginal), herpes, bacterial (acne-like)
- A maculo-papular rash
- Night sweats
- General lymph-adenopathy of the posterior cervical, axillary and epitrochlear gland. The glands are not painful but soft and palpable
- Persistent and untreatable chronic diarrhoea that last more than a month
- Oral hairy leukoplakia
- Abdominal discomfort
- Persistent headache
- Persistent cough when reactivation of TB occurs
- Opportunistic infections of various kinds

✱ *Clinical Stage 4 - The severe symptomatic phase of AIDS-defining conditions* (Systemic manifestation due to the infective process)

In the final phase AIDS has developed – 18 months to 5–10 years or longer after being infected. The symptoms of the disease become more acute and severe because the immune system deteriorates exponentially with rare persistent and untreatable opportunistic conditions and cancers manifesting. HIV-related organ damage is also manifested. Any of the following symptoms, conditions or opportunistic infections is characteristic of AIDS

- Diffuse pneumonia. Despite treatment, the pneumonia takes a long time to clear up and tends to recur
- Pyrexia – the pyrexia is intermittent or continuous and leads to serious febrility
- Weight loss ("Slims" disease). A person may lose as much as 30% - 50% of his body weight, even though diarrhoea may not be present

- Neurological complications. A progressive HIV-associated encephalopathy characterized by multiple small nodules of inflammatory cells, infected microglia and infiltrating macrophages develops with symptoms such as loss of vision, tremors, and seizures. Declining of the psychological and mental abilities of the person follows with memory loss, poor concentration, and confusion
- Peripheral neuropathy characterized by pain, numbness, and pins and needles in hands and feet
- Persistent diarrhoea. Watery diarrhoea (10–15 litres) or a large number of loose stools are passed per day. Despite antimicrobial treatment and the administering of a binding agent, the diarrhoea continues for several days
- A large spectrum of microbial diseases (acquired or re-activated). The person can become infected with any pathogen and presents with the signs and symptoms of the relevant disease
- Persistent generalised lymph-adenopathy
- Persistent oral infections – Candida and herpes
- Persistent respiratory infections
- Neoplasia manifestations such as
  - ❖ Kaposi's sarcoma - Kaposi's sarcoma is a tumour of the blood or lymphatic endothelium of the skin and, less common, of the mucosa of the mouth. It causes the person to become socially unacceptable in an early stage of the disease. Pain, oedema and respiratory problems are experienced
  - ❖ Burkitt's lymphoma (non-Hodgkin's)
  - ❖ Various other cancers such as anal-genital and liver cancers

❖ **Clinical manifestation of HIV-infection and AIDS in Children**
Children with HIV-infection and AIDS often manifest/present with non-specific conditions that are common in childhood but uncommon in uninfected children. Symptoms and signs and conditions associated with HIV-infection and AIDS in children are
- ➢ failure to thrive and weight loss due to gastro-intestinal infections or poor nutrition or opportunistic infections
- ➢ intermittent or constant prolonged fever
- ➢ oral candidiasis
- ➢ chronic diarrhoea and gastro-enteritis
- ➢ recurrent bacterial infections of the upper and lower respiratory tract, ear, urinary tract, skin, meningitis, osteomyelitis, tonsillitis, cellulitis
- ➢ lymphoid interstitial pneumonitis and other pneumonias such as Pneumocystis jiroveci pneumonia (previously known as Pneumocystis carinii) with a very poor prognosis
- ➢ anaemia, pallor, nose bleeds
- ➢ general lymph-adenopathy of the posterior cervical, axillary and inguinale glands
- ➢ hepatomegaly and splenomegaly

- skin conditions such as severe nappy rash, allergic skin eruptions, extensive seborrhoea (seborrhoeic dermatitis)
- severe herpes infections such as herpes zoster and herpes simplex
- enlargement and infection of the parotid gland (parotitis – not mumps)
- neurological abnormalities such as epilepsy, and microcephaly
- other AIDS-defining conditions such as Kaposi's sarcoma or *cytomegalovirus* infection
- complicated Chickenpox and Measles
- delay in reaching developmental milestones or loss of those already attained

Note

The clinically course of HIV-infection and AIDS in children differs significantly from that in adults as the time lap from infection to full-blown AIDS is very short. Most infants develop AIDS before the age of 5 years and die soon afterwards. The viral activity in children also differs from that in adults as the viral load increase extensively during the first weeks of life and stays very high for a year or two, after which it gradually declines, reaching a steady state by the age of 5-6 years. Rapid or slow progression of the disease may occur in children – when rapid progression takes place the infant usually dies between 6-12 months of age. When the disease progresses slowly, the child shows mild symptoms of the disease after 12 months of age and may live to reach older childhood and early adolescent years. The progress of AIDS in children is accelerated by poor nutrition and/or other medical diseases and/or other communicable diseases

❖ **Complications (Adults and children)**
- Infectious conditions that do not clear up and keep recurring, or the simultaneous presence of two or more infections
- Tuberculosis, lymph-adenopathy, herpes zoster, Kaposi's sarcoma, candidiasis, loss of weight and Pneumocystis jiroveci pneumonia
- Occurring of other STI's when the individual behaves sexually irresponsible. HIV-infection may delay the healing and cure of other STI's, resulting in the STI's becoming more severe and difficult to treat

■ **Diagnosis**
- Isolation of the virus by means of serological tests, i.e. the ELIZA test and the Western Blot test
- Clinical picture (weight loss, fever, chronic diarrhoea for more than one month – adult and child)
- It is sometimes very difficult to diagnose HIV-infection in children under the age of 18 months as the HIV-antibody test may react to the antibody transferred from the mother to the child during pregnancy. A HIV p24 PCR antigen test may be done in children younger than 18 months

■ **Prognosis**
- Very poor when the final stage AIDS syndrome has developed – 100% mortality
- Persons who are only HIV positive and show no signs of the AIDS syndrome, may live for as long as 20 years or longer when they maintain a healthy lifestyle
- When co-infected with Tuberculosis, very poor

■ **Specific healthcare interventions to be rendered**

◆ <u>**Older adolescents and adults**</u>

- The infected individual's CD4 lymphocyte count as well as viral load in the blood must be monitored on an ongoing basis as to manage the HIV-infection, all opportunistic infections and AIDS. The lymphocyte count indicates whether the immune system is compromised and whether anti-retroviral treatment must be started while the viral load is an indication of the severity of the infection and how the individual respond to antiretroviral therapy

- HIV-infected individuals must undergo regular clinical assessment - a physical examination that include the monitoring of weight; monitoring of the clinical stage of the disease; screening for tuberculosis; checking for treatment adherence as well as the screening for any side-effects of treatment; and the screening of the mental health of the individual. The necessary laboratory tests must also be done at the same time

- Chemotherapy – When eligible for treatment according to protocol, anti-retroviral therapy (ART) has to be started and taken life-long. Adherence to anti-retroviral therapy must be encouraged to avoid the development of drug resistance strains and drug failure. Individuals who develop Tuberculosis while on treatment, must continue their anti-retroviral therapy while simultaneously taking the anti-tuberculosis treatment as prescribed

- As anti-retroviral therapy reconstitutes (strengthens/enhances) the immune system of the HIV-infected individual, the risk to become co-infected with tuberculosis (TB) is dramatically reduces. But, regardless of this fact, regular screening (preferably on a monthly basis) must still be done to determine whether the HIV-infected person is free of tuberculosis. As the Immune Restitution Inflammatory Syndrome (IRIS) mostly occurs within the first 3-6 months after starting with anti-retroviral chemotherapy (with improved immune function a previously occult opportunistic infection is unmask that presents with an unusually aggressive inflammatory response or causes a paradoxical deterioration/worsening of an existing opportunistic disease and is as such not an indication of drug failure nor a drug side-effect), all HIV-infected persons are at risk for the reactivation of latent TB lesions especially during the first 6 months of therapy – hence, it is critical to ensure systemic screening for latent TB before initiating anti-retroviral therapy (ART). Accordingly, TB Preventive Therapy (TB prophylaxis) must always be offered to all HIV-infected persons – whether TB free or showing latent TB on testing – but only after active TB has been excluded

- Where one of the partners is infected, a condom must be used. Sexual abstinence is not necessary

- Individuals suffering from HIV/AIDS must receive comprehensive, holistic and culturally congruent physical, emotional, socio-cultural and spiritual healthcare. The general health of the individual must be promoted to strengthening the immune system as to keep the infected person as long as possible healthy, to prevent opportunistic infections, to treat all infections and health-related problems as soon as possible, and to improve the general health of the individual by using anti-retroviral therapy

- Treating all infections as and when they develop. Encourage all infected individuals to be voluntary vaccinated with influenza vaccine annually prior to the influenza season
- Encourage exercise, rest and relaxation
- Ensure that the infected individual eats a balanced and nutritious diet (macro-nutrients, micro-nutrients and minerals as well as enough proteins, fats, carbohydrates and fibre) and is well hydrated. Malnutrition and micro-nutrient deficiency result in a higher HIV load (especially when also suffering from co-infection with TB [pulmonary tuberculosis]). Supplement vitamins and mineral trace elements together with Probiotics can boost the infected individual's immune system
- Maintain good personal hygiene. Advise the person regarding skin care. Wash the skin with saline water (salt added to wash water) and use only natural soaps such as glycerine soaps. Avoid harsh soaps containing caustic soda or soaps containing bacterial killing/germicidal agents as it acts as an abrasive stripping the skin of its normal defence flora barrier as well as destroying the normal horny skin defence layer. Because simultaneously the high concentration of salt on the skin is inhibited, the fatty secretions on the skin is decreased and the natural acidity of the skin is altered, the skin becomes susceptible to severe and recurrent skin infections that are bacterial, fungal and viral in nature
- Ensure sufficient rest periods
- Give health information to the infected individual about protecting himself/herself against infections transmissible from fellow-men or contaminated vehicles
- Support the person psychologically by means of counselling. Keep stressful situations to a minimum and teach the person how to handle stress. Help the ill person to join support groups in his/her area/district and have a positive attitude to life
- Render symptomatic and supportive healthcare as necessary. Family members must be encouraged to become part of the care-rendering team
- Isolation (excluding contact isolation) is not necessary. The ill person who is admitted to hospital can be cared for in any ward (not necessarily a single bed ward), on condition that none of the other ill healthcare users suffer from infections. A single bed ward is recommended though, to protect the ill person against infections. In this case, care has to be taken to prevent the ill person from feeling rejected and lonesome. Isolation is also not necessary at home, though precautionary measures must be taken when any family member suffers from any infectious condition
- Contact isolation is extremely important - gloves have to be worn when handling blood, secretions and excreta from the infected person as well as standard precautionary measures when handling blood, secretions and excreta from any individual (whether healthy, ill, contact or carrier)

- Home care - the care-givers have to be taught how to prevent infection. Support the care givers and help them to join support groups for care givers in their area/district
- Support the dying person and his/her family and friends – before, during and after death
- Arm individuals, families, and communities with the relevant information they need to know about HIV and AIDS as to deal with stigmatization and to deal with the disease like any other long-term chronic condition
- Dual HIV-positive monogamous couples/polygamous families as well as monogamous couples/polygamous families where only one partner is infected, must plan their family. The medical advice given for conception, pregnancy and child rearing must be strictly followed
- Men must be involved in intervention programmes to reduce heterosexual transmission of HIV
- Gender issues, especially reducing violence against women and children, must be addressed on national, regional and local level
- Post-exposure prophylaxis for HIV-infection must be started as soon as possible following alleged penetrative sexual abuse, ideally within one (1) hour after exposure but not later than 72 hours post-exposure. Duration for prophylaxis is 28 days. All survivals of sexual assault must receive prophylaxis treatment and counselling. Follow-up of HIV-status of the individual must be done at 6 weeks, 3 months and 6 months. Prophylaxis has to be stopped when the exposed individual test positive on the HIV DNA PCr test or HIV ELISA test after 18 months or when the perpetrator is HIV ELISA negative

♦ **Children (12 months and older) and young adolescents**
   ◈ Care of the HIV-positive child is the responsibility of the parent(s) because they need care, attention, security, love, nurturing, acceptance, and a supportive home environment as to fulfil their individual bio-psycho-social and educational needs
   ◈ The specific healthcare and support needed by the child/adolescent can be provided at the primary healthcare service delivery level
   ◈ Encourage parent(s) [biological/foster/adopted/same gender] and guardians to have the HIV-positive child vaccinated according to the Expanded Programme on Immunization [EPI-SA Schedule] for Childhood Vaccination
   ◈ When HIV-infected children have been exposed to measles, they must be given additional immunoglobulin. All HIV-infected children who are admitted to hospital must receive measles vaccine as an additional dosage to the normal vaccination routine. Varicella immunoglobulin must be given within 96 hours to all HIV-infected children who have been exposed to chicken pox and/or shingles. All HIV-infected children must receive the influenza vaccine yearly. Health information to be given to the caregiver(s)

of the infected child regarding the protection of the child against infections transmissible from other children/fellow-men or contaminated vehicles

◈ HIV-infected children must undergo regular clinical assessment, namely, monitoring of growth (including weight and length) and bio-psycho-social development; vaccination; nourishment, hydration, and feeding that includes vitamin supplementation and deworming; screening for signs and symptoms of opportunistic infections, tuberculosis, and persistent diarrhoea; screening for signs and symptoms of anaemia; assessment of adherence to treatment protocol, response to treatment regime and side-effects of treatment; and assessment of the clinical stage of the disease. The necessary laboratory tests must be done at the same time

◈ With every routine clinical assessment of the HIV-infected child, the caregiver(s) must be counselled and psychosocial support given. Also, all other family members must receive treatment and healthcare when necessary

◈ All common childhood infections must be managed early and effectively according to the Integrated Management of Childhood Illnesses (IMCI) guidelines. Children with severe pneumonia, malnutrition and TB must be tested for HIV-infection

◈ Because orphans and abandoned children are at special risk of HIV-infection, their HIV-status must thus be established before being considered for adoption or fostering. All other children who have been wet-nursed or breastfed by a woman of unknown or HIV-positive status must be tested for HIV-infection. All siblings of children diagnosed as HIV-infected must be tested for HIV-infection as well as all children whose father and/or mother have been diagnosed as HIV-positive and died

◈ Ensure that all caregivers of HIV-positive children who are receiving ambulatory care know how to tell when the child is becoming ill and needs urgent attention of a healthcare provider

◈ All HIV-infected children must receive nutritional support as their nutritional status are impaired which can lead to growth failure. Feeding problems such as poor appetite, sores in mouth, vomiting and nausea as well as malnutrition (mild and severe) must be managed according to protocol

◈ Access to social grants for HIV-infected children must be facilitated

◈ As all ill children are likely to suffer from pain when ill, the ill HIV-infected child must be kept comfortable and pain-free

◈ Home care (at home or in a hospice) of the terminally ill child must be encouraged as to limit hospital admissions or to prevent long duration of hospital stay. Unnecessary drug treatment must be stopped and only medication to keep the child pain-free and comfortable must be given. Parents/caregivers must be reassured and counselled and assisted to perform the necessary non-invasive culturally required dying/death rituals. Emotional support must be provided to the dying child and the grieving family. Where available, refer the dying child and his/her family to palliative home based care services in the community. Help the parents/caregivers to make a decision as to the preferred place of death – home or hospice or hospital. After the death of the ill child, provide or refer the family for bereavement support and sibling care

◈ As HIV and AIDS present one of the greatest threats to the wellbeing and lives of children, children can be tested for HIV-infection without the consent of the parent(s) when it is in the best interest of the child. Consent for testing can be given by

   ✓ the child self when over the age of 12 years or when younger than 12 years if the child is of sufficient maturity to understand the benefits, risks, and social implications of such test

   ✓ the parent(s) or primary caregiver

   ✓ the provincial head of the Department of Social Development

   ✓ the designated child protection organization arranging the placement of the child

   ✓ the person in charge of a hospital under specific circumstances

   ✓ the children's court

Subject to Section 132 of the Children's Act, Act no 38 of 2005, a child may be tested without consent for HIV-infection to establish whether a healthcare worker may have contracted HIV-infection due to contact with any substance from the child's body that may transmit HIV during a medical procedure OR any other person may have contracted HIV-infection due to contact with any substance from the child's body that may transmit HIV, provided the test has been authorised by a court

◈ Disclosing his/her HIV-positive status to the individual child must always be in the best interest of the child. However, disclosure of their positive HIV-status to children needs to take place before adolescence as children has the right to participate in decisions about their own healthcare

◆ **The HIV-positive learner/students in educational institutions**

  ◈ **Learners/students cannot be refused admission** to any educational institution (day care centres, play groups, pre-primary schools, primary schools, secondary schools or tertiary institution) on his/her HIV-positive status

  ◈ The **HIV-positive learner/student can partake in all** academic, sport, cultural and recreational activities provided by the specific educational institution. All officials, educators and other staff attending the specific activity must adhere to standard precautions set out for the management of HIV/AIDS when a learner/student is injured

  ◈ During **periods of sicknesses resulting in absence** from school/ educational institution, special arrangements must be made to help learners/students with their studies

  ◈ Parents of learners or adult learners/students **may voluntary inform** the educational authorities regarding their child's HIV-positive status/student's own HIV-positive status

◈ Educators **may not discriminate** against any HIV-positive learners/ students in the classroom or on the play grounds or on/in the property of the educational institution

◈ All **HIV-positive learners/students must abide by the set Code of Conduct and rules** of the educational setting. Disciplinary steps can be taken against the HIV-positive learner/student when defaulting

◆ **The HIV-positive adult employee in the occupational setting**

◈ The **necessary policies regarding chronic medical conditions** (including HIV/AIDS) as well as early retirement due to ill health must be in place in all occupational settings

◈ It is the **choice of the individual employee self whether to disclose/not to disclose** to the employer that he/she is suffering from a chronic medical condition (being HIV-positive/suffering from AIDS). When the employee does not disclose his/her HIV-positive status to the employer, the employer has however no obligation towards the employee to make any arrangement to accommodate the HIV-positive employee as long as possible in the post/ position he/she is employed in, for example, adjustment to the task/job description

◈ Employers **may not demand** pre-employment HIV-testing without the necessary consent granted by the Department of Labour

◈ HIV-positive employees **may not be excluded** from any benefits provided by the employer such as bonuses, housing subsidy/allowance, medical aid funds and/or pension scheme or any other labour-related practices in place. (Please note that the employer only acts as a go-between regarding medical funds in the sense that the employer only deducts the subscription fees of the medical fund from the employee's salary and pays it over to the medical fund. The HIV-positive employee must however abide by the rules and regulations as set by the medical fund he/she belongs to. Also note that no legal grounds exist for any employer to provide a medical fund or a pension fund/scheme or a housing subsidy/allowance for employees)

◈ Employers must deal with any grievance related to chronic medical conditions in an efficient and effective manner in order to manage chronic medical conditions effectively in the workplace

◈ Employers **may not discriminate** against any HIV-positive employee, for example, withholding of promotion, withholding of skills development, and much more. The necessary policies must be in place in all employment situations as well as a code of conduct to direct the behaviour of employer and employees towards one another

◈ All employees **has the right to voluntary testing and counselling** (pre-test and post-test) without the consent of the employer. An employee does not need to inform the employer of the results of the testing and his/her HIV-status. When the employee informs the employer of his/her HIV-positive status, it is done voluntary and the employer must keep this information confidential

◈ All employees suffering from chronic medical conditions (including HIV/AIDS) have the same rights and duties/obligations to fulfil towards the employer as all other employees

◈ When the employee suffering from HIV/AIDS becomes too ill to work, special arrangement must be made with the employer, for example, changes made in task description, early retirement due to ill health. When the HIV-positive employee becomes incapacitated to work any longer, constructive dismissal on the grounds of incapacity is legally allowed. However, dismissal on the grounds of only being HIV-positive is legally forbidden

◈ All employees suffering from HIV/AIDS are governed by the agreed policy and procedure regarding sick leave. Employees suffering from HIV/AIDS must abide by the prescribed ruling

◈ It is the **responsibility of all employees in sensitive occupations** (for example, healthcare industry, emergency services, security industry such as the police service, etc.) **to strictly adhere to the Standard Precautions and to prevent stick injuries.** When an injury on duty does occur, the individual employee must follow the set protocol(s) for HIV-related injuries

◈ **All HIV-positive employees must take responsibility for their own health and safety** and abide by all rules set for a safe occupational environment by the employer. Disciplinary steps can be taken against the HIV-positive employee when defaulting

◈ All HIV-positive employees **must adhere to the set Code of Conduct, Service Contract, rules and policies** in the occupational setting. Disciplinary steps can be taken against the HIV-positive employee when defaulting

◈ HIV-positive employees **may not use their HIV-positive status as justification for non-performance of their duties** as set out in their task description/job description. HIV-positive employees can, however, be dismissed grounded in justification of non-performance of duties

◆ <u>**Specific healthcare interventions to prevent mother-to-child-transmission**</u>

<u>NOTE</u>

<u>THE MANAGEMENT OF HIV-POSITIVE PREGNANT WOMEN MUST ALWAYS BE USED TOGETHER WITH THE OBSTRETIC POLICIES AND PROTOCOLS APPLICABLE. FOR EXAMPLE, WHEN SITUATIONS SUCH AS MASSIVE BLEEDING, ECLAMPSIA, PRE-TERM BIRTHING, ETC. ARISES, THE IMMEDIATE SAFETY OF THE MOTHER AND CHILD TAKES PRECEDENCE OVER THE GUIDELINES FOR THE MANAGEMENT OF HIV-POSITIVE PREGNANT WOMEN AND WOMEN GIVING BIRTH</u>

<u>AS HIV/AIDS DOES NOT "POSES A PUBLIC HEALTH THREAT" TO THE HEALTH OF THE PUBLIC AS IN, FOR EXAMPLE, EXTENSIVELY AND COMPLETELY DRUG-RESISTANT TUBERCULOSIS, THE BILL OF HUMAN RIGHTS AND THE PATIENTS RIGHTS CHARTER ARE APPLICABLE IN THE CARE RENDERING TO THE MOTHER AND CHILD SUFFERING FROM HIV/AIDS. THE HIV-POSITIVE MOTHER/PREGNANT WOMAN HAS THE RIGHT TO REFUSE ANY ANTI-RETROVIRAL DRUGS OFFERED TO HERSELF OR HER BABY DURING THE ANTENATAL, INTRA-PARTUM AND POSTNATAL PERIOD. DO NOT PUT PRESSURE ON THE MOTHER/PREGNANT WOMAN</u>

TO TAKE ANY ANTI-RETROVIRAL DRUGS WHEN IN LABOUR AND NOR MAY HEALTHCARE PRACTITIONERS OR BIRTH ATTENDANCES DISCRIMINATE AGAINST HER ON THE BASIS OF HER DECISION. Based on the "opt-out" decision (refusal of treatment) of the mother, anti-retroviral drugs may not be administered after delivery (in labour ward, in the nursery, in the neonatal intensive care unit) to her child without her written or her verbal consent. But, under the Children's Act, No 38 of 2005, when it is in the best interest of the child, the child may receive HIV-prophylaxis treatment (infant's right to receive protection against acquired HIV). Counselling of the mother prior to instituting the Children's Act, No 38 of 2005, must have taken place

- ■ **Antenatal healthcare to be rendered to pregnant women**
    - ❖ All pregnant women must receive care according to the set protocol
    - ❖ All HIV-positive pregnant women must be informed and counselled (no less than 4 times) about infant feeding options in the context of HIV. All HIV-infected pregnant women must be counselled to **exclusively breastfeed her baby or to feed breast milk exclusively** (breast milk given per cup feeding) to her baby for up to 6 months and then introducing appropriate complementary foods whilst continuing breastfeeding for the first 24 months of the baby's life. Exclusive replacement feeding[1] using commercial infant formula or milk banks (expressing and heat-treating breast-milk from HIV-negative mothers) must only be advised when the mother cannot breast feed her baby at all (regardless the reason thereto) or when the mother had made an informed decision to give exclusive replacement feeding to her baby. When giving information to mothers, the importance of cultural practices of early child parenting must always be taken in account. For example, where does the mother stay after delivery – on her own, with her own mother or with her husband's mother?; who is the head decision-maker regarding the feeding of the baby – the mother herself, her own mother or her husband's mother?; is replacement feeding (commercial infant formula)[1] culturally acceptable?; can the mother-to-be financially afford replacement feeding over a long period of time (2 years of longer)?; must the mother go back to work in a very short period of time (3-4 month) after delivery and is she prepared to express her breast milk and preheat it before giving it to her baby?; is the practice of expressing breast milk culturally acceptable?; who will be looking after her baby when she goes back to work? The pregnant woman's final decision must be documented
    - ❖ When the mother cannot breast feed her baby or when the mother had decided on replacement feeding[1], she must receive drugs to dry up her milk to prevent mixed feeding of the infant
    - ❖ HIV-negative women and mothers-to-be whose HIV-status are unknown must be advice to exclusively breastfeed/giving breast milk per cup to their infants during the first 6 months of life and continue breastfeeding/giving breast milk for at least 2 years
    - ❖ Pregnant HIV-infected women should be informed regarding support groups in her locality/district

[1] The under-mentioned advantages and disadvantages can be used as guide line for the different infant feeding options using the AFASS criteria for the final decision regarding which infant feeding option to choose

Acceptable - The mother perceives no problem in replacement feeding. Any problems perceived may be cultural or social in nature, or due to fear of stigmatisation and discrimination

Feasible - The mother (or family) has adequate time, knowledge, skills, resources, and support to correctly mix formula or milk and feed the infant up to 12 times in 24 hours

Affordable - The mother and family, with support of the community or healthcare delivery system where necessary, are able to pay the cost of replacement feeding over a long period of time without harming the health and nutrition of the family

Sustainable - Availability of a continuous supply of all ingredients needed for safe replacement feeding for up to one (1) year of age or longer

Safe - Replacement foods are correctly and hygienically prepared and stored, and fed preferably by cup

Formula feeding should only be considered when it is safe, sustainable, feasible, affordable and acceptable. When not, exclusive breast-feeding must be encouraged. Adequate support must be given to the mother on making formula feeding safe while mixed feeding (breast and replacement feeds) must be prevented (including replacement feeding at night and in public). Ensure that other family members or persons of importance possess the skills for safe replacement in case the mother is not available. Support the mother in dealing with possible stigmatization because of being HIV-positive and not breastfeeding as culturally expected of her

- **Intra-partum healthcare to be rendered to the birthing mother**

Note

HIV counselling and testing during labour is not encouraged as a last minute practice. When the mother is in early labour and there is adequate time, counselling and testing can be done. UNDER NO CIRCUMSTANCES MUST PRESSURE BE PUT ON THE MOTHER TO UNDERGO TESTING WHILE IN ESTABLISHED ACTIVE LABOUR

  ◈ Anti-retroviral drugs can be given in all stages of labour EXCEPT IF DELIVERY IS IMMINENT (THE HEAD IS CROWNING)
  ◈ When the HIV-status of a woman in labour is unknown, the necessary standard precautions must be taken as if the mother-to-be is HIV-positive
  ◈ The normal protocols regarding labour and the vaginal delivery of the baby must be followed
  ◈ When an elective or emergency caesarean section must be performed on a known HIV-positive mother, the standard protocols needed to be followed
  ◈ When the baby is born covered in meconium stained liquor, only the nose and airway of the HIV-exposed neonate must be sucked directly after birth, otherwise the neonate must be carefully wiped

- **Post-natal healthcare to be rendered to mother and child**

  <u>Care of the mother</u>
  - ❖ When the HIV-positive mother is on any anti-retroviral programme, referral to the anti-retroviral clinic/HIV-clinic service must be done and next appointment for continued treatment must be confirmed. The same applies for mothers that are not taking any anti-retroviral medicine
  - ❖ Family planning must be discussed with the HIV-positive mother as well as positive preventive measures for HIV/AIDS
  - ❖ The mother must also be routinely assessed for
    - her general health status and the health status of her breasts
    - whether she is coping with her baby and life in general
    - infant feeding practices and difficulties – when breastfeeding exclusively, the pattern of feeding, attachment and the position for breast feeding must be checked OR when using infant formula feeds, the method for cleaning utensils and preparing the formula feed must be checked
    - participation in support groups
    - adherence to the vaccination schedule for her infant
    - social security grant for her infant
  - ❖ Responsible fatherhood programmes must be implemented

  <u>Care of the infant</u>
  - ❖ Within an hour of delivery, the HIV-exposed neonate must have skin-to–skin contact with his/her mother regardless of the mother's infant feeding choice and the infant must be fed, either exclusively breastfeeding on demand/given expressed breast milk on demand or exclusively formula feeding
  - ❖ All HIV-exposed infants must be tested as per protocol and treated as per protocol
  - ❖ The feeding of the infant must be regularly discussed with the mother and the baby's growth pattern must be monitored
  - ❖ The baby must receive the necessary childhood vaccination as per protocol
  - ❖ At all visits the infant has to be clinically monitored for the following
    - growth retardation
    - oral thrush or oral sores
    - severe nappy rash
    - fever, floppiness or irritability
    - current illnesses
    - diarrhoea and coughing
    - had been in contact with persons suffering from tuberculosis
  - ❖ Any baby who had initially tested negative for HIV and who at any stage after 12 months of age, shows signs of failure to thrive or suffers from any opportunistic infections that are suggestive of HIV infection, should be tested again and then treated according to the "Integrated Management of Childhood Illnesses" (IMCI) protocols

◆ Preventive measures to be taken

➢ Mass public health information concerning the aetiology, spread and complications of HIV/AIDS and all other sexually transmitted infections. AIDS is a disease with a social stigma attached to it. Public ignorance concerning the transmission and spreading of the disease is one of the reasons why the person suffering from AIDS is ostracised

➢ Youth-friendly services must be provided at healthcare facilities, and boys and girls must be counselled regarding the dual risk of unintended pregnancies and STI's and HIV-infection

➢ All boys and girls must be informed about sexual and reproductive health issues and responsible sexual behaviour

➢ Boys and girls must be encouraged to complete their schooling

➢ Pregnant healthcare workers should not care for sick individuals suffering from AIDS since they might become infected with HIV or other viruses (for example, *cytomegalovirus*)

➢ Blood from donors and blood products must be tested for the virus and exposed to heat processes

➢ Women who are sero-positive and women who intend marrying sero-positive men, should receive fertility counselling regarding vertically trans-placental transmission of the virus to the unborn foetus

➢ Condoms should be used during intercourse to protect the sexual partner

➢ Communities as well as individuals (including learners and students) should be informed about the value of the ABC of responsible sexual behaviour to reduce the risk of infection – abstaining from sexual coitus until married (heterosexual or same gender marriages) or until a long-lasting relationship has been formed and be faithful to your partner (monogamous relationship) or partners (polygamous relationship)

➢ Everybody who is a donor of organs or tissues must be tested for the HIV-virus

➢ All individuals must be encouraged to have themselves voluntary tested for their HIV-status. All individuals must receive pre-counselling and post-counselling. When positive, anti-retroviral treatment must be commenced

➢ All traditional healthcare workers (especially the traditional birth attendants) must be educated regarding the management of HIV-positive mothers and their infants during antenatal, intra-partum, and postpartum healthcare and the feeding options available to mother and child

➢ Health information and preventive measures regarding HIV/AIDS must take the traditional African world-view in consideration. Traditional healers must become part of the multi-professional healthcare team as the they are agents of change because they are able to explain/re-explain and interpret/re-interpreted all scientifically sound interventions within African traditional cultural beliefs and the African philosophy regarding sexuality. The collective existence and the unity of the person with the community must be the underlying philosophy of the health information to be given

◆ **Measures to prevent epidemics**
  ✛ None

◆ **Implications for disaster situations**
  ✛ None

◆ **International measures**
  ✛ None

HIV/AIDS AND TUBERCULOSIS

Any individual suffering from tuberculosis can be infected with the HIV-virus when practicing irresponsible sexual behaviour or any individual suffering from HIV/AIDS-infection can be infected with *Mycobacterium tuberculosis humanis* after being in contact with a person suffering from active tuberculosis. The pathophysiology of Tuberculosis (TB)-HIV-virus co-infection in the same individual is as follows

✠ **Reactivation of a latent infection**
  Although all individuals do become infected with drug-susceptible *M. tuberculosis humanis* during their life span, complete sterilization of all lesions (lung and metastatic foci) do not takes place in some individuals and the person do not recover completely from the disease. As sterilization of the lesions is incomplete, *M. tuberculosis humanis* remains in the lesions, alive although latent. Should the person be exposed to situations of stress/infection/disease (see chapter 10, Tuberculosis - the natural endogenic cycle of tuberculosis, figure 10.1) tuberculosis reactivates spontaneously. Because the infection with the *HIV-virus* results in the progressive compromise/deterioration of the immune system, reactivation occurs spontaneously of the already existing tuberculosis infection in the body of the HIV-infected individual. Due to the fact that the immune system of the HIV-infected individual is already compromised by the HIV-infection, the mycobacterium now multiplies more rapidly to produce caseous necrotic lesions which then spill over into other sites in the lungs. Because the immune system is now further compromised, the immune system cannot contain the mycobacterium within the existing tubercles - the *M. tuberculosis humanis* thus invades the bloodstream and causes a disseminated tuberculosis infection ('miliary' tuberculosis or extra-pulmonary tuberculosis). As tuberculosis accelerates the progress of the HIV-infection to final-stage AIDS-disease, the prognosis of the individual suffering of HIV-infection and reactivated tuberculosis infection is very poor with a high fatality rate.

✠ **New Primary Acquired Tuberculosis Infection**
  Most immuno-competent individuals, who during their life span became infected with susceptible *M. tuberculosis humanis,* heal completely as the process of healing of the tubercles commences spontaneously approximately 8–10 weeks after invasion when cell-mediated immunity has been elicited. Complete sterilization of all lesions (lung and metastatic foci) takes place and the person recovers completely from the disease. The individual does not become re-infected with drug-susceptible *M. tuberculosis humanis* as long as the individual's immune

system is and stays competent. But, as soon as the individual becomes infected with the HIV-virus and the competency of his/her immune system deteriorates, the individual becomes susceptible to be infected with either drug-susceptible or drug-resistant *M. tuberculosis humanis* - a new primary acquired TB-infection in persons not known as to previously suffered from TB (see chapter 10, Tuberculosis and drug-resistant tuberculosis). The recovery rate of a new primary acquired drug-susceptible TB-infection in HIV-positive individuals is fair when diagnosed early, treatment started promptly and an aggressive treatment regime is followed over a period of time. Because the drug-resistant *M. tuberculosis humanis strain* is extremely virulent and highly transmissible (transmissible to all persons who are immuno-competent and who have acquired adaptive cell-immunity to both drug-susceptible and drug-resistant *Mycobacterium tuberculosis humanis*, to all immuno-compromised persons and to all sufferers of active TB [drug-susceptible and drug-resistant tuberculosis]), recovery of individuals suffering from HIV/AIDS and drug-resistant TB-infection is less favourable and the treatment usually last very long. The prognosis is, however, very poor and because treatment may not be effective, the fatality rate is extremely high.

Note

☑ The HIV-virus shortens the time period between the stage of pre-pathogenesis after exposure to *M. tuberculosis humanis* (drug-susceptible and drug-resistant) and the stage of the TB-infection (clinical picture of tuberculosis as active TB had developed) in a HIV-positive individual

☑ Because active TB-infection also diminishes the number of CD4-cells in the body, the HIV-viral load increases correspondingly in the infected individual, resulting in a shorten period of time before final-phase AIDS develops

☑ Miliary TB is more common in HIV-infected individuals (adults and children). Miliary TB is often under-diagnosed because of the fact that the diagnosis of smear-negative pulmonary TB-infection has increased in HIV-infected individuals. The HIV-infection changes the presentation of smear-negative pulmonary tuberculosis from a slowly progressive disease with a low bacterial load with a reasonable prognosis, to one of disseminated tuberculosis disease with reduced pulmonary cavity formation and reduced sputum bacillary load. Frequently, the lower lobes of the lungs are mostly involved from where dissemination takes place. Smear-negative miliary TB has an exceptionally high mortality rate

☑ The accuracy of diagnostic test to diagnose TB in HIV-positive individuals becomes unreliable because of the inability of the individual's immune system to mount an immune response to *M. tuberculosis humanis* and the TB-infection may present with atypical signs and symptoms. The Mantoux Tuberculin Skin Test may give a false negative test result, sputum smears may be smear-negative and chest X-rays may not show the typical TB-cavities. The diagnosis of TB in HIV-positive individuals must be based on signs and symptoms of all forms of tuberculosis, chest radiography and smear-sputum results. Non-treatment of smear-negative Tuberculosis must be prevented at all cost

☑ A higher than normal change exist that the treatment of TB in HIV-positive individuals fails altogether. The interaction between some anti-TB drugs (such as rifampicin) and some antiviral drugs in the treatment of HIV/AIDS (such as some protease inhibitors) for the same target sites may lead to the failure of the treatment for tuberculosis. Adverse reactions to anti-tuberculosis drugs (first and second line drugs) develop also more often in HIV-positive individuals. These adverse reactions may be confused with HIV/AIDS-related conditions such as peripheral neuropathy, visual disturbances, skin reactions and diarrhoea

☑ The development of drug-resistant TB (MRD-TB, XDR-TB and CDR/TDR-TB) in HIV-positive individuals ("resistance among previously treated cases") is very high and of serious concern. Drug-resistance develops because of poor adherence to TB-treatment (skipping or stopping taking medication and then starting again), inappropriate anti-TB drug prescription, irregular anti-TB drug supply, or poor anti-TB drug quality

☑ Unusual forms of Tuberculosis such as *Mycobacterium avian-intracellular tuberculosis,* are more often diagnosed in individuals suffering from final-stage AIDS

In order to provide comprehensive healthcare to all individuals suffering of HIV/AIDS, **TB preventive therapy** or **TB prophylaxis therapy** must be offered to all HIV-infected individuals to prevent active TB among HIV-infected individuals. **TB prophylaxis therapy** reduces the risk of the development of active TB in HIV-positive individuals who showed evidence of latent TB infection (as demonstrated by a positive Tuberculin Skin Test) while prolonging their survival. TB preventive therapy refers to the administering for a continuous duration period of 6 months of one or more anti-tuberculosis drugs to HIV-infected individuals with latent infection with *M. Tuberculosis humanis* in order to prevent progression to active TB disease. Essential to the TB preventive therapy is to ensure that active TB is excluded in each and every HIV-positive individual prior to starting the preventive TB therapy. All HIV-infected persons must be regularly screened for signs and symptoms of active TB, namely, current coughing, fever, loss of weight, and night sweat. All HIV-positive individuals with 1 or more signs and symptoms are considered as suspects for TB and must be further investigated for active TB as he/she is not eligible for TB preventive therapy until active TB is excluded on the basis of sputum smear microscopy, mycobacterial culture studies and investigations for extra-pulmonary TB. Individuals who test TB-negative, must be re-assessed in 3 months time and when no longer symptomatic (Tuberculin Skin Test positive [Mantoux induration <5mm]) be offered TB preventive therapy. Because HIV-infected persons who are taking anti-retroviral medication are at risk for reactivation of latent TB during the first 6 months of anti-retroviral therapy, often occurring in the setting of immune reconstitution inflammatory syndrome (IRIS), it is critical to ensure the systemic TB screening before initiating anti-retroviral therapy (ART) and during the first initial 6 months of taking ART. TB preventive therapy must not be stopped when starting ART and can be initiated any time during ART. As the benefits of TB preventive therapy outweigh the risk of active TB that are associated with spontaneous abortion and adverse perinatal outcomes, all HIV-infected females who are pregnant or fall pregnant are eligible for TB preventive therapy, provided active TB has been excluded. TB preventive therapy can also be given to all HIV-infected persons who have successfully completed their TB treatment or after a previous episode of TB, provided active TB is excluded. Because TB Preventive Therapy also benefits tuberculosis-free HIV-infected individuals, the TB Preventive Therapy must also be offered to them. Regular follow-up visits for recording of weight, ensuring adherence to therapy, providing of counselling, monitoring for side-effects of medication such as peripheral neuropathy, hepatitis, psychosis, convulsions, severe rash, and screening for active TB are of cardinal importance.

Note

> The TB preventive therapy does not aim to control TB on the population level, nor is it an alternative to the DOTS strategy for controlling TB – it is mainly a very effective intervention for preventing morbidity and mortality attributable to TB among HIV-infected individuals
> All HIV-infected individuals are to be screened regularly on a monthly basis for active TB as to intensify TB case finding among HIV-positive individuals
> As TB preventive therapy is expected to last for approximately 18 months, TB preventive therapy must be given once (1) only. The 6 months continuous treatment duration can, however, be completed over a 9 month period. When the TB preventive therapy has been interrupted for more than 3 months and the HIV-infected individual is still asymptomatic of active TB, TB preventive therapy can be restarted
> HIV-infected pregnant women, children, healthcare workers/professionals, TB contacts, miners, and prisoners are at high risk for developing active TB and will benefit from TB preventive therapy
> Tuberculin Skin Testing is not indicated when the HIV-infected individual falls within the high risk category, namely, pregnant women, children, healthcare providers (practitioners, traditional, lay), TB contacts, miners, and prisoners. Also, because the practicalities and logistics of doing a Tuberculin Skin Test are often obstacles for the provision of TB Preventive Therapy, the Tuberculin Skin Test is not required to identify HIV-infected individuals eligible for TB Preventive Therapy
> HIV-infected individuals with active liver disease or who are actively abusing alcohol are excluded from the TB preventive therapy because of the risk of hepatotoxicity
> When active TB is diagnosed, the TB preventive therapy must be immediately discontinued and active TB treatment must be started with anti-tuberculosis drugs - either first-line drugs for drug-susceptible TB or second-line drugs for drug-resistant TB

13.2   COMMUNICABLE DISEASES WHICH AFFECT THE URINARY TRACT

Although the urinary tract is one of the most common sites of infection, communicable diseases of the urinary tract is not transmissible to other persons. Most of the bacterial infections are usually acquired by the ascending route from the urethra to the bladder. The majority of infections are acute and short-live, though severe infections have serious long term sequelae. A variety of mechanical factors (for example, anything that disrupts the normal flow of urine, or the complete emptying of the bladder, or facilitates access of microbes to the bladder), will predispose a person to infection. Sexual intercourse facilitates the movement of microbes up the urethra of both women and men when preceding bacterial colonization of the peri-urethral area of the vagina of women had taken place or had colonized the glans penis or urethra of men. When the urinary tract is parasitized by worms/flukes such as the Schistosomes, a systemic reaction associated with allergy symptoms occurs.

13.2.1 Bacterial infection of the lower urinary tract

The most important communicable bacterial infection of the urinary tract is caused by bacteria that are not related to those specific pathogens causing sexually transmitted diseases (STI's) although the bacteria are transmitted by sexual intercourse.

13.2.1.1 NON-GONOCOCCAL URETHRITIS

Non-gonococcal urethritis is an acute infection of the urethra caused by various pathogens (the pathogens are not related to those specific infectious agents that cause sexual transmitted infections)

Epidemiological data

Geographic distribution
Occurring world-wide

Causative pathogen
Various pathogens of which *Chlamydia trachomatis, Mycoplasma hominis, genitalium* and *Ureaplasmas urelyticum* are the most important. The infectious agents colonize the genital tract of healthy sexually active men and women

Incubation period
1–3 weeks, sometimes longer

Mode of transmission
Sexual intercourse

Period of infectiousness (communicablity, transmission)
As long as the pathogens are present in the individual's body

Reservoir
Humans – healthy, sexually active males and females

Intermediaries
None

Carriers
None

Immune status
No immunity with memory is elicited

Susceptibility and resistance of host
All individuals who are sexually active are susceptible

Pathogenesis
The pathogens colonize the genital tracts of healthy, sexual active men and women and gain entry into the body via the urethra. As the pathogens have developed specialized attachment mechanisms, it is not washed out by urine during micturition.

A defined peptide on the bacterial pili binds to a carbohydrate polymer on the urethral cell and is then induced to engulf the cell (parasite-directed endocytosis). The short urethra of females is a more effective deterrent to infection than the male urethra where the pathogens remain in the moist area beneath the foreskin of uncircumcised males. The infection of the urinary tract is acute and characterized by a rapid onset of dysuria, urgency and frequency of micturition. The urine is cloudy due to the presence of pus cells (pyuria) and bacteria (bacteriuria) and may also contain blood (haematuria). Recurrent infection of the lower urinary tract may occur.

❖ **Clinical manifestation**
- Dysuria and frequency of micturition
- Clear muco-purulent discharge
- Low backache
- Men in particular tend to contract non-gonococcal urethritis
- Many women are symptomless, although urethritis and cervicitis may develop
- Non-gonococcal urethritis may present without any symptoms

❖ **Complications**
- Infertility
- Conjunctivitis in the new-born infant (silver nitrate eye-drops or an antimicrobial eye ointment do lend protection when administered to the eyes of the new-born infant directly after a vaginal delivery)
- *C. trachomatis* may also cause pneumonia in new-born babies
- In men prostatitis, epididimitis, urethral constriction and Reiter's syndrome (urethritis, conjunctivitis and arthritis) may occur
- In women urethritis, cervicitis, proctitis and salpingitis develop
- Conjunctivitis may occur in both genders

■ **Diagnosis**
- Urethral discharge together with signs and symptoms
- Midstream urine sample
- Urethral smear (men) or cervical smear (women)

■ **Prognosis**
- Good when treated immediately and chemotherapy has been taken as prescribed

■ **Specific healthcare interventions to be rendered**
- Chemotherapy – antimicrobial drugs (pregnancy and breastfeeding are contra-indications for administering tetracycline)
- Using of condoms during sexual intercourse
- Oral sexual activity should be discouraged

◆ **Preventive measures to be taken**
- ➢ Tracing of contacts and treating them
- ➢ Sexual health information re the ABC of responsible sexual behaviour
- ➢ Using of condoms during sexual intercourse (particularly where monogamous or stable polygamous sexual practices are not maintained)

◆ **Measures to prevent epidemics**
  ⬓ None

◆ **Implications for disaster situations**
  ⬓ None

◆ **Compliance with international measures**
  ⬓ None

13.2.2 Helminthic (digenetic trematodes/flukes) infections of the urinary tract

Several species of flukes (a worm) only mature in humans, developing in the intestine, lungs, liver and blood vessels. All flukes have an indirect lifecycle involving stages of larva development in the body of an aquatic snail and completing the lifecycle in humans. Humans are parasitized when they come in contact with water containing the parasitized larvae released from the snails which then penetrate through the skin of the individuals and parasitize them.

13.2.2.1 BILHARZIA (SCHISTOSOMIASIS)

Bilharzia is a fluke parasitaemia of the bladder or the intestines characterized by haematuria or melaena and allergic symptoms due to the antigens released by the eggs

---

Epidemiological data

Geographic distribution
Bilharzia occurs mainly in Africa, Asia and South America. In South Africa it is endemic along the eastern coast as far south as Knysna. Rivers that run dry during the summer months are reasonably free from infesting. Irrigation schemes which ensure permanent water increase the possibility of infesting

Causative pathogen
Schistosoma, a blood fluke. Various species cause schistosomiasis, namely,
　　Schistosoma haematobium (urinary schistosomiasis)
　　Schistosoma mansoni (faecal schistosomiasis)
　　Schistosoma japonicum (intestinal schistosomiasis) – occurring largely in Japan and the
　　Philippines

Incubation period
4-6 weeks after penetration

Mode of transmission
Humans are infected when their unprotected skin comes into contact with water infested with cercaria (larvae), or when they drink infested water

Period of infectiousness (communicability, transmission)
Parasitized hosts can transmit bilharzia for as long as viable eggs are passed in the urine or faeces. This can encompass the entire lifetime of an adult fluke which may be as long as 25 years. In most

---

cases the eggs live for a few hours only. Infested snails can release parasitized cercaria for many months. Bilharzia is not directly transmissible between persons

Reservoir
Humans are the main hosts

Intermediaries
Vectors - The freshwater snail, namely, Bulinus africanus species for *S. haematobium* and Biomphalaria species for *S. mansoni*, is the intermediate host for the fluke. The water has to be warm enough and slow-flowing or stagnant to harbour the snails. There should be grassy verges surrounding dams or streams for the snails to live on. The freshwater snail encysts the cercaria in the life cycle of the Schistosoma

Carriers
None

Immune status
No immunity with memory is elicited

Susceptibility and resistance of host
Everyone is susceptible

Life cycle of the Schistosoma

As all digenetic trematodes must pass through a mollusc intermediate host to complete their larval development, the sexual reproduction of the schistosoma thus occurs in the human host and the asexual reproduction of the fluke occurs in the freshwater snail.

When a person comes into contact with cercariae infested fresh water (for example, by standing, walking, swimming or playing) the free swimming cercariae suck onto the skin of the individual and release an enzyme which dissolves the skin that allows the cercariae entry into the body. (Cercariae do not enter the body through broken skin or mucosa but penetrate the skin to enter the dermis). During penetration the cercariae lose their tails to become schistosomulae. The schistosomulae migrate to the bloodstream via the lymph vessels from where they migrate to the lungs. After 4-18 days the schistosomulae develop into larvae. The larvae migrate, via the bloodstream, to the liver where they become sexually mature flukes and mate. The mature flukes now migrate to the small blood vessels surrounding the bladder and bowel tract where they live for 3-5 years, although this period may be as long as 30 years. (The female fluke can attain a length of 20 mm.) Microscopically small eggs with sharp acanthi are laid within 6-12 weeks and the eggs migrate to the inside of the bowel, rectum, and bladder. The cycle is completed when eggs that have been laid by the female flukes, move across the wall of the bladder or gut and leave the body (see figure 13.1).

The parasitized individual excretes the eggs of the schistosomes in urine or faeces. When the person defecates on dry land, the eggs of *S. mansoni* are viable for seven days and can be washed into dams and rivers by rainwater. The eggs of *S. haematobium* must be urinated directly into fresh water to ensure that they will hatch. As soon as the eggs reach water, the miracidia hatch within half an hour. Miracidia are oval in shape and have cilia with which to swim. They live for approximately 24 hours but are harmless within 8-10 hours. The miracidia penetrate their chosen snails as soon as possible and within an hour of penetration the miracidia form sporocysts. The sporocysts migrate to the snail's liver and form cercaria within six weeks. The snail encysts the cercaria and releases the infective cercariae for months. The cercaria dies within 12-48 hours unless they find a human host.

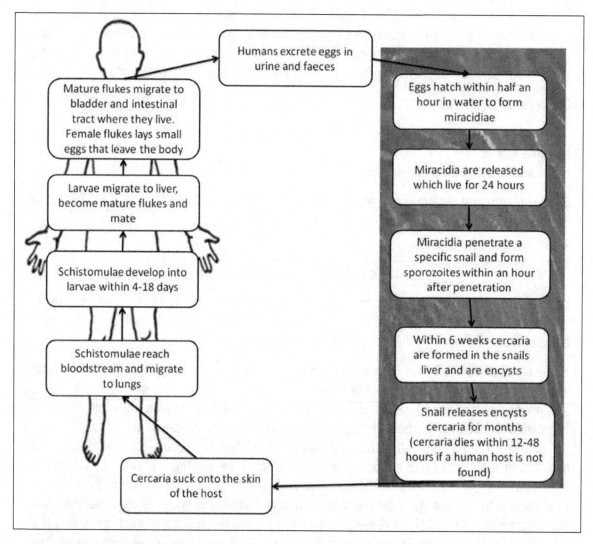

Figure 13.1 A schematic representation of the life cycle of the schistosomes

Pathogenesis

The different stages of the development of the schistosomes are each associated with pathologic changes, collectively affecting many body systems. Three syndrome entities, namely, dermatitis, Katayama fever and chronic fibro-obstructive lesions are identifiable and are associated with the various stages of development (that is, cercariae, mature flukes and egg production) in the human host. The cercariae, when penetrating the skin, elicit a dermatitis (papular-pruritic rash) which becomes more severe on repeated re-infection. The developmental stages of the schistosomulae are associated with the onset of allergic symptoms (fever, eosinophilia, lymph-adenopathy, spleno- and hepatomegaly, diarrhoea). As soon as the female schistosomes start laying eggs, the most severe pathology arises because the body became hypersensitive to the antigens released by the eggs when they pass through the tissues to the outside world, or become trapped in other organs such as the liver, lungs and central nervous system (the eggs are swept away in the bloodstream spreading to different organs). Egg production, *per se*, is therefore associated with pathologic changes affecting many body sites. Acute bilharzia, characterized by pyrexia (Katayama fever) now develops. When urinary schistosomiasis develops, the movement of eggs through the bladder wall causes haemorrhage and inflammation (the same happens when the eggs move through the intestinal wall). In the chronic stage of the disease, the bladder wall/intestinal wall becomes inflamed and infiltrated. Granulomas are formed as a delayed hypersensitivity reaction around the eggs in the tissues and polyps develop that may become malignant. When urine flows through the ureters that are blocked, hydro-nephrosis develops. Due to the emboli formed by the eggs, tissue damage occurs. This is followed by collagen deposits and connective tissue formation. The granulomas in the pre-sinusoidal capillaries and the connective tissue lesions cause severe obstruction of the flow of blood in the liver, and together with extensive hepatic portal (liver) fibrosis, results in hepatic portal hypertension. As a consequence, hepato-splenomegaly develops and collateral connections form between the hepatic vessels, while fragile oesophageal varicous-veins develop. The collateral circulation leads to eggs being washed into the capillary bed of the lungs.

❖ **Clinical manifestation**
  ✱ **Acute bilharzias**
    • A papular-pruritic dermatitis develops within 24 hours where the cercariae penetrated the skin
    • The so-called Katayama fever develops within 4-8 weeks. The onset is acute with rigor, diaphoresis, headache and a cough. Katayama fever lasts a few weeks before clearing up. (Please note that Katayama fever does not occur in *S. haematobium*, although the cough does)
    • Haematuria or melaena stools develops
    • Aching muscles are a common feature
    • Abdominal pain and diarrhoea may also develop

  ✱ **Chronic schistosomiasis**
    • Many parasitized persons are asymptomatic
    • Lethargy and fatigue develop, accompanied by drowsiness and poor concentration. (The waste products excreted by the flukes into the host's bloodstream contribute to the malaise)
    • In *S. mansoni* parasitaemia stomach ache and diarrhoea develop
    • When the eggs invade the bladder or colon, haematuria (*S. haematobium*) and melaena stools (*S. mansoni*) occur intermittently
    • Anaemia develops due to loss of blood
    • *S. mansoni* parasitaemia leads to hypertension due to liver involvement with splenomegaly and hepatomegaly

- In *S. haematobium* parasitaemia obstruction of the flow of urine occurs with urine retention, hydro-nephrosis and uraemia

❖ **Complications**
- Pulmonary schistosomiasis that present with signs and symptoms of COR pulmonale
- Cerebral schistosomiasis
- Hydro-nephrosis and uraemia

■ **Diagnosis**
- The presence of ova in urine or in stool specimens and in rectal or bladder mucosa biopsy specimens
- Urine collection must be done between 12:00 and 15:00 when the largest number of eggs is present in the urine. The bladder is emptied by 11:00 after which the urine is collected. The first and last parts of the urinary flow are collected
- Skin and complement fixation tests indicate antibody against flukes

■ **Prognosis**
- Fair to good
- When the parasitized person is not treated, a severe schistosomiasis develops and the disease may be fatal

■ **Specific healthcare interventions to be rendered**
- Chemotherapy – antimicrobial drugs
- Symptomatic and supportive
- In endemic regions, children who perform poorly at school should be thoroughly examined for anaemia as well as bilharzia. Children seldom complain about haematuria/melaena but rapidly develop anaemia due to the chronic loss of blood. Due to the anaemia their concentration is lowered, leading to poor performance at school

◆ **Preventive measures to be taken**
- ➢ Control of snails in streams and dams by promoting a flourishing birdlife (wild geese and waterfowl) and by removing the vegetation along the banks of streams and dams
- ➢ Environmental measures must be applied, namely,
    - ◈ provision of the necessary washing facilities to eliminate washing in water streams
    - ◈ public health information regarding the dangers of swimming in rivers and streams
    - ◈ provision of toilet facilities to eliminate urination and defecation in rivers and streams
    - ◈ protection of high-risk persons by wearing rubber boots (Wellingtons) and gloves and drying themselves thoroughly with a rough towel after contact with infested water
    - ◈ boiling of water for drinking purposes

❖ hygienic disposal of excreta and health information in this regard

◆ **Measures to prevent epidemics**
- None

◆ **Implications for disaster situations**
- None

◆ **Compliance with international measures**
- None

13.3 KEY NOTES

SEXUAL TRANSMITTED INFECTIONS

❏ Pathogens transmitted sexually include all groups of microbes except the rickettsiae and flukes.

❏ STI's are becoming more widespread in the community rather than remaining confined to high risk groups.

❏ No vaccines are available for STI's although antimicrobial drugs are used for treatment.

❏ Transmission of STI's depends solely on human behaviour which is notoriously difficult to influence and change.

❏ Vertically transmission from mother to child occurs in certain STI's with serious sequelae in the child.

❏ Individuals can suffer from more than one STI at the same time and as no immunity with memory is elicited, can be re-infected and re-infected ad infinitum.

❏ Sexually transmitted pathogens are becoming drug resistant.

❏ Prevention and control of STI's depends on sexually responsible behaviour (the ABC of responsible sexual behaviour) and children must be educated thereto.

❏ The long intervals between the onset of infectiousness and disease and infections without visible symptoms, increases the chances of transmission.

URINARY INFECTIONS

❏ Most urinary infections are acute episodes of infections without sequelae.

❏ Non-gonococcal urethritis may develop in healthy sexually active individuals of both genders.

❏ The digenetic trematodes (flukes) causing schistosomiasis is transmitted through an aquatic snail. The flukes cause a chronic parasitaemia characterized by hemorrhages, inflammation and hypersensitivity to the antigens released by the eggs. The consequences of the pathogenesis of the parasitaemia are very serious.

Chapter 14

ZOONOTIC DISEASES

Vector-borne and multisystem infections transmitted from animals to humans

Humans live in daily contact, directly and indirectly, with a variety of animal species, both vertebrate and invertebrate, not only sharing a common environment, but also a common susceptibility to certain pathogens. The ability to transmit infections acquired from animals to humans poses a constant threat of zoonoses. The degree to which animal contacts transmit infection depends on the type of environment (rural/urban, tropical/temperate, and hygienic/unhygienic) and on the nature of the contact. Close contact is made with vertebrate animals used for food or kept as pets as well as with invertebrate animals adapted to live and feed on the human body. Less intimate contact is made with many other species which nevertheless transmit pathogens equally well. Some zoonotic diseases such as Yellow fever have been known for centuries, whereas others such as Marburg haemorrhagic fever have been recognized more recently.

Animal-transmitted diseases in man are zoonotic infections that are transmitted to man – infections transmitted from birds/animals/insects/reptiles to humans. The relevant bird/animal/insect/reptile is infected with the pathogen and suffers from the zoonotic form of the infection. The individual is infected when he/she eats/drinks infected animal product, or is bitten, or scratched, or stung, or came in direct contact with the sick animal/bird or the animal's excreta, or in the case of birds, their feathers and/or droppings. The individual may also become infected when inhaling the pathogen. Some animal-transmitted diseases are not transmitted to other human beings, while those infections that colonize profusely in the lungs of the infected persons, are transmitted by airborne infected droplets when the infected individual coughs, sneezes, talks, sings or spits.

For convenience, animal-transmitted infections can be divided into categories, namely, those infections involving arthropods and other invertebrate vectors and those transmitted directly from vertebrates (zoonoses). The Epidemiological Data of animal-transmitted diseases depends on the frequency and the nature of contact between the vertebrate/invertebrate and the human host. The recent trend to keep exotic pets (especially reptiles, exotic birds and mammals) raises the risks of zoonotic infections as these animals and birds carry a wide range of pathogens that could be transmitted under the right conditions. The diagnosis of infections under these circumstances is very, very difficult when the healthcare provider does not know of such animals being kept as pets.

14.1 VECTOR-BORNE ZOONOTIC DISEASES

Many arthropods such as mosquitoes, biting flies, bugs, fleas and ticks feed on human blood and tissue. Insects, ticks, fleas and mites (the bloodsuckers) are the most important arthropod vectors spreading infection. In the past as well as today, insects, fleas and lice have been responsible for the most devastating epidemic diseases such as plaque, typhus and malaria. The distribution and Epidemiological Data of vector-borne zoonotic diseases are determined by the climatic conditions that allow the vectors to breed and the microbe to complete its development in the body of the vector. Some diseases are therefore purely tropical or sub-tropical diseases while others are much more widespread.

Arthropods transmit a wide variety of pathogens of all major groups, from viruses (arboviruses) to bacteria, rickettsiae, protozoa and worms. Heavy infections can build up causing a severe infectious condition. Arthropods cause diseases directly by their feeding and indirectly by transmitting infections. Contact with arthropods can be temporary or permanent. Blood feeders such as ticks and lice, feed for long periods on humans and reproduce on the body or in clothing, while the scabies mite lives permanently on man. Blood–feeders have mouthparts adapted for penetrating the skin in order to reach blood vessels or to create small pools of blood. The ability to feed in this way provides access for pathogens to gain entry through the skin or directly into the blood. The mouthparts act also as a contaminated hypodermic needle, carrying infection between individuals. Vector-borne zoonotic diseases on the other hand are transmitted by blood-feeding arthropods. These vectors inject the pathogen into humans when they take a blood meal.

14.1.1 Infections caused by Rickettsiae

Rickettsiae are small Gram-negative bacteria rods that live as parasites in blood-sucking arthropods and propagate via vertically transmission. Transfer of the *Rickettsiae* to the vertebrate host on which the arthropod lives, occurs mostly "accidental" as this transfer is not necessary for the survival of the rickettsiae. The infected arthropod does not appear to be adversely affected. The *Rickettsiae* are not transmitted from person to person.

14.1.1.1 TICK-BITE FEVER

Tick-bite fever is an acute systemic disease that persists in the human body for a long period or becomes latent

Please note - Humans contract tick-bite fever after being bitten by a tick that suffers from the zoonotic disease "tick fever". Humans cannot contract tick fever as tick fever has a stable cycle of infection due to vertical transmission (trans-ovarially) that only occurs in ticks

Epidemiological Data

Geographic distribution
Mainly prevalent in Africa

Causative pathogen
Rickettsiae conorii variety pijperi

Incubation period
10–12 days, sometimes as long as 6–18 days

Mode of transmission
Being bitten by a tick that is infected with *Rickettsiae conorii var. pijperi* causing tick fever in the tick
Person-to person transmission does not take place

Period of infectiousness (communicability, transmission)
No transmission occurs between humans. The tick is infected life-long

Reservoir
Ticks. The tick suffers from zoonotic tick fever and when the infected tick (particularly the larvae called pepper ticks) bites a person to suck blood, the person is infected and becomes sick. Vertical transmission (trans-ovarially) occurs in ticks only

Intermediaries
Vectors - Ticks

Carriers
None

Immune status
No immunity with memory is elicited

Susceptibility and resistance of host
All persons are susceptible

Pathogenesis

After the person has been bitten, the *Rickettsiae* multiply in the vascular endothelium. A papule develops at the point of entry that later suppurates. The abscess forms a black scab – the eschar. Rickettsaemia develops due to vasculitis in the skin, central nervous system and liver. The regional lymph nodes enlarge followed by a general lymph-adenopathy during the next 4–5 days. The Rickettsaemia in the liver; the skin and the central nervous system leads to hepatitis, maculo-papular skin rash, fever and headache.

❖ **Clinical manifestation**
   ✽ Prodromal signs similar to those of a cold are present for a couple of days
      • The bite of the tick causes a small abscess with a black centre – an eschar. (Only about 50% of all cases show an eschar)
      • The regional lymph nodes are enlarged

- Pyrexia of 40^0C–$40,5^0$C develops
- By the third day a rose-coloured maculo-papular skin rash appears on the entire body
- Ocular pain occurs as well as the development of petechiae
- The disease lasts for approximately 10–14 days

❖ **Complications**
- Thrombosis
- Oedema of the affected limb
- Pulmonary embolism and circulatory haemorrhages that can be fatal

■ **Diagnosis**
- History of being bitten by a tick
- Clinical picture
- Positive serological reaction

■ **Prognosis**
- Good

■ **Specific healthcare interventions to be rendered**
- Chemotherapy - administering of antimicrobial drugs
- Supportive and symptomatic

◆ **Preventive measures to be taken**
Reducing exposure to the vector by
➤ Wearing protective clothing outdoors
➤ Examining the body for ticks after walking or sleeping outdoors. Removal of ticks by hand (particularly in the ears, neck, groin, legs and hairy parts such as beard or hair)
➤ Spray socks, shoes and the hems of trousers or skirts with a tick-repellent
➤ Do not sleep on the ground during the months between October and April in the southern hemisphere
➤ Do not camp near areas where herbivorous animals graze
➤ Medical treatment after having been bitten by a tick

◆ **Implications for disaster situations**
- None

◆ **Compliance with international measures**
- None

14.1.1.2   TYPHUS

Typhus is an acute systemic disease caused by lice infected with *Rickettsiae* and is characterized by pyrexia and a typical skin rash

---

Epidemiological Data

Geographic distribution
Occurring world-wide. Epidemic typhus cannot maintain itself unless enough persons are infested with *Rickettsiae* infected lice, and as such is associated with poverty, war, and poor personal hygiene

Causative pathogen
Rickettsiae prowazeki (epidemic)
Rickettsiae typhi (endemic)

Incubation period
7-14 days

Mode of transmission
* Epidemic typhus - Bite of the *Rickettsiae* infected louse. The louse becomes infected by either biting a person suffering from typhus or by naturally contracting the *Rickettsiae* during its lifetime. The *Rickettsiae* multiply in the gut epithelium of the louse and are excreted in the faeces of the louse. When the louse bites, humans are infected when the bite is scratched and the faeces penetrate the skin through the site of the bite or through superficial cuts or abrasions. Infection may sometimes occur through the inhalation of dried faeces in dust
*Endemic typhus - Bite of the *Rickettsiae* infected rat flea

Period of infectiousness (communicablity, transmission)
No person to person transmission occurs
Epidemic typhus cannot maintain itself unless enough persons are infested with lice.

Reservoir
Humans and lice – pediculis corporis
As long as the louse is infected (lifelong) or as long infested humans serve as reservoir

Intermediaries
Vector - The louse Pediculosis humanis variety corporis

Carriers
None

Immunity status
No immunity with memory is elicited

Susceptibility and resistance of host
Everyone is susceptible, children in particular. Persons who have had previous attacks may contract a mild degree of the disease

---

Pathogenesis

After gaining entry into the body, the *Rickettsiae* multiply at the site of the bite and then spread in the blood to infect the vascular endothelium in the skin, the heart, central nervous system, muscles, and the kidneys. Because of the multiplication of and peri-vascular infiltration by *Rickettsiae*, leakage and thrombus formation follows. The vascular lesions in the skin cause the typical skin rash while the vascular lesion in the brain causes headache. The myocardium may display identical vascular lesions. The thrombus formation in the capillaries, arterioles and small venas may cause gangrene.

❖ **Clinical manifestation**
  ✻ **Epidemic typhus**
    • One (1) week after being bitten by the louse (no eschar is manifested), the infection commence suddenly with flu-like symptoms and pyrexia (39°C – 40°C)
    • A persistent headache develops fluctuating in intenseness and duration
    • A macular to maculo-papular rash appears from 4-7 days later or 5-9 days later, spreading across the entire body
    • Unproductive cough with an increased respiratory rate
    • When the infection is serious, the ill person develops meningo-encephalitis with stupor, severe hypotension, peripheral vascular collapse, renal failure, and meningo-encephalitis with delirium and coma followed by death
    • Convalescence may take months
  ✻ **Endemic typhus**
    • The disease is similar to epidemic typhus, but is less severe

❖ **Complications**
  • Secondary bacterial pneumonia
  • Toxaemia
  • Renal failure
  • Cardiac failure and peripheral vascular collapse
  • Gangrene of limbs that results in the amputation of the limb
  • In some individuals the rickettsiae are not eliminated from the body on clinical recovery and remain in the lymph nodes. The infection can reactivate after as long as 50 years to cause Brill-Zinsser disease. The individual now acts as a source of infection for any lice that may be present

■ **Diagnosis**
  ▪ History and presence of lice on the body
  ▪ A positive Weil-Felix test

■ **Prognosis**
  ▪ Children under the age of 10 - good
  ▪ Adults – 10% mortality rate
  ▪ Persons over 60 years – 50% mortality rate
  ▪ Untreated epidemic typhus has a mortality rate as high as 60%

■ **Specific healthcare interventions to be rendered**
  ▪ Chemotherapy – antimicrobial drugs

- Supportive and symptomatic
- Delousing of the infected person and all other persons who have had intimate contact with the ill person
- Contacts must be kept under observation for a period of 2 weeks

◆ **Preventive measures to be taken**
  - Outbreaks must be monitored
  - Personal hygiene must be encouraged
  - Overcrowding in refugee camps, prisons, military complexes and other places must be prevented
  - Prophylactic treatment to be given to high-risk persons
  - Regular delousing campaigns have to be undertaken

◆ **Measures to prevent epidemics**
  - Regular delousing of individuals in refugee camps, kept in detention, in military complexes, in prisons or of other persons running a high risk of being infected
  - Strict adherence to school exclusion regulations

◆ **Implications for disaster situations**
  - Epidemic typhus spreads rapidly amongst large groups of persons

◆ **Compliance with international measures**
  - None

14.1.2   Infections caused by Borrelia

Borrelia is Gram-negative spirochetes consisting of an irregular spiral that is highly flexible and move by rotating and twisting.

14.1.2.1   RELAPSING FEVER (BORRELIA RECURRENTIS)

Relapsing fever is an acute disease characterized by recurrent febrile episodes of pyrexia and spirochaetaemia

---

Epidemiological Data

Geographic distribution
Occurring world-wide

Causative pathogen
Borrelia recurrentis - transmitted by infected lice on the human body
Borrelia duttonii - transmitted by ticks. *Borrelia duttonii* is particularly prevalent in South Africa

Incubation period
Eight (8) days (3-10 days)

Mode of transmission
Being bitten by a *Borrelia* infected louse or tick and then rubbing the bite area over
Squashing/crushing of a *Borrelia* infected louse or tick over a wound or cut

---

Period of infectiousness (communicability, transmission)
The disease is not transmitted from one person to another

Reservoir
Infected tick or louse. Once ticks/lice are infected, the tick/louse is infected for life
Humans act as hosts for the louse, Pediculus humanis (epidemic form)
Rodents act as hosts for the tick of the genus Ornithodoros (endemic form)

Intermediaries
Vectors - <u>Lice</u> - As the *Borrelia* multiply in the body of louse, the *Borrelia* is introduced into the bite wound when the bite areas are rubbed and the louse is crushed. Because lice are transmitted from person to person, epidemic outbreaks of louse-borne relapsing fever can occur. *Borrelia* is transmitted trans-ovarially from generation to generation in lice
<u>Ticks</u> - In ticks, the *Borrelia* are transmitted trans-ovarially from generation to generation. Ticks also survive up to 14 years between blood-feeds which helps to maintain the endemic cycle of tick-borne relapsing fever

Carriers
None

Immunity status
No immunity with memory is elicited. When relapses occur, immunity may be mediated but wanes over time

Susceptibility and resistance of host
Everyone is susceptible. The condition is prevalent where poor hygienic conditions, overcrowding and poor socio-economic circumstances prevail

---

Pathogenesis

The *Borrelia* multiply in the louse/tick and gains entry into the human body when tick/louse bites are rubbed over or the infected louse/tick is crushed and the *Borrelia* are introduced into the bite wound. On gaining entry into the body, the *Borrelia* multiplies locally at the site of entry and then disseminate into the blood. The *Borrelia* multiply in the bloodstream (incubation period of 3-10 days) and a spirochaetaemia develops with chills and fever lasting 3-5 days. Antibody (agglutinating and lytic) is formed during the acute phase of the disease. The *Borrelia* is cleared from the blood by the antibody just before the onset of the a-febrile phase, but spreading has already taken place to the spleen, liver and kidneys where further multiplying occurs. Under "pressure" of the adaptive immune response, a new antigenic serotype emerges that is free to multiply and course a fresh febrile episode. (Antigenic variation involves switching of variable proteins on the bacterial surface. The result is that a single cloned *Borrelia* can spontaneously give rise to more or less 30 serotypes.) The a-febrile period last about a week before there is a second attack of fever. As soon as a relapse occurs, the new antigenic type of *Borrelia* appears in the blood once more. Generally there occur 3-10 or more such episodes. With each relapse more specific antibody are formed until the disease clears up. A more serious illness can occur when there is extensive growth of *Borrelia* in the spleen, liver and kidneys.

619

❖ **Clinical manifestation**
  ✹ **Febrile phase**
  - The febrile phase lasts for 3–6 days
  - The onset is sudden with rigor, pyrexia, muscular aches, aching joints, photophobia, and a cough
  - An erythematous rash appears on the trunk for a day or two
  - Epistaxis, haematuria, haemoptysis, haematemesis, splenomegaly, and neurological impairment with coma, cranial nerve paralysis, hemiplegia, meningitis, and convulsions may develop
  - The pyrexia drops abruptly with a crisis and the ill person may collapse due to hypotension and shock
  ✹ **A-febrile phase**
  - The a-febrile phase lasts 7–10 days after which the febrile phase re-occurs
  - Sweating and weakness are typical signs and symptoms during this period
  - With each relapse the symptoms are less severe
  ✹ **Relapses**
  - 3-10 or more such episodes of diminishing severity can occur
  - When there is extensive borrelia growth in the spleen, liver and kidneys, a more serious disease occurs

❖ **Complications**
  - Toxaemia
  - Shock
  - Liver failure
  - Myocarditis
  - Death

■ **Diagnosis**
  ▪ History
  ▪ Clinical picture
  ▪ Isolation of the spirochaete in a blood culture during the febrile-phase (rigor, headache, myalgia)

■ **Prognosis**
  ▪ Good, when treated with antimicrobial chemotherapy
  ▪ Mortality with endemic (tick-borne) relapsing fever is less than 5%
  ▪ Mortality with the epidemic form (louse-borne) may be as high as 40% or higher

■ **Specific healthcare interventions to be rendered**
  ▪ Chemotherapy – antimicrobial drugs
  ▪ Symptomatic and supportive
  ▪ Delousing
  ▪ Extermination of ticks

◆ **Preventive measures to be taken** (also see preventive measures for tick-bite fever)
  ➢ Health information regarding control of lice and ticks
  ➢ Improved personal and environmental hygiene
  ➢ Protecting of persons who sleep outdoors
  ➢ Regular disinfesting of floors and walls of huts and houses in rural areas and where unhygienic conditions prevail

◆ **Measures to prevent epidemics**
  ♣ Outbreaks of epidemics in humans can occur in unhygienic circumstances (where persons rarely wash and when clothes are not changes, for example, in wars and natural disasters) where large numbers of persons can be bitten by the infected lice in order to suck blood. Outbreaks can be terminated by delousing campaigns, improvement of personal hygiene, and maintaining of environmental health and hygiene. Burning of dirty and infested clothes are necessary

◆ **Implications for disaster situations**
  ♣ Louse-borne relapsing fever spreads rapidly amongst large groups of persons

◆ **Compliance with international measures**
  ♣ None

14.1.3 Infections caused by the protozoan - Plasmodium

The protozoan that affects the haemopoietic system, the *Plasmodium*, is a single-cell animal that specifically parasitizes the haemopoetic (blood), liver and nervous systems of the human host as an intracellular parasite. As an intracellular parasite, the protozoan has evolved many sophisticated strategies to avoid the responses of the host. The *Plasmodium* is transmitted by the parasitized female Anopheles mosquito when biting the human host. Due to the fact that the *Plasmodium* reproduces asexual in humans, a rapid increase in the numbers of the *Plasmodium* can take place in the parasitized individual. When the host's defence mechanisms are impaired as in young children, *Plasmodium* parasitaemia is more pathogenic in young children as in adults. *Plasmodium* parasitaemia is not life threatening but leads to ill health because the *Plasmodium* causes rupture of red blood cells resulting in anaemia and thrombocytopenia.

14.1.3.1 MALARIA

Malaria is an acute to chronic protozoan parasitaemia characterized by cyclic attacks of fever, excessive perspiring and exhaustion

Epidemiological Data

Geographic distribution

Endemic in Asia, Latin America and Africa. Malaria is the most widespread protozoan infection in Africa – it is estimated that more than 150 million inhabitants of Africa are suffering from Malaria at any given moment and an estimated 29% of the world's population is living in malaria-infested areas that are increasing rapidly.

The incidence of Malaria in the RSA is rising and it is endemic in Mpumalanga, Limpopo, Northwest and KwaZulu-Natal

The dispersal of the eggs, larvae, and pupae of the plasmodium is carried out primarily through sea routes worldwide, whereby, over large distances, the eggs, larvae, and pupae are transported around in combination with water-filled used tyres and cut flowers. The transport of mosquitoes in personal vehicles, delivery trucks, and trains also plays an important role, as with sea transport, in the further dispersal of the plasmodium

Causative pathogen

The protozoan, *Plasmodium*, of which four species exist, namely, *Plasmodium falciparum* (the most virulent); *Plasmodium vivax*; *Plasmodium ovale*; and *Plasmodium malariae*. *Plasmodium falciparum* is the most common cause of malaria in the RSA. The *Plasmodium* is an intracellular parasite and obtains nutrients from the host's cells by direct uptake or by ingestion of the cytoplasm. The *Plasmodium* infiltrates mainly the liver and erythrocytes (sometimes the brain cells) and evades the host's defence mechanisms by being an intracellular parasite that is removed from direct contact with antibody, complement and phagocytes - although the antigens of the *Plasmodium* may be expressed at the surface of the parasitized cells which then can be target for cytotoxic effectors. The *Plasmodium* also shows polymorphism in dominant surface antigens. The different species of *Plasmodium* are becoming drug- and insecticide resistant. The *Plasmodium* also lives in the red cells in the blood of many birds, reptiles and mammals

Incubation period

Plasmodium falciparum: 6-14 days (average 12 days)
Plasmodium vivax: 12-17 days (average 14 days)
Plasmodium ovale: 9-18 days (average 14 days)
Plasmodium malariae: 14-30 days (average 14 days)

Mode of transmission

Horizontally - Bite of an parasitized female Anopheles mosquito
    Blood transfusions
    Communal use of syringes by drug addicts
Vertically - Trans-placental (very rare)

Period of infectiousness (communicability, transmission)

In individuals who had received no treatment, the human is still parasitized for a month after they were declared clinically asymptomatic. Parasitized mosquitoes are infectious for their total life-span that lasts a month

Reservoir

Humans. The parasitaemia is transmitted from one person to another by the female Anopheles mosquito

Intermediaries

Biological Vectors - The female Anopheles mosquito

Epidemiological transition of the Anopheles mosquito has taken place as the species has successfully adapted to cooler regions. In temperate regions the Anopheles mosquito now hibernates over winter while in colder regions the eggs from the different species of the Anopheles mosquito are more tolerant to cold, snow and temperatures under freezing point. Even adult Anopheles mosquitoes now survive in the cold in suitable microhabitats throughout winter

Carriers

Untreated asymptomatic parasitized individuals are life-long carriers

Immunity status

Although cell-mediated and antibody-mediated immunity is elicited over a period of time, it does not last long. Re-infection can occur. In endemic regions, clinical malaria is limited to young children. Adults are usually immune with asymptomatic, low-grade parasitaemia and an enlarged spleen. Natural passively-acquired immunity is present for a few months in new-born babies of an immune mother. Foetal haemoglobin also partially protects babies during the first few months of life

Susceptibility and resistance of host

All persons of all ages are highly susceptible to malaria. One attack of malaria does not elicit immunity with memory; therefore, persons who were treated with anti-malarial drugs may become infected again. Multiple infections may be simultaneously present in the same individual (for example, *Plasmodium falciparum* and *Plasmodium vivax*). Persons living in endemic areas develop partial immunity with memory to a specific *Plasmodium* and its subspecies

Lifecycle of the Anopheles mosquito harbouring the *Plasmodium*

Anopheles Gambia breeds in small pools of water regularly filled up by rain water and heated by the sun. Anopheles funestus breeds in fresh flowing water in permanent streams to which it is endemically restricted. The female Anopheles mosquito serves as intermediate host to complete the sexual reproductive cycle of the *Plasmodium*. The Anopheles adult mosquito hibernates in dark, warm moist places. Certain species hibernate in the egg stage. The eggs of the female Anopheles mosquito hatches in warm weather within 2-3 days of having been laid. The larvae live in the water and feed on tiny plants and insects. Within 10 days the larvae change into cocoons, and after 2-4 days they have grown to adult mosquitoes which can fly a distance of 1,6 km from where they were hatched. The female Anopheles mosquito rests with its tail in the air, a characteristic which distinguishes it from the Culex mosquito which rests with its tail parallel to the surface of its resting place. Another characteristic of the female Anopheles mosquito, also called the "silent killer", is that it does not buzz around a person's head at night irritating the individual – the person is mostly not aware of the presence of the female Anopheles mosquito and sometimes unaware of having been bitten as the individual's reaction to the bite of the female Anopheles mosquito may not be as pronounced as with other blood-sucking insects. The female Anopheles mosquito lives for 30 days or longer, while the male mosquito, feeding off vegetation, only lives for 10-20 days. Within a week or more after biting a parasitized individual to suck blood (the parasites are present in the blood of an infected individual), the female Anopheles mosquito can parasitizes other persons.

The lifecycle of the *Plasmodium* takes place in man and in the mosquito and consists of three stages that are characterized by alternating extra-cellular and intracellular forms. The lifecycle commences when female and male gametocytes develop from a sub-population of merozoites in the blood of the parasitized host (the *Plasmodium* forms sexual cells, the gametocytes, instead of dividing). The gametocytes are present in the blood of the parasitized host and are thus sucked up by the female Anopheles mosquito during a blood-feed as the female Anopheles mosquito requires blood to nurture her eggs. The gametocytes mate in the intestinal tract of the mosquito forming gametes. The fertilized eggs, known as zygotes, develop into oocytes/ookinetes containing thousands of sporozoites. The oocytes rupture within ten days, releasing sporozoites which migrate to the salivary glands of the mosquito. When the parasitized female Anopheles mosquito bites a person (see fig. 14.1) the sporozoites in the saliva from the parasitized mosquito are injected into the bloodstream of the relevant individual commencing the pre-erythrocytic stage as the saliva of the female Anopheles mosquito effectively block the haemostasis system of the human individual because vascular constriction, blood clotting, platelet aggregation, and angiogenesis are negatively affected. Alteration of the immune system also takes place as the saliva of the female Anopheles mosquito induces inflammation with suppression of interleukin-2 and inferon-production, a shift in cytokine expression, and inhibiting of T-cell and B-cell proliferation. The sporozoites migrate, via the bloodstream, to the liver where they enter the parenchyma cells of the liver. In the liver, tissue schizonts are formed and when the schizonts rupture, merozoites are released that penetrate the erythrocytes within a few minutes, initiating the asexual blood or erythrocytic stage. Some merozoites remain in the liver to lie dormant as tissue hypnozoites (the hypnozoites causing the relapses when rupturing). In the erythrocytes, the merozoites mature into trophozoites forming erythrocytic schizonts - the cycle being completed when the mature trophozoites in the erythrocytic schizonts release merozoites back into the circulation. This cycle can last for months or even years without involvement of the liver. The sexual stage is initiated when a sub-population of the merozoites matures into male and female gametocytes within the erythrocytes. The lifecycle now repeats itself.

The duration of the parasitaemia is dependent on the continuous presence of the exo-/pre-erythrocytic stage. *Plasmodium falciparum* has a low recurrence incidence (less than a year) since the *Plasmodium* cannot survive as hepatic schizonts. Hepatic schizonts of *plasmodium vivax* and *Plasmodium ovale* can survive for approximately three to five years, while the hepatic schizonts of plasmodium *malariae* can survive for 20-50 years.

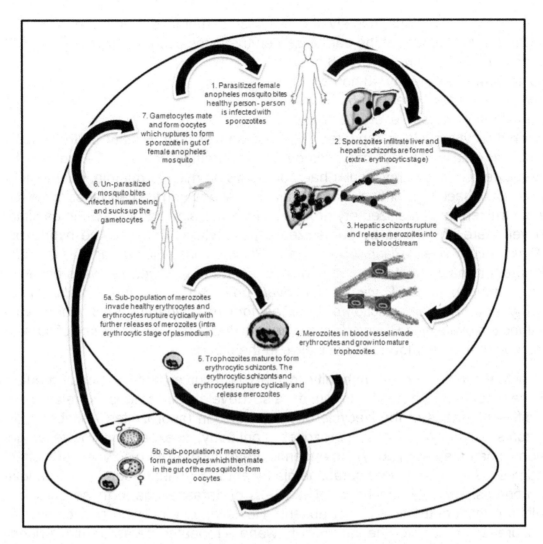

Figure 14.1 Schematic representation of the life-cycle of the plasmodium

Pathogenesis

When the female Anopheles mosquito bites a human being, it injects the sporozoites in its saliva into the subcutaneous capillaries of the host. From here the sporozoites migrate to the liver and infiltrate the hepatic parenchyma cells where they mature and multiply to form hepatic tissue schizonts in the hepatic tissue (the symptomless exo-erythrocytic or pre-erythrocytic stage). At this stage the parasitized individual does not yet feels sick.

After a week or two the hepatic tissue schizonts rupture, releasing thousands of merozoites into the bloodstream (asexual blood stage or erythrocytic stage). The merozoites within minutes penetrate into the erythrocytes where they mature within 8 days (or even so long as several months) into trophozoites forming erythrocytic schizonts which again release merozoites. When all parasitized erythrocytes simultaneously rupture, toxins formed by and waste material of the plasmodium as well as merozoites are released into the bloodstream, resulting in the typical signs and symptoms of malaria, namely, the manifestation of fever and a feeling of being ill. These cyclic rupture of the parasitized erythrocytes occur as follows

Plasmodium falciparum - every 48 hours
Plasmodium vivax - every 48 hours
Plasmodium ovale - every 49-50 hours
Plasmodium malariae - every 72 hours

The erythrocytic cycle is repeated with invasion of new healthy erythrocytes by merozoites on a continuous basis without the liver being involved. The rupture of the erythrocytes causes intravascular haemolysis giving rise to anaemia, haemoglobin-anaemia and haemoglobinuria. Cardiac failure ensues when the capillaries of the heart are obstructed by parasitized erythrocytes. In cerebral malaria the brain capillaries and veins are obstructed by parasitized erythrocytes. Because the hypnozoites of *Plasmodium vivax, Plasmodium ovale, Plasmodium malariae* and *Plasmodium falciparum* remain latent for months or even years in the liver, relapses occur – *P. falciparum* up to 1 year, *P. vivax* and *P. ovale* up to 3-5 years, and *P. malariae* up to 20-50 years. The re-surrection of the *Plasmodium falciparum, Plasmodium vivax, Plasmodium ovale,* and *Plasmodium malariae* is due to the re-emergence of parasites (*Plasmodium*) at very low levels still alive in the blood

The actual mechanism of immunity to malaria involves both antibody-mediated and cell-mediated immunity. Immunity also develops in stages correlating with the different stages of the lifecycle of the protozoan (sporozoites - antibody; liver schizonts - cytotoxic T-cells; merozoites - antibody; asexual erythrocyte stage – antibody; gametes – antibody). In endemic areas children who survive early attacks becomes resistant to severe parasitaemia by about 5 years of age. Parasite levels fall progressively until adulthood. The levels of parasitaemia in these parasitized adults are most of the time low or absent. However, one (1) year spent away from exposure is sufficient for the immunity to wane – repeated parasitaemia is needed to maintain immunity.

❖ **Clinical manifestation**
The clinical picture depends on the age and immune status of the parasitized person as well as on the parasite specie. Symptoms are associated exclusively with the asexual erythrocytic stage and range from a fever to a fatal cerebral or renal disease

✳ **Acute malaria**
The acute stage occurs when the parasitized erythrocytes simultaneously rupture releasing merozoites that were formed by the erythrocytic schizonts Acute malaria is characterized by
- Cyclic periods of fever and rigor (an elevation of the body temperature to 40^0C-42^0C) as well as headache, followed within hours by diaphoresis and a lowering of body temperature when the erythrocytes rupture (Falciparum malaria – every 48 hours; Vivax malaria – every 48 hours; Ovale malaria – every 49 to 50 hours; Malariae malaria – every 72 hours). These cyclic periods may be preceded by continuous pyrexia for several days

- Myalgia, aching wrists, gastro-intestinal symptoms such as vomiting and dehydration as well as exhaustion/tiredness may develop because of hypoglycaemia followed by delirium and coma
- Anaemia and jaundice develop because of the loss of red blood cells. Severe anaemia is caused by the destruction of both parasitized and non-parasitized erythrocytes by either the plasmodium or the body self
- Body organs like the kidneys, liver and spleen may fail due to the flood of waste materials and blood clotting in capillaries to a point where the body can no longer cope
- Parasitaemia with *P. falciparum* is frequently fatal during the first 2-3 weeks. Parasitaemia with *P. vivax, P. ovale* and *P. malariae* are normally self-limiting if no re-parasitaemia occurs

✱ Chronic malaria

When the parasitaemia is not treated and no complications occur, immunity is elicited when antibody are developed

- Individuals suffering from chronic parasitaemia have low-grade parasitaemia but are asymptomatic
- Natural recovery follows within a year in falciparum malaria, within four years for vivax malaria and within 2–3 years for malariae malaria

❖ Complications

When a serious parasitaemia exists as in falciparum malaria, some of the most severe complications may be fatal, such as

- **Blackwater fever** – because of massive red blood cell destruction and haemolysis, immune-complex glomerulo-nephritis (an immuno-pathologic condition) develops with haemoglobinuria, obstruction of the glomeruli, acute tubular necrosis and anuria. Immuno-complex glomerulo-nephritis develops when immune complexes are formed together with complement activation and the complexes escape removal by the phagocytes of the reticulo-endothelial system and become lodged in the tissues or blood vessels attracting complement and neutrophils. The release of lysosomal enzymes results in local damage, which is particularly serious in the small blood vessels, especially in the renal glomeruli. Jaundice and anaemia are also present
- **Cerebral malaria** - when parasitized erythrocytes cross the brain barrier, headache and neck stiffness develop progressively, followed by convulsions and confusion. The person becomes drowsy and lapse into a coma, followed by death. Neurological impairments such as aphasia and paralysis may also develop
- **Acute and chronic splenomegaly** occurs particularly in *P. vivax, P. ovale* and *P. malariae*
- **Severe anaemia** develops due partly to the destruction of red blood cells and partly to dyserythropoiesis in the bone marrow
- **Death** – *P. falciparum* is frequently fatal during the first 2–3 weeks due to a variety of complications. Complicated *P. falciparum* mostly occurs in children 6 months to 5 years, in pregnant women (primigravidae) and non-immune persons (for example, tourist) of any age

■ Diagnosis

- History and clinical picture of fever, anaemia, splenomegaly and/or cerebral signs in a individual could conceivably be malaria
- Blood is taken for blood smears preferably during a rigor attack. A negative result does not necessarily mean that the person is free of malaria, since the annular forms of the *Plasmodium* that are being investigated, periodically disappear. Smears must therefore be repeated. "Dip stick" testing helps to make early rapid diagnosis possible in especially non-immune persons (infants, travellers from malaria-free areas, and victims of malaria epidemics)
- The presence of parasites in the blood of an ill person from an endemic area does not mean malaria is the cause of the present disease because the parasitaemia may be asymptomatic

■ Prognosis

- Good, when the ill individual receives treatment and no complications develop
- Cerebral malaria, however, has a high mortality rate
- Pregnant women and young children are at a higher risk for developing severe complications
- Parasitized individuals who has had a splenectomy are at a higher risk for rapidly progressive malaria
- HIV-infected non-immune adults (i.e. individuals whose childhood were spend in areas where malaria does not occur) are at a higher risk for severe malaria and their risk increases when their CD4+ T-cell count is low

Note

- ◈ Because the symptoms of malaria closely resemble those of influenza, malaria may be misdiagnosed
- ◈ Because jaundice may be present in malaria, an erroneous diagnosis of viral hepatitis can be made
- ◈ Signs and symptoms of malaria may develop quite a while after leaving the malaria area – thus reducing the suspicion of malaria to the detriment of the ill person
- ◈ Immunity is only acquired under conditions of frequent parasitaemia – immunity does not prevent parasitaemia but decreases the severity of the parasitaemia whereby the rate of recovery is increases. Because immunity is *Plasmodium* species specific, immunity is lost when a person leaves the malaria area. Immunity is also transferred from mother to infant (natural passively-acquired immunity) but lasts only for 3-6 months. Foetal haemoglobin partially protects infants during the first few months
- ◈ A parasitized individual can suffer from more than one species of *Plasmodium* simultaneously, making diagnosis of the different species difficult. As anti-malaria drugs deal only with the erythrocytic stage and not the hepatic stages of the disease, the Vivax and Ovale species that have dormant liver stages, often do not get treated initially. When two or more species are present in the blood and one or two species are not identified, malaria can sometimes flare up again many months later. Once the different species have been identified, the liver stage can be successfully treated

■ Specific healthcare interventions to be rendered

- Chemotherapy – anti-malarial drugs such as schizonticides, chloroquine and amodiaquine. Parasitized individuals must be encouraged to complete the course of treatment (especially the oral drugs) since the *Plasmodium* has developed drug-resistance against anti-malarial drugs and because of the inadequate drug levels in the blood, the *Plasmodium* is allowed to multiply and to develop, resulting in full blown malaria. The chemotherapy must be taken according to the prescribed method as these agents are only effective as prescribed. Any haphazard use or inappropriate use makes the drugs totally ineffective. When serious side-effects occur, medical help should be sought and the drug be discontinued. Mild nausea, occasional vomiting or loose stools are not adequate reasons to stop taking the oral anti-malarial drug. Simplicity in the drug regimen improve compliance and once a parasitized individual is compliant on one specific drug regimen and is tolerating it well, do not transfer to another drug regimen as the likelihood is high for developing side-effects due to the introduction of a different drug.

Oral chemotherapy is used for uncomplicated malaria while intravenous or intramuscular treatment for severe malaria. Combination therapy (artemisinin-based combination drug-therapy) is being advocate to delay the onset of resistance. Resistance must also not be confused with a lack of compliance, a prescription for an inadequate dosage, and a re-infection with a new or same species. When an individual suffering from malaria vomits within one (1) hour after an oral dosage, the dosage must be repeated

- When necessary, blood transfusion is to be given
- When renal failure develops, haemodialysis is to be done
- Supportive therapy to be given with bed rest for fever and other symptoms
- Intake and output must be measured to detect kidney failure
- Measures must be taken to counteract hyponatraemia and hypoglycaemia
- Complications to be observed and the necessary care to be initiated
- Hospital care is required for cases of severe malaria and cerebral malaria

◆ Preventive measures to be taken

Preventive measures are based on vector control, health information, chemo-prophylaxis and other measures

➤ Vector control aimed at mosquito eradation

- ◆ Extermination of mosquito larvae and pupas must be done on a continuous basis. Initially oil combined with spreading agents was sprayed on water surfaces to smother larvae and pupae. This practice is no longer being used. Insecticides are now used weekly to destroy larvae. Breeding places can be destroyed by drainage and filling up with soil. Protecting of natural predators like droganflies and larvae-eating fish as well as habitat modification and trapping can also be used for mosquito control
- ◆ Mosquitoes have to be destroyed on a continuous basis. During the summer months the walls and ceilings of houses must be sprayed on the inside with a long-acting insecticide which is effective for six months. (Mosquitoes are adept in infiltrating and can find their way into residences via de-activated air conditioning units). Control of adult mosquitoes is maintained throughout the year and is considered the most important

preventive measure because of the increasing resistance of the plasmodium to chemotherapy

- Avoid sleeping near mosquito harbouring areas such as swamplands, marshes and areas of thick vegetation. Also avoid drinking alcohol in such excess that awareness of risk situations is diminished, i.e. falling asleep outdoor in the open particularly in warm and hot localities or during wet and warm periods. Remember, high minimum night temperatures induces the developmental phase of the plasmodium within the mosquito

- Prevent mosquito bites by having homes made mosquito-proof; sleeping under impregnated and treated mosquito-netting; wearing clothing that protect the whole body (fully covering arms and legs when outdoors between sunset and sunrise) particularly after sundown; and using mosquito repellents (spraying for insects and applying mosquito repellent to the body)

- Insect repellents. Use insect-repellent agents in the form of lotions, sticks and sprays. Apply liberally on all exposed skin surfaces after sunset. Flying insect spray can be used indoors together with body-applied agents. (Note that DEET-based mosquito-repellent agents can have harmful effects [Diethyl-meta-toluamide {DEET} mosquito-repellent agents])

- Avoid braais (barbecues) and other recreational activities outdoor such as parties after sunset

- The use of long lasting insecticide treated nets (ITN's) by pregnant mothers and children under the age of five (5) years is recommended

> **Health information**

- The public has to be made aware of the fact that malaria can be prevented. The myths around malaria (chemoprophylaxis must not be taken as it will masks the symptoms, malaria cannot be cured, take only chemoprophylaxis while in a malaria area, and "I was not bitten, so I am stop drinking anti-malaria chemoprophylaxis") must be de-mystified as travellers to and inhabitants in malarial areas are at a high risk of contracting a dangerous and life-threaten form of malaria

- Pregnant women and young children under 5 years of age as well as immune-compromised HIV-infected persons are high risk travellers to malarial areas and should not travel into such areas

- The perpetuation of the parasitisation of mosquitoes by already parasitized persons who are relatively immune to malaria and does not fear the disease, is an extremely serious problem. When these persons do not take precautions against mosquito bites, they parasitize the mosquitoes when they are bitten. In this way, the life-cycle of the plasmodium is maintained. These individuals must be informed to prevent mosquito bites at all cost by strictly adhering to both environmental and personal preventive measures

- All travellers to malaria areas (including malaria-free areas) must give a full travelling history when feeling ill and seek medical help immediately when they develop fever and a flu-like illness

➢ **Chemoprophylaxis**

Short-term chemoprophylaxis is indicated for all persons who are visiting an endemic region for a limited period, while long-term chemoprophylaxis is used for persons living in endemic malaria regions

- The taking of short-term chemo-prophylactic drugs is extremely important for visitors to high-risk areas. The course of these drugs must be started a week before the visit, maintained during the stay and kept up for four weeks after the visit has ended. Prophylactic drugs that prevent malaria are known as schizontocides and become active once the Plasmodium has entered the erythrocytes, a process that does not occur until 10 to 14 days after being bitten by the parasitized mosquito. When the drug is stopped before the four (4) weeks has lapsed after leaving the malaria area, the drug level in the blood will be too low to kill off the plasmodium. Pregnancy is a contra-indication

- Long-term chemoprophylaxis is obtained by means of a parenteral depot compound, such as Camolar. An injection of this drug renders a person reasonably insusceptible for a period of four (4) months

Please note

1. Travellers should take the chemoprophylaxis according to the prescribed method as these agents are only effective as prescribed. Any haphazard use makes them totally ineffective. When serious side-effects occur, medical help should be sought and the drug be discontinued. Mild nausea, occasional vomiting or loose stools are not adequate reasons for stopping the anti-malarial drug

2. Simplicity in regimen improve compliance and once a individual is compliant on one prophylactic regimen and is tolerating it well, do not transfer to another regimen as the likelihood of the development of side-effects, due to the introduction of a different drug, is increasing

3. Individual risk assessment is important when deciding what advice to be given. The advice to be given will vary with the season. Of importance are the other measures to be taken to minimize exposure to infection, especially protection from being bitten while asleep. Medical help must promptly be sought when symptoms develop. Citronella repellents is poorly effective and sonic buzzers are useless

4. As cure is not always possible, malaria must be prevented at all cost. **DO NOT STOP PROPHYLAXIS ON THE BASIS OF HEAR-SAY OR QUASI- OR PSEUDO-EXPERTS. THE SERIOUSNESS OF MALARIA WARRENTS TOLARATION OF TEMPORARY AND MILD SIDE-EFFECTS**

◆ **Other preventive measures to be taken**

➢ Resistance to chemotherapeutic drugs must be continuously monitored. In particular, attention has to be given to promoting health behaviour that prevents non-compliance of treatment. Knowledge of malaria has to be spread in communities and the health behaviour as well as the attitude of sick and healthy persons and communities towards malaria have to be monitored

➢ Endemic regions should preferably be visited during the dry season or when the rainfall is relatively low. Persons who are considered high-risk cases such as pregnant women, children under the age of 5, persons over the age of 60, and persons whose immunity is suppressed due to illness, are advised not to visit endemic regions

◆ **Measures to prevent epidemics**
   ⯇ The inhabitants of endemic areas must be made aware that there will be an increase in the prevalence rate of malaria (more new malaria cases) after heavy rains. There is a correlation between an increase in the number of mosquitoes and a high rainfall in the environment. Vector control has to be intensified. Communities must be encouraged to take part in the control programmes against mosquitoes. Industries and the private business sector as well as all other social institutions must be encouraged to maintain a healthy environment to prevent mosquitoes from hatching
   ⯇ Close cooperation has to be negotiated with neighbouring countries regarding existing preventive programmes as well as the planning and implementation of new programmes. The involved countries must do regular evaluation of all control programmes
   ⯇ A system of supervision must be implemented for all immigrants (legal as well as illegal) entering the country from endemic regions
   ⯇ Blood-safety must be instated to ensure a malaria-free pool of voluntary blood donors while blood transfusion due to malaria-related anaemia needs to be reduced
   ⯇ To effectively control malaria, good cooperation between the public, the private and the traditional healthcare sectors must be maintained. Of utmost importance is to educated traditional and lay healthcare providers regarding
      ♦ Recognition of malaria according to the signs and symptoms
      ♦ Referring for the necessary treatment and acting as supervisor overseeing the treatment protocol
      ♦ Health information to be given to all healthcare users (whether healthy or sick) – especially regarding adhering strictly to all preventive measures
      ♦ Maintaining of a healthy environment including the eradication of mosquitoes

◆ **Implications for disaster situations**
   ⯇ None

◆ **Compliance with international measures**
   ⯇ None

14.2 MULTISYSTEM ZOONOTIC DISEASES

In multisystem zoonotic diseases, a non-human vertebrate host is the reservoir of the infection and humans are mostly incidentally involved. A stable life cycle of the pathogen usually occurs in the natural animal host-reservoirs and a harmless persistent lifelong infection is caused in the animal. The human host, however, is not essential for the microbe's lifecycle or for its existence in nature. Quite often, the ecology of the physical-biological environment where the animals live is disturbed or the infected animal(s) is purposely removed from its natural habitat by man himself.

The zoonotic origin of some of these infections/diseases is sometimes less clear. Some infections is acquired either by direct contact with the reservoir host (for example, arbovirus from apes) or from an arthropod-vector (rat flea from plague-infected rats).

Vertebrate animals transmit many pathogens directly to humans by a variety of different routes that include contact, inhalation, bites, scratches, contamination of food or water, and ingestion as food (animal meat and infected animal products). When transmission of the pathogen from animal reservoir to humans take place, it causes a severe to fatal illness in humans characterized by haemorrhage, capillary damage, haemo-concentration, and collapse followed by death. Few multisystem zoonotic diseases are effectively transmitted from human to human, but, when transmission between humans does occur, it gives rise to a more serious-to-fatal disease with an extremely high mortality rate. Transmission between humans takes place when the lungs of the infected human have been seeded with the pathogen due to the haemo-concentration of the pathogen [dissemination of the pathogen into the blood has taken place followed by profuse multiplication of the pathogen in the blood]. A viraemia/bacteraemia/toxaemia develops in the lungs, leading to broncho-pneumonia due to the profuse growth of the pathogen in the lungs. Direct horizontally transmission, via infected droplets, now takes place between persons (person-to-person transmission). Transmission between persons also occurs via infected human blood, tissue fluids, and secretions such as sputum (large numbers of the specific pathogen is present in the sputum). Transmission is also multi-host, in so far that the pathogen can be transmitted from person to person by an intermediary vector, or directly from vertebrate(s) to humans. Hence, in all multisystem zoonotic infections, all body systems in humans are affected (the infection is not localized only to one system of the body) and the infection is extremely seriously and can be fatal.

14.2.1   Multisystem zoonotic diseases caused by bacteria

Most bacteria exist as free-living microbes and only a relatively few species cause disease. Bacteria are single-celled prokaryotes and their DNA is not contained within a nucleus. Their cell wall is a key structure in their metabolism, virulence, and immunity. Flagella enable bacteria to move in their environment while pili enable them to attach themselves to other bacterium or to host cells. The rate at which bacteria grow and divide depends in large on the nutritional status of their environment – in a rich medium like blood it can divide in identical daughter cells within 20-30 minutes whereas the same process is much slower (1-2 to 24 hours) in a nutritionally depleted environment. When introduced into a new environment, bacterial cell division occurs rapidly after an initial period of adjustment, followed by a slowing of cell growth and then a decline as nutrients are depleted and toxic products accumulate.

14.2.1.1 BRUCELLOSIS (MALTA FEVER, MEDITERRANEAN FEVER, UNDULANT FEVER OR ABORTUS FEVER)

Brucellosis is acute or sub-acute disease characterized by repeated attacks of rigor, pyrexia, weakness and painful muscles and joints

---

Epidemiological Data

Geographic distribution
Occurring world-wide, particularly in hot countries

Causative pathogen
Brucella, an animal pathogen, is a non-motile coccobacillus adapted to intracellular replication. The more virulent specie, *Brucella melitensis*, infects sheep and goats while *Brucella suis* infect mostly pigs with *Brucella abortus* infecting cattle and *Brucella canis* infecting dogs. *Brucella abortus* is the most common kind of brucellosis found in South Africa

Incubation period
5–35 days or even longer

Mode of transmission
Horizontally from animals to humans
- Through direct contact with the tissue, blood, urine, vaginal secretions, placenta and aborted foetuses of infected animals (via abrasions in the skin or mucosa of the alimentary tract or via the respiratory tract)
- Indirectly through the ingestion of infected meat, un-pasteurized milk that is infected and cheese made of infected milk (no contact with infected animal)

Period of infectiousness (communicability, transmission)
The disease is not transmissible between humans

Reservoir
Animals – cattle, goats, pigs, sheep and dogs. In cows and she-goats, the Brucella localizes in the placenta causing contagious abortion as well as infecting the mammary glands from where the pathogen is shed for long periods in milk. Brucella is also present in all uterine discharges, faeces and urine

Intermediaries
None

Carriers
None

Immune status
No immunity with memory is elicited

Susceptibility and resistance of host
Everybody is susceptible. It would appear that children suffering from the disease are less severely affected than adults

---

Pathogenesis

After the *Brucella* have gained entry into the body via abrasions in the skin, or via the alimentary tract on ingestion, or via the respiratory tract, the *Brucella* is phagocytised by the phagocytic cells and then disseminates to the local and regional lymph nodes, the thoracic duct and the blood where it multiplies (bacteraemia phase). The reticulo-endothelial cells of the reticulo-endothelial system (lymph nodes, liver and spleen, bone marrow and lymphoid/lymphatic tissue) are also infected. As the *Brucella* does not die off after being phagocytised, the *Brucella* survives for prolonged periods in these cells. Because of the presence of *Brucella* in the reticulo-endothelial cells, an intermittent bacteraemia cyclically occurs. The result is a granulomatous inflammatory reaction with epithelioid and giant cells, central necrosis and peripheral fibrosis.

❖ **Clinical manifestation**
   ✹ **Acute brucellosis**
   - After an incubation period of 1-3 weeks, the disease begins gradually (sometimes sudden) with malaise, rigor, intermittent pyrexia (periods of pyrexia can last for weeks, alternating with periods without any pyrexia), diaphoresis, arthralgia and myalgia
   - The cervical and axillary lymph nodes are enlarged but not painful
   - Splenomegaly and hepatomegaly develops
   - Relapses occur and the sick person sometimes suffers from depression, insomnia and irritability
   - The disease may last from a few weeks to years
   ✹ **Sub-clinical brucellosis**
   - When the sick individual does not recover within a few weeks or months, the disease becomes chronic (being sick for more than one year) and sub-clinical
   - Tiredness, aches and pains, anxiety, depression and occasional fever develops
   - Relapses and remissions frequently occur

❖ **Complications**
   - Complications of bacteraemia usually develop during the acute stage of the disease, namely endocarditis, hepatitis, nephritis with renal failure, osteomyelitis, meningitis or encephalitis
   - Quite often the disease becomes chronic

■ **Diagnosis**
   ▪ History of working with sick animals, their meat and tissues; or ingesting infected meat, un-pasteurized milk (cow or goat) that is infected, and cheese made of infected milk
   ▪ Serological tests
   ▪ Specific agglutination tests

- ■ **Prognosis**
  - ▪ Good

- ■ **Specific healthcare interventions to be rendered**
  - ▪ Chemotherapy - antimicrobial therapy that is administered orally or intravenously
  - ▪ Supportive and symptomatic
  - ▪ Health information to all persons working with cattle, sheep, goats and pigs regarding the disease as well as the products originating from these animals. These workers have to wear protective clothing
  - ▪ Pasteurization, or sterilization, or boiling of cow/goat milk

- ◆ **Measures to prevent epidemics**
  - ✦ Vaccination of all herds of cattle and goats
  - ✦ Elimination of infected cattle and goats either through isolating them or by slaughtering them
  - ✦ Regular inspection of dairy farms (this also applies to goats that are milked)

- ◆ **Implications for disaster situations**
  - ✦ None

- ◆ **Compliance with international measures**
  - ✦ None

14.2.1.2 PLAGUE

Plague, also known as the Black Death, is an acute systemic disease causing a diffused haemorrhagic septicaemia in the body. The *Yersinia pestis* infiltrates all organs and tissues in the body and cause a variety of symptoms

---

Epidemiological Data

Geographic distribution
Occurring world-wide. In localized regions in the RSA plague is endemic among rodents in the wild

Causative pathogen
Yersinia pestis – a Gram-negative rod with a surrounding anti-phagocytic capsule that is associated with virulence

Incubation period
Bubonic plague 2–7 days
Pneumonic plague 2–3 days, sometimes a few hours

Mode of transmission
From animals to humans via the bite of infected rat fleas (bubonic plague)
Directly from one human to another human via airborne infected droplets (septicaemic and pneumonic plague)

Period of infectiousness (communicability, transmission)
For as long as *Yersinia pestis* is present in the body of the infected animal. In favourable circumstances fleas can be infected for weeks or months

---

Reservoir

Rodents such as rats, mice, hares, rabbits, squirrels, gerbils, and all other carnivorous rodents are the sylvatic reservoirs for plague. Rodents mostly suffer from a generally mild infection. These rodents (both rural and urban) have a stable flea cycle and only a few deaths occur. This stable endemic flea cycle serves as the long-term reservoir for the pathogen *Yersinia pestis*. As soon as the stable endemic flea cycle is broken, the disease spreads rapidly. Infected fleas on the dead/dying infected rodents flee from the dying/dead rodent and bite humans, cats and dogs to suck blood. Also, when humans come in contact with the infected fleas on cats and dogs, the *Yersinia pestis* is spread to humans. Humans now become the reservoir for *Yersinia pestis* (see fig. 14.2). The urban rat is the most important source of plague in humans and plague outbreaks in humans has at times decimated populations and influenced the course of history

Intermediaries

Vectors - The exopsylla cheopsis-rat flea. The rat flea carries the *Yersinia pestis* from rat to rat and from rat to humans. The rat flea leaves the body of the sick rodent after sucking up the *Yersinia pestis* infected blood of the sick rodent, for example, rat. Because *Y. pestis* multiplies profusely in the blood that was sucked up, clotting of blood occurs in the lumen of the gut of the flea leading to the blockage of the anterior section of the digestive canal of the flea. When any warm-blooded host is bitten by the flea, the flea regurgitates thousands of *Yersinia pestis* into the puncture. Fleas bite more than once in order to suck up blood

Vehicles - Contaminated articles, surfaces, fomites

Carriers

None

Immune status

On recovery immunity with memory is elicited with all *Yersinia pestis* bacilli being eliminated from the body

Susceptibility and resistance of host

All persons of all ages are susceptible

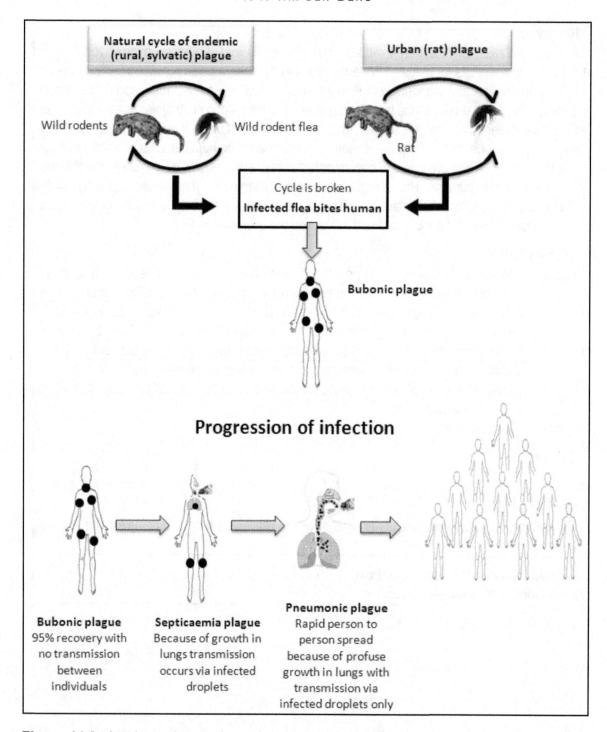

Figure 14.2 A schematic representation of the spread of plague from rodents to humans and between humans

Pathogenesis

Yersinia pestis produces a number of virulence factors, namely, an anti-phagocytic capsular antigen, endotoxin, and various other protein toxins. Because the *Yersinia pestis* has a surrounding anti-phagocytic capsule, the *Yersinia* multiplies at the site of entry into the skin, from where it disseminates via the lymphatic drainage system to local and regional lymph nodes (the clinical site of bubonic plague). Because of the inflammatory response and haemorrhaging in the lymph nodes, the nodes enlarge to form "buboes". The buboes develop in the lymph nodes nearest to the site where the individual was bitten – when bitten on the feet or legs, the buboes forms in the lymph nodes in the groin, or, when bitten on the hands or arms, the buboes forms in the lymph nodes in the axilla. A bacteraemia follows quickly that is characterized by purulent, necrotic and haemorrhagic lesions in the lymph nodes. Signs now develop of a general toxaemia of the body such as hypotension, oliguria, changed levels of consciousness and sub-clinical disseminating intravascular coagulation. At this stage, plague is not transmissible between persons.

In 95% of cases of bubonic plague, the inflammation response is limited to the lymph nodes and does not spread to the rest of the body. As soon as *Y. pestis* spreads via the blood to the other organs in the body, septicaemic plague has set in. A generalized bacteraemia of the whole body characterized by purulent, necrotic, haemorrhagic lesions in all organs of the body, toxaemia and septicaemia are present. Owing to the profuse seeding of the lungs (multiplication of *Y. pestis* in the lungs) by *Y. pestis*, plague is now rapidly transmitted by means of airborne infected droplets from person to person inducing pneumonic plague (see fig 14.2). Pneumonic plague is a rapid progressive infection of the lungs and other body sites characterized by fever, respiratory distress and death within hours/days after being infected.

❖ **Clinical manifestation**
  ✹ **General signs and symptoms of all forms of plague**
   • Moderate toxaemia with remitting pyrexia
   • Abdominal pain, nausea, vomiting, constipation followed by a bloody diarrhoea
   • Purulent or vesicular or haemorrhagic skin lesions appear all over the body
   • The more serious the disseminated intra-vascular coagulation, pneumonia and meningitis become, the more restless, apathetic and anxious the ill person becomes
   • Convulsions, coma, followed by death
  ✹ **Bubonic plague**
   • The characteristic buboes (enlarged lymphatic glands) in the drainage area of the lymph nodes (armpit or groin) appear usually 2–6 days after being bitten by the infected flea
   • The sick person is seriously ill and the lymphadenitis is extremely painful
   • The lungs of the ill person have not yet been seeded by the *Yersinia pestis*. When this condition is treated within 24 hours, the ill person recovers within 72 hours. No transmission between humans occurs at this stage
   • When not treated, the *Y. pestis* spreads rapidly, via the blood, through the body, leading to septicaemia, haemorrhagic illness (bleeding from all organs) and multisystem involvement (spleen, liver, lungs, and central nervous system)
   • Though the sick person may not appear to be very ill, he/she dies soon as a result of septicaemia

- Because of the septicaemia, profuse bacterial growth in/seeding of the lungs take place and transmission via infected droplets (airborne transmission) occurs rapidly between persons (person-to-persons)
- During an epidemic a mild form of the disease develops without any visible typical signs and symptoms. The ill person recovers without treatment

✱ **Septicaemic plague**
- Signs and symptoms of septicaemia with severe ecchymosis
- Progressive cardiac failure with respiratory and circulatory collapse
- Haemorrhagic pneumonia develops because of the profuse bacterial growth of *Y. pestis* in the lungs. Transmission of the disease to other persons now occurs through airborne infected droplets when sneezing, talking, and coughing
- Death follows quickly

✱ **Pneumonic (pulmonary) plague**
- This is the most fatal fulminating form of plague. The lungs are primarily involved
- Treatment has to commence within 18 hours in order to prevent death
- A severe cough, pyrexia (40^0C and higher), tachycardia, an intensive headache, haemoptysis, and exhaustion are present
- The ill person dies within hours to days after being infected
- **The disease is now only transmitted by means of airborne infected droplets. An epidemic culminating in a pandemic follows soon that spreads extremely rapidly**

✱ **Meningeal plague**
- Meningeal plague is a rare but an extremely serious complication of bubonic or septicaemic plague
- The signs and symptoms are similar to those of cerebrospinal meningitis with an intensive headache and neck stiffness
- Convulsions, vestibular-cerebellar symptoms, and coma typically occur followed by death

❖ **Complications**
- Disseminated intravascular coagulation
- Pneumonia
- Meningitis

■ **Diagnosis**
- Clinical picture
- A history of exposure to fleas of rodents with marks of flea bites on the body
- Identification of *Y. pestis* in blood cultures and/or fluid aspirated from lymph nodes, and/or sputum monsters

Note - **The diagnosis of plague can be problematic as the typical buboes are not always present, particularly in septicaemic and pneumonic plague. When plague has not been diagnosed for years in endemic and other localities, laboratory staff may not be familiar in the identification of the of the *Y. Pestis* pathogen. An epidemic of fleas,**

a sudden decrease in the activities of rodents, or the appearance of a number of dead rodents should give good warning of the possibility of an imminent outbreak of plague

■ **Prognosis**
  ▪ 60–90% of persons with untreated bubonic and septicaemic plague die
  ▪ In pneumonic plague the mortality rate is mostly 100%

■ **Specific healthcare interventions to be rendered**
  Medical treatment
  ▪ In order to be effective, medical treatment has to commence within 14 hours after the signs and symptoms have appeared. There should be no waiting for the results of laboratory tests before antimicrobial treatment is started. Chemotherapeutic treatment should at least be given for a period of 10 days
  ▪ Plague antiserum has to administered
  ▪ Antimicrobial and other drugs are to be administered
  ▪ Sedatives and analgesics are to be administered
  ▪ A drug regime consisting of a combination of antiserum and antimicrobial drugs is effective for seriously ill person
  Specific healthcare interventions
  ▪ High grade barrier isolation in a specialized unit
  ▪ Incineration of all secretions (including faeces since the spread may occur via toilets)
  ▪ Symptomatic treatment of shock, pyrexia and convulsions
  ▪ Administering of large quantities of fluids and intravenous transfusions
  ▪ Disinfesting/de-flea-ing of fleas and/or burning of the ill person's clothing immediately on being admitted to hospital

◆ **Preventive measures to be taken**
  ➢ Notification of all cases (including contacts) immediately according to law
  ➢ All contacts are to be isolated for a period of six (6) days. Their temperature should be taken twice daily and antimicrobial therapy must be administered. When the condition of a contact deteriorates, he/she should be hospitalized and isolated in a high grade barrier unit
  ➢ Tracing of infected cases and contacts in the relevant community. The movement of inhabitants should be restricted in order to control fleas
  ➢ Vaccination of all high-risk groups (for example, elderly persons, healthcare providers, military personnel and field workers). Vaccination lasts effectively for six months
  ➢ Prophylactic treatment with antimicrobial drugs of all inhabitants in communities where plague had broken out
  ➢ During an epidemic, the public should be advised that any person who feels unwell, should report immediately to a healthcare service delivery point
  ➢ All community members must adhere to all measures for the disinfesting of fleas
  ➢ Rodents must be eradicated as part of the surveillance programme in a community

> Buildings and homes in suburban and rural areas should be made rat-proof and strict environmental hygiene must be maintained
> Carcasses of dead animals (particularly rodents) have to be buried, burnt, or covered with soil as soon as possible
> The cycle of transmission, rodent→flea→human has to be severed by all possible means
> All refugees/survivors in disaster areas have to be examined regularly for flea bites
> **Extremely strict adherence to all medical and other healthcare interventions as well as to Standard Precautions and Transmission-based precautions in all healthcare establishments**
> **Strict adherence to all preventive measures**

◆ **Short-term control measures during an outbreak**
  • Severing of the transmission cycle of rodent→flea→human by eradicating of rodents
  • Notification of the District Health Authority and the National Department of Heath that an outbreak had occurred
  • Protection of all medical and field personnel by wearing the necessary protective clothing and masks
  • Early diagnosis and treatment of cases and high grade isolation of ill persons
  • Placing contacts (even entire communities) under quarantine. The service of the National Defence Force can be called in to enforce all quarantine measures
  • Tracing of cases and chemotherapeutic treatment to be given to all contacts
  • Implementing measures for disinfesting of fleas and eradication of rodents
  • Informing of public that an outbreak of plague had occurred and the measures the public have to take to prevent being bitten by fleas
  • Implementing of control measures at airports, harbours and land custom control facilities regarding the departure of all persons to other countries
  • Immediate notification of the World Health Organization by the National Department of Health that plague has broken out in humans in South Africa

◆ **Long-term control measures**
  • Surveillance programmes to be implemented to prevent further outbreaks
  • Continuous eradication of rodents and measures for disinfesting of fleas to be maintained as part of the surveillance programme
  • Health information to be given to the public regarding the prevention of plague
  • Regular submission of epidemiological reports, for example, compulsory veterinary reports regarding epidemic outbreaks of the natural cyclic endemic plague under rodents as well as the compulsory reporting by all farmers of occurrences of the natural rodent plague on their farms
  • Rodent control must be strictly adhered to at all airports and harbours as well as in cities, towns, informal settlements and rural areas
  • Ships and aircrafts have to be certified free of rats before they are allowed to enter any harbour or airport

◆ **Measures to prevent epidemics**
  ⬦ Reporting of the occurrence of natural and urban/rural outbreaks of rodent plaque

◆ **Implications for disaster situations**
  ⬦ Pest control to be instated during disaster situations

◆ **Compliance with international control measures**
  ⬦ When an outbreak of plague occurs on another continent or in a country on the Africa continent, **every person** (tourists, immigrants and citizens of the RSA) arriving from the region(s) concerned must be monitored for the prescribed period, regardless whether they have entered the RSA by car, ship or aeroplane
  ⬦ No sick person may leave any specific country (e.g. the RSA) after plague has been diagnosed
  ⬦ All travellers (leaving or arriving) are to be examined by health officials at harbours, airports or overland custom facilities and all arriving travellers/immigrants/citizens are under obligation to notify the healthcare authorities of any symptoms of ill health or influenza occurring within six (6) days of their arrival
  ⬦ When a traveller/immigrant/citizen leaves a country where an outbreak of plague had occurred and becomes ill on an aeroplane, he/she has to be isolated immediately (in the country of arrival) and all the other passengers are treated as contacts. These measures are also applicable when an outbreak of plague occurs on board a ship. Eradication of rats in the hold of ships and disinfesting of the hold of aeroplanes should be done immediately
  ⬦ Vaccination against plague cannot be demanded by the country of entry
  ⬦ All international health regulations have to be complied with by both the country of exit and country of entry

14.2.2 Multisystem zoonotic infections caused by viruses

A wide range of different viruses exist that are transmitted by animals to humans. The arboviruses are mostly transmitted by arthropods such as ticks, mosquitoes and sand flies. The arboviruses multiply in the arthropod vector, and for each virus there is a natural cycle involving vertebrates (various birds or mammals). The virus enters the arthropod when the latter takes a blood meal from the infected vertebrate. The virus then passes through the gut wall to reach the salivary gland where replication takes place. Once this has happened, 1-2 weeks after ingestion of the virus, the arthropod becomes infectious and then transmits the virus to another vertebrate during a blood meal. The arboviruses tend to replicate in vascular endothelium, the central nervous system, the skin and muscles and cause therefore multisystem infections in animals and humans.

The arena virus infections on the other hand, are transmitted to humans in rodent excreta (faeces and urine). Arena viruses cause a harmless lifelong infection in rodents with continuous excretion of the virus in the urine and faeces of an apparently healthy infected animal. Humans infected from this source, develop a severe febrile to fatal zoonotic disease. Arena virus infection is diagnosed by serology, virus isolation or viral genome detection carried out in special laboratory centres. The virulence of the virus increases when transmission of the virus from one person to another person takes place. Transmission from a sick person to healthcare providers and employees occurs via blood, tissue fluids and airborne infected droplets resulting in a more serious disease being contracted. Haemorrhaging, capillary damage, haemo-concentration, collapse and death follow.

Please note
Travellers from world-wide regions with fevers of unknown origin must be isolated in high barrier specialized care units because the incubation period of 3-21 days would allow an infected individual to carry infections, caused by viruses of zoonotic origin, from and to any place in the world. Fellow travellers are viewed as high-risk contacts

14.2.2.1 VIRAL HAEMORRHAGIC FEVERS - DENGUE FEVER, CONGO FEVER, MARBURG FEVER, EBOLA FEVER, LASSA FEVER AND RIFT VALLEY FEVER

Haemorrhagic fevers comprise a group of acute diseases which is highly infectious and transmissible and is characterized by pyrexia and haemorrhages in all body organs and tissues. Of importance is to exclude other causes for the symptoms and to obtain a thorough history that includes other signs and symptoms, recent travelling and camping, insect exposures, and contact with animals such as game (large and small) and livestock. The onset of the infection manifests with signs and symptoms similar to that of influenza (headache, sore throat, muscular aches, and pyrexia) as well as an erythematous maculo-papular rash and disseminated intravascular coagulation. Diffuse haemorrhage occurs in all body organs as the infection runs its course. Haemorrhage may present as haematemesis (vomiting blood) and/or melaena (passing blood in faeces) and/or a petechial/purpuric rash or ecchymoses and/or bleeding from the nose and gums and/or bleeding from vena-puncture sites, and/or menorrhagia in women.

Neither prophylactic vaccines nor any antimicrobial treatment are available for these communicable diseases. The mortality rate of these diseases is extremely high. When the person does not die, recovery usually takes place within two weeks. These group of communicable diseases constitute a serious risk to all healthcare providers and other employees in healthcare establishments as the different viruses are transmitted to humans via blood, fomites and airborne infected droplets (when seeding of the lungs had taken place and profuse growth of the pathogen in the lungs had occurred). Veterinarians who have to do autopsies on infected animals are also at risk to be infected. High grade barrier care in a specialized unit has to be instituted and the care has to be rendered by specialized trained healthcare personnel. No visitors (family and friends) are allowed.

The Epidemiological Data of the various haemorrhagic fevers are discussed in table 14.1 while the pathogenesis, clinical manifestation, complications and diagnosis of each disease is individually explained. The healthcare to be rendered as well as measures to be instituted to prevent epidemics, the implication for disaster situations and international measures to comply with are given as one for all the various haemorrhagic fevers.

Table 14.1 EPIDEMIOLOGICAL DATA OF HAEMORRHAGIC FEVERS

DENGUE FEVER	EBOLA FEVER (EBOLA VIRUS DISEASE)	LASSA FEVER	CONGO FEVER (CONGO-CRIMMEAN HAEMOR-RHAGIC FEVER)	MARBURG FEVER	RIFT VALLEY FEVER
Geographic distribution					
Tropical and subtropical regions	Africa	West-Africa	Africa, Asia and South-East-Europe	Africa and Europe	East-Africa and South Africa. Epizootics are associated with years of unusually heavy rainfall and localized flooding
Causative pathogen					
Small RNA viruses which cause disease during the period of viraemia. The viruses are believed to change to aerosol infectivity when the lungs of the infected person becomes seeded					
Dengue virus - a flavivirus	*Ebola virus* – a filovirus. Four strains exist, namely, Ivory Coast, Reston, Sudan, and Zaire	*Lassa virus* - an arenairidae virus	*Nairo virus* - an arbovirus (bunya virus)	*Marburg virus* – a filovirus	*Phlebovirus* – a Bunyaviridae virus
Incubation period					
4-8 days	4-16 days	6-21 days	1-6 days	4-21 days	2-7 days
Mode of transmission					
Bite of an infected mosquito	*Inhalation of airborne infected droplets from animals *From one person to another	*Ingestion or *inhalation of pathogen, or *penetration of the mucous membranes by pathogen	*Bite of an infected tick *Person–to-person transfer through contact with infected blood and infected body	* Inhalation of airborne infected droplets from animals *From one person to another	*Bite of an infected mosquito *Through handling of infected tissues (when slaughtering

through contact with infected blood, body fluids, urine and body secretions *Transmission by infected droplets when virus seeds the lungs	*Excreta (urine) of rodents penetrate skin through cuts, abrasions when in direct contact *Trans-mission by infected droplet when virus seeds the lungs *Person-to-person transfer through contact with infected blood and infected body excretions or secretions	excretions/ secretions *Transmission by infected droplets when virus seeds the lungs	through contact with infected blood, body fluids, urine and body secretions *The virus has also been isolated in semen *Transmission by infected droplet when virus seeds the lungs	and butchering as well as when assisting with animal births) and/or when handling carcases of animals that died from the disease (during conducting of veterinary procedures or when disposing of carcasses or animal foetuses) *Inoculation (via wound from an infected knife or needle stick) *Injuries or contact with broken skin *Inhalation of infected aerosols during slaughtering of infected animals *Ingesting of unpasteurised or uncooked milk of infected animals

Period of infectiousness (communicability, transmission)					
For as long as the virus is present in the blood (viraemia)	For as long as the virus is present in the blood (viraemia)	For as long as the virus is present in the blood (viraemia)	For as long as the virus is present in the blood (viraemia)	For as long as the virus is present in the blood (viraemia)	For as long as the virus is present in the blood (viraemia)
Reservoir					
Monkeys	Unknown , but could be primates, guinea pigs or bats	Rodents such as the bush rat, M. natalensis	Rodents, hares, birds, ticks, cattle, sheep , goats, and ostriches	Unknown but could be primates (small and large)	Enzootic to big game, sheep, goats, cattle and camels
Carriers					
None	None	None	None	None	None
Immunity status					
Antibody –mediated immunity is elicited on the first infection. Subsequent infections neutralize the antibody and enhance the ability of virus to infect the monocytes with an increased release of cytokines in the circulation	Unknown	Secondary attacks occur	Immunity with memory is elicited	Unknown	Unknown

Intermediaries Vectors or vehicles					
Vector - Mosquitoes - *Aëdes aegypti *Aëdes albopictus *Aëdes polynesiensis Aëdes scuttelaris	**Vector** – None **Vehicle** – Infected secretions, contaminated needles and syringes	**Vehicle** Urine of infected rats	**Vector** - Ticks (Hyalomma species) **Vehicles** – *Infected secretions of infected persons * Infected secretions of infected livestock	None	**Vectors** - Various species of mosquitoes such as the Aëdes, Culex, and Erethma- poditis mosquito
Susceptibility and resistance of host					
Everybody is susceptible	Everybody is susceptible	Everybody is susceptible	Everybody is susceptible	Everybody is susceptible	Everybody is susceptible High risk persons are herders, farmers, abattoir workers and vetenarians

❖ **Pathogenesis and clinical manifestation of the different haemorrhagic fevers**

✱ **DENGUE FEVER**

  ❖ Pathogenesis

  The *Dengue virus* replicates in monocytes and in the vascular endothelium. Vascular congestion and increased vascular permeability lead to oedema and haemorrhages which in turn lead to loss of plasma volume. This results in electrolytic imbalance. Bleeding time is prolonged and thrombocytopenia occurs. When Dengue haemorrhagic shock sets in, the mortality is high

  ❖ Clinical manifestation

  *Sudden onset with malaise, pyrexia, nausea and vomiting

  *Headaches and influenza-like symptoms

  *Sometimes a macular-papular rash appears

  *Haemorrhaging occurs by the second or third day

  *Shock out of proportion to haemorrhaging

❖ Complications
Shock
Death due to haemorrhage

■ Diagnosis
History of international travelling or national travelling in tropical areas or living in tropical areas
Clinical manifestations
Virus is isolated in blood specimen, throat swabs, and in urine and stool specimens

✱ EBOLA FEVER (EBOLA VIRUS DISEASE)

❖ Pathogenesis
After gaining entry into the body, the *Ebola-virus* replicates in the cells of the reticulo-endothelial system. Within days viraemia with pyrexia develops. Capillary damage takes place leading to loss of erythrocytes and plasma. A mild thrombocytopenia is present. Haemorrhages occur in all the organs and tissues of the body

❖ Clinical manifestation
*Flu-like syndrome with pyrexia, headache, arthralgia and myalgia
*Sore throat, vomiting and nausea, diarrhoea
*Conjunctivitis and chest pains
*Maculo-papular rash covering the entire body
*Abdominal pain and hepatic dysfunction
*Dehydration and significant wasting occur as the disease progresses
*Neurological involvement manifested by delirium and/or coma
*By the fifth day haemorrhages occur in organs and in body tissues due to thrombocytopenia

❖ Complications
Shock
Death due to haemorrhage

■ Diagnosis
History of international travelling or national travelling in tropical areas or living in tropical areas
Clinical manifestations
Virus is isolated in blood specimens

✱ LASSA FEVER

❖ Pathogenesis
After gaining entry into the body, the *Lassa-virus* replicates in the cells of the reticulo-endothelial system. Within days viraemia with pyrexia develops. Capillary damage takes place leading to loss of erythrocytes and plasma. A mild thrombocytopenia is present. Haemorrhages occur in all the organs and tissues of the body

❖ Clinical manifestation
  *Gradual onset with non-specific symptoms such as anorexia, diarrhoea, vomiting, abdominal pain, dysphasia
  *Neurological signs such as headache, and general malaise
  *Within days a sore throat develops (pharyngitis and/or laryngitis with an exudate)
  *Retrosternal pain (pulmonary and chest pain with coughing)
  *Conjunctival infection (conjunctivitis)
  *Arthralgia of joints and back ache
  *Temperature rises gradually
  *Progressive oedema of the face and neck
  *Proteinuria
  *Hepatic dysfunction
  *By the second week the symptoms worsen and a hypovolemic hypotension develops as well as vasoconstriction, decreased renal excretion, pulmonary oedema and ascites
  *Massive haemorrhages occur with myocarditis or cardiac failure
❖ Complications
  Shock
  Death due to haemorrhage
■ Diagnosis
  History of international travelling or national travelling in tropical areas or living in tropical areas
  Virus can sometimes be isolated in blood, throat and urine specimens

CONGO FEVER (CONGO-CRIMEAN HAEMORRHAGIC FEVER)
❖ Pathogenesis
  After gaining entry into the body, the *Congo-virus* replicates in the cells of the reticulo-endothelial system. Within days viraemia with pyrexia develops. Capillary damage takes place leading to loss of erythrocytes and plasma. A mild thrombocytopenia is present. Haemorrhages occur in all the organs and tissues of the body. Resolution of the condition leads to the formation of virus specific antibody
❖ Clinical manifestation
  *Sudden onset with rigor, headache and epigastric pain, conjunctivitis, nausea, vomiting, diarrhoea, anorexia and loss of muscular strength
  *Conjunctivitis and pharyngitis occur 3-7 days after being infected
  *Neurological signs such as photophobia, sharp mood swings, confusion and aggression. After 2-4 days the agitation can be replaced by depression and lassitude
  *Pyrexia (39^0C-41^0C) with tachycardia develops
  *Hepatitis and hepatomegaly as well as thrombocytopaenia and leukopenia
  *Haemorrhages (petechiae, progressive ecchymosis and other bleedings) occur in all the organs and tissues of the body 3-6 days after onset of disease

*Multiple organ failure develops due to shock

*Death usually occurs due to organ failure (hepato-renal and pulmonary) and haemorrhages during the second week of disease

*When the ill person recovers, improvement generally begins on the ninth or tenth (9-10th) day after onset of the disease

❖ Complications

Shock

Death due to haemorrhage

■ Diagnosis

History of international travelling or national travelling in tropical areas or living in tropical areas

Clinical manifestations

Virus is isolated in blood specimens

Culture of cerebro-spinal fluids and tissue

✸ MARBURG FEVER

❖ Pathogenesis

After gaining entry into the body, the *Marburg-virus* replicates in the cells of the reticulo-endothelial system. Within days viraemia with pyrexia develops. Capillary damage takes place leading to loss of erythrocytes and plasma. A mild thrombocytopenia is present. Haemorrhages occur in all the organs and tissues of the body

❖ Clinical manifestation

*Onset is sudden or gradual with pyrexia myalgia and arthritis

*Abdominal pain, nausea and vomiting occur, followed within 2-3 days by severe diarrhoea, a dry cough and chest pains

*A maculo-papular rash appears on the trunk (chest, back, and stomach) roughly 5 days after the onset of the symptoms. The rash spreads to the entire body with eventual desquamation

*The symptoms increase in severity and progress to include jaundice because of liver failure, pancreatitis, and severe weight loss

*Massive haemorrhages occur from the sixth (6th) day due to thrombocytopenia resulting in shock, multi-organ failure, and death

*Encephalitis may develop with delirium

❖ Complications

Shock

Death due to haemorrhage

■ Diagnosis

History of international travelling or national travelling in tropical areas or living in tropical areas or working with primates living in equatorial areas

Clinical manifestations

Virus is isolated in blood specimen and throat swabs

* ## RIFT VALLEY FEVER
  * ❖ Pathogenesis
    After gaining entry into the body, the virus replicates in the cells of the reticulo-endothelial system. Within days a viraemia with pyrexia develops. Capillary damage takes place, leading to loss of erythrocytes and plasma. A mild thrombocytopenia is present. Haemorrhages occur in all the organs and tissues of the body
  * ❖ Clinical manifestation
    The clinical picture has a highly variable clinical manifestation and the disease lasts for a few days only. Recovery is slow. In most cases the infection is asymptomatic or mild with severe illness in just over one percent of infected persons
    * ➢ Mild illness
      *Flu-like syndrome with pyrexia, headache, arthralgia and myalgia that last for 4-7 days
    * ➢ Severe illness
      *Sudden onset with chills, pyrexia, headache, myalgia
      *A biphasic fever occurs that lasts about 7 days
      *Photophobia and pain in the eyes due to congestion of the conjunctiva, optic neuropathy resulting in ocular (retinal) disease
      *Nausea and vomiting, abdominal fullness and pain
      *Bradychardia
      *Necrosis of the parenchyma cells of the liver, hepatitis and hepatomegaly
      *Viral haemorrhagic fever
      *Encephalitis
      *Massive haemorrhages in organs and tissues appear 2-4 days after onset due to interferon response associated with disseminated intravascular coagulation, micro-angiopathic haemolytic anaemia and intravascular deposition of fibrin thrombi
      *Within 3 to 6 days oliguria, anuria and renal failure follows, culminating in death
  * ❖ Complications
    Ocular disease
    Meningo-encephalitis (loss of memory, intense headache, hallucinations, confusion, disorientation, vertigo, convulsions, lethargy and coma)
    Severe neurological complications (sensory and motor)
    Hepatitis
    Shock
    Death due to haemorrhage

  * ■ Diagnosis
    History of direct or indirect contact with the blood or tissues of infected animals or being bitten by a mosquito
    Clinical manifestations
    The virus is present in the blood within three days of onset of disease

■ Specific healthcare interventions for all haemorrhagic fevers

There is no vaccine, preventive prophylactic medication or chemotherapeutic agents available for the treatment of most haemorrhagic fevers. Nosocomial transmission to hospital staff or other ill healthcare users often occur

- **The ill person is cared for in a high-grade isolation unit and the principles of Standard precautions, transmission-based precautions and high barrier isolation rendering, must be strictly adhered to. Negative pressure is maintained in the room-isolator or bed-isolator. In this way the sick individual is effectively isolated from the environment. Since this isolation is an unusual experience for the sick person and his/her family, special care in this regard has to be given according to their needs**
- Specific supportive and symptomatic rendering of care to maintain renal function, fluid and electrolyte balance and combating haemorrhage/shock and multi-organ failure; to handle neurological alterations and convulsions, and to prevent alteration in nutritional status
- Blood transfusions as medically prescribed
- Plasma transfusions containing antibody and/or antimicrobial drugs
- All excreta, garbage and consumables are sealed in bags and are either sterilized or incinerated. Sterilized excreta and waste water are disposed off in the sewage system
- Terminal disinfection includes the fumigation of the room and all non-disposable equipment and the incineration of disposable equipment
- After death, all bodies must be handled and buried according to the prescribed legislative regulations
- If necessary, cultural customs regarding the death of a person (such as keeping the clothes of the deceased person) must be modified to prevent the spread of the disease

◆ General preventive measures to be taken

- ➢ **Strict high grade isolation of ill individuals with no movement of the sick person allowed between rooms or departments. Only the minimal highly specialized trained staff should have contact with the ill person. Only disposable equipment must be used; cleaning must only be done with hypochlorite solution, while nothing should be removed from the room – all waste should be immediately incinerated as clinical waste**
- ➢ High-risk contacts (such as family members) are placed under quarantine at home or in the hospital where the sick individual is cared for and are monitored for early signs and symptoms of the disease. (Personnel who were in direct contact with the sick individual are also treated as high-risk contacts)
- ➢ All other contacts (for example, travellers on the same aircraft or in the same vehicle) must be traced and monitored. Their temperature must be taken twice daily and should they present with any of the signs and symptoms, they have to be immediately hospitalized

> If the ill person was cared for in a general ward before isolation measures were taken, all other sick persons, staff and visitors are also treated as high-risk contacts. When deemed necessary, the ward must.be closed and fumigated

> Extremely strict standard infection control measures to be applied as to prevent nosocomial transmission in health care establishments

◆ **Specific preventive measures to be taken**

Dengue Fever - Control of mosquitoes

Ebola Fever - Environmental hygiene

Lassa Fever - Environmental hygiene
  Control of rodents

Congo Fever - Health information regarding wearing protective clothing when walking or sleeping in the veld
  Also see preventive measures for tick-bite fever

Marburg Fever - None known

Rift Valley Fever - Control of mosquitoes and zoonotic vaccination of animals

◆ **Measures to prevent epidemics**

- Extremely strict adherence to all school exclusion regulations
- Extremely strict adherence to Standard precautions, transmission-based precautions and high grade barrier isolation
- Extremely strict adherence to all legislative measures
- Cultural practices have to be overruled where necessarily
- **When any haemorrhagic fever/infection is suspected, high grade barrier care must be immediately instituted until blood and other serological tests indicate the contrary**

◆ **Implications for disaster situations**

- None

◆ **Compliance with international measures**

- All persons **who presents with pyrexia** entering the RSA (whether by land, sea or air) must receive medical treatment and be considered as suspect cases and treated as such until evidence to the contrary is proven. These persons must immediately be placed in strict isolation until the results of the necessary blood tests are known
- Co-passengers are treated as high-risk contacts and are placed under quarantine for the prescribed period of time
- All suspected/sick cases must be immediately reported telephonically to the Communicable Disease Units of the District Health Authority, the Provincial Department of Health and National Department of Health that has to notify the World Health Organization

14.2.3 Multisystem zoonotic infections caused by other biotypes of protozoa

Protozoa, single-celled animals, parasitized all major tissues and organs in the body such as the central nervous system, the blood, liver, intestines, skin and urinal-genital tract. *Protozoa* parasitized body tissues and organs as intracellular or extracellular parasites. Both the intracellular and extracellular *protozoa* parasites have evolved many sophisticated strategies to avoid host responses. *Protozoa* parasitized humans via a variety of routes such as vector-borne, sexual activity, indigestion and vertically via trans-placental in-utero transmission. Because *protozoa* reproduction is asexual in humans, rapid increase in numbers in the parasitized individual can take place. When the host's defense mechanisms are impaired as in the foetus and young children, some *protozoa* are most pathogenic in young children. Most protozoan parasitaemia is not life threatening and more often the pathology is caused by the responses of the host.

14.2.3.1   TOXOPLASMOSIS

Toxoplasmosis is an acute to chronic protozoan parasitaemia. The protozoan becomes an intracellular parasite in macrophages, muscle cells, epithelial cells, brain cells and the endothelium of the circulatory system

---

Epidemiological Data

Geographic distribution
World-wide

Causative pathogen
Toxoplasma gondii – a protozoan. The *T. gondii* is intracellular specie that parasitizes the macrophages, epithelial cells, brain and muscle. The *protozoa* obtain their nutrients from the host's cells by direct uptake or by ingestion of the cytoplasm. The *T. gondii* survives particularly in macrophages and has evolved a variety of devices to evade or inactive the harmful effects of intracellular enzymes, reactive oxygen and nitrogen metabolites

Incubation period
Uncertain, but mostly 10 days

Mode of transmission
Horizontally - Direct ingestion of uncooked or partially cooked meat containing the cysts of the *Toxoplasma*.
Faecal-oral through contact with faeces (particularly cat faeces)
Contact with soil contaminated by infected cat faeces - the cysts of the *Toxoplasma* wherein the protozoan live, can stay alive for as long as a year in soil
Vertically - Trans-placental from the mother to the unborn foetus in-utero

Period of infectiousness (communicability, transmission)
Not transmitted between persons

Reservoir
Mammals such as cats; dogs; pigs; sheep; rodents; chickens; and pigeons. Cats are the general reservoir

---

Intermediaries
None
Carriers
None
Immune status
It is not entirely certain that one infection elicits immunity with memory
Susceptibility and resistance of host
All persons are susceptible

Pathogenesis

When the *Toxoplasma gondii* is ingested by a person, the *protozoan* gains entry into the body via the gastro-intestinal tract and becomes an intracellular parasite when phagocytised by the macrophage of the lymph nodes, liver and spleen. The *protozoan* is not killed off by the macrophage as the protozoan has developed a variety of strategies/devises to avoid immune recognition and inactivate the harmful effects of intracellular enzymes, reactive oxygen and nitrogen metabolites. The *protozoan* live and multiply intracellular in the host's cells (asexual reproduction) and obtains its nutrients from the host's cells by direct uptake or ingestion of cytoplasm. As the *protozoan* are removed from direct contact with complement and phagocytosis as well as antibody, the antigens of the *protozoan* can be expressed at the surface of the parasitized host's cells - thus, becoming the target for the cytotoxic effectors of the host's adaptive immune system. The *protozoan* may also become encapsulated in the affected cell. In the latter case the *Toxoplasma* remains in the body for years resulting in recurrent mild inflammatory responses. When the encapsulated cyst ruptures, however, a serious inflammation response follows. The general reaction of the body on invasion by the *protozoan* is the formation of granuloma which is very effective although complications set in when the granuloma occur in sensitive tissues of the body such as the brain and the eyes.

❖ **Clinical manifestation**

Toxoplasmosis is manifested as either an acquired condition or a congenital disease

✱ **Acquired toxoplasmosis**

When toxoplasmosis is acquired by ingestion, the course of the disease is as follows

- In most of the cases the person remains asymptomatic and the disease is diagnosed by means of serological tests only
- Most of the clinically observed parasitized individuals manifest with enlarged lymph nodes, particularly the posterior cervical lymph nodes
- Myalgia, pyrexia, sore throat, headache and a maculo-papular rash develop
- An acute and potentially fatal form of the acquired disease may develop that is characterized by pyrexia, skin rash, myocarditis, pneumonia and meningo-encephalitis (very rare)

* **Congenital toxoplasmosis**

The *protozoa* possess the ability to cross the placental barrier and are thus transmitted vertically from the mother who suffers from an asymptomatic parasitaemia, to her baby. Spontaneous abortion, prematurity or still-birth may occur. When the baby is born alive, the baby is usually asymptomatic at birth, but after several weeks/months/years lesions develop mainly in the brain and the eyes. The most common lesions and conditions occurring are chorioretinitis, strabismus, blindness, deafness, epilepsy, hydrocephaly and microcephaly. The organs in the body may also be afflicted which lead to hepatomegaly, splenomegaly, pneumonitis and a skin rash. Most of the individuals suffering from congenital toxoplasmosis are asymptomatic

❖ **Complications**

The infected person may be ill for months or even years and complications such as choroiderotinitis, encephalitis and meningitis can develop

■ **Diagnosis**

Serological tests and isolation of *Toxoplasma gondii* or its presence in tissue biopsy, smears, or the sediments of body fluids (direct microscopy)

■ **Prognosis**
- The prognosis of good or poor depends on the virulence of *Toxoplasma gondii*, the susceptibility of the parasitized person and the organs that are affected
- When congenital toxoplasmosis is diagnosed, the prognosis is poor
- In acquired toxoplasmosis the prognosis is good when a person presents with only lymph-adenopathy
- In most cases the condition clears up within a month and because the disease is self-limiting, anti-microbial chemotherapy is not always necessary

■ **Specific healthcare interventions to be rendered**
- Chemotherapy - antimicrobial drugs
- Supportive and symptomatic

◆ **Preventive measures to be taken**
➢ Treatment of parasitized mothers during pregnancy in order to prevent congenital toxoplasmosis by having all mothers who keep cats as pets, undergo Toxoplasma-serological tests
➢ Washing of hands thoroughly after cleaning the litter box of a cat
➢ Pregnant women should not clean the litter box of cats
➢ Children's playing facilities should be covered when not in use and the sand must be treated once weekly with a disinfection solution
➢ Uncooked or partially cooked meat should not be eaten

◆ **Measures to prevent epidemics**
- None

◆ **Implications for disaster situations**
  ╇ None

◆ **Compliance with international measures**
  ╇ None

14.3   KEY NOTES

❑ Disease transmission by animals, birds, reptiles (domestic, farming, wild and exotic) and insects (vectors) has major implications for humans and the pathogen.

❑ Zoonotic vector-borne and multisystem infections are maintained naturally in a reservoir of non-human vertebrates or invertebrates.

❑ In multisystem zoonotic diseases humans are infected mostly incidentally (for example, from rodents, domestic pets, exotic pets, etc.) while in vector-borne diseases man is infected when arthropods feed on human blood.

❑ As human blood is an inhospitable environment for the animal/avian/insect/reptilian pathogen, the pathogen must make a remarkably complex transformation in a very short time to require the necessary subtle evasion mechanisms to survive.

❑ In man, infection with animal/avian/insect/reptilian pathogens often results in death as humans have not previously experienced the specific virulent antigen.

❑ Human-to-human transmission seldom takes place in zoonotic diseases, but when the lungs of human beings becomes seeded by the pathogen from animals/birds/insects/reptiles, transmission by airborne infected droplets may lead to epidemics and pandemics.

❑ Although strong immune responses are mounted, it often leads to immuno-pathological complications. Antimicrobial therapy is not always successful and no vaccines (with a few exceptions) are available for this group of diseases.

❑ Vector control is very difficult and the zoonotic origin of some of these infections is less clear.

BIBLIOGRAPHY

About Infectious Diseases. XDR TB is Extensively Drug Resistant Tuberculosis. http://www.archives.healthdev.net/stop-tb/msg00841.html (Accessed on 9/5/2007).

ALERCON, K., KOLSTEREN, P.W.W, PRADA, A.M. et al. 2004. Effects of separate delivery of zinc or zinc and Vitamin A on haemoglobin response, growth, and diarrhoea in young Peruvian children receiving iron therapy for anaemia. American Journal of Clinical Nutrition, 80:1276-1282.

AVENTIS PASTEUR. 2004. ACTACEL ACELLULAR. 1 June.

AVENTIS PASTEUR. 1998. COMBAcct-HIB. September.

AZIZ, M.A. AND WRIGHT, A. 2005. The World Health Organization/International Union against Tuberculosis and Lung Disease Global project on Surveillance for Anti-Tuberculosis drug resistance: A Model for other Infectious Diseases. Clinical Infectious Diseases, 41:258-262.

BARCLAY, L. AND MURATA, P. 2007. Children Born Prematurely Need Comprehensive Treatment. American Family Physician, 76:115

BASTIAN, I. AND COLEBUNDERS, R. 1999. Treatment and Prevention of Multidrug-resistant Tuberculosis. Drugs, 58 (4):633-661, October.

BLŐNDAL, K. 2007. Barriers to reaching the targets for tuberculosis control: multidrug-resistant tuberculosis. Bulletin of the World Health Organization 85(5):387-390, May.

BRATZLER, D.W., CHRISTIAENS, B.P., HEMPSTEAD, K., AND NICHOL, K.L. 2002. Immunization for Elders. The Journal of Law, Medicine and Ethics, 30(3. Supplement):128-134, Fall.

CAMARON, N. 2006. Why do we Immunize Children? – An approach to Parents who are Uncertain or Object. Professional Nursing Today, 10(6):30-36, November/December.

CLARK, M.J. 1999. Nursing in the Community. Stamford: Appleton and Lange.

COOKE, R.A. 2008. Infectious Diseases. North Ryde: McGraw-Hill Australia Pty.

CULLINAN, K. AND MAKHAYE. 16 April 2007. South Africa: locking Up XDR TB III healthcare users is Extreme. http://allafrica.com/stories/200704160503.html (Accessed on 5/9/2007).

CUTILLI, C.E. 2006. Do Your III healthcare users Understand? Providing Culturally Congruent Patient education. Orthopaedic Nursing, 25(3):218-224. May/June. http://www.nursingcenter.com/prodev/ce_article.asp?tid=649983 (Accessed on 17/04/2009).

DALTON, J. 1983. Leprosy – a curable disease. Nursing Times. 79(40):57-59.

DAO, M. AND MEYDANI, S.N. 2009. Micronutrient Status, Immune Response and Infectious Disease in Elderly of Less Developed Countries. Sight and Life Magazine, Issue 3/2009:6-15.

DEBBIE, J.G. 1988. Rabies: an old enemy that can be defeated. World Health Forum, 9:536-541.

DE LANGE, M. 2006. Tuberculosis and the emergence of drug resistance. Professional Nursing Today, 12(4):18-21, July/August.

DENNILL, K. 2008. Managing the TB tsunami in South Africa. Professional Nursing Today, 12(4):18-21, July August.

DENNILL, K. 2008. Meeting maternal and child survival targets in South Africa through prevention of mother-and-child transmission of HIV. Professional Nursing Today, 12(6):39-43, November/December.

Department of Health. 1977. The Health Act, Act 63 of 1977.

Department of Health. 1998. Regulation R.1411 of 23 September 1966 regarding rodent infestation. Regulation R.703 of 30 June 1993.

Department of National Health and Population Development. 985. Recognition and management of viral haemorrhagic fevers. National Institute for Virology, March.

Detention of ill healthcare users with extensively drug-resistant tuberculosis (XDT-TB). Position statement by the South African Medical Research Council (SAMRC). http://www.mrc.ac.za/pressreleases/2007/1press2007.htm (Accessed on 5/9/2007).

Dialogue on diarrhoea. 1987. No. 31. United Kingdom: Bourne Offset Ltd. December.

Dialogue on diarrhoea. 1990. No. 43. United Kingdom: Bourne Offset Ltd. September.

Dialogue on diarrhoea. 1991. No. 44. United Kingdom: Bourne Offset Ltd. March.

Dialogue on diarrhoea. 1991. No. 45. United Kingdom: Bourne Offset Ltd. June.

Dialogue on diarrhoea. 1991. No. 47. United Kingdom: Bourne Offset Ltd. December.

Dialogue on diarrhoea. 1992. No. 50. United Kingdom: Bourne Offset Ltd. September.

ESS, S.M. AND SZUCS, T.D. 2002. Economic Evaluation of Immunization Strategies. Clinical Infectious Diseases. Travel Medicine, 35:294-297, August 1.

Extremely drug-resistant TB emerges. http://www.hindu.co./seta/2006/09/28/stories/2006092800121500.ht (Accessed on 5/9/2007).

Facts about dietary supplements: Zinc. http://www.dietary-supplements.info.nih.gov/factsheet/cc/zinc.html (Accessed on 7/8/2006).

FEUDTER, C., AND MARCUSE, E.K. 2001. Ethics and Immunization policy: Promoting dialogue to sustain consensus. Paediatrics, 107(5):1158-1164, May.

FOX, M.D. 2001. Resident's column: a resident's view of the ethics and morality of immunization. Paediatrics annals, 30(7):422-423, July.

FREE STATE PROVINCIAL GOVERNMENT, HEALTH. 2007. Health support circular no 3 – Tuberculosis management program.

GANDY, M. AND ZUMLA, A. 2003. The return of the WHITE PLAGUE. London. Verso.

GETAHUN, H., HARRINGTON, M., O'BRIEN, R. AND NUNN, P. 2007. Diagnosis of smear-negative pulmonary tuberculosis in people with HIV infection or AIDS in resource-constrained settings: informing urgent policy changes. The Lancet, 369:2042-2049, June 16.

GLATTHAAR, E. 1982. Tuberculosis control in South Africa. Suid-Afrikaanse Mediese Tydskrif. Special edition. November.

GLATTHAAR, E. 1991. Tuberculosis. Pretoria:J.L. van Schaik

GlaxoSmithKline. (s.a) PRIORIX™

GlaxoSmithkline. 1997. Infarix. 20 August.

GlaxoSmithkline. 1999. Hiberix. 24 March.

GlaxoSmithkline. 1999. Trantanrix-HB. 23 March.

GlaxoSmithkline. 2002. HAVRIX1440 and HAVRIX JUNIOR. 30 November.

GlaxoSmithkline. 2002. Varilrix. 14 May.

GlaxoSmithkline. 2006. Rotarix. 23 January.

GlaxoSmithkline. 2008. Infanrix[R] hexa. February.

GRACIANO, F. 2010. The Dance of Climate Change and Hidden Hunger. Sight and Life Magazine, Issue 3/2010:55-60.

GRIFFITHS, C., STURDY, P., BREWIN, P., BOTHAMLEY, G., ELDRIDGE, S., MARTINEAU, A., MACDONALD, M., RAMSAY, J., TIBREWAL, S., LEVI, S., ZUMLA, A., FEDER, G. 2007. Educational outreach to promote screening for tuberculosis in primary care: a cluster randomized controlled study. Lancet, 369:1528-1533, May 5.

HINMAM, A.R., ORENSTEIN, W.A., WILLIAMSON, D.E., AND DARRINGTON, D. 2002. Childhood immunization: laws at work. The Journal of Law, Medicine and Ethics, 30(3. Supplement):122-127, Fall.

HOBFOLL, S.E. AND LILLY, R.S. 1993. Resource Conservation as a Strategy for Community Psychology. Journal of community Psychology, Vol 21:128-146, April.

Inflammation. http://en.widipedia.org/wiki/Inflammation (Accessed on 4/30/2013).

INGLIS, T.J.J. 2007. Microbiology and Infection. Master medicine. 3rd edition. London: Churchill Livingstone – Elsevier.

ISAACS, D. 2004. Should Australia introduce a vaccine injury compensation scheme? Journal of Paediatrics and Child Health, 40(5/6):247-249, May/June.

ISAACS, D., KILHAM, H.A., AND MARSHALL, H. 2004. Should routine childhood immunizations be compulsory? Journal of Paediatrics and Child Health, 40(7):392-396, July.

JANSE van RENSBURG, Y. 2008. Patient isolation with minimal resources. Professional Nursing Today, 12(6):16-17, November/December.

JAMIESON, A. 2006. Malaria prevention and treatment. Professional Nursing Today, 10(6):4-7, November/December.

KAPLAN, C., TURNER, G.S. AND WARREL, D.A. 1986. Rabies: the facts. 2nd edition. Oxford:Oxford University Press.

KRANTZ, I., SACHS, L. AND NILSTUN, T. 2004. Ethics and vaccination. Scandinavia Journal of Public Health, 32:1403-1498, (translated in English by Taylor and Francis. Health Sciences, 172-178).

KU, C., BESSER, J., ABENDROTH, A., GROSE, C., ANDARVIN, A.M. 2005. Varicella-Zoster Virus Pathogenesis and Immunobiology: New Concepts Emerging from Investigations with the SCIDhu Mouse Model. Journal of Virology, 79(5):2651-2658. March.

LACHMAN, S.J. 1991. The emergent reality of heterosexual HIV/AIDS. Republic of South Africa: Lennon Ltd.

LEATHARD, H.L., AND COOK, M.J. 2009. Learning for holistic care: addressing practical wisdom (phronesis) and the spiritual sphere. Journal of Advanced Nursing, 65(6):1318-1327.

Lectin pathway. http://en.wikipedia.org/.wiki/Lectin_pathway (Accessed on 4/27/2013).

Leprosy mission (the). (s.a.) Leprosy: a guide for professional workers.

MAHLANGU, F. 2009. We can cure this disease. Nursing Update, 33(8):26-27, September.

MAKGATHO, M.L. 2010. Mind your health. Nursing Update, 34(6):42-43, July.

MANT, D., and MAYON-WHITE, R. 2007. Tuberculosis: think globally and act locally. Lancet, 369:1493-1494, May 5.

MARIN, G. 1993. Defining Culturally Appropriate Community Interventions: Hispanics as a Case Study. Journal of Community Psychology, Vol 21:149-159, April.

MEDPHARM STAFF WRITER. 2006. What you should know about nausea, vomiting and traveller's diarrhoea. Professional Nursing Today, 10(6):16, November/December.

MIGLIORI, G.B.; ORTMAN, J.; GIRARDI, E.; BESOZZI, G.; LANGE, G.; CIRILLO,,D.M.; FERRARESSE, M.; DE LACO, G.; GORI, A.; RAVIGLIONE, M.C. AND SMIRA/ TBNET STUDY GROUP. 2007. Extensively drug-resistant Tuberculosis, Italy and Germany. Emerging Infectious Diseases, 13(5):1-3 (letter), May. http://www2a. cdc.gov/ncidod/ts/print.asp (Assessed on 5/16/2007).

MIMS, C., DOCKRELL, H.M., GOERING, R.V., WAKELIN, D., ROITT, I. AND ZUKERMAN, M. 2004. Medical Microbiology. 3rd edition. Philadelphia: Elsevier-Mosby.

MONATH, T.P. 1975. Lassa fever; review of epidemiology and epizootology. Bulletin of the WHO, 52:577-590.

MONATH, T.P., CASALS, J. 1975. Diagnosis of Lassa fever and the isolation and management of ill healthcare users. Bulletin of the WHO, 52:707-713.

MONSHI, B AND ZIEGLMAYER. V. 2004. The Problem of Privacy in Transcultural Research: Reflections on an Ethnographic Study in Sri Lanka. Ethics and Behavior, 14(4):305-312.

Multidrug-resistant Tuberculosis Fact Sheet – American Lung Association site. http:// www.lungsa.org/site/pp.aspx?c=dvLUK90Oe&b=35815&printmode=1(Accessed on 3/6/2006).

MWINGA, A. s.n. Drug-resistant tuberculosis in Africa. Annuals New York: Academy of Science. p.106-112.

National Department of Health. South Africa. National Health Act, No. 61 of 2003.

National Department of Health. South Africa. 2009. Expanded Programme on Immunisation – EPI (SA). Revised Childhood Immunisation Schedule from April 2009.

National Department of Health. South Africa. 2009. New EPI Vaccines Guidelines.

National Department of Health. South Africa. 2010. Guidelines for Tuberculosis preventive therapy among HIV infected individuals in South Africa. South African National AIDS Council.

National Department of Health. South Africa. 2010. Clinical Guidelines: Prevention from Mother-to-Child Transmission. South African National AIDS Council.

National Department of Health. South Africa. 2010. Guidelines for the Management of HIV in Children. South African National AIDS Council.

National Department of Health. South Africa. 2010. Clinical Guidelines for the Management of HIV and AIDS in Adults and Adolescents. South African National AIDS Council.

NATHANSON, E; LAMBRECTS-VAN WEEZENBEEK, C.;RICH, M.L.;GUPTA, R.; BAYONA, J.; BLÖNDAL,K.; CAMINERO, J.S.; CEGIELSKI, J.P.; DANILOVITS, M.; ESPINAL, M.A.; HOLLO, V.; JARAMILLO,E.; LEIMANE, V.; MITNICK, C.D.; MUKHERJEE,J.S.; NUNN, P.; PASECHNIKOV, A.; TUPASI, T.; WELLS, C. AND RAVIGLIONE, M.C. 2006. Multidrug-resistant Tuberculosis Management in Resource-limited Settings. Emerging Infectious Diseases, 12(9):1389-1397, September.

Natural killer cell. http://en.wikipedia.org/wiki/Natural_killer_cells (Accessed on 4/23/2013).

NIEUWVELD, R.W. *et al.* 1982. Drug-resistant malaria in Africa. Suid-Afrikaanse Mediese Tydskrif, 62(6):173-175, July 31.

Nursing Update. 2007. Meningitis - knows the signs and symptoms, 31(4):54-56, May.

Nursing Update. 2007. Yellow fever inoculation alert. 31(10):14-15, September.

Nursing Update. 2009. The fight against TB. Vol. 33(2):25-29, March.

Nursing Update. 2009. Unite against TB. Vol. 33(2):32-33, March.

Nursing Update. 2009. African haemorrhagic fevers. Vol. 33(2):36-39, March.

Nursing Update. 2009. Alternative medicines set to be regulated. Vol. 33(3):12, April.

Nursing Update. 2009. Cross-border crisis in Humanity. Vol. 33(3):22, April.

Nursing Update. 2009. Health Awareness Month – make a difference. Vol. 33(3):30, April.

Nursing Update. 2009. Polio-eradation - a global effort. Vol. 33(3):52-55, April.

Nursing Update. 2009. The silent killer. Vol. 33(3):56-59, April.

Nursing Update. 2009. Polio set-back in Africa calls for traveller vaccination boosters. Vol. 33(8):7, September.

Nursing Update. 2009. The entire population is protected. Vol. 33(8):12-13, September.

Nursing Update. 2009. Swine Flu Update. Vol. 33(8):26-27, September.

Nursing Update. 2009. Pregnant Women and Novel Influenza A (H1N1) Virus: Consideration for Clinicians. Vol. 33(8):28-29, September.

Nursing Update. 2009. World record for healthy hands. Vol. 33(10):7, November.

Nursing Update. 2009. AIDS is not a death sentence. Vol. 33(10):24-25, November.

Nursing Update. 2010. Extensive drug-resistant tuberculosis and health care workers (article 1). Vol. 34(3):26-27, April.

Nursing Update. 2010. The silent killer. Vol. 34(3):58-61, April.

Nursing Update. 2010. Extensive drug-resistant tuberculosis and health care workers (article 2). Vol. 34(4):30-31, May.

Nursing Update. 2010. Pandemic Alert. Vol. 34(4):32-34, May.

Nursing Update. 2010. Personal protection (article 3). Vol. 34(5):24-25, June.

Nursing Update. 2010. HIV/Depression. Vol. 34(6):23-27, July.

Nursing Update. 2010. TB control in the working environment (article 4). Vol. 34(6):28-29, July.

Nursing Update. 2010. TB/HIV cannot be fought alone. Vol. 34(7):42, August.

Nursing Update. 2010. Returning TB-free people into society. Vol. 34(8):32, September.

Nursing Update. 2011. Working together (with Traditional Healers). Vol. 35(3):25-27, March.

OBERLEAS, D. and HARLAND, B.F. 2010. The True story of Zinc Nutrition and Homeostasis. Sight and Life Magazine, Issue 2/2010:13-19.

OLLÉ-GOIG, J.E. 2006. Editorial: The treatment of Multi-drug Resistant Tuberculosis – a return to the pre-antibiotic era? Tropical medicine and International Health, 11(11):1625-1628, November.

PATHOGENESIS of VARICELLA ZOSTER VIRUS INFECTION. http://virology-online.com/viruses/VZV2.htm (Accessed on 6/8/2013).

PAVERD, N. 1988. Crimean-Congo haemorrhagic fever: a nursing care plan. Nursing RSA/Verpleging RSA, 3(4):33-34, April.

PHIPPS, W.J., SANDS, J.K. AND MAREK, J.F. 2003. Medical-Surgical Nursing – Concepts and Clinical Practice. 7th Edison. St Louis: Mosby, Inc.

PROFESSIONAL NURSING TODAY. 2008. Landmark study confirms the importance of home and personal hygiene in reducing infectious diseases. Vol. 12(4):28, July/August.

RACING AGAINST AN AIRBORNE KILLER. http://www.results.org/website/article.asp?id=2540&printFriendly=1 (Accessed on 5/9/2007).

RAMAZANI, A. AND PROSEVITA, B.P. 2006. A campaign to raise awareness of and combat vitamin A deficiency. Sight and life. Newsletter 1/2006:23-24.

RAVIGLIONE, M.C. 2007. The new Stop TB Strategy and the Global Plan to Stop TB, 2006-2015. Bulletin of the World Health Organization, 85(5):327, May.

Reader's Digest. 2006. Looking after your body - Your personal guide to successful ageing. China: Leo Paper Products Ltd.

ROWLAND, K. Totally drug-resistant TB emerges in India. http://www.nature.com/news/totally-drug-resistant-tb-emerges-in-india (Accessed on 6/1/2013).

SAARI, T.N. and the Committee on Infectious Diseases. 2003. Immunization of Preterm and Low Birth Weight Infants. American Academy of Paediatrics 112(1):193-198, July.

Sanofipasteur. 2009. Complete Childhood Vaccination Schedule. South Africa.

Sanofipasteur. 2009. Catch-up Vaccination Schedule. South Africa.

Sanofipasteur. 2009. Tetraxim.

SHARMA, S.K. AND MOHAN, A. 2009. Multidrug-resistant Tuberculosis. A Menace that Threatens To Destabilize Tuberculosis Control. CHEST, 130(1):261-272, July.

SIGHT AND LIFE MAGAZINE. 3/2009. Supplement.

SIMPSON, D.I.H. 1978. Viral haemorrhagic fevers of man. Bulletin of the WHO, 56(6):819-832.

SKIN LESIONS.   http://medical-dictionary.thefreedictionary.com/Skin+Lesions (Accessed on 4/29/2013).

Smithcline Beecham Pharmaceuticals. 1996. Primary care manual. Johannesburg: Jacana.

SPIER, R.E. 2004. Ethical aspects of the methods used to evaluate the safety of vaccines. Vaccine, 22:2085-2090.

SOUTH AFRICAN DEVELOPMENT COMMUNITY. 1999. Protocol of Health

STELLENBERG, E.L. AND BRUCE, J.C. 2007. Nursing practice – medical-surgical nursing for hospital and community. Philadelphia: Churchill Livingstone Elsevier.

STEVENS, M. 2009. Tuberculosis – a women's health issue. Nursing Update, 33(2):30-31, March.

STEVENS, M. 2010. Women's private battle with HIV. Nursing Update, Vol. 34(7):42, August.

[stop-Tb] STATEMENT: XDR-TB – Open letter to Dr. Manto Tshabalala-Msimang. http://www.archives.healthdev.net/stop-tb/msg00841.html (Accessed on 5/9/2007).

Time Magazine. 1988. Stop that germ – the battle inside your body. Vol. 21:52-58, May 23.

THURNHAM, D. 2008. Handling Data when Inflammation is Detected. Sight and Life Magazine, Issue 2/2008:49-52.

THURNHAM, D. 2009. Selenium – Some Notes on Immune function and recent Cancer Trials. Sight and Life Magazine, Issue 2/2009:49-56.

THURNHAM, D. 2009. Micronutrient Deficiencies and affluence. Sight and Life Magazine, Issue 3/2009:56-61.

THURNHAM, D. 2010. Should organically Produced Foods be Healthier than Conventionally Grown Foods? Sight and Life Magazine, Issue 2/2010:30-38.

Totally drug-resistant tuberculosis. http://en.wikipedia.org/wiki/Totally_drug-resistant_tuberculosis (Accessed on 6/1/2013).

"Totally drug-resistant" tuberculosis spreads in South Africa as researchers warn global outbreak would be 'untreatable'. http://life.nationalpost.com/2013/02/12/totally-drug-resistant-tuberculosis-spreading-in-South Africa (Accessed on 6/1/2013).

TRUTER, I. 2008. A therapeutic approach to coughing. Professional Nursing Today, 12(4):37-42, July/August.

TUPASI, T.E., GUPTA, R., QUELAPIO, M.I.D., ORILLAZA, R.B., MIRA, N.R., MANGUBAT, N.V., BELEN, V., ARNITO, N., MACALINTAL, L., ARABIT, M., LAGAHID, J.Y., ESPINAL, M., FLOYD, K. 2006. Feasibility and Cost-effectiveness of Treating Multidrug-Resistant Tuberculosis: A cohort Study in the Philippines. Plos Medicine, 3(9):1587-1596, September.

ULMER, J.B. AND LUI, M.A. 2002. Ethical Issues for Vaccines and Immunization. Nature Reviews – Immunology, 2(4):291-296.

UPLEKAR, M. AND RAVIGLIONE, M.C. 2007. The "vertical-horizontal" swing debates: time for the pendulum to rest (in peace)? Bulletin of the World Health Organization, 85(5):413-414, May.

URDAN, L.D.; STACY, K.M. AND LOUGH, M.E. 2006. Thelan's Critical Care Nursing. Diagnosing and Management. 5th edition. St Louis: Mosby Elsevier.

van den BERG, R.H. AND VILJOEN, M.J. 1989. Oordraagbare Siektes: 'n Verpleegkundige Perspektief. Pretoria: HAUM Opvoedkundige Uitgewery.

van DYK, A. 2005. HIV/AIDS care and Counselling - a multidisciplinary approach. 3rd edition. Cape Town: Maskew Miller Longman (Pty) Ltd.

VELLA, E.E. 1978. Lassa fever and Marburg disease. Occurrence, origins and diagnosis. Royal Society of Health Journal, 98(4):150-152. August.

VERWEIJ, M. AND DAWSON, A. 2004. Ethical principles for collective immunization programmes. Vaccine, 22(23/24):3122-3126, August.

WHARTON, B.A., PUGH, R.E. AND TAITZ, L.Z. *et al.* 1988. Dietary management of gastro-enteritis. British Medical Journal, 66(20):450-452, February 13.

WEEKLY EPIDEMIOLOGICAL RECORD. 2006. Addressing the threat of tuberculosis caused by extensively drug-resistant Mycobacterium tuberculosis. No. 41, October.

WHO. 1986. Expert committee on rabies. Technical Report: Series 709. Geneva.

WHO. 2001. A human rights approach to tuberculosis. Guidelines for social mobilization. The Stop TB Partnership Secretariat. Geneva.

WHO. 2004. Anti-tuberculosis drug resistance in the world. Report no 3. Geneva.

WHO, UNICEF AND THE NATIONAL DEPARTMENT OF HEALTH, SOUTH AFRICA. 2005. Integrated management of childhood illness.

WHO, UNICEF AND THE NATIONAL DEPARTMENT OF HEALTH, SOUTH AFRICA. 2005. IMCI complementary course on HIV/AIDS (introduction).

WHO. 2006. Guidelines for the programmatic management of drug-resistant tuberculosis. WHO/HTM/2006:361.

WHO. The Global Plan to Stop TB 2006-2015. The Plan sets out actions for Life – actions towards a world free of TB. http://www.who.int/tb/features_archive/globalplan_to_stop_tb_/en/print.html (Accessed on 6/21/2007).

WHO. 2006. Addressing the threat of tuberculosis caused by extensively drug-resistant *Mycobacterium tuberculosis* in The Weekly Epidemiological Record, No 41, 13 October.

WHO. Drug- and Multidrug-resistant Tuberculosis (MDR-TB). http://www.who.int/tb/dots/dotsplus/en/ (Accessed on 3/6/2007).

WHO. Emergence of XDR-TB. WHO concern over extensive drug resistant TB strains that are virtually untreatable. http://ww.who.int/mediacentre/news/notes/2006/np23/en/print.html (Accessed on 5/9/2007).

WHO. XDR-TB: extensively drug–resistant tuberculosis. May 2007. www.who.int/tb Stop TB Department.

WHO. Anti-tuberculosis DRUG RESISTANCE in the world. Third Global Report. The WHO/IUATLD global project on anti-Tuberculosis Drug Surveillance 1999-2002.

WHO report 2007. Global tuberculosis control – key findings.

Wyeth. 2005. Prevenar:Pneumoccal Conjugate Vaccine, 7-Valent. 11 May.

XDR-TB in South Africa. http://www.news-medical.net/print_article.asp?id=21469 (Accessed on 5/9/2007).

Yellow fever – inoculation alert. 2007. Nursing Update, 31(10):14, November.

ZIMMERMAN, R.K. 2007. Recent changes in influenza vaccination recommendations, 2007. The Journal of Family Practice, 56(2):S12-S17, February.